HurstReviews

NCLEX-PN®
Review

HurstReviews

NCLEX-PN®
Review

**Marlene Hurst, RN, MSN,
FNP-R, CCRN-R**

President
Hurst Review Services
Brookhaven, Mississippi

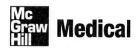

New York   Chicago   San Francisco   Lisbon   London   Madrid   Mexico City
Milan   New Delhi   San Juan   Seoul   Singapore   Sydney   Toronto

Hurst Reviews: NCLEX-PN® Review

2 3 4 5 6 7 8 9 0   QPD/QPD   12 11 10 9

Set ISBN 978-0-07-148430-5
Set MHID 0-07-148430-2
Book ISBN 978-0-07-154577-8
Book MHID 0-07-154577-8
CD ISBN 978-0-07-154578-5
CD MHID 0-07-154578-6

This book was set in Minion by International Typesetting and Composition.
The editors were Quincy McDonald and Robert Pancotti.
The production supervisor was Catherine Saggese.
The illustration manager was Armen Ovsepyan.
Project management was provided by Madhu Bhardwaj, International Typesetting and Composition.
The designer was Alan Barnett; the cover designer was David Dell'Accio.
Cover photo: Veer.
Quebecor World, Dubuque was printer and binder.

This book is printed on acid-free paper.

Library of Congress Cataloging-in-Publication Data

Hurst, Marlene.
   Hurst reviews : NCLEX-PN review / Marlene Hurst.
     p. ; cm.
   Includes index.
   ISBN 978-0-07-148430-5 (pbk. : alk. paper)
   1. Practical nursing—Examinations, questions, etc.   2. National
Council Licensure Examination for Practical/Vocational Nurses—Study
guides.   I. Title.   II. Title: NCLEX-PN review.
   [DNLM: 1. Nursing Care—Examination Questions.   2.
Nursing—Examination Questions.   WY 18.2 H966h 2008]
RT62.H87 2008
610.73076—dc22
                          2007031604

CONTENTS

CONTRIBUTORS

Dana M. Armstrong, RNC, MSN
Associate Degree Nursing Instructor
Hinds Community College
Nursing Allied Health Center
Jackson, Mississippi

Amanda K. Boyanton, RN, BSN, MSN, CDFS, CFNP
Family Nurse Practitioner
River Oaks Hospital
Emergency Department
Flowood, Mississippi

Wanda Todd Bradshaw, RNC, MSN, NNP, PNP, CCRN
Assistant Clinical Professor
Duke University School of Nursing
Durham, North Carolina

Patricia L. Clutter, RN, MEd, CEN, FAEN
Emergency Department Nurse and Consultant
St. John's Regional Health Center
Springfield, Missouri;
Med-Ed
Strafford, Missouri

Christine R. Duran, APRN-BC, DNP, CNS, CCTN
Clinical Nurse Coordinator
Hematological Malignancies & Blood and Marrow
Transplant
University of Colorado Hospital
Aurora, Colorado

Amy Martinez Garcie, MSN
Nurse Practitioner
DeSoto Regional Health System
Zwolle Rural Clinic
Zwolle, Louisiana

Autumn Langford, RN, BSN, CCRN
Hurst Review Services
Brookhaven, Mississippi

Lisa Lathem, RN, BSN, CIC
Infection Control Nurse
St. Dominic-Jackson Memorial Hospital
Jackson, Mississippi

Joahnna D. Evans Songer, RN, CCRN, CLNC
Co-Founder and Lead Consultant
Songer, Valdivia & Associates Legal Nurse
Consultants
Visalia, California
ICU and CVICU Nurse
Community Regional Medical Center
Fresno, California
Kaweah Delta Intensive Care Unit
Visalia, California

Cassandra Lynn Hall Valdivia, RN, BSN, LNC
Quality Management Clinical Coordinator
Community Medical Centers
Fresno, California
Co-owner and Lead Consultant
Songer, Valdivia & Associates Legal Nurse
Consultants
Visalia, California

PREFACE

Hello, nursing students! My name is Marlene Hurst, President and owner of Hurst Review Services and author of this book. Hurst Review Services, which is based in Brookhaven, Mississippi, opened its doors in 1988 when I began my new teaching job at a major university. As I began to teach nursing students, I quickly realized how much additional help they needed while in nursing school. Actually, I figured that out during my days as a nursing student, but at that time I just assumed that I was the only one struggling to survive nursing school! Today, my passion to help nursing students still rings true, and this desire motivated me to write this book for you.

I love to make difficult nursing concepts fun and easy to understand! I believe that if students are relaxed, they will learn and retain more information. I've always said that nursing isn't meant to be difficult: it's meant to be understood! My specialty is guiding students to a true understanding of the "why" of nursing content. If you understand "why" you are performing a specific nursing intervention, you will understand the related nursing concepts. On the other hand, if you blindly perform skills without knowing why they are required, you will never understand how nursing really works.

I know that many of you bought this book to help you pass the NCLEX-PN® examination. No sweat! This book is designed to help you PASS the FIRST time. The book takes difficult nursing content and breaks it down into core concepts that are easy to understand. It also includes specific test-taking strategies and practice questions. If you read this book and use it exactly as I've suggested, you will pass the NCLEX-PN® the first time! For those of you who have purchased this book to help you survive nursing school or exit exams, you won't be disappointed either.

I'll bet you're thinking "What makes her different from any other nurse authors?" Well, for starters, while I was director of a nursing program, my wonderful faculty and I always achieved a 100% pass rate on the NCLEX-PN® examination! I also have a solid nursing background. Once I graduated from nursing school, I began working in the intensive care unit at a very large hospital. When I interacted with the nursing students during their clinical days, I knew that teaching was what I really wanted to do! So I bit the bullet and went back to school while working full time. I completed my master's degree in nursing as an adult and family nurse practitioner and also became certified in critical care nursing. During my nursing career, I have worked as a nursing instructor, assistant professor of nursing, staff ICU nurse, charge nurse, emergency department clinical nurse specialist, and director of a nursing program.

I hope that this book helps you to achieve your dream—and makes your life easier in the process—whether it is to survive nursing school, pass exit exams, or whip the NCLEX-PN® the first time!

You may visit me at www.hurstreview.com to say "hello" or to receive information about how Hurst Review Services can visit your school to conduct a NCLEX® review for you and your classmates.

Best of luck,
Marlene Hurst
President, Hurst Review Services

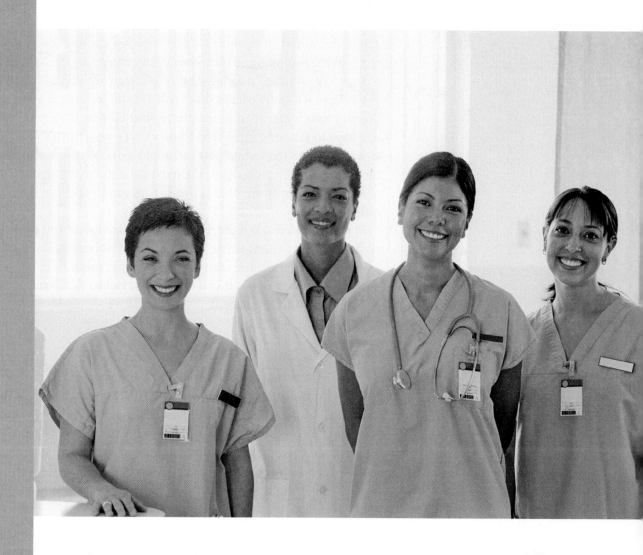

CHAPTER

1

Let's Get It Started in Here!

LET'S GET IT STARTED IN HERE!

This is where you need to play the song "Let's Get It Started in Here" by the Black Eyed Peas to get you pumped-up!

Now don't think because this is the first chapter that you can skip it. You must read it in order to understand how we will work together to achieve NCLEX® success. This book parallels the same successful approach I use when teaching NCLEX® Review classes. This chapter serves as the beginning of your journey in conquering the NCLEX®!

So, you've finished nursing school. What an accomplishment! Can you believe it's really over? I'll bet you are still walking around feeling like you have a care plan to turn in to your clinical instructor! Now you have to take one more test! I know that's very frustrating. You're anxious to take the test, so you can get to work to help buy that new car you've already picked out. Or, maybe the nurse manager at your new job or a family member is pressuring you to take the test sooner rather than later.

Maybe you have taken the test five times already and you feel there is no hope for you. Guess what? There is hope! Just because a student may have to take the test more than one time doesn't mean he or she isn't going to be a great nurse. If you follow this book and do what I say, you will achieve NCLEX® success!

✚ Don't assume anything

Some of you may assume that passing nursing school and the NCLEX® predictor tests assures your ability to pass the NCLEX®. Your teachers have probably emphasized that NCLEX® tests for *minimum* nursing competency. You may be saying to yourself, "Surely, I'm *minimally* competent." Unfortunately, these things may set you up for false reassurance.

Pretend it's new!

Let me emphasize one important point: NCLEX® is not like any test you have ever taken. Your safest approach to this test is to pretend you are starting your very first IV, and you have to remember each step you learned in the clinical learning laboratory in order to successfully insert the IV. Doing something for the first time can be very scary, but I will help you to overcome those feelings as far as NCLEX® is concerned.

✚ What's the good news?

Yes, there is good news! You can pass the first time if you CHOOSE. Achieving success in anything requires the investment of *time*. I'm not advocating weeks and weeks of studying. I'm encouraging you to study this book thoroughly, so that you can walk into the testing center with a level of confidence that will propel you to pass the FIRST time!

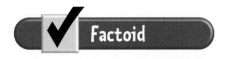

NCLEX® is not like any test you have ever taken!

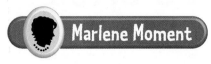

My goal is for **you** to pass NCLEX® the **first** time!

WHAT'S THE NCLEX®, AND WHY DO I HAVE TO TAKE IT?

Look at it this way: This could be the most important test you ever take! Let's look more closely at the NCLEX® and why it is important.

✛ Define time

The NCLEX®, or National Council Licensure Examination, is a test that determines if you have the minimum level of knowledge necessary to practice nursing safely. The test is written by nurses with advanced degrees and clinical expertise in each specific area of nursing.[1]

✛ What exactly does "practice nursing safely" mean?

The American Nurses Association (ANA) developed a standard set of protocols to guide nurses in making decisions regarding the care of clients.[2] Nursing in its basic form provides care to clients in order to help them achieve specific goals to return them to wellness, to return them to an adapted state of wellness, or to help the client die with dignity and peace.[2] Practicing these services without causing harm to the client, **or** the lack of practicing these services, at the very least, is what NCLEX® considers as the minimum level of knowledge needed to practice nursing safely.[1] In other words, nurses are safely helping clients return to the level of self-care or wellness before their illness. That was deep!

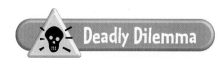

Here's the Deal

Don't let distractions or a long list of client needs supersede the safety of any client!

✛ Applying your knowledge

Passing the NCLEX® does not include learning and memorizing a never-ending amount of content. Instead, the key is to take what you DO know and apply it to concepts you may never have heard of. How? Don't worry; we'll work through this together. This concept of applying your knowledge will prevent you from panicking at the sight of a question that asks you about some unfamiliar disease. I have successfully used this method of writing test questions since I began teaching in schools of nursing in 1988. You will learn how to methodically work through this type of question and confidently select the correct answer.

CASE IN POINT Imagine you work on a medical-surgical unit. You are given your assignment of six acutely ill clients. Do you know every detail listed in your clients' charts? Of course not! But, you are still responsible for caring for these clients. What do you do? Do you rush to the computer on your unit to look up the etiology of every disease your clients have? No way! You implement what you do know by applying basic principles of safety to prevent harm to your clients. We will use this same approach with NCLEX® test questions.

Deadly Dilemma

If you've never heard of a disease or illness that is presented on the NCLEX®, then no one else has either! This is most likely a distracter that the NCLEX® Lady has cooked up!

✚ Don't believe everything you hear

There is a rumor floating around that if you don't know the answer on a standardized test, pick "C." That is simply untrue; it will not help you pass this particular exam. The key to passing the NCLEX® is to take the knowledge you **do** know and **apply** it to new and different concepts.

What the NCLEX® Lady Thinks

The NCLEX® Lady views you, the test-taker, as a new nurse with only two weeks of vast nursing knowledge. This should be a relief that you do not have to know everything about nursing! We aren't trying to make 100% on this test. We got over that compulsion a long time ago! However, you want to approach this test as if you are a brand new nurse, not an experienced nurse. In fact, if you approach the test like you are an experienced nurse, you will scare the NCLEX® Lady! This book will show you how to think like a new nurse.

✚ Will taking a million practice tests help me pass?

Many of you have been told you need to take a million practice tests in order to pass the NCLEX®. Your friends have been smothering you with study guides, workbooks, and CDs. Your plan is to memorize these questions. Bad move! No matter how many questions you memorize, NCLEX® has many thousands more waiting for you. This book will show you how to answer the test questions in a way that makes the NCLEX® Lady very happy.

CORE CONTENT AND THE NCLEX®

You will hear me refer to "core content" many times in our journey together. I have a complete on-line review of core content on my website (if you need a review), **www.hurstreview.com.** Let's take a brief look at core content, because it will be a key factor in your test preparation.

✚ Define time

The core content is the information you must know *without a doubt* and *without hesitation* if you wish to pass the NCLEX® the first time.

✚ Without a doubt and without hesitation

Heavy words! So, what exactly is the core content that I should know without a doubt and without hesitation? The core content that I will keep referring to is information such as fluids and electrolytes or acid–base balance.

CASE IN POINT Let's take a look at an example that includes core content that you should know without a doubt and without hesitation.

The nurse is caring for an 8-hour postop thyroidectomy client. Which client symptom should concern the nurse the most?

1. Slight twitch of the left arm.

2. Depressed patellar reflex.

3. Blood pressure of 136/83 mm Hg, pulse of 72 beats/min, respiratory rate of 18 breaths/min.

4. Occasional premature ventricular contractions (PVCs) noted per the monitor.

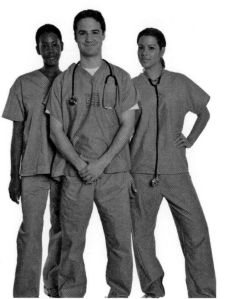

Let's use a step-by-step process to answer this question.

• Step #1: Did you know that while reading this question your main focus should include **hypocalcemia?** To answer this question, you have to use multi-logical thinking. You have to be knowledgeable about a thyroidectomy and the related complications. Remember: NCLEX® questions usually focus on actual or potential **problems** that can occur. There aren't many "happy" NCLEX® questions. Note: After a thyroidectomy there is a chance the surgeon could accidentally remove the parathyroid glands.

• Step #2: Now you need to know about the parathyroids. Parathyroids increase serum calcium. So, if a couple of the parathyroids are accidentally removed, then the serum calcium goes down. Next, focus on how fluctuations in calcium affect the body. If the serum calcium is raised, then the body will be sedated. If the serum calcium is lowered, the body will be tight or contracted. This is my simple way of looking at it.

• Step #3: What can tightened or contracted muscles lead to? Seizures. When that arm starts to twitch, you should worry and assume the worst: the client may be headed toward a seizure. The client's patellar reflex is depressed due to the effects of general anesthesia. Also, if the calcium drops, the reflexes increase—not decrease. The vital signs remain normal. Okay, I know the PVCs worried you, but the answer choice said "occasional." You'll want to watch this to make sure the PVCs do not increase. This is not highly unusual; many people have occasional PVCs.

• Step #4: Now we have arrived at the correct answer, #1. Muscle twitching is a specific sign you must watch for in the care of the post-thyroidectomy client.

See how your knowledge of core content was needed in order to answer this question?

+ More good news

Once again, the good news is you do not have to know everything in the world about nursing to pass the NCLEX®. It is not necessary to reread every class note or textbook. Remember, the NCLEX® Lady thinks of you

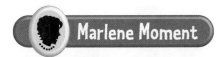

Marlene Moment

You will never be more motivated than you are right now to study for the NCLEX®! Now is the time to take action to pass the test so you may get on with your life!

as someone with only two weeks of vast nursing knowledge! Every test question stems from core content. This book will provide you with many opportunities to refresh your core content knowledge and put this knowledge into practice with test questions.

SUMMARY

I'm excited about this opportunity to help you achieve your goal, and hope you will not only learn, but actually enjoy studying with me. My successful approach is unique, so it is important for you to pay close attention to every word in this book. **Now let's get it started in here!**

References

1. National Council of State Boards of Nursing. *NCLEX Examinations*. Available at: **www.ncsbn.org.** Accessed October 25, 2006.

2. American Nurses Association. *Nursing: Scope and Standards of Practice*. Introduction. Washington, DC: ANA; 2004.

Bibliography

American Nurses Association. *Nursing: Scope and Standards of Practice*. Washington, DC: ANA; 2004.

Huber D. *Leadership and Nursing Care Management*. 2nd ed. Philadelphia: Saunders; 2002.

Hurst Review Services. Available at **www.hurstreview.com.**

National Council of State Boards of Nursing. Available at **www.ncsbn.org.**

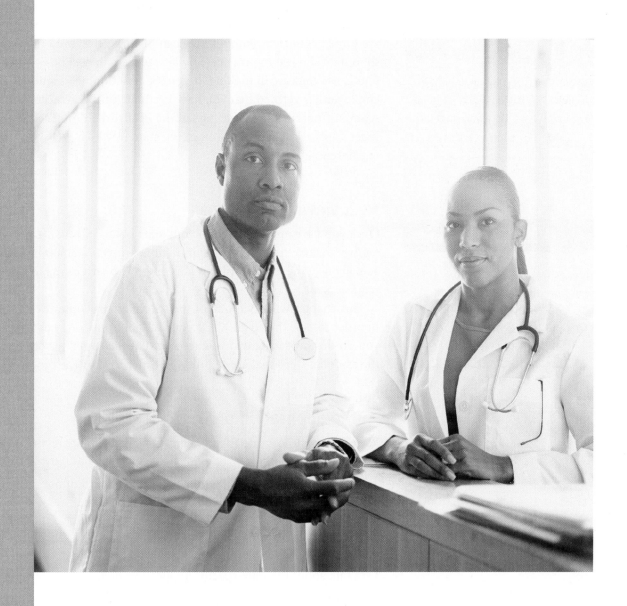

CHAPTER

2

The Process You Must Go Through

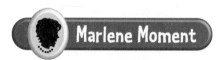

Hurst Hint

The NCLEX® Candidate Bulletin will become your favorite handout in the next few weeks. Be aware that the guidelines may change each year.

Marlene Moment

There is usually a 3- to 6-week wait from the time you submit your application to the time you take your test. Sometimes longer. Sometimes shorter.

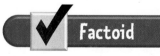

Factoid

You and your friends may decide to travel to another state to take your exam, so you can take a small vacation and have some fun after the test is over!

THE PROCESS YOU MUST GO THROUGH

First, you must graduate from an accredited school of nursing before you are eligible to take the NCLEX®! I know it sounds ridiculous, but there are some people who think if they can just pass the "test," then they should be allowed to practice in whatever field they choose. Fortunately, that is not the case in nursing. If you are functioning as a nurse, your employer has verified that you have graduated from an accredited school of nursing and have passed the licensure exam. Second, you must apply for licensure through the state in which you wish to be registered.[1]

✚ Reviewing the steps

Once you have applied through your state board of nursing, you can register to take the NCLEX® examination, but you will not be allowed to actually take the exam until you have met the board of nursing eligibility requirements.

This chapter will review all of the specific steps you must go through in order to take the NCLEX®. If your school of nursing has instructed you on this process, great! You are ahead of the game! If not, these are the essential steps that are required in order to start the process!

✚ The application process

You will have to complete two applications prior to taking the NCLEX® examination.

1. State-specific application (from your state's board of nursing)
2. NCLEX® examination registration and application[1]

State-specific application

Let's talk about the state-specific application first.

• You must submit the state-specific application to the board of nursing in the state or territory where you wish to be licensed. This application is usually given to you during your last semester of nursing school. If you do not wish to be licensed in your state, it is your responsibility to contact your desired state of licensure to obtain their specific application. Some states may even have the application online. If so, just follow the instructions to the letter![1]

• This is your licensure application—not the application to take the NCLEX® examination. *Also, your board of nursing may have an application deadline, so be sure to verify this date.*

• Just because you fill out the state-specific application does not mean you can't TAKE the test in another state. You can. For example, if I want to be licensed in Mississippi, but my girlfriends and I want to take the test in New Orleans, Louisiana, because we want to go and have some fun after we finish . . . we can.

- Each individual state has its own criteria that affect the application process (e.g., criminal background check). Make sure you read the application carefully and follow all of the directions![1]

- Your results will be sent to YOUR state board where you requested licensure, no matter in which state you physically take the exam.[1]

- When the state board receives your application, they will send a card or e-mail confirming receipt. In some states, you have to send your permanent transcript as well. Many times the deans or directors of nursing programs will send all applications and transcripts to the state board of nursing at one time.[1]

- You have to send money with each application. The fee may vary from state to state. However, the fee you send to the National Council to take the NCLEX® examination is $200. The fee you send to your particular state is for actual licensure. If you wish to take your test at an international testing site, then you will be required to pay an additional international scheduling fee of $150. In addition, a "value added tax" may apply. These fees are due when a testing candidate schedules the examination appointment.[1]

NCLEX® exam registration and application

Administration of the NCLEX® is performed by Pearson Professional Testing Centers. The testing centers are located throughout the United States and its territories. They also have some international testing centers. The addresses and locations of the testing centers are on the NCLEX® Candidate website. That web address is: **www.ncsbn.org.** You will first need to click the NCLEX® Examinations link from the left menu. On the next screen, choose the NCLEX® link from the left menu. Then choose Scheduling and Locations from the submenu.[1]

METHODS OF APPLICATION

There are several ways to complete your NCLEX® application. We will review these to help you decide which route is easiest for you. All three methods of application require a completed applicant Candidate Bulletin. (See "Phone" for instructions on how to get a Candidate Bulletin.)

✚ Phone

You can complete your NCS Pearson application by phone by calling NCLEX® Candidate Services (1-866-49-NCLEX; 1-866-496-2539 for U.S. candidates). Other numbers are available at **https://www.ncsbn.org/718.htm.** Before you call, you need to complete the mail-in registration form, which is in your Candidate Bulletin. If you do not have the Candidate Bulletin, just go to **www.ncsbn.org.** You will first need to click the NCLEX® Examinations link from the left menu. On the next screen, choose the NCLEX® link from the left menu. Then choose Candidate Basic Info from the submenu and open the Candidate Bulletin from the right screen. Print it out. **Fill it out.** Have your credit card ready and make the call![1]

Hurst Hint

You may find that a testing center in another state has an opening at a time that is more convenient for you. You may decide to take a road trip to take the test. Cool!

Hurst Hint

Follow your state-specific application process to the letter!

Marlene Moment

You do not want anything to slow down the application process (e.g., overdue books in the library, transcripts from other schools you may have attended that never were sent, fines). My problem at graduation was the 58 unpaid parking tickets I had accumulated!

Factoid

Have your credit card ready! Visa, MasterCard, and American Express are accepted.

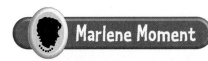

Marlene Moment

You can **always** call the NCSBN to request a Candidate Bulletin.

✚ Web

You can register on-line at **www.pearsonvue.com/nclex.** You will have to answer questions, of course! Have your VISA, MasterCard, or American Express ready to roll![1] NOTE: You will need the Candidate Bulletin for reference.

✚ Mail

You can register by snail mail. You must enclose a certified check, a cashier's check, or money order (at the time of this writing money orders are still being accepted) made payable to the National Council of State Boards of Nursing for $200 in U.S. dollars. You must use a U.S. bank. Personal checks, cash, credit cards, foreign currency, stamps, receipts, or any proofs of payment are not accepted. So don't even ask. You must also enclose your completed registration form, which is found in the Candidate Bulletin. Mail your payment and registration form to:

NCLEX Operations

P.O. Box 64950

St. Paul, MN 55164-0950

Be sure to affix your signature to the registration form. DO NOT PRINT your name.[1]

✚ Final check

Please check your completed application several times. If ANYTHING is missing from the application, or if the money isn't correct, the NCLEX® people are going to send it back to you without a doubt and without hesitation! Ha!

If you provide an e-mail address at the time of registration for the NCLEX®, you will receive all further correspondence from Pearson VUE only through e-mail. (This is true no matter if you registered by phone, mail, or online.) Be careful. If you are not one who checks your e-mail regularly, or if you are moving and your e-mail address will be changing, you may reconsider providing it. If an e-mail address is not provided, then all correspondence with Pearson VUE will be via U.S. mail.[1]

✚ Making changes

If you decide to change the state in which you wish to be licensed AFTER you have registered to take NCLEX®, you must contact NCLEX® Candidate Services. You will have to pay $50 for any changes you wish to make. If you select the wrong test (maybe you clicked NCLEX-RN and meant to click NCLEX-PN), then you must follow the same procedure as above. When you register, you must give your name EXACTLY as printed on the picture ID you will use at the testing center. If your name, address, or e-mail address change, you must submit this information to your board of nursing and request a new Authorization to Test (ATT) from the NCLEX® Call Center (the phone number for your specific Call Center is located in your handy Candidate Bulletin). The name on the

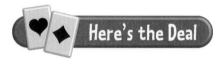

Marlene Moment

I would send the registration form by certified mail, so as to have a signed receipt indicating your information was received. Keep this document in a safe place.

Here's the Deal

Don't forget to check and recheck your completed application.

ATT must match the name on your ID you will use at the testing center. We will talk more about the ATT shortly.[1]

✚ Registration information checklist

The following checklist will help you through the registration process. When registering for the NCLEX®, be prepared to supply the information shown in Table 2-1.

Table 2-1. Registration Information Checklist for the NCLEX®

Item	Comments
✓ Name of exam you wish to take	To ensure that you are selecting the correct test.
✓ Your name	Full name exactly as it appears on your picture ID.
✓ Mother's maiden name	The name given to your mother at birth. They only want your mother's last name. Do not give her full name.
✓ Your date of birth	Month, day, and year.
✓ Sex	Used for statistical purposes only.
✓ Social Security number	This is optional, but some boards of nursing use this information to connect your NCLEX® results to your application.
✓ Ethnic information	Used for statistical purposes only.
✓ Telephone number	They may need to call you. ☺ Provide home, mobile, and work numbers.
✓ Have you taken NCLEX® before?	Yes or No answer.
✓ Have you ever taken the NCLEX® examination to qualify for the same license for which you are now applying?	Yes or No answer.
✓ Have you ever taken the NCLEX® examination to qualify for a different license than the one for which you are now applying?	Yes or No answer; maybe you are an LPN who is now taking the RN exam. They want to know this. They will ask if you have used any other last name during the registration process or while applying for licensure with your state board of nursing. They will also want to know the last date you used this name.
✓ Your maiden name	Your birth name.
✓ Another last name you have used, if any	Name used immediately prior to present name.
✓ Last date above name used	Data collection.
✓ Primary language spoken	Used for statistical purposes only.

(Continued)

Table 2-1. Registration Information Checklist for the NCLEX® (*Continued*)

Item	Comments
✓ Education Program Code	This is a 5-digit code you can find in your trusty Candidate Bulletin; international candidates can find their program code here as well.
✓ Date graduated from nursing school	This is to make sure you are taking the test within the appropriate time frame. This info is double-checked against your school's information.
✓ Commission on Graduates of Foreign Nursing Schools (CGFNS) number	They will want your CGFNS certification number.
✓ From which board of nursing you have requested licensure	So they will know where to send your results.
✓ Current mailing address and email address	Please refer to your Candidate Bulletin for very specific information regarding mailing addresses, especially for international students.

From the Candidate Bulletin at National Council of State Boards, available at **www.ncsbn.org**. Accessed October 25, 2006.

NOW YOU ARE ELIGIBLE TO TEST

Now that you have provided all the information possibly known to man and have completed all the appropriate documentation, you are ready for the test. The following are a few other items that are important to know about this process.

- You will have 365 days for your board of nursing to determine your eligibility. If they do not find you eligible during this time-frame, you must wait until your current registration expires before re-registering. If you try to register a second time during this 365-day waiting period, your second application will be processed and denied and your money will not be refunded.

- Once you have met the eligibility requirements for your state, you will get an ATT. This form may arrive by mail or e-mail. If you have not received your ATT within 2 weeks of registration, please contact NCLEX® Candidate Services for further information.

- Be sure to check your name on your ATT to make sure it is correct. If it's not, then you need to write or call your board of nursing. The name on the ATT must exactly match the other form of identification you plan to take. If it doesn't match, then you have to bring legal documentation of the name change. The only legal documents accepted in regard to this issue are a marriage license, divorce decree, and/or court action legal name change documents. All documents must be in English and must be the **original** document. If you need to make a legal name change, address change, or e-mail address change, you must contact your board of nursing. You cannot do this at the testing center.

- There will be a candidate number on your ATT. You must have this number to schedule your exam.

- You can now register to take NCLEX® by phone, mail, or online. The website and phone number will be on the ATT or in your Candidate Bulletin.

- This is the website: **www.pearsonvue.com/nclex**

- If you choose to register by phone, the numbers are listed in the Candidate Bulletin.

- Along with your ATT you will receive a list of testing centers from which to choose.

- If you require special testing accommodations, you must call your state board of nursing and NCSBN. You may not schedule the exam online. You must do this **prior** to registering for the NCLEX® exam.

- If at any point you have questions, just review the Candidate Bulletin for phone numbers and for specific information regarding the registration process or scheduling process.[1]

✦ Timing is everything

Once you have your ATT, you are entitled to a testing date within 30 days of your initial call. You do not **have** to take the exam within 30 days, but you do have a set time-frame in which you must take your test. This is decided upon by each state. Some states give you 90 days to take your test and some give you up to a year.

Keep these points in mind:

- The scheduling personnel will do their best to give you the testing time you want.

- If you miss your time-frame, you have to start the process all over again.

- Your time-frame will not be extended if you go past the deadline.

- When scheduling your test, select a time that is good for YOU!

If you need to reschedule your appointment, you must visit **www.pearsonvue.com/nclex** or call NCLEX® Candidate Services. **This must be done at least one full business day prior to your appointment.**[1]

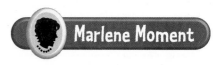

Marlene Moment

If you are not a morning person, don't take the 8:00 AM time slot to test. Okay?

✦ Keeping up with your ATT

Be sure to keep your ATT in a safe place. I know, this is just something else to keep track of, but the ATT is very important.

- Once you have set the testing date and time, write it on your ATT. You will receive an official confirmation.

- If you have any questions about registering to take the NCLEX®, the ATT, a lost ATT, or you want more information about acceptable identification, just go to the NCLEX® candidate website: **www.pearsonvue.com/nclex.**

- For general information, go to **www.ncsbn.org** or e-mail them at: **NCLEXinfo@ncsbn.org.**[1]

Table 2-2. Acceptable and Unacceptable Forms of Identification

Acceptable identification	Unacceptable identification
✓ Your identification must be printed in English-language letters	Any language other than English
✓ Your identification must not be expired	Expired identification
✓ You must have identification with a recent photograph and signature signed in English	The ID photo does not resemble you
✓ Drivers license (with photo and signature)	Learner permit
✓ State/province identification card (with photo and signature)	Library card
✓ U.S. military identification (with photo and visible signature, not imbedded)	School ID
✓ Passport (with photo and signature)	
✓ National identity card (with photo and signature)	

Information from National Council of State Boards of Nursing. Available at: **www.ncsbn.org**. Accessed October 25, 2006.

✚ Proper identification at testing

The testing centers will only accept certain forms of identification. The following information is vital.

- Make sure you have proper identification.
- You must have a photo ID with signature and your valid ATT when you go to the testing center. If you go to the testing center without either of these, you will be asked to leave ☹. You will now have to re-register and pay the exam fee of $200 again. If you paid the international scheduling fee of $150, you will have to pay this again as well.

Table 2-2 details acceptable and unacceptable forms of identification as deemed by the NCLEX® people.

SUMMARY

Now that you are registered to take the NCLEX®, you need to set aside some specific times to study for the exam. We will be discussing how this test is different from all the others you have taken in nursing school, so studying is very important. Remember our goal is to pass the NCLEX® the first time!

Reference

1. National Council of State Boards of Nursing. NCLEX Examinations. Available at: **www.ncsbn.org.** Accessed October 25, 2006.

Bibliography

Hurst Review Services. **www.hurstreview.com.**

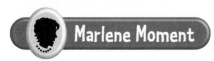

Marlene Moment

If you gained 50 pounds in nursing school, then you will need to have a new picture made. Your ID picture must look like the current you!

Marlene Moment

On any form of identification, check the date to make sure it has not expired, or it will not be accepted.

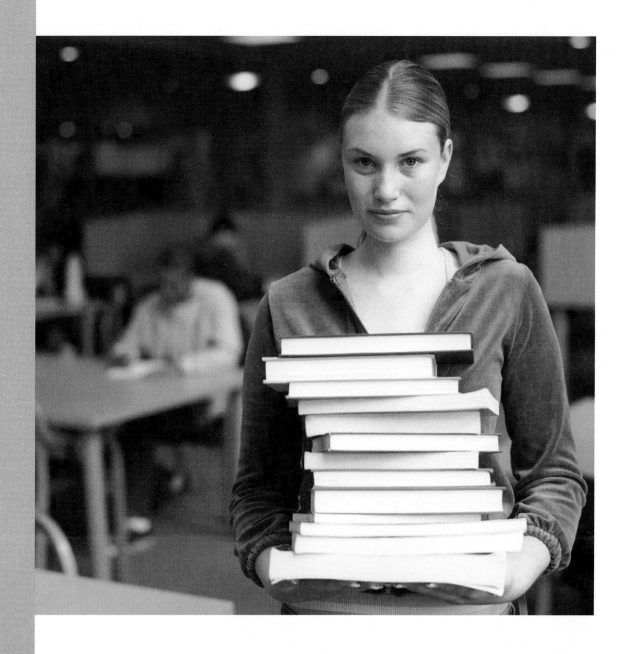

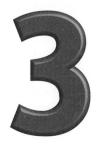

How Is This Test Different?

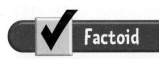

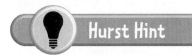

HOW IS THIS TEST DIFFERENT?

You will soon see this test is different in many ways from the nursing school exams you are accustomed to taking. That's okay. This isn't the first nor will it be the last time you encounter something new and different in nursing. The purpose of this chapter is to show you how the NCLEX® is different so you can adapt easily and pass THE FIRST TIME! Here are some ways the NCLEX® exam is different.

✚ Computer-adaptive testing

If you want the exact explanation of how computer-adaptive testing (CAT) is used, let me refer you to this site: **www.ncsbn.org.** You will see "NCLEX®" on left side of screen, click on this; click on NCLEX®; click on Candidate Basic Information; then you will see "Computerized Adaptive Testing Overview" at the top, middle of screen. Click here to read everything you ever wanted to know about CAT.

The main points I think you need to understand about this form of testing are as follows:

* The test is constantly changing according to the way YOU are answering the questions.[1]

CASE IN POINT If you get a question right, your next question will either be of the same level of difficulty or it may be a higher level of difficulty. If you get an answer wrong, the level of difficulty will drop down. If you get the next answer right, the level of difficulty goes back up again.

* Everybody's test is different. How can this be? In nursing school everybody had the same test.

✚ The test plan

There is a NCLEX® test plan, which we will be reviewing in more detail in Chapter 5. The test plan is broken down into many different **areas.** Each area covers several testing topics. On **YOUR** test you will receive a required percentage of questions from each area. Everyone who takes the exam is required to get the same percentage from each area. However, because there are so many different potential testing topics listed under each area, you and your nursing school buddy may get totally different test questions from the same area.[1]

✚ How is the NCLEX® graded?

In nursing school, your course syllabus or policy manual documented what grade you had to make to pass. This number began to RULE your life. You soon learned to fight for this number. You did anything to get that extra test point.

* Maybe you got all of the students in your class to sign a petition rebelling against a particular test question.

- Maybe you found documentation from many sources to prove your teacher wrong (oh, what joy!).

- Maybe you held a class meeting to rebel against a certain test.

✚ Your fight is over

These items should encourage you.

- NCLEX® is not graded by a score.

- Here we get into subtest scores, role delineation studies, calibrations on an interval scale, ordinal scales, Rasch definition of measurement, and invariant factors. You know, the more I think about all that, the more I'd better just stick to the simplest way of understanding grading. However, I do not discourage you from visiting **www.ncsbn.org** to check out psychometrics.[1]

- Basically, as far as passing is concerned, you have to show the NCLEX® Lady you are more **consistently** right than wrong when answering test questions.

- At a minimum, you have to get more test questions RIGHT than WRONG.

- Now, I know what you are wondering. How many more right than wrong, Aunt Marlene? I don't know, but by the time I'm finished with you, you'll be getting so many more right than wrong this won't EVEN be a concern anymore. So, let it go! Set that thought free!

- I know some of you are still fighting this concept of more "right than wrong." I'm going through this whole scenario, and then at the end you're still going to ask, "What do you have to make on this exam to pass? Just give me the number and I'll make it."

- NCLEX® is looking to see if you are more consistently RIGHT or more consistently WRONG when you answer questions!

✚ Let's pretend

Let's look at some different scenarios regarding how you pass—or yes, I must say it . . . fail.

- Scenario #1: You are the student that studies just like I tell you to. You do everything just like Aunt Marlene has outlined. You even speak with a southern accent. You go into that testing center with a certain amount of knowledge that you know without a doubt and without hesitation. You are going to miss some questions. That's okay. You can miss questions and still pass! Hallelujah! Remember, we gave up on trying to make 100% on the bed-making and hand-washing test! In spite of all of this, you are going to get the majority of answers right. You won't FEEL like you are getting any right, because if you study my way, you are going to move into the high-level questions quickly. High-level questions make you feel inferior, inadequate, and incompetent. They make you feel like you have taken your test too soon! But you haven't, because you have Aunt Marlene in your head and in your heart.

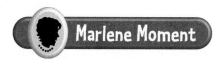

Marlene Moment

Anything! I'll do anything to get those 2 extra points! (To be said in desperation.)

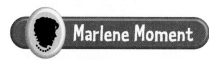

Marlene Moment

It took me three times to pass the math test (and I've never made a drug error, thank you) in nursing school, so I know I can't understand in-depth NCLEX® psychometrics. I'll leave that to the experts!

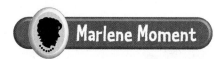

Marlene Moment

Nursing school wouldn't have been any big whoop if all I had to do was get more right than wrong! Well, NCLEX® is a little more complex than this, but I'm all about simplifying things.

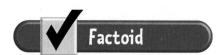

Factoid

NCLEX® is not graded like nursing schools exams where you have to make a certain score to pass.

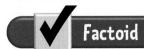

Marlene Moment

If you study Marlene's way, but you still feel like you don't know anything on the exam . . . you are passing! Weird, huh?

✔ **Factoid**

If you answered the minimum number of questions and ended up not passing the exam, you have a lot of work to do! Aunt Marlene will help you PASS NCLEX®!

Hurst Hint

When you take the entire test you have a 50-50 chance of passing.

---

* There is no doubt in my mind that if you study properly instructed, you will move into the high-level questions quickly. The computer will shut off at the minimum number of questions required to show competency (passing). You are going to sit there and wonder "Why did my computer just turn off? I wasn't ready for it to shut off." You are going to go home and tell everyone you know you failed—this is a defense mechanism you use innately to prepare family members and significant others for the worst—and then you'll worry, worry, and worry. However, you will find out you passed! Not only did you pass, you ACED that NCLEX®! Who would have ever thought it!

* Scenario #2: You are the student who did fine in school. Nursing school didn't really stress you like it did other people. You may be thinking things like, "This is my second degree anyway, and nursing is mainly common sense. My family has had every disease I've ever studied." You bought some study questions you found on eBay and you've memorized them (all 6500 to be exact). In addition, you already have a job in the neurological (neuro) intensive care unit (ICU). NCLEX® only tests for **MINIMUM** competency anyway. You say, "Surely, I'm minimally competent or they wouldn't let me work in the neuro ICU. Basically, I'm just ahead of this game."

* So here you go to take NCLEX® . You answer questions and you don't feel badly about the exam. Your computer shuts off at the minimum number of questions and you are out of there! You go to work that night and everyone is asking you about it. Basically, you tell them, "It wasn't that bad, but who knows?"

* Later, you get the test results and they are definitely NOT what you expected.

* Scenario #3: You are so happy to be out of school. All of your family came to graduation. Everybody is just SO HAPPY you finally finished something! You've been so busy moving, starting a new job, or maybe even getting married! You even participated in an NCLEX® review course held at your hospital. There's just been so much going on! Now NCLEX® day is here. You sit down at your computer and begin. A couple of hours have gone by and you've taken a snack break. You are on question number 68. You think: "Surely I'm getting close to finishing." Two more hours go by and you are just exhausted, but at least you have picked up your test-taking pace a little. Now you are at question number 200. You keep working at it until you end up taking the whole test. You can't believe it. You took the WHOLE test! What in the world does this mean?

* What it means in a nutshell is this: You kept the computer confused the whole time you were testing. Not at any point did you convince the computer that you were more consistently right or wrong. Therefore, the computer just kept giving you another question in an effort to figure you out.

Understanding the why

If you do not understand the "Why?" behind causes, signs and symptoms, nursing interventions, and medical interventions then you will have a very hard time answering NCLEX® questions correctly. You need to develop an inquisitive mind. Knowing "Why" is the KEY to answering critical thinking questions correctly.

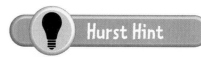

Hurst Hint

The more "Why's" you know, the more you understand, the less you have to memorize, and the greater the chance you will pass NCLEX® the first time.

THE TEST QUESTIONS ARE DIFFERENT

When you took a test in nursing school, you basically knew what topics were going to be covered. For instance, you may have had a cardiac and respiratory test. This test may have had 25 cardiac questions and 25 respiratory questions. Hopefully, you had specific notes to study, a thousand pages to read, a handout, and a copy of the instructor's Power Point slides. The questions were specific to the cardiac and respiratory topics. During NCLEX® you will not read a question and say, "This is a cardiac question." You will more likely say, "Hmmmm, there are a lot of things going on with this client."

CASE IN POINT A question may ask you about a 50-year-old client who undergoes in-vitro fertilization for her infertile daughter. During the delivery, the client develops congestive heart failure (CHF), which leads to a premature newborn. Okay, so I went a little crazy, but my point is this: NCLEX® questions will require you to use your knowledge of many subjects to generate one answer. You will have to use multi-logical thinking. Relax. I will show you how to deal with test questions later. I'm just laying the groundwork now. The questions on NCLEX® are written at a high level. You will be expected to comprehend, analyze data, and make critical decisions regarding client care.

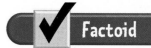

Hurst Hint

Who knows what topic will be covered on the next NCLEX® question? NCLEX® is an **integrated exam,** and we're going to show you how to get ready for it!

Factoid

NCLEX® questions are going to have several different topics rolled into one, and you will have to use multi-logical thinking to generate a correct answer.

SUMMARY

So, that's how the test is different. Don't worry. The majority of students still pass the first time and you can, too! Just keep reading and studying with me and we will get the job done. Now we are going to dispel some common NCLEX® myths!

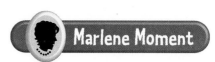

Marlene Moment

I doubt very seriously you will get any questions that are knowledge based. You know, the kind of questions where you could memorize the "handout" and pass?

Reference

1. National Council of State Boards of Nursing. NCLEX Examinations. Available at: **www.ncsbn.org.** Accessed November 10, 2006.

Bibliography

Hurst Review Services. Available at: **www.hurstreview.com.**

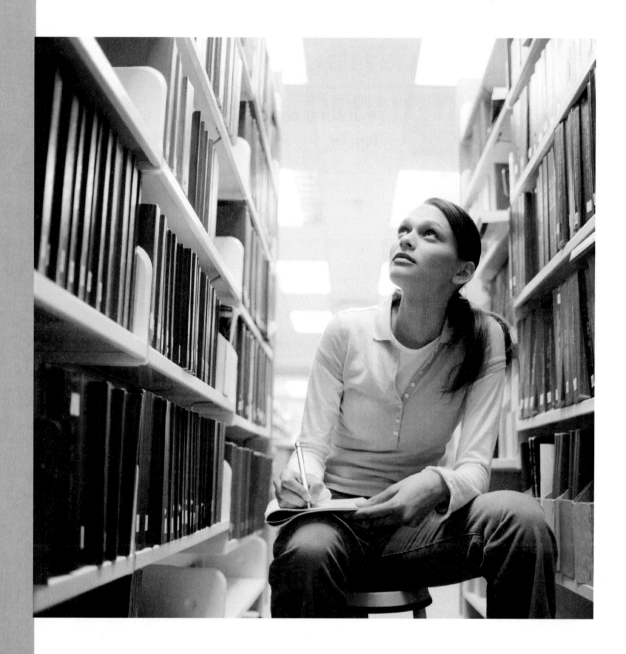

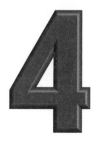

CHAPTER

4

NCLEX-PN®—Fact or Fiction?

NCLEX-PN®—FACT OR FICTION?

There's a lot of buzz out there about NCLEX®. Some of it is fact and some of it is fiction. Let's sort it out!

✛ Testing center

There are some points regarding the testing center that we need to clarify.

✔ Factoid

If you get the whole test, this is because of the way you answered the questions.

Every once in a while they just pick someone at random and give them the whole test.	Fiction.	They are not allowed to do this.

♥♦ Here's the Deal

The people at the testing center have no idea whether you passed the exam or not once you've completed your exam.

The people at the testing center know if I failed or passed.	Fiction.

The people who work at the testing center are experts on NCLEX®.	Fiction.	Case in point: The people who work at the testing center administer lots of test. Not many people, even in nursing, understand how NCLEX® works. Don't rely on the people who administer the test to answer any questions about anything. I do not mean that disrespectfully, but NCLEX® is just a different ballgame.

✛ Testing

There are a lot of myths out there regarding the test. Let's dispel them now.

The first few questions are most important.	Fiction.	You can miss the first 15 questions and still pass!
		Understanding the why: Maybe you were so scared when you started the exam, you were missing questions right and left. Then you settled down and started getting more questions right than wrong. You can still pass! This is why you must understand how the test works!

| You can't predict whether you passed or failed based on your last exam question. | Fact. | Many people think if you got your last question right you passed, or if you got your last question wrong you failed.

Case in point: This just isn't so! Your last question may have been a pilot question that does not even count anyway. |

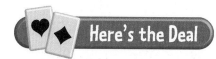

You have as much time as you need on each question. You have a total testing time of 5 hours for the NCLEX-PN®.

| I have only one minute per question, so I had better hurry! | Fiction. |

| I can't skip questions like I did in school. | Fact. |

You must answer the question displayed on the screen prior to moving to the next question.

| There are pilot questions on the exam, but I won't know which ones they are. | Fact. | Understanding the why: Yes, there are pilot questions and you will NOT know which ones they are.

These are questions that do not count toward your score in any way. They are placed on the test to ensure they are valid questions. Each question, before it is used as a real question, is tested in this manner. The NCLEX® people are test question experts and they invest a lot of time, effort, and brain power to ensure each question is fair, valid, and statistically sound. This is actually a blessing. |

| Essay questions are being used now. | Fiction. | Get real! Not happening! Do you think they want to read a bunch of essays? They'd never get all the tests graded! |

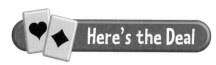

You will never be asked to select an answer outside your scope of practice.

| All questions will require an answer within my scope of practice. | Fact. |

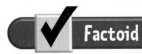

NCLEX® questions are at the application level and higher.

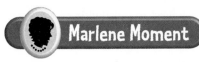

When you are questioned about an unfamiliar topic, you must remain calm! Be aware that this is the way that every nursing student across the country feels. You can still pass this exam!

Most of the questions on NCLEX® are either "knowledge based" or "comprehension."	Fiction.	Case in point: Those days are over. You will have to use more problem-solving skills to select the right answer. That's why you better stick with Aunt Marlene.

If I get a question on something I've never heard of, I shouldn't waste time on that question. I should click "C" and move on to something else.	Fiction.	The next question could be something you've never heard of and the question after that one as well! Remember, the exam addresses basic nursing care, even though you may have never heard of the disease or drug addressed in the test question.

The test is searching for your weakness.	Fiction.	Get real! The computer does not have a soul. The computer isn't psychic. The computer can't look at you and say, "Look at her. She doesn't know anything about crutch walking. Give her all crutch walking questions!" There is a test plan and the computer has to give you a certain percentage of questions from each area of the test plan. However, students always feel like they get more questions addressing their weak areas. If you get one question on counting peri-pads for a postpartum client and you know NOTHING about peri-pads, I promise you are going to tell all your friends: "The whole test was about peri-pads. Just study peri-pads!" Especially if you are a male student.

The higher the level of question, the worse you feel and the better you are doing.	Fact.	Think about it. A very high-level question will bring on some degree of stress. This is a good thing, because that means your hard studying has paid off.
		Marlene's rule: When you are asked a higher-level question, this means you have fewer questions to answer and the greater the likelihood you will pass!

If I get two questions that seem almost identical, this is the computer giving me a second chance so I should change my answer from the way I answered the first time.	Fiction.	This is pure coincidence. Do not change your thinking process if you believe you are right.

✚ Grading

Because the NCLEX® is not graded like other exams, there are some issues that we need to clear up.

I must make an 80 on the exam to pass.	Fiction.	Remember, you are being graded on how consistently you answer questions correctly or incorrectly. This is a good thing. You have to get more right than wrong. You can do that! Now you are wondering, "How many more question do I need to answer right than wrong?" I don't know, but you can do it. The majority of students who take the exam do. YOU CAN TOO!

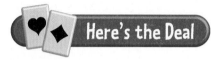

The test is not graded like your tests in school.

You can't pass if you take the whole test.	Fiction.	Yes, you can! In this scenario, the entire test is evaluated to see if you were consistently right or consistently wrong.

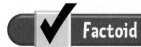

You can still pass if you take the entire test.

If your computer doesn't cut off at 85, that means you are doing poorly on your test.	Fiction.	Yes, many times the computer *does* cut off at 85 questions. When this happens, you have either passed or failed. We know this much without a doubt. But when it goes PAST 85 questions what does it mean? It means YOU'RE NOT failing!!!!! You are still in the ballgame. You have to look for the positive. If you were not passing, the computer would cut off. Because the test is still giving you questions, this means the computer hasn't completely made up its mind about you yet. At this point you know you are getting more answers right than wrong, or the computer would have already cut off!

If the computer goes past 85 questions, you know you are close to passing.

| The number of questions your test ends on can in no way predict whether you pass or fail. | Fact. | Refresh your knowledge: There is no way to predict whether you passed or failed by the number of questions you answer on your exam. The only way you can use this number is after you have gotten your results, and who cares then? For instance, if the computer cuts off at 85 and you passed the exam, this tells you that you passed with a high degree of difficulty. This tells you that you got to the high-level questions. If your computer cuts off at 205 and you pass, this means you were vacillating between passing and failing to the bitter end. You were basically keeping the computer confused! Finally, you got enough right answers—more than wrong ones—to prove to the computer that you are minimally competent to care for clients. Now, if your test cut off at 85 and you did not pass the exam, you flunked the test big time! The computer was just waiting to reach 85 questions, so it could cut off and rest. The computer already knew by number 85 that you were getting way more wrong answers than right ones . . . to the point it wasn't *even* going past 85. If the computer cuts off at 205 and you fail, this means you *barely* failed. You were so close to passing. Hey, if you have to fail, this is the way to fail. Now, what about all those numbers in between? Again, you can't make a judgment about how you did on your test based on the number of total test questions you get until AFTER you get your score. |

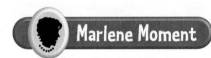

Instead of spending a lot of time trying to figure out how you did, just go and relax—or worry—whichever you choose.☺

✚ Test content

Now we have some specific "content" myths we need to bust.

| As most new nurses go to work in areas of maternity and pediatric nursing, the bulk of the test will come from these content areas. | Fiction. | Case in point: Most new nurses go to work in acute-care environments, and the majority of their clients are adults and the elderly. When I say acute care, that may mean critical care, medical-surgical units, pulmonary units, etc. In my opinion, the major focus of the test is focused on medical-surgical nursing. |

Only the latest and greatest information or research will be tested on NCLEX®.	Fiction.	Understanding the why: New information has to be studied by the NCLEX® personnel first. They will make sure the new information is a "standard" across the country prior to testing it on the actual test. I always think of NCLEX® as being a little behind the times in terms of research findings.

✛ NCLEX® policies

You need to be aware of some of the NCLEX® policies. Let's take a look at these.

The test is easier in different states.		Fiction.

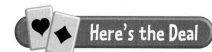

Factoid

The test is the same in every state, country, and province. The passing standard is the same everywhere.

If I decide to wait on taking my test, my money will be refunded.	Fiction.	No, it won't!

The testing people won't let you take but certain breaks at certain times.	Fiction.	You just have to remember your time is ticking during the breaks. Yes, there are designated break times, of which your computer screen will alert you.

Here's the Deal

You may take a break whenever you like. Just raise your hand and follow proper procedure.

✛ Timing

Here are some very important points regarding timing that we need to analyze.

When I see my time is almost up, I should start clicking "C" and hope for the best.	Fiction.	Pathway to destruction: This is a sure way to promote an unsuccessful outcome, and has nothing to do with knowing nursing content. You must think about it like this: I must be doing okay or the computer would not still be going. If I were failing, the computer would have shut down already. For the computer to still be giving me another question I haven't failed yet, so I can still pass! The computer has not made a pass or fail decision about me (it's not convinced about me one way or the other). That's why I am still getting questions.

You are going to blow it if you start clicking option "C." When you start clicking C, odds are you going to start making yourself get more questions wrong than right. So what do you do?

Marlene's rule: Calm down. Slow down. Take it one at a time at a pace where you can think sensibly. This is a higher-stress time because you know the clock is ticking. This is where you must get a hold on your emotions and control the situation as best as you can. Speed testing is not the right thing to try at this point. If you are devastated and having a panic attack, you would be better off just to sit there and let the computer tick down until it cuts off (assuming there are only 4 to 5 minutes left).

| If you run out of time you automatically fail. | Fiction. | Case in point: You can still pass. However, you will only be graded on the last 60 questions you answered. If you were consistently right on the last 60 questions, you passed. If you were consistently wrong on the last 60 questions, you failed. This is the very reason you should not start clicking "C" when you see yourself running out of time. |

✚ Studying

You've already heard me say how important it is to study the right way. Check out these pointers on studying.

| If I memorize five NCLEX® books and answer 5000 questions, I will pass. | Fiction. | Get real! I guarantee the NCLEX® people have every NCLEX® book you have. Do you think they are going to administer a test where all one has to do to pass is memorize? No. In fact, they are doing everything they can to make sure this doesn't happen. If all you had to do was "memorize" to pass, just think of how many unsafe nurses would be out there. They want nurses who can think on their feet in unfamiliar situations. THINK being the key word here! |

I have NCLEX® study materials from three of my friends who took NCLEX® and all three of them passed. So if I study this material, I will pass too.	Fiction.	Case in point: How do you know that? You may not have the same knowledge base as those students. You do not know what else they did to prepare. You are giving yourself a false reassurance. I'm not saying NOT to study those items; I'm saying you are an individual and each person has strengths and weaknesses. Can you pass the first time? Yes, you can!

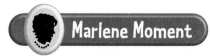

I'm not going to study my med-surg book because some of that information may not be NCLEX®-like.	Fact.	Good move. Besides, you do not have time for that unless you just want to look at the pictures and shaded boxes like you did in school. Let me give you an example: under appendicitis in your textbook it may say "cleansing enemas are given pre-op." Not NCLEX®-like! This action will scare the NCLEX® people, because you could rupture the fragile appendix.

It's not wise to study with experienced nurses when preparing for this exam.	Fact.	That's exactly right. Clinical alert! Remember, the way an experienced nurse answers questions (even a nurse who has only been out of school for 1 year) is totally different from the way a brand new nurse should answer a question. You'll see what I'm talking about when we start looking at practice test questions later in this book.

✚ To succeed or not to succeed

I already know you want to pass the *first* time! Assess this data to ensure your success.

If I had a 4.0 GPA in nursing school, I shouldn't have any trouble on NCLEX®.	Fiction.	Who knows? Path to destruction: This kind of thinking is definitely setting you up for false reassurance. I don't know what kind of questions were on your exams in nursing school. There's just no way to know. I'm not trying to be negative, just realistic; I've seen just as many straight A students do poorly on boards as C students have done well. Remember, studying for NCLEX® is like starting over. The playing field is level at this point. Your past grades do not matter. What matters is how you choose to study to prepare from this point on.

I've seen some really questionable people pass boards so I know I can pass because I'm smart!	Fiction.	We've all seen (or been the student) that just barely got by each semester. We've all seen (or been the student) that prayed for that extra half of a point to ensure passing that semester. How do these students pass boards? Well, here's my philosophy: When you've possessed a severe knowledge deficit throughout nursing school, you've been aware of this shortcoming for quite a while! You've known this was an issue. You've needed to go the extra mile to survive the process. If you can relate to this, as I can, what do people like us do? Well, first, we have no sense of false reassurance. We know that we will have to *overcompensate* in our studying to pass NCLEX®, and we do so!

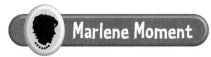

Marlene Moment

The number 1 reason people fail NCLEX® is due to the nursing diagnosis: **knowledge deficit.**

The number one reason people are unsuccessful on NCLEX® is test anxiety.	Fiction.	Wrong! They are unsuccessful because they do not know the core content. If you use the core content the proper way, you will pass. The best cure for test anxiety is being prepared the proper way!

I've worked in a hospital before, so I'm sure this will help me on NCLEX®.	Fiction.	Marlene's rule: You better forget what you've seen in the hospital. Why? Because what you've seen in the hospital may not make the NCLEX® people real happy. Remember the NCLEX® hospital is perfect. Your hospital is not. Sorry!

It's a good idea to take a medication for anxiety or something like a beta-blocker to keep you calm during the test.	Fiction.	Bad idea. The only way I would take a medication for anxiety is if the doctor had prescribed it AND I had been on it for a while. I certainly would not recommend taking any medication for the first time the day of the test. You just do not know how it will affect you. Now, let's get the beta-blocker thing straight!

Clinical alert! Okay, so a beta-blocker belongs in the class of drugs that decreases your output of epinephrine and norepinephrine (your stress hormones, your catecholamines). If you take a beta-blocker, you will stay cool as a cucumber because you will be unable to release these hormones. This is still not a good idea unless the medication is something you have been on for other reasons. Why? When you take a beta-blocker your heart rate slows down. Therefore, your cardiac output drops. When your cardiac output drops, then you do not have as much blood flowing to your brain. I do not think test day is the day to alter the amount of blood going to your brain! Okay? Okay.

SUMMARY

I hope we've dispelled some myths and rumors that you've heard throughout nursing school regarding the NCLEX®. You need to have correct information in your brain prior to taking the exam. The more you understand the exam, the better you will do. Next, we'll study the actual NCLEX® Test Plan.

Bibliography

Hurst Review Services. Available at **www.hurstreview.com.** Accessed November 5, 2006.

National Council of State Boards of Nursing. Candidate Bulletin. Available at: **www.ncsbn.org.** Accessed November 5, 2006.

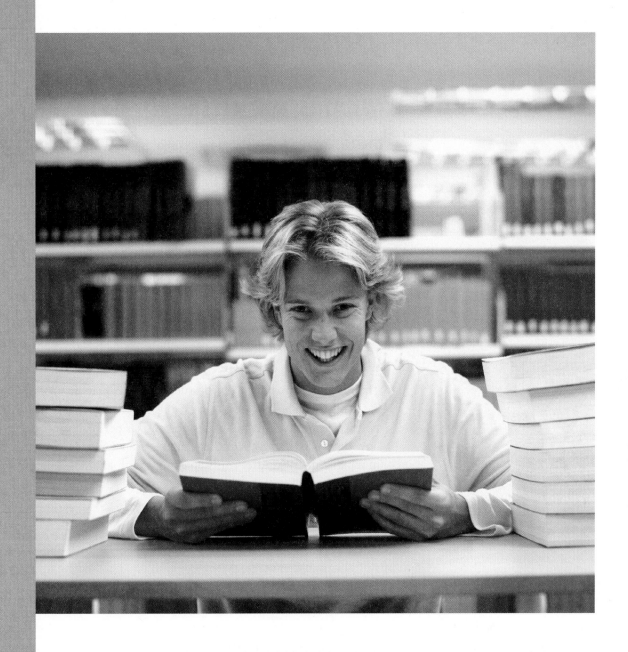

CHAPTER

5

Let's Make Sense of the Test Plan!

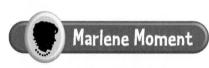

Factoid

Remember, the National Council of State Boards of Nursing is in the business of protecting the public. Therefore, the NCLEX-PN® ensures that only SAFE NURSES are allowed to practice.[1]

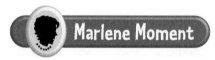

Marlene Moment

From the data collected in the surveys, a new baby test plan is born!

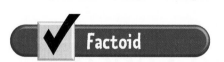

Marlene Moment

Don't get hung up on this test plan, because we are going to break it down for you to help make it simple.

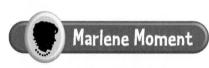

Factoid

The percentages listed in the table can vary by plus or minus 3%. If 8–14% of your test is on infection control, that means the actual percentage could really be as small as 5% or as much as 17%.[1]

LET'S MAKE SENSE OF THE TEST PLAN!

You're going to like this chapter. It's a quickie! The test plan for the NCLEX-PN® can be very confusing. But we are about to make sense of it all.

WHAT IS THE NCLEX-PN® TEST PLAN?

The NCLEX-PN® Test Plan for licensed practical nurses is a document that outlines the content that may be tested on the NCLEX-PN® exam. This document is developed by the National Council of State Boards of Nursing. The test plan is structured so that it defines the abilities and competencies the new graduate should be able to perform in any setting.[1]

✚ Why do they have a test plan?

The National Council takes great consideration when preparing this very important test. They do not just pull questions from out of the blue and put them on the exam. Therefore, they have a specific **test plan** to help determine what specific nursing knowledge is to be tested.[1]

✚ Where do they get the test plan?

The National Council conducts studies every 3 years in an effort to determine which skills nurses are using in their first 6 months of practice. It determines what activities new nurses perform **most frequently,** how these activities impact client safety, and what **areas** new nurses work in most frequently. After this step, an in-depth analysis is completed, which helps define entry-level nursing for **this** day and age.[1]

Here's the breakdown

Let's look at the percentages for each category that will be on the test (Table 5-1).

Table 5-1. Percentages of Categories on the NCLEX-PN®

Safe effective care environment	
• Coordinated care	11–17%
• Safety and infection control	8–14%
Health and promotion maintenance	**7–13%**
Psychosocial integrity	**8–14%**
Physiological Integrity	
• Basic care and comfort	11–17%
• Pharmacological therapies	9–15%
• Reduction of risk potential	10–16%
• Physiological adaptation	12–18%

From National Council of State Boards of Nursing. Test Plans. **www.ncsbn.org.** Accessed September 17, 2007. In April 2008, The test plan percentages will change slightly. Here's how:
1. The category "Coordinated Care" will comprise 12–18% of the exam (this is a slight increase from 11–17%)
2. The category "Physiological Adaptation" will comprise 11–17% of the exam (this is a slight decrease from 12–18%)

Basically, everything else is the same!

✛ What's in every category?

Integrated processes! Now I know you are asking, "what does integrated processes mean?" Well, let me tell you. Throughout the NCLEX-PN® exam you will find four major client needs categories; these are the integrated processes. The integrated processes are intertwined into each exam question. The processes are:

- Nursing process
- Caring
- Communication and documentation
- Teaching and learning[1]

CASE IN POINT The Registered Nurse teaches skin care to a client who is receiving external radiation therapy. Which of the following client statements would alert the nurse that further teaching is indicated?

1. I will use a mild soap to wash the area.

2. I will handle the area very carefully.

3. I will limit my exposure to the sun.

4. I will wear loose clothing over the site.

The correct answer is #1: I will use a mild soap to wash the area. The client receiving external radiation should avoid soap, lotions, and powders over the site. The **integrated process** used in this question is "teaching and learning."

✛ How does the test plan affect me?

It's all about YOU, isn't it? Yes, it is right now!

- Your test will come directly from the test plan.
- This does not mean you will get questions that address everything that is on the test plan.

SUMMARY

Okay, so NCLEX-PN® has a test plan. We've got that straight. We will analyze it to the letter in Chapter 12. So for right now, just be happy there is a documented plan that we can use to study together. Now that we've had a quickie test plan review, let's start looking at some real strategies for testing that actually work!

Reference

1. National Council of State Boards of Nursing. Test Plans. **www.ncsbn.org.** Accessed November 9, 2006.

Bibliography

Hurst Review Services Website at **www.hurstreview.com.**

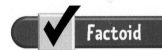

The latest and greatest test plan was implemented for the NCLEX-PN® in April 2005.

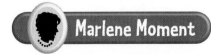

Don't worry. Aunt Marlene's got you covered.

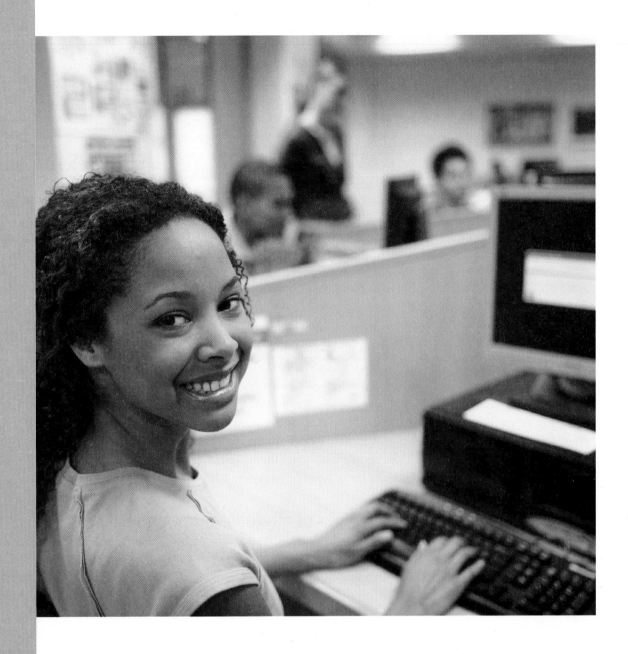

6 Basic Test-Taking Strategies

BASIC TEST-TAKING STRATEGIES

The basic test-taking strategies we will discuss in this chapter will help you to read the question stem and understand what the NCLEX® Lady is looking for in an answer. Then you'll be able to use your knowledge of core content to give the NCLEX® Lady just what she wants!

ALTERNATE FORMAT QUESTIONS

Let's go ahead and talk about "alternate format" (formerly called "innovative items") style questions first, so we can put this issue behind us. The majority of your test, if not all of it, will be multiple-choice questions. So, multiple-choice questions are the type of questions you must master. However, I know you are still worried about this "other" style of question. Now, let's get something straight. It doesn't matter how a question is stated—if you know your core content properly, you will get the question right more times than not, and that's the name of the game. If you understand the principles of congestive heart failure, it shouldn't matter how a question on this topic is stated. You'll be able to select the correct answer based on your knowledge of the core content. You can also go to **www.ncsbn.org** (click on NCLEX® Examinations, then click NCLEX®, Candidate Basic Info, then click Information Regarding Alternate Item Formats) to check out these questions directly from the people who write them. Your Candidate Bulletin will also have examples of these types of items.

✚ Types of alternate format questions

The types of alternate format questions you will encounter include

- Select all that apply
- Hot spot
- Fill in the blank
- Charts or exhibit items
- Drag-and-drop items.

Let's review these different test question formats to help you make sense of it all.

Select all that apply (also called multiple-response item)

With this style of question, you will be provided with a scenario and a list of potential answer options. You will know this is an alternate format question because it will actually say "select all that apply" after the stem of the question. You will have more than four options. Just break each selection down by pretending each statement is a true or false statement.

Something else that makes this question look different is that BOXES will appear before each numbered answer, so you can check the boxes you want. You will have to choose one or more answers.[1]

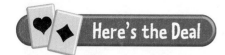

You may see more than one or two of these types of items on your test. No stress!

Hot spot

The example I like to use to demonstrate this type of question involves a motor vehicle accident (MVA) victim who seems to have some difficulty remembering. If you are asked to pick the lobe of the brain that is responsible for memory, you will be shown an image of the lobes of the brain. Move the mouse around until you get to the lobe of the brain that is responsible for memory.[1]

Fill in the blank

To answer this type of question, you will have to type a number into the blank space. For example, you may be asked to calculate intake and output (I&O) or medication dosages. Only numbers go in the blank . . . no milliliters (mL) or ounces (oz), etc. You may have to type in a decimal point if appropriate. Nothing but numbers and decimal points are allowed in the blanks. Not even units of measure.[1]

Charts or exhibit items

You will be given a scenario with a chart or an exhibit. You will study the chart or exhibit to properly answer the question. In addition, you may see the word "Tab" that you have to click on to get further information.[1]

Drag-and-drop items

For this type question, you will be asked to prioritize nursing actions. You decide which step you would take first, second, and so on. The answer you put in the blank may look like 614352 (you're saying I would do #6 first, #1 second, and so on).[1]

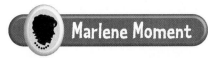

Marlene Moment

You know, some topics are just easier to test with this new style of test questions rather than using multiple-choice questions.

> ### What the NCLEX® Lady Thinks
>
> I want to constantly develop better ways to assess a new nurse's competency. I'm a techie diva! I want to use the diverse test-taking technology that's out there by including it on the NCLEX®.

✚ General points for alternate format items

Keep these general points in mind when answering alternate format type questions.

- They don't count any more or any less than a multiple-choice item.
- They're either right or wrong, just like a multiple-choice question.
- No partial credit will be given on an alternate format item.
- These items will not affect your pass rate.
- Having a degree in computer engineering is not necessary to select the right answer.

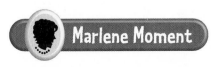

Marlene Moment

In my opinion, you could probably miss this entire style of question and still pass.

THE GOLD STANDARD: THE MULTIPLE-CHOICE QUESTION

In my opinion, now is the time to focus on what you will see the most of on NCLEX®—multiple-choice questions. It's kind of like my philosophy on memorizing 200 individual drugs. You could learn the whole *Physicians Desk Reference* (PDR) and only get 4 drug questions. Think how long it would take you to memorize the PDR and think of how much fun that would be! Or, you can spend 4 hours reviewing the major classes of drugs and get on with life. The smart thing to do (especially now that you have time constraints) is to focus on what you will see the most of: the multiple-choice question.

This type of question is presented as a scenario with four answer choices. Circles are present in front of each numbered answer selection. You will only be allowed to select one answer.[1]

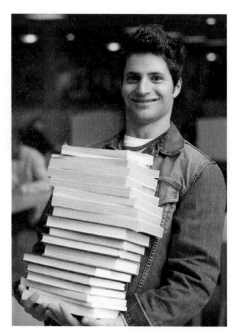

✚ Strategies for platinum success

There are several strategies that need to be reviewed first in order to come to the correct test answer. Let's take a look at these strategies more closely.

Break it down!

Here's one of my favorite ways to break down a test question. Let me show you.

- Read the stem (scenario) and figure out what the PROBLEM is.
- Read the stem and figure out what you are supposed to be worried about even if everything sounds great.
- What is the WORST thing that can happen in this scenario?
- Once you've got an idea about what the problem is, then select an answer that fixes the problem.

CASE IN POINT   If the problem is HEMORRHAGE, then you should not select an answer like "assess the vital signs." Why? Because "assessing" the vital signs does not FIX the PROBLEM or stop the hemorrhage.

Trash 'em

There are times when you will know immediately an answer is wrong.

- Look for answers that you know are wrong without a doubt and without hesitation, and throw them in the trash compactor! Why waste precious time on things you know are wrong?

I'm on the disorient express

There are going to be times during this exam when you feel like you just don't know what to do. Let's see if these strategies help.

1. What if I read a question and I have absolutely no idea what they are asking for? The first thing to remember is this: **If you are baffled,**

bewildered, or discombobulated, so is every other nursing student in the country! Don't come unglued. Let's blitz, drive, and score because I've got a game plan:

- Imagine yourself at the bedside in this scenario.
- Do I have any idea about what I'm supposed to be WORRIED about?
- Read the answers for a tip-off. You might find a Jordonesque (as in Michael Jordon, the famous basketball player!) answer.
- Then if all else fails, pretend each answer is written on a separate index card; then select which answer (if it were all by itself) sounds the safest as an independent statement all alone.

2. What if all 4 answers are beckoning my call? When all 4 answers look good, it's either a high level question or we don't know our core content on this topic. Hey! You can't know everything. It's not uncommon for all 4 answers to look inviting. Be aware going into this exam that this feeling is going to occur. If it's happening to you, it's happening to every other nursing student who is taking this test. You can still pass! The key is not to get psychodramatic. Keep your game face on, do your best, and move on!

Answer advancer

Here's some advice on "answers" that may help you in your moment of need.

1. It's a fact: The answer you want will never be there (just like in nursing school) no matter how long you stare at the computer screen. That's okay. Everybody feels the same way. I know that's not very therapeutic of me, but if everyone who takes the test feels just like you, and the majority pass, then YOU can too!

CASE IN POINT If I asked you, "What does the skin feel like when someone starts going into shock?" I'll bet you would immediately say, "cold and clammy!" See? Everybody knows this! The NCLEX® people already know that every nursing student around the world knows this is the answer. So WHY would they want to waste their time writing questions about things they already know YOU know? That's why they are going for the less obvious answers. They want to make the questions harder and also higher level. Examples of less obvious answers would be: decreased $PaCO_2$, shallow depth of respirations, and paste-like mucous membranes.

2. A question that asks for a "nursing action" may mean you need to select an answer where you are performing an assessment or implementing a specific nursing action. Remember assessment and implementation are two separate phases of the nursing process. Nursing action doesn't mean you have to pick a nonassessment–related answer as assessment IS an action. You have to read the scenario and figure out where you are in the nursing process prior to selecting an answer.

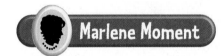

Marlene Moment

It helps to know you are not alone in feeling frustrated because the answer you want so badly is not staring you in the face. If the answer is not obvious to you, it's not to anyone else, either.

Hurst Hint

It is safer to pick a "nursey" answer because this test is about what the nurse thinks or does . . . not what the other health care team members do (even though these team members are very important).

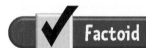

Factoid

Pain never killed anybody. I'm not saying pain is not important; it does need to be dealt with immediately. Prior to selecting the "pain" answer, look for an item that is more life threatening (increasing intracranial pressure, shock, or hypoglycemia).

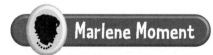

Marlene Moment

If Aunt Marlene is your client, you had better be taking care of her pain stat! But, that's after you pass NCLEX®!

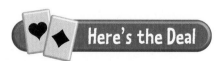

Here's the Deal

If someone is in the emergency department (ED) with an acute onset of gout, I don't think airway is an appropriate answer.

Check out these points below for some tight clarification!

* You have to make sure a proper assessment has been done first.
* After you read the stem (scenario), you will know if a proper assessment has been performed. Then you can move on to an implementation answer.
* If an assessment has already been described in the stem of the question, please do not pick an assessment answer. Move on, girl, to the next phase of the nursing process—implementation!
* If your client describes what is wrong, this is the client's assessment, and the client isn't the one trying to get a nursing license. You need to perform your OWN assessment prior to moving to implementation.

3. When you have answers such as "call the supervisor" or "call the dietician," you have to be suspicious. Why? Because the NCLEX® Lady would prefer YOU do something to help the patient directly.

CASE IN POINT Don't pick answers that refer your client AWAY from your care. Don't give YOUR work to someone else. I'm not saying we do not get other members of the health care team involved, but if the answer sounds like you are completely referring the client away, do not pick that answer!

4. Stay away from restraints, wheelchairs, and drugs (especially invasive drugs) as long as you can when choosing an answer. The NCLEX® Lady does not like nurses who tie people down or nurses who run to the medication cart for every little thing.

Mesmerizing maslow

Remember Maslow and his little triangle from your first week of nursing school? Well, here he is again!

1. Just because someone is in pain does not mean they are about to die. Pain is considered to be a higher-level need. Higher-level needs come later. Remember, YOU need to deal with the life-threatening problem first, and you can send someone else to deal with the pain. Now if it's pain as with a myocardial infarction (MI), that's a whole different ballgame!

2. Airway isn't always right! I bet I'm the first one to tell you that!

CASE IN POINT "My toe hurts!" says the ED client. "OK, let me check your airway," says new nurse. "I don't think so!" says the nursing instructor.

3. Don't let the stem of the question trick you.

4. You'll score more points with "physiological" answers than "psychosocial" answers.

CASE IN POINT

Physiological = administer medication to restore normal bowel flora, therefore decreasing episodes of explosive diarrhea.

Psychosocial = evaluate and identify individual coping behaviors in regard to explosive diarrhea.

If you had to choose between these two options, go for the physiological answer. The physiological answer is a lower-level need. Lower-level needs must be met first.

The hospital and the hospitalist

These strategies deal specifically with the hospital and the physician.

1. You already have the order! Don't sit there and say, "Oh, I wonder if I have to have an order for that?" If it's an option, you have an order. Don't fight it!

2. Do not use what you have seen in the hospital as a test-taking strategy. Many times what you have seen does not have the NCLEX® seal of approval.

3. "Call the physician" answers: I would be careful of this answer. Now don't get me wrong. There are times when calling the physician is the ONLY thing you can do. Just make sure there is not a nursing answer you can select that will help the client or problem first, prior to selecting this answer. However, don't just pick any answer to avoid selecting, "call the physician." Sometimes this will be the answer because the physician is the only one who can FIX the problem (based on the four options given).

Medication fixation

All students fear drug questions. Here's a rule that may help if you are in a bind.

* General Rule: Drug + Side Effect = Problem.

Unless you are an expert on the particular drug listed in the question, this is a safe way to select an answer. Don't sit there and wonder if those side effects are normal or expected unless you are very knowledgeable about that particular drug.

Don't be scared

There's no need to fear, Aunt Marlene is here. Here are a few strategies to make you less afraid.

1. Don't be afraid to select an answer that says "sit with the client."

CASE IN POINT #1 Most students look at an answer like this and say, "I don't have time to do this. I have other clients to take care of." No, the only client you have to worry about is the one on the screen, and if this is the best option, DO IT, no matter how unrealistic it sounds.

2. Don't be afraid to select an answer just because you've never seen it done. If it's safe, consider it to be a reasonable option.

CASE IN POINT #2 Have a Parkinson's disease client pretend there are imaginary lines on the floor when walking. You may think that sounds weird, but this is okay because it will force the client to focus on picking

Hurst Hint

If in the stem of the question there is no indication of breathing problems, do NOT select an answer to help breathing (elevate the head of the bed, etc.), as it would not be applicable.

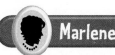

Marlene Moment

Client says, "My bowels haven't moved in a while." New nurse says, "Let me elevate your head to help you breathe better." NCLEX® Lady says, "I don't think you're going to get a license!"

Marlene Moment

It it's an answer option, you already have an order. Go for it!

Marlene Moment

The NCLEX® hospital is an awesome place to work! This hospital has all the staff you need, all the equipment you need, an excess of time in which to complete tasks, and every office and department is always open. And finally, the only client you have to worry about is the one on the computer screen! (And the NCLEX® hospital pays well, too!)

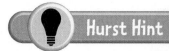

Hurst Hint

If there is something that you can do to help the PROBLEM, do that prior to calling the doctor. The catch is that your action must be helping the problem.

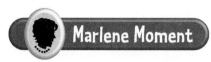

Marlene Moment

Just go ahead and assume the worst client outcome, and select the answer that is the most life threatening.

up his feet when walking rather than shuffling. When you help the client focus on picking up his feet, this decreases the number of falls.

CASE IN POINT #3 Would you rather your client with Parkinson's wear well-fitting sneakers or hot pink furry house slippers? Now here are the thoughts that are going through your head: hot pink furry house slippers!? That is so ridiculous! Now think back to Parkinson's . . . shuffling gait. You put grippy sneakers on that client, and when he shuffles, he is going to grip the floor and fall! Now he has a head injury, broken hip, and Parkinson's disease! That's not nice! Nursing student says, "But they taught us in the first semester of nursing school to beware of slippery shoes due to the likelihood of a fall." Hey! You have to be flexible and work with the answers you have no matter how off the wall they sound! The slippery shoes will actually help the Parkinson's client with a shuffling gait glide along the floor more easily. The art of becoming flexible with your knowledge is imperative and shows you are moving into higher level thinking.

Compliant client

Now we have some tips that deal specifically with the client.

1. Client first, equipment later.

CASE IN POINT #1 Your client is post-prostatectomy. He is complaining of bladder spasms. What should you assess first?

* The bladder for distension.
* The catheter tubing for kinks.

You know you are going to do both, but if you use this strategy you will assess the bladder for distension first, as this answer is client centered.

2. We've all heard, "Treat the client, not the monitor."

CASE IN POINT #2 This is a handy little tip to know if you have a client with pulseless electrical activity (PEA). In other words, she has a rhythm on the monitor and everything looks groovy up there. If you assume the client is okay because she has a pretty rhythm on the monitor, you have just let somebody die. (You aren't going to get a license like that!) This client has electrical activity showing up on the monitor, but no pulse. The electrical part of the heart is working, but the pump has stopped. This is why we must treat the client, not the monitor.

CASE IN POINT #3 Your client has just gone into ventricular tachycardia. You run into the room ready to defibrillate. But when you get in the room, the client is sitting up in the bed flipping the TV remote watching "Deal or No Deal." You'd better not shock them, or you are not going to get a nursing license in the mail! You can have V-tach with a pulse! So let's treat the client, not the monitor.

I'm seeing things

Sometimes when students read questions, lots of other thoughts start coming into their minds. Let's see if we can remedy this.

1. Stop reading into questions. If you find yourself saying "What if?" that should be a red flag that you are about to read into a question. Read the question and figure out what you are WORRIED about. Then select an answer that best addresses your worry.

2. Don't freak out if you get a question with a graphic or picture. So you have a cute picture to look at. No big deal. Just stay focused on the question. This question is not weighted any differently than any other question.

3. With every question, pretend you are in the scenario. Start analyzing every question by saying, "I'm taking care of a client who . . . ." This makes it real.

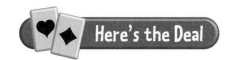

Read the question and figure out what you are WORRIED about. Then select an answer that best addresses your worry.

Trail mix

Let's now discuss the various situations you may encounter on the exam.

1. If the test writer goes to the trouble of including a time-frame, then this information has been put there to help you select a correct answer (late symptoms, early post-op, and early shock symptoms verses late shock symptoms).

2. Teaching questions: answer them no differently than you would any other question.

   If you understand your core content, then you will know what to teach the client.

3. Your whole test could ask questions about clients who are pregnant.

   This does not mean you are being tested on maternity nursing explicitly. I can write you a med-surg test and every client could be pregnant. The reason I mention this is that if you start getting lots of pediatric questions, you may panic and think you didn't study this area enough. I promise you the question is about general client care, not just pediatrics. You've got to be prepared for this ahead of time, so that when you start feeling like you are getting only obstetric (OB) related questions or only pharmacology questions you can regain your composure and realize this is simply not the case. Now if the question is about growth and development in a 2-year-old . . . that's different.

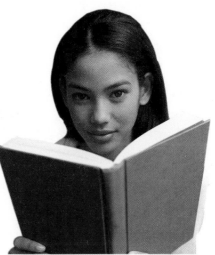

4. What if I feel like I need more information to answer the question? This means you've probably encountered a high-level question. The less information you have in the stem of the question, the higher the level of question. So be happy you are in the high level and keep on doing what you're doing. You must be doing something right or you wouldn't be there!

5. What if I can narrow it down to two and can't decide? This is so common. One of two things is happening. You've either encountered a higher-level question or you haven't studied the content thoroughly. This happens to everyone and it will happen to you, too but you can still pass the exam. So what do you do? Study Chapter 7, "How to Tackle a Priority Question," and do my on-line review to make sure you know your core content." Each of these will help you with these questions.

ANCIENT, BROKEN-DOWN, FOSSILIZED, MOTH-EATEN STRATEGIES

Why don't these strategies work anymore? Because NCLEX® test writers are experts in writing test questions; they don't use old tricks over and over. But go ahead and read them so they will be in your brain. These are the ones you are most familiar with anyway:

1. Repeated words: If there is a certain word in the stem (the first part of the question) and you see the same word in an answer . . . this is probably the answer.

2. Opposites: When two answers are opposite of each other, then one of these is probably the answer. Example: Increase the infusion rate or decrease the infusion rate.

3. Odd man wins: The answer that is the most different from the others will usually be the answer.

4. Umbrella answer: This is the answer that includes more.

CASE IN POINT Check blood pressure (BP) versus check vital signs.

The umbrella answer is "check vital signs," because it covers more information and includes something from another answer.

5. Absolutes: Nothing in nursing is absolute because every client is different. You learned quickly in nursing school when an answer said "always or never" that this was usually wrong. NCLEX® likes answers with words like "frequently" or "sometimes." The minute you say NEVER, then the physician is going to allow the client to do something you just told them they should NEVER do. Other good words that leave you some breathing room are: usually, potentially, normally, commonly, partial, might, nearly, almost, may, should, generally, occasionally, could, seldom, and often.

Hurst Hint

Leave yourself some breathing room when selecting answers. Don't back yourself into a corner.

What the NCLEX® Lady Thinks

I'm going to try my best to avoid writing a question where an old "strategy" is all that is needed to answer a question correctly.

SUMMARY

You will find these strategies handy when you start practicing test questions, and I promise to re-emphasize them along our journey together. Remember, however, the more you know your core content, the fewer strategies you will need to select the correct answer. Preparing for NCLEX® is like putting together a big puzzle, and you and I are going to put the entire puzzle together, TOGETHER.

Reference

1. National Council of State Boards of Nursing. Available at: **http://www.ncsbn.com.** Accessed October 30, 2006.

Bibliography

Hurst Review Services. Available at **http://www.hurstreview.com.**

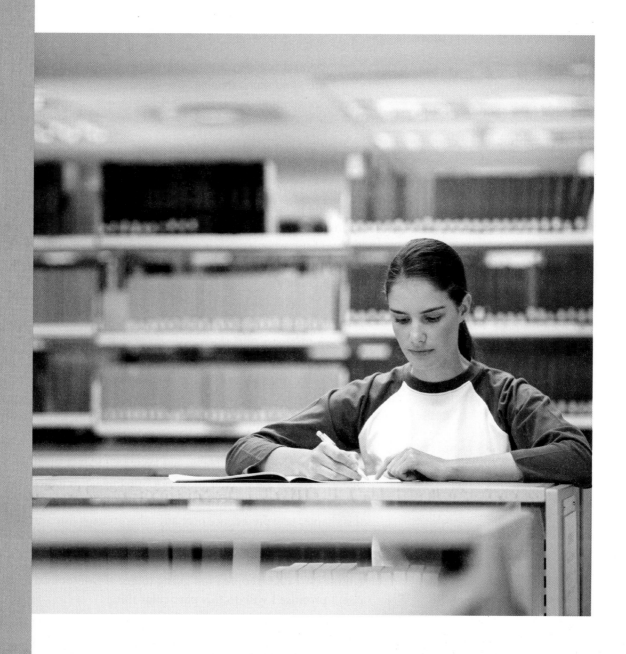

CHAPTER

7

How to Tackle a Priority Question?

HOW TO TACKLE A PRIORITY QUESTION?

WARNING: This chapter will change your testing life!

I wanted to talk about priority questions separately, because they seem to give students so much trouble. We will first go over some basic strategies for these types of questions and then practice what we have learned. Remember, this type of thinking does not come overnight, so be patient!

✚ Mustn't hate

Most students hate questions that have the word "priority." That's okay; we are going to learn how to deal with these right now because you will be seeing a lot of these types of questions on NCLEX®. I have some guidelines I use when answering priority questions. Not all guidelines are applicable for every priority question, but as we practice you will learn how these guidelines will help.

1. First, you need to realize the word "priority" changes everything. Priority does not necessarily mean "What would I do first." This is what confuses students the most!

Define time

Priority means if I do not do one of the following, my client could die or experience significant harm.

2. To be perfectly honest, even when the question does ask "What would you do first?" you have to remember what NCLEX® is all about: **keeping people alive.** NCLEX® is all about not bringing harm to people. Even when the question asks "What would you do first?" the strategies listed in this chapter take precedence over any other strategy listed anywhere else.

3. Ask yourself the following questions: When given four options, what's the ONE thing I'd better do? What's the one thing I'd better tell the NCLEX® people I am going to do? If I do not do anything else, I promise I will do this particular thing.

4. When you select your answer, you are COMITTED to it! You can't say, "Well, I was going to do that other stuff, too. I just thought I should have done this first."

5. When selecting an answer: think killer answer!

Define time

A killer answer is an answer that will bring death or some form of harm to a client. You can "kill" someone physiologically or psychologically.

✚ NCLEX® practice question

Here's a quickie example that incorporates all of these guidelines:

The nurse is aware that the most serious side effect of the tocolytic terbutaline sulfate (Brethine) is:

1. Respiratory depression

2. Pulmonary edema

3. Hypertension

4. Renal failure

Refresh your knowledge

What's a tocolytic? What's terbutaline sulfate (Brethine)? If you don't know, you may miss this question. Most everyone knows Brethine is a bronchodilator—a drug that promotes breathing, but in this scenario it is being given as a tocolytic. Tocolytics relax the uterus. You know that drugs can be given for various things. Now the question said "the most SERIOUS side effect."

* Once you look at the answer you should be thinking "pick the KILLER answer." However, the answer has to be applicable. For instance, renal failure (answer #4) will kill you but has nothing to do with this drug, so this answer is out. (It's not applicable.)

* You probably looked at respiratory depression (answer #1) and thought "That's It! Airway is always right!" Not if it's not applicable. Bronchodilators (Brethine) HELP you breathe. So answer choice #1 is out.

This leaves choices #2 and #3.

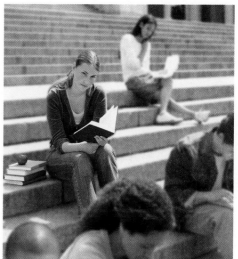

* Everybody knows that, in general, drugs that promote breathing pump up the vital signs, thus making people nervous and jittery. So, answer #3, hypertension, is still in the ballgame.

* Now let's look at answer #2. Is this answer possible? An answer must be POSSIBLE in order for you to consider it. Could pulmonary edema even happen with this drug?

Refresh your knowledge

When you give this type of drug, the heart rate is probably going to go up. When the heart rate goes up too high, the ventricles do not have as much time to fill with blood, so cardiac output goes down. The same amount of blood remains in the cardiac system, so this blood has got to go somewhere. If it's not being pumped forward (remember the cardiac output has dropped), then the blood is going to start to go backward into the lungs. Therefore, pulmonary edema could occur.

* This answer is applicable. Now we have 2 correct answers: #2 and #3. Pick the KILLER answer. Using this strategy, answer #2 makes the most sense. This strategy will help when you narrow it down to two answers. This may leave you feeling like you are just guessing between the remaining two answers. This is another common predicament students find themselves in. This study guide will teach how to pick the most correct answer. Read on . . . .

✛ How do you want the NCLEX® lady to think of you?

Now I'm going to present more plots to impress the NCLEX® Lady plus help you prevail over perplexing priority predicaments.

* Every time you select an answer on NCLEX® you are sending a message to the NCLEX® people about the kind of nurse you are. They are sizing

you up and deciding what kind of nurse you will be by the answer you choose. You are sending a vital message with each answer you select.

- You've got one shot at letting the person who wrote the question know that you know what nursing action to take.

- Once you select your answer, that does not mean you are NOT going to do the other options as well (especially if all four answers are correct and applicable). It just means you'd better make sure the NCLEX® people know you will do "*this*" if you do not do anything else. There is no place on the side of the computer screen for you to send notes explaining your answer.

- You have no opportunity to explain your answer to the NCLEX® people. They have to judge you by the answer you select. Once you select your answer you can't leave the NCLEX® people wondering, "I wonder if he knew to do this as well." So you have to get into the habit of deciding "Would I rather the NCLEX® people know that I knew to do this thing versus that thing?"

✚ Fix the problem

There are many ways to conquer priority predicaments. Let's take a peek.

- A good little tip is to try to figure out the WORST possible thing that could happen to the client based on the data given in the question. Then select an answer that most directly ATTACKS OR FIXES the problem.

Understanding the why

Understanding the why will keep you from selecting answers like "assess the vital signs." Doesn't assessing the vital signs sound like a safe and reasonable tactic? Yes! Why does this answer sound so good? Because it has been drilled into your head "assessment is the first phase of the nursing process!" But if someone is hemorrhaging, how will assessing the vital signs fix the PROBLEM? It won't. This concept is very important. I'm not saying you are not going to assess the vital signs; I'm saying you need to show the NCLEX® people you know how to keep people alive. This is a great example of how answering questions on nursing school tests is slightly different than on the NCLEX®!

THE PRIORITY INTERVENTION QUESTION

A priority intervention answer has some specific characteristics:

1. You are NOT selecting an answer like pulmonary edema or renal failure because these aren't nursing interventions.

2. You ARE selecting a nursing intervention that takes precedence over all other interventions.

3. The intervention MUST be done in order to keep the client ALIVE even if ALL of the answers list interventions that must be performed immediately.

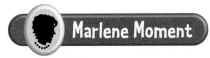

Marlene Moment

It's not like nursing school, where after a test you can pen your teacher up in her office and say "Oh, you're going to listen to my rationale because I need these 2 points!"

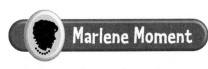

Marlene Moment

You have only one shot at letting the NCLEX® Lady know that "If I only do ONE thing, I PROMISE to do this and I KNOW to do this."

EXAMPLES OF PRIORITY QUESTIONS

Let's look at some examples to make these points come to light. This first question is an example of a priority intervention question.

✚ NCLEX® practice question

A client has returned from a routine colonoscopy. The client is complaining of a small amount of abdominal discomfort. The client informs the nurse that he passed a drop of blood. Which action takes priority?

1. Taking the vital signs

2. Instructing the client to remain in the bed

3. Calling the physician

4. Administering PRN pain medication

Slow down and chill out

You need to read this information slowly and with an open mind! This type of thinking is a MUST if you want to pass NCLEX®!

Are you worried?

First let me ask you something: Based on this data, are you worried or not worried about the client? You'd better be worried to death because this is NCLEX® we are taking!

Marlene's rule

A question will not be a question on NCLEX® unless there is something wrong with the client—something you should be worried about. There are no happy NCLEX® questions!

Don't crash on me

Now don't panic, but the answer is #3. Okay, go ahead and have a panic attack and then read on. I've already told you this kind of thinking does not occur overnight.

Think worst circumstance

When you read the data, what is the worst thing(s) that could happen with this client? You may be saying, "I don't know. Doesn't sound like much of a problem to me. He is just having a little discomfort and a drop of blood never hurt anyone."

NCLEX® DEADLY DISTRACTER You just fell into the NCLEX® trap. This kind of thinking is exactly what the NCLEX® people fear you will have when you become a nurse. In the NCLEX® people's eyes, with that attitude, you just brushed off client symptoms and complaints. This is a no-no! You are a brand new nurse who must view everything as a problem. You can't go wrong thinking like this. Even if it's not a problem, in the end you still offset a *potential* problem. Be *overly cautious*.

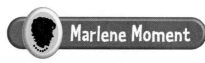

Marlene Moment

By the time I'm finished with you, we'll both have a peptic ulcer, unless you already have one from nursing school.

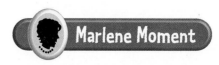

Marlene Moment

You might get on people's nerves thinking like this, but WHO CARES? We're gonna pass NCLEX® and save lives!

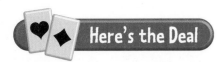

Here's the Deal

Assume all test question scenarios are set up to trick you into thinking nothing is going on with the client that can't wait a little while.

Be a pessimist

You'd better ASSUME THE WORST to keep yourself and your client out of trouble when answering NCLEX® questions.

When you assume the worst, you are forced to at least rule out life-threatening situations first.

CLINICAL ALERT! You may feel like you are overreacting thinking like this. It's better to overreact and possibly save somebody's life then to underreact and miss something big. Again, I want you to be overly cautious. We are trying to keep people alive.

- Let me re-emphasize that the questions will be worded to make you think "This situation is no big deal. I'll just sit back and watch the client for a while."

What the NCLEX® Lady Thinks

The NCLEX® Lady thinks you are going to brush off little subtle hints. Now that you have been forewarned, are you? No! You going to pretend, with each question, something horrible is happening to the client! Hey, I didn't have to go to nursing school to know something is wrong when I see a large amount of bright red blood coming from a client! In the end if I did overreact, and nothing major is going on with my client, I still did the right thing.

- Now let's get back to figuring out what is the worst thing that could happen in this scenario. Based on the data (small amount of discomfort and a drop of blood post-colonoscopy), the worst thing that could occur is hemorrhage or perforation of the intestine due to the procedure.

CLINICAL ALERT Just because you only see one drop of blood doesn't mean there's not a lot of blood concealed inside the peritoneum.

But I'm not a doctor

Now I know what you are saying. Nurses are not supposed to diagnose. But you do need to understand the why of medical situations in order to pass NCLEX®.

UNDERSTANDING THE WHY You have vast nursing knowledge, so use it.

- You aren't going to call the doctor and say, "We have a perforation here, and I've notified the surgical team." You are just using your knowledge to help you make the right decisions for your clients and to pass NCLEX®!

- Even if you didn't think about perforation or hemorrhage you still should have at least known the following:

   1. You're taking the NCLEX®.

   2. There's a problem.

3. There are symptoms in this scenario.

4. Can you **fix** the problem with the options you have been given?

5. No, you can't.

Back it on up

Let's go back to some of the guidelines we have reviewed with these two complications in mind.

1. If the problem is hemorrhage or perforation, which answer will attack/fix the problem? Now hold that thought. Let's look at the answers individually.

   - Answer #1: Taking the vital signs. In your nursing student brain you are saying things like assessment is the first phase of the nursing process, or you have to take the vital signs before you call the doctor! (I know you are thinking this because the first thing the doctor is going to ask is "What are the vitals?")

   - But I want to ask you something: Tell me how taking the vital signs FIXES hemorrhaging or perforation? It doesn't.

2. Go back to another one of my guidelines: Once I pick my answer I'm COMMITTED to it. That's it. You can't do anything else.

KILLER ANSWER You are telling the NCLEX® people (to be said very humbly): "NCLEX® Lady, I promise, when I have a client who is hemorrhaging or who has a perforation I will, without a doubt, take their vital signs over and over and over. This is the ONE thing I will do. I'm COMMITTED to this. I will take them over and over and watch the blood pressure go down, down, down . . . to zero.

   - No! I am not saying that taking the vital signs is inappropriate, but the question did not ask what data the doctor was going to ask you for first. The question asked which intervention takes priority. In other words, what MUST be done (out of the four options I have been given) to keep this client alive? Select an answer that is the closest to fixing the problem and keeping the client alive.

MARLENE'S RULE This is the way you should think about all NCLEX® questions. If you do not tell the NCLEX® people anything else in this scenario, you had better let them know you know how important it is to notify the physician.

DON'T LEAVE THEM WONDERING When you click answer choice #1 and move to the next question, you leave the NCLEX® Lady wondering, "Was the student going to check the vital signs and then call the physician, or did the student think this was all that was needed?" The answer did not say "Check the vital signs and then call the physician." You wished it had said that, didn't you?!

BUT MARLENE! Now I know what you are battling with. The first thing the physician is going to ask me when I call her is "What are the vital signs?"

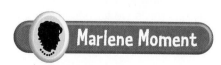
Marlene Moment

Never leave the NCLEX® Lady wondering if you were going to take action to save the client's life.

- Real world nursing: Yes, in the real world you would immediately check the vital signs and then call the physician. But once again, this is a PRIORITY question, and the word "priority" changes everything.
- NCLEX® nursing: The word "priority" in this question means "If I can only do ONE thing, what is the ONE thing I should do to keep this client alive?" Even if you do not know the vital signs when you call the doctor, you still did the right thing as far as NCLEX® is concerned. You knew to hurry and notify the physician of this problem, as calling the physician is the only one (out of these four options) that can FIX the problem.

Get real! If the arm were bleeding profusely from a laceration, you would say, "Uh-oh, the client is hemorrhaging; I need to apply pressure!" Because in this situation the problem is hemorrhage and the appropriate intervention to attack/fix the problem is to hold pressure. However, in my sample test question, applying pressure and fixing the perforation are not options! How are you going to hold pressure on a bleeding intestine?

DEADLY INSTANT MESSAGING Talk about the popularity of instant messaging! Let's look at some answers that immediately send a message about the kind of nurse you might be.

- Answer #2: Instructing the client to remain in bed.

You are not painting a NCLEX®-like image of yourself by selecting this answer!

CASE IN POINT Imagine yourself in this situation saying, "Sir, you have either perforated your colon or you are hemorrhaging. I do not know which one it is, because I am a new nurse. See, it says on my badge GN (graduate nurse), which means I haven't passed the NCLEX® yet. You need to stay in bed because in a little while you are going to start feeling dizzy from shock, which may cause you to fall down. Okay? I'll be back in a little while to check on you. Here's your call light if you need me."

KILLER ANSWER How did this answer attack either problem? Remaining in the bed does not stop bleeding and it doesn't fix a perforation. That's why you must not select answer #2.

- Answer #4: Administering PRN pain medication.

Now you have really scared the NCLEX® people! You are telling them that when you have a client who is hemorrhaging or who has a perforation, you are going to medicate them. How does pain medicine fix the problem? It doesn't. It makes everything worse.

CLINICAL ALERT! The pain medicine is going to mask the client's symptoms. The client is going to fall asleep *permanently*, but at least he will die pain-free. Because the physician ordered the medication, it must be okay, right? No!

MARLENE'S RULE Stay away from selecting a "drug" answer for as long as possible on this test!

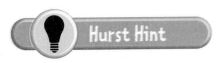

Just because we have an order doesn't mean we have to implement it!

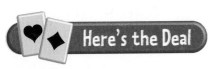

You never give pain medication until you know for sure what's wrong with the client.

THE BOTTOM LINE We are getting closer to an answer, so hang in there.

- Answer #3: Calling the physician. It has been pounded into your head in nursing school to never pick "call the physician."

MARLENE'S RULE If there is something you can do to fix the problem, do this first and then notify the physician.

- In this situation, there was no option you could do right then that fixed the problem. The only person who can fix the problem is the doctor.
- Yes, there are things that could be done, but they won't help the client. These things *delay* the treatment.
- If we assume the worst about this situation, the client goes back to surgery and the doctor rushes to get there.

  Real world nursing: Okay, here we go. You call the physician. The first thing she asks is, "What are the client's vitals?" You say, "I don't know, but you'd better hurry up and get here!" Now the physician is mad because you didn't relay the vitals. That's okay. This type of thinking is for a specific test! NCLEX® does not care if the physician is mad. In the real world, you would quickly take the vitals and then call the physician. But, NCLEX® isn't like the real world. Sorry. Hey, aren't you glad you read this prior to taking your test! I am!

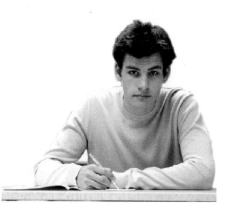

MAKE THE NCLEX® LADY VERY HAPPY Now when you select this answer, the NCLEX® people can breathe a sigh of relief. Even if it comes to pass that neither problem is occurring, you still acted correctly while preventing harm to the client. Yes, the physician could get mad because you called her about a drop of client blood, but who cares! You're trying to pass a test in which the major focus is keeping people alive. So you are going to overreact at times. This is much safer than underreacting or using your 2 weeks of vast nursing knowledge and judgment to just sit back and watch the client for a while.

REFRESH YOUR KNOWLEDGE Even if you don't consider hemorrhage or perforation, you still should follow this principle: When a client goes for a procedure and they come back with symptoms or complaints they were not having before the procedure, you have no choice but to assume the worst!

CLINICAL ALERT!

Procedure + Symptoms = Something Bad.

Be proactive: Ask for help. Let the physician tell you to just watch the client. It's not your place to make these kinds of judgment calls.

TIME FOR ANOTHER PRIORITY PREDICAMENT

Now, let's tackle another question and learn to think Aunt Marlene's way!

✚ NCLEX® practice question

The nurse is caring for a 30-week primagravida who is receiving magnesium sulfate IV for premature contractions. The nurse is monitoring hourly urine output. The first hour, urine output is 180 mL. The next hour, the urine output has decreased to 140 mL. Based on this data, which action should take priority?

1. Notifying the physician
2. Documenting the urine output on the flow sheet
3. Reporting the decreased urine output to the Registered Nurse
4. Reassess the urine output in 15 minutes

Meditate

Think about it and select an answer. Use the previous guidelines we have already discussed.

FIRST THINGS FIRST Are you worried or not worried? You'd better be worried! (I'm glad we've got that straight!)

CORE CONTENT REVIEW As with any exam question, you have to know the core content. Do you know the action of magnesium sulfate? Do you know why the nurse is monitoring hourly output?

- Is the data about the urine output decreasing important? If you do not know, then you do not know your core content. If you do not know your core content, it will be very difficult to answer this question. If you want to hear me discuss core content, then get on my website at **www.hurstreview.com** and get busy! The only problem is, you will have my southern accent when you finish!

Now let's review the core content needed to answer this question:

REFRESH YOUR KNOWLEDGE

- Magnesium sulfate (also known as mag-sulfate, Mg, $MgSO_4$) acts like a sedative on the body. You know how a sedative makes you feel. If you want to get fancy, you can say mag-sulfate acts like a central nervous system depressant. Whatever.

- Yes, there's a reason you were given the quantity of the hourly output. If it were not important, then it would not be in the question. Anything that is in a question has been put there for a reason: to help guide you to an answer.

- Monitoring hourly output is a must when administering mag-sulfate. The only way excess magnesium can be excreted from the body is through the kidneys. So we need to make sure our client keeps a good output to rid the excess magnesium.

- Now you are looking at the numbers the exam question offers: 180 mL down to 140 mL.

- Most nursing students think: "This looks like pretty good urine output to me. I don't worry until it drops to around 30 mL/hr. So the kidneys are working pretty well."

Dissection time

Now, let's analyze the answers.

- Answer #1: Notifying the physician. There is nothing wrong with this answer, but is there something I can do first that will HELP the client? Notice I said HELP the client and the problem. So let's hold off on this answer choice right now.

- Answer #4: Reassessing the urine output in l5 minutes. I know what you are thinking: "Assessment is the first phase of the nursing process!" I've heard this since nursing school. Even if it's not the right answer I can argue with my teacher long enough to get 2 points on my exam.

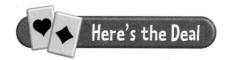

You're through with nursing school. You are now dealing with a different test that is asking a PRIORITY question.

STORY TIME Before I go any further, I must tell you a story. While you are reading this I want you to pretend there is spooky music playing in the background. When you get to the testing center, someone is going to be waiting for you at the front door, holding the door open, and saying (in a low, scary voice), "Welcome to my testing center." Let me tell you a little about this person. His name is Newt. Newt the negligent knucklehead who's never going to be a nurse! Newt wants to be a nurse, but he failed hand-washing twice, hung an IV antibiotic his very first day of clinical, and wore mustard colored suede shoes to the hospital. So needless to say, he didn't stay in nursing school long. Newt grew bitter over the years due to his failure. Because he couldn't get work as a nurse, he started working as a private sitter for hospital clients, and he also got a job at the testing center on the side! Newt likes to walk around the testing center to tempt NCLEX® test-takers into selecting wrong answers because he doesn't want nurse graduates to succeed!

When you are being tempted by something, are you more easily tempted by things that look good or things that look bad? We are tempted by things that look good! Newt looks good and can make any answer sound so good! That's why all four test answers are going to look good to you. That's Newt tempting you. Now, do you think Newt wants you to do nice things or mean things to your clients? Mean things! He either wants you to kill someone, hurt someone, or at the very least leave permanent residual damage! We've got to learn to fight Newt, the NCLEX® dream annihilator! Well, you can rest assured he's no match for Aunt Marlene and her no-nonsense approach to nursing! Rest assured that one answer selection is good and three are Newtish.

DEFINE TIME Newtish describes an answer that Newt would like you to select because it will bring about death, hurt, or permanent residual damage to your clients. Newt can cause NCLEX® failure.

- When you select answer #4, you are sending this message to the NCLEX® people: "I know something's wrong with my client (because this is NCLEX® world), but I don't know what it is. I'll be back in l5 minutes!"

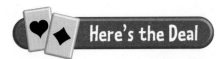

When you walk into this client's room, Newt and the client are flipping the remote through the television channels. You and your insecure self are tempted to listen to Newt because he is very cute, cunning, and clever. Newt says, "Go on little new nurse. I'll watch your client. I'll be right here by her side." You slowly leave the room saying, "I'll be back in just 15 quick minutes. What can happen in 15 minutes?" A lot can happen in 15 minutes!

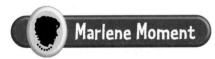

Sing this tune made famous by Roberta Flack: Killing her slowly with magnesium, killing her slowly with magnesium. Lah, lah, lah."

MARLENE'S RULE Never delay treatment! Delaying treatment will always be wrong. If you are being asked a question about something, you know something is wrong with the client, or it wouldn't be a test question. You need to do something right now! The NCLEX® people want you to deal with problems at once. Do not delay!

REFRESH YOUR KNOWLEDGE Magnesium acts like a sedative; it is excreted from the body by the kidneys. When the client's urine output has dropped, the body retains magnesium. What will excess magnesium do to respirations? Decrease them. You just let your client get 15 more minutes worth of magnesium. Now when you come back in the room, your client is cyanotic!

* I didn't have to go to nursing school to know something's wrong now! Now even the housekeeping lady in the room is saying, "Girl, you better do something!"

* You've got to learn to pick up on problems EARLY so there will be more time to save your client's life. Newt won with #4! This answer is incorrect, because receiving 15 more minutes of magnesium could potentially kill the client!

Now we have answer choices #2 and #3 left.

* For those of you who selected answer # 2, I'm worried about you because you are still sending an ugly message to the NCLEX® Lady.

* You are not showing the NCLEX® people that you are going to be proactive. You are showing them you are not aware of ANY client complication; you are just going to go about your usual routines.

* How does documenting the urine output on the flow sheet FIX the problem?

The message

The message you are sending is very lame. The message is, "All I know to do is document the hourly outputs."

Answer #3 is the safest answer for the client.

MARLENE'S RULE On NCLEX®, I can do whatever I have to do within my scope of practice to save a client's life, limb, or vision!

CASE IN POINT If a client's blood pressure (BP) drops significantly while receiving a nitroglycerin infusion, you will not hesitate to report this change at once to the RN, will you? No!

EXPERIENCE DOESN'T HELP An experienced nurse may handle this situation differently than you. For example:

* An experienced nurse may say, "I'm going to check some other things first before I report to the RN."

* A more experienced nurse may check the respirations, BP, and reflexes and then decide what to do next.

- An experienced nurse has more refined judgment skills than you have at this point.

- Remember, you are a brand new nurse, so you have to be overly cautious and alert the RN to any problems at once. The RN will decide, in this situation, what needs to be done next. But if you do not know your core content, you will be oblivious to potential client problems.

- The bottom line is this: You let the NCLEX® people know that you know (1) how magnesium affects the body, (2) to be concerned about the DECREASE in the urine output even though the numbers are good, and (3) to report this change at once to the RN because it could have life-threatening implications.

NCLEX® DEADLY DISTRACTER I realize the urine output numbers in the practice question are good. The testing folks will give you good numbers to make you think nothing is wrong with the client. The key in this test question is that there was a DECREASE in the client's output.

CLINICAL ALERT! When a client is receiving magnesium intravenously, you never want the urine output to drop; you actually want the urine output to increase to make sure the excess magnesium is being excreted.

OTHER WORDS THAT MEAN PRIORITY

In general, I like to think that all questions are priority questions, whether that particular word appears or not. However, there are other words that mean the exact same thing as "priority." Here they are, showing how they may be placed in a test question:

- What is the most IMPORTANT action?
- The most IMPORTANT action would be?
- The BEST action would be to?
- The BEST response would be?
- Your INITIAL response or action would be to?
- What would concern the nurse the MOST?
- What should be your FIRST ACTION?
- The most ESSENTIAL nursing action would be?
- Your IMMEDIATE response should be?
- The nurse's NEXT action should be?
- The PRIMARY or VITAL nursing action would be to?
- The BEST action is?

SUMMARY

Priority questions are going to hurt your brain! But just like anything else, with practice, you can master these questions. This way of thinking may be a little different from what you are accustomed to, but remember, we are trying to pass a specific test. I assure you these strategies will get you to the right answer more times than not, and that adds up to a nursing license!

Bibliography

Hurst Review Services. Available at **http://www.hurstreview.com.**

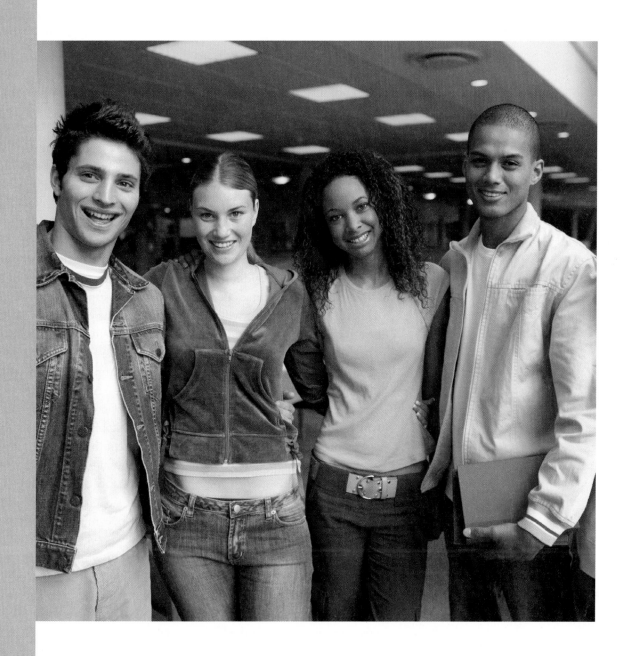

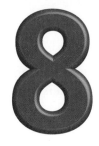

Management and Delegation

MANAGEMENT AND DELEGATION

I'm sure many of you have heard this: "There are a lot of management and delegation questions on NCLEX®." You're stuck wondering how to study specifically for this content. It's easy to study a topic like congestive heart failure (CHF). You review the definition, pathophysiology, signs and symptoms, and treatment to get an understanding of this concrete subject. However, management and delegation can be vague topics. In your career you will encounter varied theories on management and delegation. In this section, I will help you master the management and delegation questions you will definitely encounter on NCLEX®. Note: I am not re-teaching a management or leadership course.

You may ask yourself, "Why do I have to know this type of content? I'm a new nurse and I'm not going to be managing or delegating anything." The studies conducted by the National Council of State Boards of Nursing show new nurses do manage activities, supervise others, and delegate every day.[1] You will be working with many members of the health care team as soon as you begin employment in a hospital. Therefore, this content will be a part of your exam, as NCLEX® tests specifically for the skills and knowledge NEW nurses use most frequently during their first 6 months of practice. If you do not know how to manage, delegate, supervise, and prioritize care, this could affect client safety, which in turn could affect whether you pass NCLEX® or not.

You may find these types of questions difficult because in school you may have just listened to a lecture on this content—you may not have been tested on this specific material. You probably didn't get a lot of opportunities to manage or delegate to other people during clinical. Most students are happy when they just get their meds given on time during clinical!

Over the years I have heard students say, "The whole test was on management and delegation." Just study that content. How? The truth is you must understand the core content of nursing prior to even attempting management and delegation-style questions. Let's make this as simple as possible and start with the basics of delegation.

![Factoid]

Factoid

Delegation is defined as transferring to a competent individual the authority to perform a selected nursing task in a selected situation.[2] The nurse retains accountability for the delegation. Let's look at the five rights of delegation.

DELEGATION

Delegation is an integral part of your nursing career. Let's take a closer look at how NCLEX® approaches this topic.

✚ The five rights of delegation

The National Council of State Boards of Nursing has instituted the Five Rights of Delegation.[3] You must understand these five rights before delegating:

1. The right task

2. The right circumstances

3. The right person

4. The right direction/communication

5. The right supervision/evaluation

✛ Guidelines for selecting the right task

Here we have some guidelines and questions you may ask yourself when selecting the right task on NCLEX®.

1. Is it a task that reoccurs in daily care? For example, AM care and routine vitals signs occur in daily care.

2. Is nursing judgment required? If nursing judgment is required, then you have to delegate this task to someone who is qualified or retain the task for yourself. For example:

   * Your nursing judgment is required to determine a client's need for a PRN medicine. Therefore, you would not delegate this task to the UAP.

   * Ambulating a client who is postop total hip replacement requires special knowledge and judgment versus ambulating a postop abdominal hysterectomy client.

3. Is the potential for risk minimal? Does the potential for harming the client exist if the task is delegated? For example:

   * What is the potential for harm in inserting a Foley catheter in a client who is in labor versus inserting a Foley catheter in a client with a prostate condition? The catheter insertion is most likely uneventful in the labor client, whereas the prostate client could have an obstruction or resistance, which could put this client at harm.

   * What is the risk potential in turning a newly admitted nursing home client with pneumonia as opposed to an ED client who was involved in an automobile accident? Turning the nursing home client should be uneventful and predictable, whereas turning the ED client could result in exacerbating head or spinal injuries.

CLINICAL ALERT Any time you are inserting a Foley catheter into a male patient, you cannot be careful enough. It is very common for the tubing to get tangled in the urethra. You can insert the Foley tubing all the way down to the balloon insertion port and think, "Surely, the end of this tubing is in the bladder!" If you do not get urine return, you do not know for sure if the catheter is in the bladder. If you blow up the balloon in this situation, you WILL tear the urethra. This happens frequently in the hospital setting. This is why nurses must educate their staff on proper catheter insertion to eliminate doing harm to clients!

4. Are the results predictable? If the scenario entails setting up a client's lunch tray, the task is different for the client who is 1 hour post-heart catheterization (heart cath) versus the client who is admitted with fever of unknown origin (FUO). The task is predictable for the client with a fever as opposed to the heart cath client. Why? The client who is post-heart cath could bleed if the head of the bed is raised too much

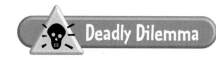

Deadly Dilemma

The LPN/LVN needs to be sure the RN is present or at least close by if the LPN/LVN is about to ambulate a postop client for the first time. There are too many things that can go wrong with a client in this situation.

whereas the outcome of setting up a lunch tray for the client with FUO is typically uneventful.

5. Does the task have a standard or unchanging procedure? Does the hospital have a procedure for this task? Is there an outlined and detailed checklist of how to perform this task? In standard procedures which are documented in the hospital's policies and procedure manuals, the expected outcome is known.

✚ Guidelines for selecting the right circumstances

Every client's circumstances are different.

1. Does the complexity of the task match the competency of the delegatee?

 - Does the person to whom I am delegating the task have the proper training? Is this person competent to perform the task? The bottom line is that you need to know your staff's level of competency. The right circumstances include knowing the employee's history, background, and capabilities. A LPN that is pulled from the well-baby nursery to help on an orthopedic floor is not familiar with the routine task of ambulating postop orthopedic clients. The staff member should only be assigned to those clients who are within the employee's scope of knowledge and expertise.

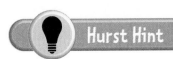

Hurst Hint

Anytime a nurse is floated to an unfamiliar area and is given a client assignment, consider him to be a brand new nurse all over again no matter how many years of nursing experience he has.

CASE IN POINT   The well-baby nursery employee should be assigned a client with a deep vein thrombosis (DVT) rather than a client in pelvic traction. Why? Any nurse should be able to take care of a client with a DVT, but caring for someone in pelvic traction requires specialized knowledge more so than a DVT. The safest way to think of this scenario is to consider the well-baby nursery employee as a new graduate nurse.

2. Is supervision readily available?

 - Delegate to a newly graduated nurse only those procedures that she has performed routinely. Supervise any new skills such as discontinuing a tube feeding or setting up a sterile field. You know a new nurse can perform these tasks, but she may not have had much experience.

✚ Guidelines for selecting the right person

You'll be working with several different levels of personnel with varying degrees of expertise. Let's pick the right person for the job.

1. What is the competency level of the delegatee?

 - Selecting the right person requires the same considerations as those listed above when we discussed the right circumstances. Make an attempt to delegate the task to the lowest trained staff, while maintaining proper client care and safety.

- The employee's scope of practice, licensure, and expertise should be considered when delegating. An example is assigning discharge instructions for a client with a urinary tract infection who has only one antibiotic prescribed, as opposed to the client who is discharged post-neurosurgery with specific instructions cautioning against sneezing, sniffing, and snoring. The second client requires a nurse of greater competency because the post-neuro client could rupture a suture line or have increased intracranial pressure, which could be fatal. The LPN should realize the second client is out of his scope of practice due to the complexity of the situation.

✚ Guidelines for selecting the right direction/communication

Communication is an element of delegation we cannot forget. Some staff members may require more direction than others.

1. Have you been specific in your communication?
   - Did you tell the delegatee:

     The client's name and information?

     The specific data that needs to be collected?

     The specific manner in which the data should be collected?

     How long the data collection will take?

     The expected results?

     Specific client instructions or limitations?

     What the possible complications are?
   - Have you explained the possible negative outcomes?

     The time-frame in which to report back?

✚ Guidelines for selecting the right supervision/evaluation

You can't delegate and forget it. You must follow up.

- Did you monitor the performance?
- Did you receive or give feedback?
- Did you intervene when needed?
- Did you document properly?

Recap

Okay, now that we have gone over the five rights of delegation in detail, let's recap the biggies here:

- Delegate to staff members who have been taught properly and can perform the task in a safe manner.
- If the staff members have not been taught properly or if you have concerns, you must supervise the task.

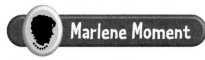

Marlene Moment

Selecting the right person requires the same considerations as those reviewed when we discussed the right circumstances. Make an attempt to delegate the task to the lowest trained staff, while maintaining proper client care and safety.

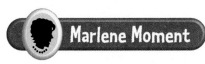

Marlene Moment

I know what you are thinking: "Nobody ever has time to ask all of those questions! If I asked a nursing assistant all of those questions prior to delegating they would tell me to just go do it myself!" I understand where you are coming from, but you must remember something: The NCLEX® hospital is a perfect hospital. You have all the time in the world to ask anything you need. In the real world, you get to know the people with whom you are working. You learn who you need to explain more to and you learn who has more expertise. NCLEX® world or not, you have to always make sure the person you are delegating to knows what they are doing prior to doing it. If it takes asking 15 questions, then ask 15 questions. Then if you STILL aren't sure, GET UP and go with the staff member to watch and teach them. This is your DUTY and RESPONSIBILITY!

- Supervision does not necessarily mean to stand by the delegatee's side unless it is the first time the task is being performed.
- Make sure you follow up and evaluate the delegatee's performance after the task is completed.

✚ Let's get the names straight

In the ever-changing health care environment, delegation is critical for each level of client care. From the top down, management and staff alike delegate and re-delegate tasks to free time and personnel to perform more complex functions. It is essential to know the correct titles, educational backgrounds, and abilities of those assigned to work with you as well as those assigned to work for you.

Who is who?

Unlicensed assistive personnel (UAP) are those who may help perform specific tasks for the client and the nurse. The nursing assistant (NA), the certified nursing assistant (CNA), orderlies, and the unit secretary are considered UAPs. The licensed practical nurse (LPN) and the licensed vocational nurse (LVN) are simply different names for the same educational background and may be called one or the other depending on the state in which you are working.

Look at Table 8-1 to get a quick idea of who is who.

✚ RN delegation

Understanding delegation requires knowledge of several areas. We will begin to review some of these areas here. See Table 8-2.

Table 8-1. Who's Who in Nursing Management

UAP	LPN/LVN	RN
• Education of the UAP may be an in-house, on-the-job training program or an accredited program at a medical facility or local college.	• Education of the LPN/LVN ranges from 12 to 24 months.	• Education of the RN includes an accredited program with an associate or baccalaureate degree.
• Skills taught are basic nursing skills such as hygiene, vital signs, and I&O.	• Skills taught in addition to basic nursing skills are basic pathophysiology, pharmacology, and nutrition.	• Skills include basic nursing tasks as well the primary responsibility of the nursing process, i.e., complex nursing assessment, diagnosis, planning, implementation, and evaluation.
• Passing test is required for certification. Local Nurse Practice Acts (NPA) and the facility guidelines may allow additional tasks such as venipuncture, blood glucose monitoring, or Foley catheterization.	• Passing the State Board of Nursing exam for practical nurses is required prior to practicing. The NPA of certain states allow additional IV certification for LPN/LVNs.	• Passing the State Board of Nursing exam for registered nurses is required prior to practicing. Additional certification may be obtained for expertise in specific client populations.
• Operate under the direct supervision of licensed personnel.	• Operate under the direct supervision of the registered nurse.	

Table 8-2. Delegation Guidelines for RNs and LPNs

Staff to whom RNs may delegate	Staff to whom LPNs may delegate
1. Licensed vocational nurse (LVN)	1. Another LPN
2. Licensed practical nurse (LPN)	2. UAP
3. Unlicensed assistive personnel (UAP) • Nursing assistant (NA) • Medication technician (MT)	3. Ancillary health care team member
4. Ancillary health care team members: • Unit secretaries • Client transporters	

✛ How do I know what tasks can be delegated?

Let's look at what skills are appropriate for which employee. The lists of tasks below are general lists and are not all inclusive. Do not memorize these lists. There is some variation from state to state, and NCLEX® does not test on state-specific material. Don't forget the focus of the REGISTERED NURSE is assessment, diagnosis, planning, implementation, and evaluation. Although all nursing personnel may take part in the nursing process, it is the primary responsibility of the registered nurse.

For RNs only

The registered nurse is the leader of the team and is responsible and accountable for providing client care. Here are just a few of the many responsibilities that the RN possesses:

- Performing head-to-toe assessment including complex and/or routine vital signs.
- Administering basic and advanced life support.
- Assessing—data collection and analysis.
- Diagnosing—identifying and prioritizing client problems.
- Planning—stating expected outcomes and methods for achievement.
- Implementation—interventions to achieve expected outcomes.
- Evaluating—analysis of plan of care and client outcomes.
- Caring for invasive lines (examples: peripherally inserted central line (PICC), Swan-Ganz catheter, arterial lines).
- Feeding clients with oral or swallowing problems.
- Administering blood and blood product transfusions.
- Titrating medications based on specific client needs and physician orders.
- Performing extensive or complex dressing changes or wound care.
- Teaching of clients and families (example: discharge teaching to parents caring for a child with a ventriculoperitoneal shunt).[4]

Remember, RNs can do anything listed in the LPN/LVN section, too.

The licensed practical/vocational nurse

The LPN/LVN has completed a program study and has successfully passed the NCLEX-PN® exam. Here we have a group of commonly performed duties of this health care provider:

- Taking routine vital signs.
- Providing basic life support.
- Bathing, giving oral hygiene, and changing bed linens.
- Turning and positioning.
- Administering enemas, digital fecal removal.
- Administering medications via PO, NG, PEG, IM, Z-track, intradermal, SQ, suppository, topical, and sublingual routes. Medication administration via the intraurethral route is not within the LPN/LVN's scope of practice.
- Administering instillations in the eyes, ears, nose, buccal muscosa, and rectum.
- Administering enteral or tube feedings.
- Monitoring blood glucose.
- Oral suctioning.
- Feeding clients without any oral or swallowing problems.
- Performing simple dressing changes (example: dry gauze dressing).
- Inserting and removing Foley catheters.
- Caring for ostomies.
- Administering respiratory treatments.
- Providing postmortem care.
- Inserting rectal tubes.
- Removing sutures and staples.
- Caring for newborns including cord care, vital signs, and feeding.
- Performing noncomplex procedures requiring sterile technique.
- Documenting the care given to the client and the client's response to that care.
- Updating an initial assessment; the data that is collected by the LVN must be validated by the RN.
- Reinforcing the teaching performed by the RN.
- Teaching from a standard care plan, noncomplex teaching (examples: simple diabetic teaching, simple dressing changes).[4]

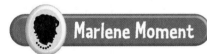

Marlene Moment

Be aware that prior to ANY discharge teaching, an ASSESSMENT must be done by the REGISTERED NURSE.

The unlicensed assistive person (UAP)

The unlicensed assistive person (UAP) provides support services to the licensed nurse during client care. Let's look at some of the tasks they can perform.

- Obtaining routine vital signs. *Did you catch the word "routine?"*
- Bathing, providing oral hygiene, changing bed linens.
- Turning and positioning.

- Feeding clients <u>without</u> any oral or swallowing problems.
- Providing basic life support.
- Providing postmortem care.
- Ambulating (in stable/noncomplex clients).
- Obtaining height and weight measurements.[4]
- Assisting with elimination.
- Monitoring input and output (I & O).
- Administering soapsuds enemas.
- Assisting with general activities of daily living (ADLs).
- Obtaining specimens (such as a clean catch or midstream urine specimen, or stool specimen).
- Transferring clients with the use of proper body mechanics.
- Documenting and reporting information related to client care to the RN/LPN.
- Reporting unusual observations and symptoms reported by the client or observed to the RN/LPN.
- Administering gastrostomy feedings (NO NG TUBE FEEDINGS).
- Utilizing proper communication techniques (introducing self; listening to the nurse/client; resolving conflicts or initiating resolution; giving/receiving feedback).
- Prioritizing tasks (per the direction of the RN or LPN/LVN).
- Handling complaints (report to appropriate personnel).

The UAP cannot perform any invasive or sterile procedures or assist in client teaching.[4]

✛ Times when you should question delegation

There are times when you need to re-evaluate to determine if delegation is appropriate. Here are some red flags:

- If the staff member does not know how to perform the task.
- If a client's condition has changed.
- If appropriate resources are not readily available.
- If the RN or LPN is not readily accessible for backup.
- If the employee is working in a new area or with different types of clients than they are accustomed to caring for.

MARLENE'S GENERAL RULES FOR ANSWERING MANAGEMENT AND DELEGATION QUESTIONS

Now we will review rules that will help you answer NCLEX® management and delegation questions. You will find I have divided the rules into management rules and delegation rules.

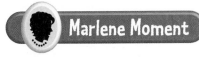

Marlene Moment

Remember, the nurse is still responsible for proper instruction, supervision, and evaluation of the client and accurate documentation. You retain accountability for the task you delegate.

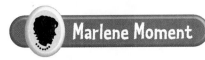

Marlene Moment

Just because an employee has been floated to a different area or does not like to care for an unpleasant/difficult client, does not create an unsafe situation. However, remember if a UAP/LPN/LVN has floated to a different area there may be activities on this unit that will be new to the floated staff member. They are not familiar with this area and may not be updated on the appropriate standards and procedures for these clients. For example, an LPN/LVN who works in the surgical unit is floated to postpartum and has been asked to bind a postpartum client's breast since the client does not wish to breastfeed. YOU, the LPN who routinely works on the postpartum unit, should perform this task. The **floated** LPN/LVN will not be familiar with observing for engorgement; therefore, she may not bind the client's breast appropriately.

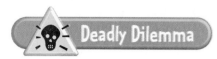

This can be tricky, as not all complex clients are unstable. A client can be complex and stable at the same time.

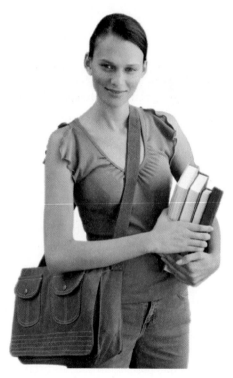

Marlene's rules

Now we will review the mainframe for management mastery.

1. Determine which client to see first.

- Choose the more acute, unstable client.

Define time

Unstable client = the client who is medically fragile who requires increased level of care, emergency interventions, and monitoring for fluctuating vital signs. Examples of unstable clients: a client with low blood sugar or a client with sudden changes in routine neuro checks.

CASE IN POINT #1 A 36-year-old single mother with four children is discharged home after a right mastectomy. She has a lot of physiological and psychosocial problems causing her to be a complex client, but she is STABLE. **She has been discharged home! If you have to pick between a stable and an unstable client on NCLEX®, go for the unstable client first.**

CASE IN POINT #2 You may think that a client with chronic lung disease is unstable because of airway. But if there is no information in the question to make you think the client is in any acute distress, hold off going to see that client first while you examine the other options. Remember, it took this client a long time to develop chronic lung disease.

CASE IN POINT #3 What about a client with a cerebrovascular accident? The client sounds like he's critical, but look at the data. When did the stroke happen? Is he having any acute changes RIGHT NOW? All I'm saying is that a client can have a diagnosis of chronic lung disease or a cerebrovascular accident and still be stable.

- Consider how long a client has had a condition. It takes years to develop diseases such as diabetes or chronic lung disease. Consider what the data is saying about that client RIGHT NOW, AT THAT MOMENT.

CASE IN POINT #4 Of the following two clients, which one requires your immediate attention?

- A newly diagnosed diabetic who awakens with a quarter-sized foot ulcer. Pedal pulses are present but weak. The morning glucose is 200 mg/dL.

- Vital signs are obtained on a postpartum client who delivered 12 hours ago. Four hours post-delivery her blood pressure is 118/70 mm Hg. Now her blood pressure is 140/80 mm Hg.

The second client requires immediate attention. Possible seizure due to eclampsia is more life threatening than a foot ulcer.

Refresh your knowledge

Always watch for any increase in the blood pressure, especially in the first 48 hours post-delivery. You should report this change in blood pressure immediately to the RN.

- Look at the **complexity of the client.** Which client has the most possible complications?
- The client who has the most problems is another good rule of thumb to remember when determining who you should see first.
- Remember that all clients will sound critical in each test question answer option. NCLEX® does this on purpose, so don't get upset.
- Just because someone is in pain does not mean that they are about to progress to death.

  Pain never killed anyone!

  We do take pain seriously. But beware: There could be another answer that is a better option to choose here.

  The pain of a myocardial infarction indicates a much more life-threatening situation than routine postop pain.

  Let's consider postop pain. It is the nurse's responsibility to determine if the client's pain is routine or if it is a sign of a more life-threatening complication. If it is the latter, report this to the RN immediately. The UAP is not trained to determine if pain is routine or due to a possible complication.

- Assess the most critical client first: Such as someone with a head injury whose neuro checks are fluctuating or an OB client who has a prolapsed cord (each of these would be examples of life-threatening situations).

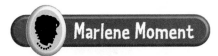

Marlene Moment

Always remember, you should assess the client with a life-threatening problem first before visiting your other clients.

CASE IN POINT #5 You have two clients on your home health route who need to be seen today. Who would you go see first? (We are assuming the NCLEX® question specifically stated the LPN is certified in intravenous therapy.)

- The client complaining of postop hip replacement pain.
- The diabetic client who is scheduled for a fasting blood sugar.

What's the worst case scenario?

Okay, here we go. What is the worst possible scenario that each client can experience?

- The client with postop hip pain could be suffering from hip dislocation.
- Picture the diabetic client, sitting there waiting for the nurse to come to draw their fasting blood sugar. They are fasting! They are just sitting and waiting . . . and waiting . . . and waiting. What is happening to their blood sugar while they are waiting for the nurse to arrive? It's dropping! Could this client's blood sugar drop out the bottom? Yes!

Out of these two situations, which one is more life threatening? The diabetic client who is scheduled for a fasting blood sugar! So this is the client who needs attention first! Even if the hip has dislocated it will not **kill** this client.

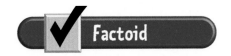

Factoid

Don't forget, NCLEX® **IS ABOUT KEEPING PEOPLE ALIVE.**

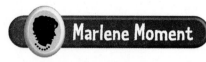

If all the clients are having changes in their condition, then you must consider how fast those changes are occurring. Ask yourself, *"Which client do I have the least amount of time to work with?"* In other words, which client is in the most immediate danger?

Real-world nursing: Now the most perfect answer in this situation is to call the diabetic client, tell them to eat something, and inform them you will draw the fasting blood sugar tomorrow, thus enabling you to go see the client who is in pain. But of course, the most perfect answer will never be an option on NCLEX®.

2. The LPN/LVN should never assume the care of an unstable client. Another way to think of an "unstable" client is like this:

An unstable client is the client who is most likely to have **a change** in their condition.

CASE IN POINT # 6 Your client has a head injury; the intracranial pressure (ICP) is being monitored. The client has noticeable pupillary changes. Is this an immediate concern?

Refresh your knowledge: When "head things" start happening, they happen FAST and can bring DEATH quickly if they are not acted upon immediately. This assessment finding requires immediate action. Pupillary changes are a sign that ICP is increasing, which could lead to a rapid death. The RN should retain this client during the assignment-making process. If the client is stable initially under the LPN's care but suddenly has a change in status, then the LPN must report this situation immediately to the RN.

3. A new admission is considered unstable, otherwise this client would not have been admitted in the first place. The RN should retain this client for herself. An LPN/LVN should not be solely assigned a new admission in the hospital setting.

4. When making assignments you must consider how much care each client is going to require.

5. The registered nurse has the <u>ultimate</u> responsibility and accountability for the management of client care, but the LPN/VN must be responsible & accountable too.

Define time

Responsibility is the obligation present when you take on an assignment.[4]

Define time

Accountability occurs when one is responsible for the actions and inactions of oneself and others.[4]

If a licensed nurse delegates inappropriately, or if an UAP performs an unauthorized task, either may lead to action being taken against one or both staff members.

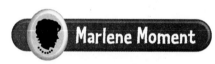

Unlicensed personnel are there to help the RN/LPN/LVN, not to replace them. When a task is delegated to an UAP, the UAP is not allowed to redelegate the task.

MORE ON DELEGATION

The RN is required to oversee the activities of the unit and in some cases all RN staff share the client load equally. In other situations, an RN delegates **tasks** to a team of LPN/LVNs and UAPs while overseeing the unit. In long-term care settings, the LPN/LVN may be the delegator.

✚ Marlene's delegation rules

You are described as the most diplomatic and discerning delagator due to your distinct desire to designate tasks according to the following directives:

1. The registered nurse, who assesses the clients' needs and develops the plan of nursing care, should be the primary delegator and should determine which tasks are appropriate or not to delegate.

   - The registered nurse retains accountability.
   - The registered nurse has a higher degree of accountability when delegating to a UAP than when she assigns tasks to another RN. The same is true when the LPN delegates to another LPN or UAP.

2. It is inappropriate to delegate the core activities of nursing: the initial client assessment, establishing a nursing diagnosis, establishing nursing care plans, and evaluating a client's progress toward achieving a goal.

3. Communication issues:

   - It is appropriate to have the delegatee repeat your instructions, especially if you are not convinced that they understand the task at hand.
   - The delegatee should be encouraged to ask questions. Listen to the delegatee. This may cue you in to areas that need further investigation or where the delegatee may need further assistance.
   - The LPN/LVN provides feedback when he deems necessary. This is an essential part of nursing care.
   - Be specific when you speak! Provide clear directions and expectations of how you want the task to be performed and define the findings you wish reported.

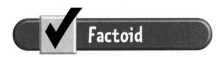

Factoid

No part of the nursing process should be delegated.

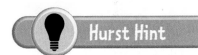

Hurst Hint

According to the National Council of State Boards of Nursing, inadequate communication is the most frequent reason delegated activities are not completed as expected.[3]

CASE IN POINT "Please get Mr. Smith's temperature" is not as specific as, "Please get Mr. Smith's temperature while I get his blood from the blood bank." (This statement places a time-frame on the task.)

"Be sure to tell me if Mr. Jones' blood sugar is too high" is not as thorough as, "Please let me know immediately if Mr. Jones' blood sugar is over 240 mg/dL."

4. Always keep cost-effectiveness in mind.

   - Delegation is an effective way of managing costs on a unit.
   - Referring to the guidelines for selecting the person for delegation and choosing the appropriate person for the appropriate task will benefit the client, the caregiver, and the organization as a whole.

5. The UAP/LPN/LVN should act as the RN's eyes and ears when the RN is not present.

   - The delegatee should ask for help when he is unsure about a client's situation and should alert the RN to unusual observations or unexpected results.

6. It is the RN's responsibility to help the UAP/LPN/LVN accomplish nursing activities.

CASE IN POINT The same activity may differ in each situation (feeding a healthy client who has two broken arms is different than feeding a client who has dysphagia; bathing a weak client is not the same as bathing a client who is severely burned).

7. You must assure the availability of adequate resources including supervision.

   • Always consider how much supervision will be required to safely accomplish the needed activity. Ask yourself: "Will supervision/assistance be available and readily assessable?"

Define time

Supervision occurs when a licensed nurse guides, directs, evaluates, and follows up on a delegated task.[3]

8. To delegate properly, you have to adequately plan at the beginning of each shift.

9. The more stable the client is, the more likely you will be able to delegate certain aspects of care.

CASE IN POINT A UAP or LPN/LVN may be assigned to take the routine vital signs of a client who is recovering from an elective surgery. A client who is receiving propanolol hydrochloride (Inderal) needs the LPN/LVN to take their vital signs first. Because administration of this medication entails monitoring the heart rate and blood pressure, this task cannot be delegated to a UAP as these vital signs are not "routine".

10. You may delegate a task that has a very predictable outcome.

CASE IN POINT Ambulating a client who is 3 days postop and has had an uneventful recovery is an example of a predictable outcome. It never hurts to ask the client if she is short of breath or is experiencing pain in the legs when walking, however. Remind and re-teach the UAP of these important points as needed.

11. It is essential that the task YOU delegated be **monitored and evaluated.**

   • The LPN/LVN will follow through the cycle of evaluating the client and the performance of the delegatee as well as obtaining feedback on a continuous basis. Ask yourself, "Did I get the outcome I wanted?" Evaluate the delegated action by collecting data on the client within a reasonable amount of time. You must ensure no harm was brought to the client.

12. When deciding whether to delegate a task, always consider the client's condition and the level of care the client requires.

✚ The "DO NOTs" of delegation

We have all heard of the "have nots," the "will nots," and "want nots." Now we are going to talk about the DO NOTs of delegation.

1. Do not delegate any task that requires excessive problem-solving skills. (Examples: diabetes teaching and insulin administration).

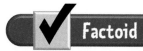

Only delegate tasks for STABLE clients.

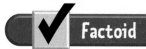

All decisions related to delegation must be based on the protection of the client.

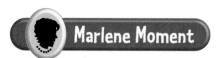

Evaluation is often the missing link in providing appropriate client care. Delegation decisions and client outcomes must be continually evaluated. YOU will need to intervene if necessary.

2. Do not delegate any task that has the slightest chance of causing harm.

   * Case in point: feeding a client who has dysphagia, because the client is at risk for aspiration. Do not delegate this task in this situation.

3. Do not accept the task of admitting a new client to your unit. It's appropriate for the LPN/LVN to assist the RN with the new admission, but not to take the complete responsibility.

   * A new admission is considered unstable and the registered nurse must assume responsibility for this client.

4. Do not delegate data collection, evaluation, or nursing judgment.

5. Do not delegate client teaching to the UAP.[4]

Marlene's rule

Do not give telephone advice, unless it's "call all!"

6. Never delegate data collection to the UAP.

7. Never delegate any task that requires nursing judgement.

   * Case in point: You are caring for a client who has just returned from a bronchoscopy. You completed your second set of vital signs 15 minutes ago, and it's now time to get your third set. Just as you are about to take your client's vitals, the nursing supervisor calls asking for your census.

   * Should you send the UAP who is assigned to your team tonight to take the third set of vital signs for you while you deal with the nursing supervisor?

     ANSWER: You must use your nursing judgment that you have been taught to determine whether the client is recovering appropriately from the bronchoscopy. The census will have to wait.

8. Do not delegate any task, no matter how trivial, if there is any chance of harm.

   * Case in point: You are working the 3–11 shift in the best nursing home in town. One of your clients is having a little trouble with swallowing. She tells you, "I feel like there is a piece of lint stuck in my throat." Do you ask the CNA to assist this client with her meal this evening?

     ANSWER: Nursing assistants feed people every day! However, if you have a client who is having difficulty swallowing, then YOU, the LPN/LVN, need to feed the client because this client is at risk for aspiration. Now, I know what you're thinking: "I see nursing assistants feed all kinds of really sick people every day in the hospital and the nursing home." So? I told you to forget what you have seen in the hospital. What you have seen in this type of setting is not always "textbook perfect."

A FEW MORE POINTS

You know I always have something else I want to tell you to help you pass the NCLEX® the first time.

   * When the answer uses the word "after," be careful!!!!!!

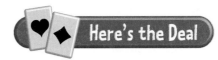

Here's the Deal

Examples of routine, simple teaching include: postop client hemorrhoidectomy teaching or application of a Foley leg bag for a post-prostatectomy client.

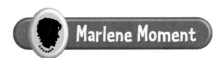

Marlene Moment

In most health care facilities, giving telephone advice is prohibited except for those trained to do so. Please don't dispense any health care advice either in person or on the phone until you know the protocol in your facility.

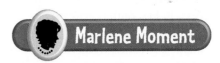

Marlene Moment

Notice how the word "after" is used. "After" would make you think *all is well, everything is okay, this client is stable.* How do you know this???

CASE IN POINT #1 AFTER a post-acetaminophen overdose the client is stable; will you assign tasks for this client to an UAP?

Think about it. First of all, the doctor would not admit the client if she thought the client was stable. If this client was stable, the physician would have discharged the client home.

Secondly, acetaminophen kills the liver, which increases the risk for bleeding. You must monitor closely for signs and symptoms of hemorrhage. Can you see how this question is so nonchalant at first? Be careful; use your nursing judgment. The word "after" may lead you to believe the worst is over.

CASE IN POINT #2 A client presents to the ED after an acute asthma attack. The client is admitted to your unit, where he is sleeping with a respiratory rate of 24 breaths per minute. A family member remains in the room at the bedside. Is this a stable or unstable client?

ANSWER: Unstable! But doesn't this client sound peaceful, sleeping soundly in their little hospital room? The family member is sitting right there at the bedside. If the client was stable, the doctor would have discharged her home. Obviously, the doctor did not deem her stable enough to go home. The client was admitted to the hospital! I know what went through your mind initially. Airway! Good job!

- Determining the nurse/patient ratio depends on the complexity and the amount of care the client requires. Ask yourself:

  1. How stable/unstable is this client?

  2. How complex are this client's needs?

Many nurses want everyone to have an equal client load. This is not always possible or correct. You may have one nurse who is assigned to five clients and another who only has two clients due to the complexity of the two assigned clients.

Assigning clients based on location is not always the ideal situation either. If we could choose exactly where and when clients are admitted, it would be wonderful. But we don't have that luxury in most situations. The clients are admitted and sent to the floor without any sense of order. It is the responsibility of the nurse in charge to assign clients based on acuity, experience of the staff, and the clinical needs of the clients. Some facilities have a system in which each client is assigned points based on the level of care and the number of tasks that need performing. This "acuity system" provides the nurse in charge with an objective tool which helps make decisions regarding staff assignments. In most cases, it can provide a fair system to distribute the workload on a unit and provide the clients with the adequate amount of staff needed.

- Be careful when you see a task intertwined with a nursing responsibility on the NCLEX®.

- You should also be careful when you see words like "experienced nursing assistant" or "experienced LPN/LVN" on the NCLEX®. This could leave you with the impression that this person is capable of doing more than they are trained to do. Don't forget, when you delegate, a task YOU *retain accountability*. Be cautious as to what task you delegate and to whom you delegate it.

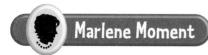

Marlene Moment

YOU, the LPN/LVN, should bathe a client if YOU are worried about possible posterior skin breakdown. A bath can also offer the time you need to talk with a client who is emotionally upset. For example: the postop radical mastectomy client or the client who is postop radical prostatectomy.

SUMMARY

Management and delegation principles can be very perplexing, especially to a new nurse. Remember, the ultimate goal is to improve the level of health for your client, or at the minimum maintain the client's comfort level to the best of your ability while holding yourself to the highest standards of care. To do so, you will have to work effectively with other members of the health care team. Now, let's move on to the nursing process!" More fun to follow!

References

1. *2005 RN Practice Analysis. Report of Findings.* Volume 21. Available at: **www.ncsbn.org/359.htm.** Accessed November 9, 2006.

2. *2005 RN Practice Analysis. Delegation: Concepts and Decision Making.* Volume 21. Available at: **www.ncsbn.org/359.htm.** Accessed November 9, 2006.

3. National Council of State Board of Nursing. Available at: **www.ncsbn.org.** Accessed

4. Heidenthal P. *Nursing Leadership & Management.* New York: Delmar Learning; 2003.

Bibliography

Hurst Review Services. **www.hurstreview.com.**

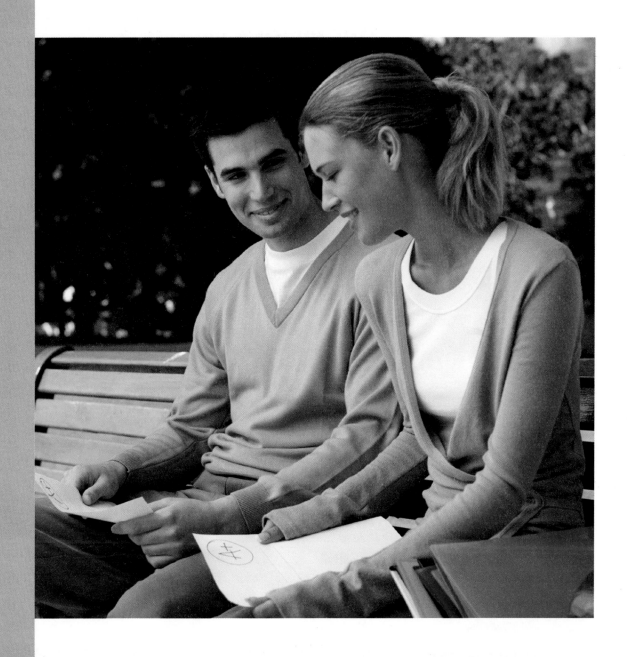

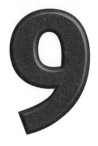

Why Do I Really Have to Understand "the Nursing Process"?

WHY DO I REALLY HAVE TO UNDERSTAND "THE NURSING PROCESS"?

You used the nursing process throughout nursing school to write care plans and to problem-solve when delivering client care. When you first started using the nursing process it was something that took quite a bit of thought, and you probably used a lot of reference books to help you understand it. Remember how long it took to write your first care plan? Now you are probably to the point where you go through the process without even knowing you are doing it.

✛ Why is the nursing process important to NCLEX®?

The National Council of State Boards of Nursing believes the nursing process is fundamental to the practice of nursing.[1] Therefore, the nursing process is integrated throughout the entire exam. This does not mean you will receive a specific question on the nursing process like you did when you took your Fundamentals of Nursing class, but the question may ask you to identify which phase of the nursing process you used to help you select the correct answer.

- If you use the nursing process appropriately, it will also help you prioritize answers more easily.

✛ Let's review the phases of the nursing process

The phases of the nursing process haven't changed! They are exactly the same as they were in nursing school:

1. Assessment

2. Analysis

3. Planning

4. Implementation

5. Evaluation

Now we are going to break down each stage of the nursing process to show you how to use this information when answering test questions.

Assessment

Assessment is the **most important** phase of the nursing process. This stage involves gathering data: physical assessment, signs and symptoms, laboratory and diagnostic test results, and information provided by the client and family members.

In nursing school, your teachers taught you **normal** physical assessment findings. Now you must look at each client individually to consider what is **normal** for **that client.**

CASE IN POINT A barrel-chest is not a normal assessment finding in an adult. However, a barrel-chest is a normal assessment finding in someone with chronic lung disease.

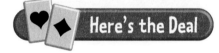

Here's the Deal

Assessment is **the most important** phase of the nursing process.

Hurst Hint

You have to understand what's normal before you can know what's abnormal.

SUBJECTIVE VERSUS OBJECTIVE DATA Let's compare and contrast subjective and objective data.

- Subjective data—data given by the client; things the client tells you.
- Objective data—data that can be observed or measured; usually obtained through physical assessment or diagnostic tests.

Analysis

Analysis, the second phase of the nursing process, occurs when you look for normal and abnormal findings in the assessment data. Next, you must go one step further to figure out what's normal for your individual client based on the client's disease process.

When you first started doing complete assessments in nursing school, you had tons of data written down about your client. As time progressed, you were able to put the pieces of the puzzle together—the pieces of the assessment data—to figure out what problems your client was experiencing. This is the point when you started to **analyze** and **interpret** the collected data.

Once you've analyzed your assessment data, you can identify actual or potential client problems and state them in the form of a Nursing Diagnosis.

Planning

Planning is the phase when you decide which client problem needs attention first—this is when you begin to prioritize your nursing care. Don't get me wrong. When you were doing your initial client assessment you may have found something right then that needed dealing with immediately . . . like an airway problem!

Planning is also the time for setting realistic client goals/outcomes and deciding which interventions are needed to obtain these goals. NCLEX® loves to see if you can correctly select the most qualified person to perform the interventions you are planning.

Implementation

You carry out the planned actions—nursing interventions—during the implementation phase. This helps the client attain the set goals/outcomes. As nurses, we have been taught specific nursing interventions based on our **own** nursing knowledge. Also, we implement some interventions based on the physician's specific order (**dependent** nursing intervention). Another part of this phase is to document what intervention you implemented, to document the client's response (during and after the intervention) to the intervention, and to share this information with the other health care team members.

Evaluation

When you **reassess** your plan of care to determine if it is working, you are using evaluation skills. You need to ask yourself, "Are the goals/outcomes I have set being met by the plan of care we, as a team, are using to bring my client back to her highest level of wellness?"

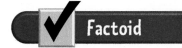

Data can be subjective or objective.

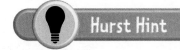

In the **analysis** phase, you may find you need **MORE** data in order to come to a conclusion about your client.

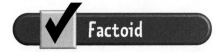

Planning is the phase where you decide what the desired outcomes **are** for your client.

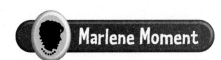

Interventions that do not require a physician's order are called **independent** nursing interventions.

Marlene Moment

As nurses, we can't do everything by ourselves, so we work with other members of the health care team. **Interdependent** nursing interventions reflect the team approach to client care.

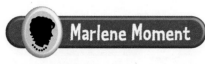

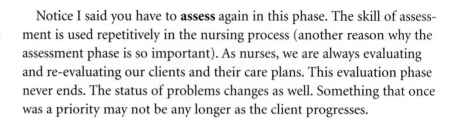

If you **reassess** the plan of care to find the goals aren't being met, . . . the client isn't progressing. You need a new care plan!

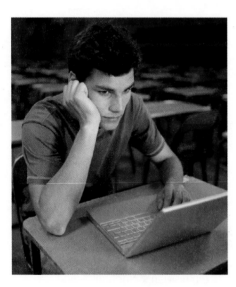

Notice I said you have to **assess** again in this phase. The skill of assessment is used repetitively in the nursing process (another reason why the assessment phase is so important). As nurses, we are always evaluating and re-evaluating our clients and their care plans. This evaluation phase never ends. The status of problems changes as well. Something that once was a priority may not be any longer as the client progresses.

LET'S LOOK AT NURSING PROCESS TYPE QUESTIONS

We will review plenty of **complete** questions later in the text. Right now, let's get an idea of how the **stem** of a question—the first part—is worded using the nursing process.

✚ Assessment stems

Following are examples of assessment stems.

1. A client is admitted to the pulmonary unit with a diagnosis of chronic obstructive pulmonary disease (COPD) with pneumonia. When taking the client's history, the nurse could expect the client to describe which of the following?

2. To determine a client's self-care ability, it is essential for the nurse to ask the family:

3. Which room would be most appropriate for the nurse to assign to the client with:

✚ Analysis stems

Here's a list of sample analysis stems.

1. A client is admitted with a diagnosis of diabetic ketoacidosis. This condition is most often exacerbated by:

2. A client presents to the emergency department with acute abdominal pain. The pain has been present for 2 days, but has increased in severity over the last 4 hours. The pain is localized in the left upper quadrant with some radiation to the back. The client has a history of alcoholism and intravenous drug use. What is the priority nursing diagnosis for this client? Or another way the above question could be posed would be: What are the client's symptoms most clearly an example of?

✚ Planning stems

Examples of planning stems follow.

1. In preparing the care plan for a client with pulmonary embolism, it is vital to include a goal that addresses the need for:

2. A client is being discharged from the hospital post-wound debridement. In planning the client's discharge, the nurse should coordinate with:

3. The nurse realizes that preparation for a thoracentesis would include:

✚ Implementation stems

Let's look at examples of implementation stems.

1. After an endoscopic retrograde cholangiopancreatography (ERCP), the nurse should ensure that:

2. While caring for a client who has intracranial pressure monitoring in place, which nursing measure is most essential for his care?

3. A client has been diagnosed with diverticulosis and has been placed on a high-fiber diet. The nurse explains that the purpose of this diet is to:

✚ Evaluation stems

Examples of evaluation stems follow.

1. In evaluating the effects of heparin, the nurse would monitor the results of which laboratory value?

2. To detect a common untoward effect of gentamycin, the nurse should assess the client for the possible development of:

3. After teaching a family member how to perform range of motion, which of the following methods would provide the nurse the best information regarding the family member's understanding of the procedure?

SUMMARY

This chapter has shown you why you must understand the nursing process in order to analyze test questions. We will practice use of this content when we practice answering test questions later in this book. Next, we are going to learn how to answer communication questions!

Reference

1. National Council of State Boards of Nursing. 2000 RN Practice Analysis Update. Available at **https://www.ncsbn.org/501.htm.** Accessed November 8, 2006.

Bibliography

Hurst Review Services. Available at **http://www.hurstreview.com.**

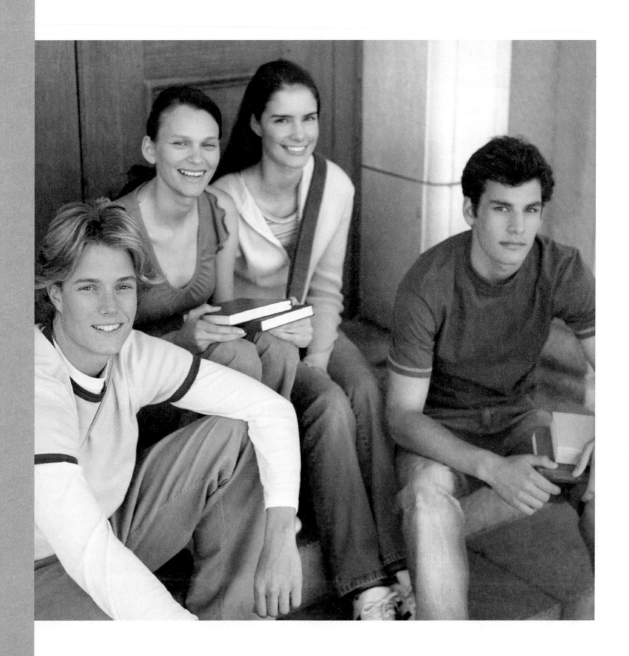

10 Everything You Ever Wanted to Know About Therapeutic Communication

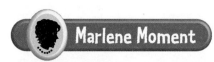

Nonverbal communication speaks just as plainly as verbal communication.

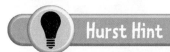

Reassure the client that anything she tells you will be kept confidential; only those involved in her direct care will access her health care information.

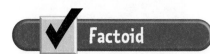

Focusing on the client leads to effective communication.

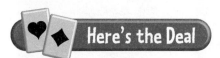

Ensuring the client's comfort level improves the nurse–client interaction.

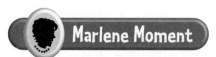

I once heard someone say, "You never learn anything if you're the one doing all the talking."

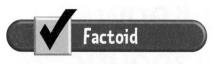

Therapeutic communication focuses on the client's feeling, concerns, and fears; not those of the nurse.

TALK IS NOT CHEAP

As a nurse you communicate with clients, their families, nurses, nursing assistants, physicians, and other members of the health care team. To communicate therapeutically means to use communication to improve the client's ability to function.[1] Communicating therapeutically is critical to being successful in your practice as a nurse. Great nurses know how to be great communicators. Communication occurs mainly verbally, but do not forget that nonverbal communication also speaks volumes. In every area of nursing, you have to communicate with others. Therefore, therapeutic communication appears **everywhere** on the NCLEX®. So let's get ready for these types of questions once and for all!

THE INTERVIEW

Valuable information can be obtained during the interview phase. There are some things you can do to ensure that you get the most accurate data during this time. Let's look at a few.

1. Appropriate time. The interview should not occur when the client is distracted by visitors, procedures such as blood draws, change of shift, or when the client is in intense pain.

2. Ensure privacy. You may need to close the door, pull a chair up close to the client, or wait until visitors have left to ask the client personal questions.

3. Proper approach. When you approach a client you should let him know who you are, what job you do for the hospital, and the reason you are interacting with him at this moment. If the visit with the client will be time consuming, let him know how long the process should take. Do not act rushed or hurried when interacting with your clients. If you are rushed, wait and talk with them once you have done whatever task it is that has your mind preoccupied.

4. Client comfort. If the patient is cold, uncomfortable, or in pain, you need to intervene before attempting long conversations, assessments, and treatments.

5. Hush and listen. Encourage the client and others to express their thoughts and feelings. Listening to the client voice her feelings will help you identify areas that require focus and further attention.

6. Use a nonjudgmental approach. As the nurse, you need to accept clients exactly as they are. A judgmental attitude is easily identified by the client and immediately blocks effective communication.

TECHNIQUES THAT PROMOTE THERAPEUTIC COMMUNICATION

Table 10-1 illustrates techniques that promote therapeutic communication.

Table 10-1. Techniques That Promote Therapeutic Communication

Therapeutic communication technique	Rationale
Face-to-face listening	Face your clients when they are speaking to you and you to them. Listen to, don't just hear, what your clients are telling you. Allow the client time to formulate thoughts . . . this may lead to questions she may have.
Nonverbal actions	Do the client's nonverbal actions match his words? Assess actions just as you do language.
Observing	Make note of client behaviors and seek the reason. Example: You seem angry today . . . .
Broad openings and general leads	These allow the client to lead the conversation and select topics that may be of concern to the client. Example: What would you like to discuss today? Example: I would like to hear more about . . . .
Open-ended questions	Open-ended questions allow more free-flowing conversation. This enables you to gather more information while keeping the client focused on important issues. Example: How are you feeling today?
Validating	Make sure you and the client are interpreting the topic and message the same way. Encourage the client's correct understanding of the topic.
Restating	Repeat what the client says to provide the opportunity for clarification if needed.
Focusing	Bring the client or family member, who may digress, back to what was originally being discussed.
Informing	Provide the client with information. Information decreases client anxiety. Most people harbor fear of the unknown.
Summarizing	State briefly what has been discussed in the conversation. Example: "During the past few minutes we've talked about . . . ."

CASE IN POINT Let's look at a couple of examples that use therapeutic communication techniques.

- Case #1: You are a home health nurse visiting a client with a history of depression and suicide attempts. Today the client is very tearful and moderately withdrawn. It is appropriate and expected for you to say, "Are you having thoughts of suicide?" You may think this approach is too blunt. You'd better be blunt in this situation to find the answer to the question even though it only requires a yes or no response. If you do not ask this question, you leave the NCLEX® people wondering if you are going to assess and prevent a possible suicide. Remember, the focus of NCLEX® is to keep people alive!

- Case #2: You are working a suicide hotline. A client calls talking about suicide. It is perfectly okay to say, "Do you have a plan?" instead of "How long have you been feeling this way?" By asking the more direct question, you can assist the client in this emergency situation in a timelier manner.

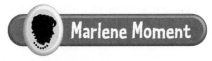

Marlene Moment

The client is not there to hear about your problems. Make the NCLEX® people happy and stay client-centered.

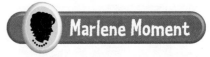

Marlene Moment

When you put on your nursing uniform you automatically assume a position of authority. Don't stand over the client looking down on him! This is mean! Show respect and compassion by getting down on his level to look him in the eyes.

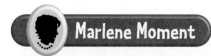

Marlene Moment

When you are inattentive, you are telling the client: "I really don't want to be in here with you. I've got to finish my charting so I can get to the mall."

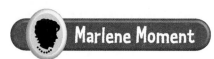

Marlene Moment

This has been the hardest habit for me to break, because I want to know "why" about everything. However, when I'm using therapeutic communication techniques, I never use the question "WHY?"

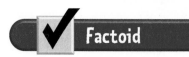

Here's the Deal

Accept it, no one wants advice. Clients want you to listen and not give advice. Also, if the client follows your advice and things don't work out the way anticipated, you may be blamed!

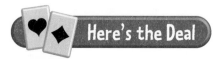

Factoid

Limit conversations to "need-to-know" information.

Hurst Hint

Remain neutral and allow your clients to express their thoughts. Do not interject your thoughts and feelings.

✚ Therapeutic communication blockers

Following are some specific blockers that may lead to poor communication with your clients. In other words, don't do these.

- Being inattentive: Constantly writing on your clipboard and never responding verbally or with eye contact to the client; straightening the room while looking in another direction. These behaviors relay the message that you are too busy to listen to the client.

- "Why?" questions: Asking the client "WHY?" causes the client to feel defensive. Asking "Why?" implies a nonaccepting and critical attitude on the part of the nurse.

- Making judgmental statements: Do not make statements that address your client's morals. Example: "You know better than to talk like that."

- Another example: "You don't smoke, do you?"

- Giving advice: This decreases the client's independence. This also may make the client feel that if he does not take your advice, you won't give him the best care possible.

- Falsely reassuring: No one knows the results of every disease, procedure, or problem. Do not reassure the client of a certain positive outcome that cannot be guaranteed.

- Belittling: Much of what clients experience in the hospital is scary to them. Don't belittle their concerns by saying things like, "Don't worry. We do this every day."

- Using close-ended questions: "Yes" or "no" answers do not promote conversation. They inhibit information gathering. Example: Do you have pain? However, close-ended questions are appropriate during life-threatening situations.

- Changing the subject: Avoiding what the client wants to talk about implies that you do not feel what she is saying is important.

- Asking excessive questions: Demanding information or asking for information that does not affect the client's care is inappropriate. Never ask for information that is not needed. Example: "So, why are you suing your son?"

- Approving or disapproving: Clients may seek your approval and try to avoid your disapproval. This is not therapeutic for the client and should not be encouraged.

CONSIDER THE CULTURE

Culture is something else to consider when communicating with your clients. Each culture is different, with its own unique communication structure. Three things to consider at this time are the communication style, use of eye contact, and meaning of touch to your client (Table 10-2).

Table 10-2. Communication Style, Use of Eye Contact, and Meaning of Touch for Different Cultural Groups

	African Americans	Asian Americans	European (White) Americans	Hispanic Americans	Native Americans
Communication Styles	Personal questions are an invasion of privacy.	Disclosing personal emotions is a sign of weakness. Silence is valued.	Silence can show respect or disrespect for someone, depending on the situation.	Dramatic body language, such as gestures or facial expression, express emotion or pain; verbal expressiveness is common.	Silence shows respect to the speaker. Body language is an important mode of communication. Expect others to be attentive when they speak and speak in low tones of voice.
Eye Contact	Rude behavior.	Disrespectful.	An indicator of trustworthiness.	Avoiding eye contact shows respect and attentiveness.	Disrespectful.
Touch	Acceptable with family and close personal friends.	Avoid touch with others during conversations. Do not like to be touched by members of the opposite sex. Touching of the head is disrespectful because the head is considered sacred.	Avoid close physical contact. Handshakes are for formal greeting.	Very comfortable with close contact. Very tactile and enjoy hugs and handshakes. Enjoy each others company and like to have family, friends, and acquaintances around.	Light hand touch is used with a greeting. Massage is used to promote bonding between infant and the mother. Touching the dead is prohibited. Like to have their own personal space.

From Delaune SC, Ladner PK. *Fundamentals of Nursing Standards and Practice*. Albany, NY: Delmar Publishers; 1998: 122–125, 286–293.

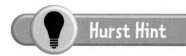

Be aware that lack of eye contact does not always indicate lack of attentiveness in all clients.

SUMMARY

Therapeutic communication is essential to quality nursing care. The nurse must be aware of effective ways of communicating and potential barriers to communication. Sociocultural differences can pose challenges for nurses. Becoming familiar with these differences can aid communication. Effective therapeutic communication among nurses, clients, and members of the health care team is vital for positive client outcomes. Start practicing your therapeutic communication techniques so you can impress the NCLEX® Lady and scare Newt away!

Reference

1. Delaune SC, Ladner PK. *Fundamentals of Nursing Standards and Practice.* Albany, NY: Delmar Publishers; 1998: 122–125, 286–293.

Bibliography

Hurst Review Services. **www.hurstreview.com.**

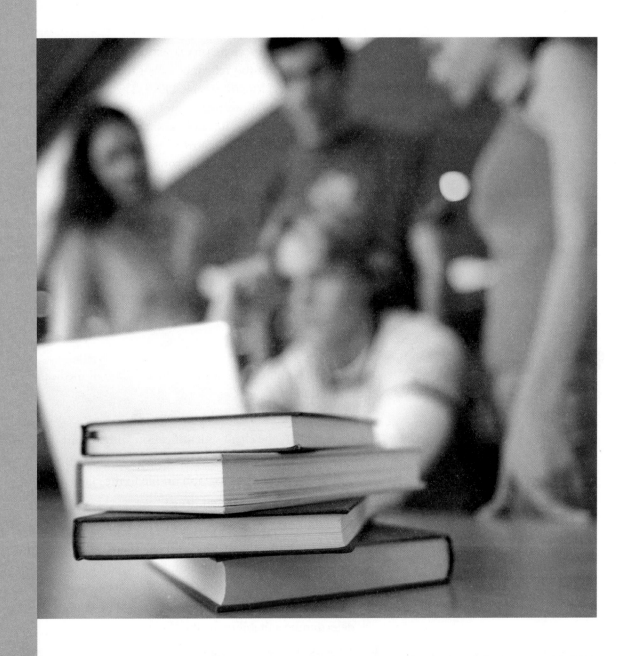

11 Pharmacology in a Nutshell

PHARMACOLOGY IN A NUTSHELL

Pharmacology content can be very stressful to a new nurse. There are so many drugs—how do you remember all of them? First of all, you do not have to know every drug to pass NCLEX®. The next rule of thumb is to investigate any medications you are not familiar with PRIOR to administering them to your client. It is not possible to memorize every single medication, but you can remember some key points about groups of medications and some of the more common drugs you are likely to see. I realize pharmacology is only one component of the NCLEX®. However, so many students are worried about "drugs" I just had to include a quickie review. In addition, many times in this chapter I discuss drugs that are administered intravenously. You and I know LPN/VN's do not administer drugs IV until they have completed a special certification course. However, you will be monitoring clients who are receiving these medications so I felt it was important to include this information as well. As always, stay within your scope of practice as a LPN/VN.

✚ You've got rights!

Let's start with a quick review of the "five rights" of medication administration.

1. Make sure you have the right person.
   - Always verify the client's identification with at least two methods.
   - Ask the client to state his name if possible, check the armband, and/or compare a photograph on file to the client.
2. Make sure you have the right drug.
   - Does the medication ordered match the medication you are preparing?
   - Is the medication appropriate for the client? Appropriateness is determined by obtaining a complete medical history, an updated medication history, and any pertinent laboratory studies.
   - Knowing the specifics of the ordered medication is also necessary in determining suitability for the client.
3. Make sure you have the right dose.
   - Is the dosage in the normal range for the client's age and size?
   - Mathematical calculations should be rechecked, and watch those decimals!
4. Make sure you are giving the drug at the right time.
   - To achieve a therapeutic blood level, medication must be given at the right time.
   - Each agency has their own policies regarding specific times for routine medications.
   - The common rule of thumb for most medicines is to give the medicine within 30 minutes of the scheduled time.
5. Make sure you have the right route.
6. Know how to correctly and safely administer the prescribed medication.
7. Never assume the route of a medication—always clarify.

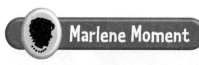

Marlene Moment

Prior to giving a medication, you should check at least three times to make sure you are right. Since you are a new nurse, you might want to check it five times. (I still do!)

Marlene Moment

Read carefully. For example, Motrin is an analgesic, not an "anal" gesic. Besides, you are not going to get a license if you try to make your client swallow their Tylenol suppository even if it is lubricated!

✚ Speculate before you medicate

There are a couple of things that need to be done before administering any medication.

- Make sure the client is not hypersensitive to the drug being given—that is, make sure your client does not have a known allergy to the medication.

- Get a complete history from your client. Look at all medications the client is taking and make sure there are no adverse drug or food interactions.

- Know why you are giving the drug and what the expected response is.

- Are there any labs or vital signs you need to check prior to administration?

- Document and report any adverse effects and counteract these effects appropriately.

- Find out if the client is pregnant or breast-feeding, as most medications are contraindicated in these women.

✚ Over-the-counter meds

Over-the-counter (OTC) medications are medications that can be obtained without a prescription, allowing clients to self-treat their ailments without seeking health care advice. Check out these points.

- Be sure to review the use of OTCs during the client's health history.

- Teach your client these medications can be harmful if not taken correctly.

- Your client should also be able to recognize contraindications and possible adverse reactions.

- Some of the more common types of OTC medications are antacids (Tums, Maalox) and acid-controlling drugs (Tagamet, Pepcid); antifungal agents (Lotrimin, Monistat); antihistamines and decongestants (Benadryl, Claritin, Robitussin); acetaminophen (Tylenol); aspirin (Bayer, Ecotrin); and ibuprofen (Advil, Motrin).

✚ Alternative or complementary therapies

Alternative or complementary therapies are nontraditional therapeutic methods such as herbal medicines, chiropractics, acupuncture, and reflexology.

- Herbal remedies need to be considered when obtaining a medication history from your client. They are available over-the-counter and used for a variety of ailments. As with any drug, herbal products can have drug or food interactions when taken with certain medications.

- Clients should be aware that even though herbs are natural substances, they can still be harmful and manufacturers of these products are not required to provide proof of effectiveness or safety.

Common herbal supplements and potential drug interactions are shown in Table 11-1.

✚ Don't take the wrong route

There are many routes to administer medication. The most common are oral (PO), topical, vaginal, rectal, and parenteral.

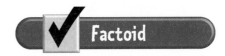

Factoid

An adverse drug reaction is when a drug or food effects the action of another, causing an unfavorable result.

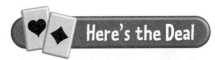

Here's the Deal

Remember prescribed drugs, over-the-counter drugs, and herbal supplements can all have adverse effects.

Table 11-1. Common Herbal Supplements and Potential Drug Interactions

Herbal supplement	Drugs herbs may interact with
Aloe	Steroids, antidysrhythmics, digitalis, diuretics, chamomile
Echinacea	Anabolic steroids, immunosuppresants
Garlic	Aspirin, anticoagulants, nonsteroidal anti-inflammatories, antiplatelets
Ginko	Anticoagulants, thrombolytics, MAO inhibitors, nonsteroidal anti-inflammatories, antiplatelets, anticonvulsants, tricyclic antidepressants
Ginseng	Warfarin, MAO inhibitors, nonsteroidal anti-inflammatories, estrogen
St. John's wort	Alcohol, antidepressants
Kava-kava	Alprazom (Xanax), CNS depressants, antiplatelets
Saw palmetto	Hormonal agents
Feverfew	Anticoagulants, antiplatelets, thrombolytics, antibiotics, nonsteroidal anti-inflammatories

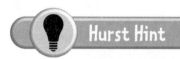

Hurst Hint

Enteric-coated or timed-released medications must be swallowed whole. Never crush or cut a tablet or capsule. Crushing or opening these medications can cause gastrointestinal irritation or drug toxicity.

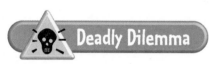

Deadly Dilemma

Never apply topical medications with a bare hand. Use a tongue blade, cotton-tipped applicator, or gloved hand to apply unless you would also like a little dose of nitroglycerin ointment.

- Oral forms of medication include tablets, capsules, sublingual tablets, elixirs, suspensions, syrups, emulsions, and lozenges. Oral medications are absorbed in the small intestine and circulate through the liver.

- Topical forms of medication are aerosols, ointments, creams, pastes, powders, foams, gels, transdermal patches, and inhalers. Ophthalmic, otic, and intranasal routes are also considered topical medications.

- When placing a transdermal patch on a client, always wear gloves, remove the old patch, and rotate sites to prevent skin irritation.

- After instilling ophthalmic drops in the client's conjunctival sac, hold slight pressure on the nasolacrimal duct for 30 seconds to prevent systemic absorption of the medication.

CASE IN POINT Atropine can be given as an ophthalmic drop to decrease inflammation. If you do not hold pressure properly, it can absorb systemically and make the heart rate go up.

My parents went to the pharmacy and all I got was this stinkin shot!

First of all, it's not parental . . . it's parenteral. Parenteral medications come in different forms that include injectable solutions, suspensions, emulsions, and powders for reconstitution.

- The most common routes of parenteral medication are intravenous (IV)—administered directly into the circulatory system; intramuscular (IM)—administered into the muscle; subcutaneous (SC)—administered into the subcutaneous tissue; and intradermal (ID)—administered into the outer layers of the dermis. The most common IV access devices are peripheral intravenous catheters (PIC line) and central venous access devices (CVAD).

* Peripheral IVs are, as the name suggests, catheters that are inserted into a peripheral vein. These are the most common IV access devices used. The four most common types of CVADs seen are nontunneled or percutaneous catheters, peripherally inserted central catheters (PICCs), tunneled catheters, and implanted ports.

   1. The nontunneled catheter is inserted by a physician into a subclavian or jugular vein to the superior vena cava. These are considered short-term and usually stay in less than 6 weeks.

   2. The PICC line may be inserted by a specially trained nurse or physician. It is inserted through the basilica of cephalic vein to the axillary, subclavian, or brachiocephalic vein or the superior vena cava.

   3. The tunneled catheter is inserted surgically by a physician. It is threaded under the skin to the subclavian vein and into the superior vena cava. These catheters have a cuff to deter migration and infection. They may be used for years.

   4. Implanted ports are inserted surgically by a physician. These catheters do not exit the skin as the preceding catheters do. Instead, the end of the catheter is connected to a small chamber that is implanted subcutaneously. Infusion through these devices requires a special noncoring needle such as a Huber-tipped needle that is inserted through the skin into the chamber.

* IV medications are often administered in the forms of IV piggybacks (IVPBs) or IV pushes (IVPs).

   1. IVPBs may come as an admixture or in an infusion bag that requires activation prior to administration. The medication is mixed in a small amount of IV solution and run intermittently by connecting to the primary IV fluids using secondary tubing. The IVPB should hang higher than the primary fluids during infusion.

   2. IV pushes are medications that are injected into a port in the primary IV tubing from a syringe. Prior to administration, IV medications should be looked up to determine a safe infusion time. Peripheral IV sites need to be monitored frequently for signs and symptoms of infiltration.

* Total parenteral nutrition (TPN) is nutritional support delivered by intravenous infusion for clients unable to tolerate and maintain adequate enteral or oral intake. It may also be called hyperalimentation or parenteral nutrition. Its contents are specified to the client's nutritional needs. It can provide calories, carbohydrates, amino acids, fats, trace elements, vitamins, minerals, and other essential nutrients. TPN can be irritable to the peripheral veins, and long-term use may cause phlebitis. CVADs are preferred for long-term TPN infusions. Laboratory studies need to be monitored closely in the client receiving TPN infusions. Some specific values to consider are glucose, electrolytes, total protein, albumin, blood urea nitrogen (BUN), red blood cell count (RBC), white blood cell count (WBC), cholesterol, hemoglobin, total lymphocyte

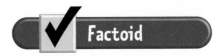
Factoid

There should be no blood pressures or blood drawn from the affected extremity of the client with a PICC. These lines can be used from several days to months.

count, serum transferring, iron levels, urine creatinine clearance, lipid profile, and urinalysis.

• Prior to administration, IV medications must be investigated for drug incompatibilities. In other words, can these drugs be mixed with the IV fluid that is already infusing? If the answer is "no," extra precautions such as flushing the IV line before and after administration need to be taken to prevent this from happening. A drug incompatibility causes a chemical change or even destruction of at least one of the medications involved, possibly creating a harmful effect to the client. Remember, a LPN/VN must have completed an IV certification class prior to administering drugs by this route.

THE BLOODY REALITY

Even though the LPN/VN is not the one primarily responsible for blood administration. You will still be caring for clients receiving blood or blood products. Therefore, we need to at least review the basics. The IV administration of blood or blood products is often done as replacement therapy for whichever blood components are deficient in the client. There are different types of blood products available and their use is dependent on the needs of the client.

• The most common types of blood products are:

1. Whole blood: can replace all blood components and increase circulatory volume.

2. Packed red blood cells (PRBCs): given to increase the oxygen-carrying capacity in the circulatory system by increasing the number of red blood cells.

3. Platelets: given to clients with bleeding disorders or platelet deficiency.

4. Plasma protein fractions (PPFs) and albumin, fresh frozen plasma (FFP): used as volume expanders and provide plasma proteins.

5. FFP, and cryoprecipitate: contain clotting factors, and are administered to clients who are hemorrhaging and lack adequate coagulating factors of their own.

• Blood products are categorized into four main groups—A, B, AB, and O. The Rh factor of a blood type is known as Rh positive or Rh negative.

• Prior to blood administration, there are some steps you need to follow.

• Blood typing and cross-matching are ordered by the physician to ensure that the client receives the correct blood type.

• A signed consent for the blood administration is required from the client.

• Blood products and clients are verified through several checks according to agency guidelines. The first check begins in the blood bank and the last check occurs at the bedside by two licensed personnel.

• Routinely, baseline vital signs are obtained prior to the blood administration and 15 minutes after the infusion begins. Again, agency guidelines dictate how often and when vital signs are obtained when administering blood.

- The client is assessed before, during, and after blood administration for potential reactions. The more common reactions are hemolytic, febrile, and allergic reactions.

1. Hemolytic reactions occur when there is an incompatibility between the donor's blood and the client's blood. It is manifested by chills, fever, headache, backache, dyspnea, cyanosis, chest pain, tachycardia, and hypotension.

2. A febrile action is caused by a sensitivity of the client's blood to the donor's white blood cells, platelets, or plasma protein. This is manifested by fever, chills, skin that is warm flushed, headache, anxiety, and muscle pain.

3. Allergic reactions are due to an antibody-antigen reaction and can range from mild to severe. A mild allergic reaction consists of flushing, itching, urticaria, and bronchial wheezing. Severe allergic reactions lead to dyspnea, chest pain, circulatory collapse, and cardiac arrest.

- If any kind of reaction is suspected, stop the transfusion immediately! Get new tubing and infuse normal saline at a keep vein open rate before notifying the physician. Observe agency guidelines for blood transfusion reactions and send the remaining blood with the tubing to the laboratory for analysis. You will need to get a urine specimen as well so a hemolytic reaction can be ruled out.

- Blood administration needs to be carefully documented. Some items to note are type of product, blood unit number, sequence number, starting time, rate, ending time, amount infused, how the client tolerated the procedure, vital signs, and verification/identification of blood product and client.

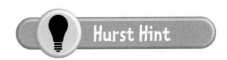

Hurst Hint

The first 15 to 30 minutes of a transfusion are critical, as this is when most reactions occur.

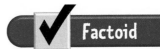

Factoid

A "Keep Vein Open" (KVO) rate is whatever your facility says it is. KVO may mean 30 mL/hr or 5 mL/hr.

PAIN MANAGEMENT

Some agencies consider pain a fifth vital sign. Pain is subjective; therefore it is whatever or wherever the client says it is. Pain is the body's way of saying "Hey! Something's wrong here!"

- Pain begins with nociceptors, which are peripheral nerve organs that react to mechanical, thermal, or chemical stimuli.

- Pain medications work by altering the impulses that interpret the stimuli as pain.

- Pharmacological management of pain is carried out by the teamwork of nurses, physicians, clients, and sometimes the families.

- The nurse's responsibility is to maintain analgesia by administering prescribed medications, assessing its effectiveness, monitoring for side effects or adverse reactions, and reporting whether the intervention is beneficial. The most effective way to make this determination is to ask the client to rate the pain prior to administering a pain medication and again after the medication is administered.

- Pain medications work best when the dose and interval between doses are specific to the client. In other words, dosage and intervals should be based on the client's needs versus a rigid standard or routine schedule.

- The client should be instructed to request pain medication before the pain gets severe in order to maintain a therapeutic serum level of the medication and to get the most pain relief.

- PCA (patient controlled analgesia) pumps are a common method of pain management for postoperative clients. Safety limits are programmed into the pump, and the client is allowed to control their own pain medication administration within these limits. This gives the client the ability to self-administer a continuous infusion of pain medication and to administer extra if there is an increased episode of pain. The client using the PCA pump should be encouraged to administer the pain medication before pain gets severe. And the client and family members should be instructed that ONLY the client is to administer the medication.

✚ Specific categories of pain medications

Some of the pain medications that will be looked at closer are nonopioid analgesics, opioid analgesics, opioid antagonists, anesthetics, and controlled substances.

Nonopioid analgesic medications

HOW DO THE NONOPIOID ANALGESIC MEDICATIONS WORK? This particular type of medication can work three different ways:

- Inhibit the stimulation of pain receptors.
- Inhibit substances that increase the sensitivity of the pain receptors in the central nervous system.
- By acting on the hypothalamus to reduce fever.

WHAT ARE NONOPIOID ANALGESICS USED FOR?

- These medications are used to treat mild to moderate pain.
- Some forms of nonopioid analgesics are used to decrease fever and/or inflammation.
- Some examples of nonopioid analgesics are salycilates (Aspirin), acetaminophen (Tylenol), and nonsteroidal anti-inflammatory drugs, also known as NSAIDS (Advil, Toradol, Anaprox).

AS A BRAND NEW NURSE, WHAT DO I NEED TO KNOW ABOUT NONOPIOID ANALGESIC MEDICATIONS?

- Because aspirin can cause gastric irritation and has some anticoagulating effects, it is contraindicated in clients with bleeding disorders or gastric ulcers.
- Aspirin should not be given to children or adolescents due to the increased risk of Reye's syndrome in these clients.
- Since these drugs are metabolized in the liver, they must be used cautiously in clients with severe hepatic disease, and those that have a history of chronic alcohol use.
- More than 4 grams of acetaminophen daily can lead to liver toxicity in any client.

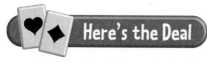

Here's the Deal

Do not give Tylenol to anyone with any type of liver problem even if the problem was in their past. This is a good NCLEX® tip. Assume the worst!

WHAT DO I NEED TO TEACH MY CLIENTS ABOUT NONOPIOID ANALGESIC MEDICATIONS?

- These drugs need to be taken with meals or after meals to prevent gastric irritation.
- If not taken with meals, take the medication with a full glass of water.
- Avoid alcohol consumption while taking this medication.
- Remain in a upright position for 15 to 30 minutes after taking medication to empty stomach. (It helps decrease GI upset.)

Opioid analgesic medications

HOW DO OPIOID ANALGESIC MEDICATIONS WORK?

- Alter the perception of pain by binding to opiate receptors in the central nervous system.

WHAT ARE OPIOID ANALGESICS USED FOR?

- These medications are used to treat pain that is not relieved by non-opioid analgesics, cough relief, and to enhance anesthesia effects.
- Some examples of opioid analgesic medications are meperdine (Demerol), morphine (MS Contin), codeine, hydromorphone (Dilaudid), and fentanyl (Duragesic).

AS A BRAND NEW NURSE, WHAT DO I NEED TO KNOW ABOUT OPIOID ANALGESIC MEDICATIONS?

- Assess blood pressure, pulse, and respirations before/during/after administration of this type of medication.
- Some adverse reactions to watch for are orthostatic hypotension, sedation, light-headedness, dizziness, hallucinations, and respiratory depression.
- Caution should be used when administering these medications to the elderly or debilitated client because they may require a lower dosage.
- Client safety should be maintained when using opioid analgesics such as placing the bedrails up, putting the bed in the lowest position, and making sure the call light is within reach.
- Naloxone (Narcan) is the antidote for an opioid overdose.

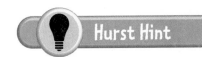

Hurst Hint

Check hospital policy regarding raising siderails as this could be viewed as a form of restraint.

WHAT DO I NEED TO TEACH MY CLIENTS ABOUT OPIOID ANALGESIC MEDICATIONS?

- This medication should be taken with food to minimize gastric irritation.
- The client needs to know what orthostatic hypotension is and how to decrease its risk of occurring by moving slowly. (Especially when changing positions from supine to standing.)
- Activities requiring alertness such as operating machinery should be avoided while taking this medication.
- Alcohol consumption should also be discouraged while taking this medication (alcohol enhances effects). Respiration could decrease to a deadly rate.

- For maximum pain management, client should be instructed to take medication before pain gets severe.

Opioid antagonists

HOW DO OPIOID ANTAGONISTS WORK?

- These medications impede (block) the effects of opioids without creating analgesic effects.

WHAT ARE OPIOID ANTAGONISTS USED FOR?

- Used to reverse the central nervous system and respiratory depression that result from an opioid overdose.
- Examples are naloxone (Narcan) and namefene (Revex).

AS A BRAND NEW NURSE, WHAT DO I NEED TO KNOW ABOUT OPIOID ANTAGONISTS?

- Administer only the amount required to reverse respiratory depression or to increase mental alertness. Any more than this can cause severe withdrawal symptoms in the client who is physically dependent on opioids.
- Some adverse reactions to watch for are nausea, vomiting, tachycardia, hypotension, hypertension, and arrhythmias.
- Immediately after opioid antagonist administration, the unconscious client may abruptly return to consciousness, hyperventilate and experience tremors.
- Repeated doses of this medication may be necessary if the effects of the opioid analgesics outlast those of the opioid antagonist.

WHAT DO I NEED TO TEACH MY CLIENT ABOUT OPIOID ANTAGONIST MEDICATIONS?

- This is typically a medication that is used in a critical or life threatening situation. The main thing to teach your client, if possible, is the purpose and effects of the medication.

Anesthetic medications

HOW DO ANESTHETIC MEDICATIONS WORK?

- These medications depress the central nervous system, causing the loss of pain perception and/or other sensations.

WHAT ARE ANESTHETIC MEDICATIONS USED FOR?

- Used to induce and maintain anesthesia for medical or surgical procedures.
- Anesthetic medications can be general or local, depending on where in the central nervous system the specific anesthetic substance acts.
- Some examples of IV anesthetics are midazolam hydrochloride (Versed), ketamine (Ketelar), fentanyl (Sublimaze), and propofol (Diprivan).
- Halothane (Fluothane) and nitrous oxide are examples of inhalation anesthetics.
- Lidocaine (Xylocaine) can be used as a local or topical anesthetic.

**AS A BRAND NEW NURSE, WHAT DO I NEED TO KNOW
ABOUT ANESTHETICS?**

- Some adverse reactions to monitor for when administering anesthetics are respiratory depression, apnea, hypotension, arrhythmias, tachycardia, confusion, nausea, vomiting, and tissue necrosis with extravasation at the IV site.

- Caution should be exercised when administering these drugs to the elderly or debilitated client.

- Atropine should be readily available during administration to reverse possible bradycardia.

- Monitor vital signs frequently.

- Hypothermia is a common side effect of inhalation anesthetics, so obtaining a temperature needs to be included when monitoring vital signs.

- Provide warm blankets and administer oxygen therapy during the recovery period to compensate for the increased oxygen demand caused by the normal side effect of shivering.

- When using a local or topical anesthetic, remember that upon application of the medication, the client loses the ability to sense cold, warmth, pain, and touch in the affected area, so client safety regarding this area is a concern until those sensations return. You must protect this area and assess it frequently.

- If a client's throat has been anesthetized, make sure the gag reflex has returned before having the client attempt to swallow food or drink.

- Naloxone (Narcan) is the antidote for an overdose of anesthetic medications and as stated earlier, reverses the actions of these central nervous system depressants.

**WHAT DO I NEED TO TEACH MY CLIENT ABOUT
ANESTHETIC MEDICATIONS?**

- The client needs to be NPO at least 8 hours prior to surgery.

- Alcohol consumption and other central nervous depressants should be avoided for at least 24 hours after receiving an anesthetic medication.

- Clients need to be educated of appropriate safety measures to take because of the possible psychomotor function impairment that can last 24 hours or longer after an anesthetic agent.

- If a local anesthetic was used, advise the client to use caution around the anesthetized area until complete sensation returns.

Sedative/Hypnotics Medications

HOW DO SEDATIVE/HYPNOTIC MEDICATIONS WORK?

- By producing a generalized depression of the central nervous system.

- The difference in these medications from previously mentioned medications is that sedative/hypnotics have no analgesic properties.

WHAT ARE SEDATIVE/HYPNOTIC MEDICATIONS USED FOR?

- Sedatives are generally used to provide sedation and hypnotics are used to treat insomnia.
- Other uses of these medications are as anticonvulsants, enhancements in treating alcohol withdrawal, enhancements of general anesthesia, or as amnesics.
- Some examples are lorazepam (Ativan), phenobarbital (Luminal), diazepam (Valium), and zolpidem (Ambien).

AS A BRAND NEW NURSE, WHAT DO I NEED TO KNOW ABOUT SEDATIVE/HYPNOTIC MEDICATIONS?

- These medications are contraindicated in clients who have uncontrolled pain or a pre-existing central nervous system depression.
- Caution should be exercised when administering these medications to the elderly or debilitated client.
- Many of these medications are classified as controlled substances, which will be discussed later.
- Supervision is required when ambulating and transferring clients after the administration of sedatives or hypnotics and client safety measures should be implemented.
- Naloxone (Narcan) is the antidote used for the overdosing of sedatives or hypnotics.

Marlene Moment

It's not smart to have an Ambien and a margarita on the rocks!

WHAT DO I NEED TO TEACH MY CLIENT ABOUT SEDATIVES/HYPNOTICS?

- If it works as it is supposed to, it MAY cause drowsiness!
- Avoid alcohol consumption and other central nervous depressants when using these medications.
- Ask for assistance before attempting ambulation or transferring.

✚ Controlled substances

Controlled substances are medications or substances that are federally regulated. They are grouped in schedules according to their potential for abuse and dependence liability.

- Schedule I has the highest abuse and dependency potential. These usually consist of illegal drugs or drugs used in research with appropriate limitations set. Examples of Schedule I substances are heroin, LSD, and marijuana.
- Schedule II substances are prescription medications that have a high potential for abuse and dependency. These medications are dispensed with a written prescription only and there are no refills allowed. Examples of Schedule II substances are hydromorphone, oxycodone, and morphine.
- Schedule III substances have an intermediate potential for dependency and abuse. They may be dispensed with a written or oral prescription

that extends no longer than 6 months. There can be no more than five refills in that 6-month period. Examples of Schedule III substances are hydrocodone and dihydrocodeine combinations.

● Schedule IV substances have less abuse and dependency potential than Schedule IIIs. They can be dispensed according to a written or oral prescription that does not exceed 6 months. These medications can be refilled six times within the 6-month period. Some examples of Schedule IV substances are diazepam, lorazepam, and zolpidam.

● Schedule V substances have little potential for abuse and dependency. These medications can be refilled as many times as the prescriber allows and some forms may be available as over-the-counter medications. Some examples of Schedule V substances are buprenorphine and diphenoxylate/atropine.

Controlled substances are kept locked in health care facilities with very stringent administration procedures. Inventory forms and guidelines of controlled substances are agency specific. They are similar in that any discrepancies in the controlled substances inventory have to be resolved immediately. Another similarity is that a second nurse is required to witness the discarding of a portion or all of a controlled substance. Both signatures are then necessary to validate the occurrence.

✛ Pain management documentation

When documenting the administration of pain medication, there needs to be more detail than simply initialing that it was given.

● Documentation needs to start with the client's description of the pain and how they rate it, using the appropriate pain scale.

● Location of the pain should be noted and vital signs obtained.

● What was done about it? Did you call the physician? What was the name of the physician? The name of the drug, dosage, and route also need to be documented. After the medication has had time to act, the pain needs to be re-evaluated to determine if it provided the intended relief.

● Obtain vital signs and have the client rate her pain.

● If pain relief has occurred, both (VS and pain) will have decreased.

● If not, then the process starts over as prescribed, until the desired result is achieved.

DRUGS BY SYSTEM

✛ Respiratory system drugs
Bronchodilators

HOW DO BRONCHODILATORS WORK?

● They relax the bronchial smooth-muscle cells causing the bronchi and bronchioles to dilate, improving airflow.

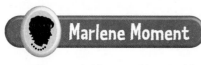

Marlene Moment

Expect your child to run like a wild animal around the house after giving them a breathing treatment!

WHAT ARE BRONCHODILATORS USED FOR?

- Used to treat bronchospasms, asthma, bronchitis, emphysema, and neonatal apnea.

- Some examples of bronchodilators are albuterol (Proventil), aminophylline (Phyllocontin), and theophylline (Slo-bid).

AS A BRAND NEW NURSE, WHAT DO I NEED TO KNOW ABOUT BRONCHODILATORS?

- Possible adverse reactions are *anxiety, nervousness,* tremors, shaking, headache, palpitations, tachycardia, hypertension, and arrhythmias.

- Contraindicated in clients with uncontrolled arrhythmias.

- Administered around the clock to maintain therapeutic level.

- Assess vital signs and respiratory status before/during/after therapy.

WHAT DO I NEED TO TEACH MY CLIENT?

- Teach the importance of taking medication around the clock.

- Encourage client to drink at least 2000 mL per day to keep secretions thin and easier to cough up. (Unless contraindicated.)

- Instruct client to seek medical assistance if respiratory status is not improved after taking this medication.

- If the client is using more than one inhaler, the bronchodilator should be administered at least 5 minutes prior to other medications to achieve maximum absorption.

Corticosteroid medications

HOW DO CORTICOSTEROIDS WORK?

- Used in the topical form through some sort of inhalant device when treating respiratory illnesses.

- Neutralize biochemical mediums that cause inflammation, thereby reducing edema that creates airway obstruction.

WHAT ARE CORTICOSTEROIDS USED FOR?

- Used to treat chronic asthma, chronic bronchitis, or allergic rhinitis.

- Examples of inhaled corticosteroids are flunisolide (Aerobid), fluticasone (Flovent), and mometasone (Nasonex).

AS A BRAND NEW NURSE, WHAT DO I NEED TO KNOW ABOUT CORTICOSTEROIDS?

- Intended for long-term management of asthma, not acute attacks.

- Adverse effects are mostly related to the respiratory system such as pharyngeal irritation, coughing, dry mouth, and oral fungal infections.

- The composition of inhaled corticosteroids typically contains smaller doses of the medication making systemic effects rare (you're not going to develop Cushing's syndrome by using inhaled steroids).

- Administer with caution in clients who are immunosuppressed, taking other corticosteroids, have clinical tuberculosis, or have other viral respiratory infections.

WHAT DO I NEED TO TEACH MY CLIENT ABOUT CORTICOSTEROID MEDICATIONS?

- Remind the client that this medication is not intended for acute respiratory attacks.
- Instruct client on the use and care of the inhaler.
- If using a bronchodilator inhalant in addition to the steroid inhalant, use the bronchodilator at least 5 minutes prior to the steroid to facilitate maximum medication absorption.
- Instruct clients to rinse their mouth after using steroidal inhalers (prevents infections in the mouth).

Antitussive medications

HOW DO ANTITUSSIVE MEDICATIONS WORK?

- Decrease coughing.
- Inhibit neural activity in the cough center located in the medulla oblongata or by anesthetizing cough receptors throughout the bronchi, alveoli, and pleura.

WHAT ARE ANTITUSSIVE MEDICATIONS USED FOR?

- There are some instances when coughing causes more harm than good in the client. Examples of these situations would be a nonproductive cough or one that hinders a client's rest or daily activities.
- Antitussives are cough suppressants and they come as opioid or non-opioid antitussives.
- Examples of antitussives are codeine sulfate (Codeine), benzonatate (Tessalon), and dextromethorphan (Robitussin DM).

AS A BRAND NEW NURSE, WHAT DO I NEED TO KNOW ABOUT ANTITUSSIVE MEDICATIONS?

- Assess breath sounds and cough prior to and during treatment with antitussive medications.
- Use cautiously in the elderly or debilitated client.
- Adverse reactions are drowsiness, drying of respiratory secretions, dizziness, nausea, vomiting, pruritis, and sedation.
- Respirations and level of consciousness should be closely monitored even more closely if administering opioid antitussives to a client that is also receiving other central nervous system depressants (can have synergistic effect).
- Drinking fluids immediately after administering this medication can offset the desired actions so the client should be instructed to wait at least thirty minutes before drinking anything.

WHAT DO I NEED TO TEACH MY CLIENT ABOUT ANTITUSSIVE MEDICATIONS?

- May cause drowsiness. Caution must be used if considering doing things that require mental alertness.
- Fluid intake should be at least 2000 mL per day to keep the bronchial secretions thin.
- Call the physician if cough persists more than 7 days.
- Consult with a health care provider prior to taking over-the-counter medications with the antitussives.
- Do not drink fluids for at least 30 minutes after taking the medication.

Expectorants

HOW DO EXPECTORANTS WORK?

- Expectoration means to cough up and spit out secretions from the respiratory tract.
- Expectorants work by thinning the sputum and bronchial secretions, requiring less effort on the clients to clear their airways by coughing.

WHAT ARE EXPECTORANTS USED FOR?

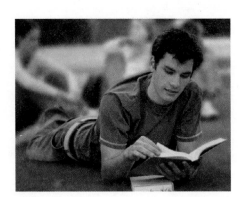

- Treat coughs related to upper respiratory tract infections.
- An example of an expectorant is guaifenesin (Robitussin, Humibid LA, and Tussin).

AS A BRAND NEW NURSE, WHAT DO I NEED TO KNOW ABOUT EXPECTORANTS?

- Adverse effects are nausea, vomiting, drowsiness, diarrhea, and abdominal pain.
- Make sure the airway is patent and have suction available. Assess breath sounds before and during treatment using expectorants.

WHAT DO I NEED TO TEACH MY CLIENTS ABOUT EXPECTORANTS?

- Maintain an adequate fluid intake of at least 2000 mL per day to keep secretions thin (makes the secretions easier to cough up).
- Consult a health care provider if cough persists for more than 7 days.
- Advise the client this medication may cause drowsiness and to exercise caution when performing tasks that require alertness.

Mucolytics

HOW DO MUCOLYTIC MEDICATIONS WORK?

- Decreases bronchial secretions by breaking down the mucous.

WHAT ARE MUCOLYTICS USED FOR?

- Treat clients with thick, abnormal mucous.
- This medication is also used as an antidote for an overdose of acetaminophen (Tylenol).
- An example of a mucolytic medication is acetylcysteine (Mucomyst).

AS A BRAND NEW NURSE, WHAT DO I NEED TO KNOW ABOUT MUCOLYTIC MEDICATIONS?

- Adverse effects are bronchospasms, stomatitis, nausea, vomiting, drowsiness, and rhinorrea.
- This medication has an odor resembling "rotten eggs."
- Exercise caution when administering this medication to the elderly or debilitated client.
- Maintain a patent airway and assess breath sounds prior to and during administration of the mucolytic medications.

WHAT DO I NEED TO TEACH MY CLIENTS ABOUT MUCOLYTIC MEDICATIONS?

- Warn the clients of this medication's odor. Encourage them to drink at least 2000 mL daily fluids thin secretions making it easier to cough them out.

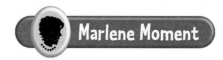

Marlene Moment

There is nothing like the smell of rotten eggs when you are sick.

Decongestants

HOW DO DECONGESTANT MEDICATIONS WORK?

- Shrink tissues in the nasal passage, promoting nasal drainage.
- Adrenergic agents cause vasoconstriction in the nasal passages, resulting in decongestion.
- The other type of decongestant would be steroids, which decrease inflammation by altering the body's immune response to antigens.

WHAT ARE DECONGESTANTS USED FOR?

- Treat nasal congestion that is as a result of the common cold, hay fever, acute or chronic rhinitis, and sinusitis.
- Some examples of decongestants are oxymetazoline hydrochloride (Afrin), pseudoephedrine hydrochloride (Sudafed), and budesonide (Rhinocort).

AS A BRAND NEW NURSE, WHAT DO I NEED TO KNOW ABOUT DECONGESTANTS?

- Some adverse effects are *hypertension,* headache, dizziness, light-headedness, drowsiness, insomnia, nervousness, mucosal irritation, and dryness.
- Observe vital signs, specifically blood pressure and pulse rate.
- If taken with an MAO inhibitor, hypertension can result.
- Overuse of decongestants can cause rebound congestion.

WHAT DO I NEED TO TEACH MY CLIENTS ABOUT DECONGESTANTS?

- Demonstrate proper medication administration, including how to avoid contaminating the container (if medication is an inhalant) during administration.
- Instruct client not to share medication container with others. Do not exceed the prescribed dosage of the medication.

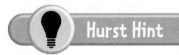

✛ Nervous system drugs

Let's get the normal stuff straight first. The function of the nervous system is to coordinate muscle activity, monitor organs, conduct and interfere with input from the senses, and initiate actions to restore homeostatic imbalances. It is made up of two parts. The autonomic nervous system, which is the homeostatic regulator of the body, controls involuntary body functions, glands, and organs. It is comprised of the sympathetic nervous system (SNS), which prepares the body for "fight or flight," and the parasympathetic nervous system (PSNS), which works to get the body back to normal after a stressful event has passed.

During a stressful event, the parasympathetic nervous system releases acetylcholine (ACh), a neurotransmitter that sends information to the effector cells by combining with cholinergic receptors. The central nervous system is made up of the brain and spinal cord. It is the processing center that receives information from certain stimuli and then determines appropriate behavior or action in response to those stimuli. Medications for the nervous system are generally directed toward either the autonomic or central nervous system, depending on what therapeutic action is desired.

Cholinergic medications

These medications are also known as cholinergic agonists and parasympathomimetics.

HOW DO CHOLINERGIC MEDICATIONS WORK?

- Stimulate the parasympathetic nervous system to bring the body back to its homeostatic state.
- Imitate the action of ACh and stimulate the cholinergic receptors, thus returning the body to its normal state.
- Cholinergic medications can be direct-acting, and bind to the cholinergic receptors; or they can be indirect-acting, preventing ACh breakdown and thus allowing more ACh at the receptor sites.

WHAT ARE CHOLINERGIC MEDICATIONS USED FOR?

- Used to treat glaucoma, bladder and intestinal function, stimulation, nonobstructive urinary retention, neurogenic bladder, myasthenia gravis, and Alzheimer's disease.
- Examples of these medications are pilocarpine (Pilocar), donepezil (Aricept), and bethanechol chloride (Duvoid).

AS A BRAND NEW NURSE, WHAT DO I NEED TO KNOW ABOUT CHOLINERGIC MEDICATIONS?

- Contraindicated in clients with enlarged prostate, possible urinary or GI obstruction, hyperthyroidism, bradycardia or defects in cardiac impulse conduction, asthma, epilepsy, COPD, hypotension, and Parkinson's disease.
- Adverse reactions are usually the result of overstimulation of the peripheral nervous system such as hypotension, headache, flushing, diaphoresis, bradycardia, increased bronchial secretions, and blurred vision.

- Drugs that may cause negative effects are anticholinergics, antihistamines, and sympathomimetics.
- Bethanechol chloride is never given by IV or IM, only by mouth or subcutaneously.
- Administer medication around the clock to maintain therapeutic blood level of the medication.
- Monitor vital signs and evaluate intended therapeutic effects of medications.
- Monitor client for signs of drug toxicity.
- Typical cholinergic effects are papillary constriction, sweating, headache, tremor, excess saliva production, diarrhea, abdominal cramps, nausea.
- The antidote to cholinergic toxicity is atropine.

WHAT DO I NEED TO TEACH MY CLIENT ABOUT CHOLINERGIC MEDICATIONS?

- Take the medication as prescribed to avoid over-medicating.
- Space doses evenly to maintain therapeutic level.
- Notify health care provider if shortness of breath, diarrhea, increased muscle weakness, or abdominal cramps occur.

Anticholinergic medications

HOW DO ANTICHOLINERGIC MEDICATIONS WORK?

- Also known as cholinergic-blocking agents, parasympatholytics, and antimuscarinic agents. Work by blocking the action of ACh at the muscarinic receptors in the parasympathetic nervous system, thereby, preventing a cholinergic effect.

WHAT ARE ANTICHOLINERGIC MEDICATIONS USED FOR?

- These medications are usually used to reverse heart block, reduce salivary and gastric secretion, induce mydriasis, decrease GI spasms, reduce motion sickness, counter enuresis, and relieve symptoms of Parkinson's disease.
- Examples of these drugs are atropine, benztropine (Cogentin), and scopolamine (Transderm Scop).

AS A BRAND NEW NURSE, WHAT DO I NEED TO KNOW ABOUT ANTICHOLINERGIC MEDICATIONS?

- These medications are contraindicated in children and clients with narrow-angle glaucoma, acute asthma, myasthenia gravis, acute cardio-vascular instability, and GI or GU (genitourinary) tract obstruction.
- Monitor for adverse reactions such as blurred vision, conjunctivitis, photophobia, tachycardia, constipation, dry mouth, and urinary hesitancy or urine retention.
- Evaluate client for therapeutic results.
- Drug interactions can occur in the client who is also taking antihist-amines, phenothiazines, tricyclic antidepressants, and monoamine oxidase inhibitors (MAOIs).

- Antacids decrease absorption of these medications.
- Overdoses of anticholinergics are treated symptomatically and with supportive therapy. The stomach is emptied by either Syrup of Ipecac or gastric lavage. Activated charcoal may also be used to remove any drug that may have already been absorbed.

WHAT DO I NEED TO TEACH MY CLIENT ABOUT ANTICHOLINERGIC MEDICATIONS?

- Ice chips, hard candy, or gum can alleviate dry mouth.
- Increased dietary fiber and exercise can reduce constipation.
- Teach client how to monitor for signs and symptoms of urinary retention.
- Client should be instructed to seek counseling from physician or pharmacist prior to taking over-the-counter medications to ensure that there are no known drug interactions.

Adrenergic agonists

HOW DO ADRENERGIC AGONIST MEDICATIONS WORK?

- Also known as adrenergics or sympathomimetics, these medications work by activating or inhibiting alpha and beta receptors that are normally activated by norepinephrine, or to stimulate dopaminergic receptors that are usually activated by dopamine.

WHAT ARE ADRENERGIC AGONIST MEDICATIONS USED FOR?

- Commonly used to treat hypotension, heart failure, asthma and allergies, mild renal failure, cardiac arrest, mydriasis, shock, preterm labor, and nasal congestion.
- Examples of these medications are albuterol (Proventil), dobutamine (Dobutrex), and epinephrine (Adrenalin).

AS A BRAND NEW NURSE, WHAT DO I NEED TO KNOW ABOUT ADRENERGIC AGONIST MEDICATIONS?

- Contraindicated in angle-closure glaucoma, severe hypertension, and tachyarrhythmias.
- Adverse side effects are arrhythmias, tachycardia, angina, restlessness, urinary urgency or incontinence, rebound stuffiness, headache, insomnia, hypertension, dry mouth, nausea, vomiting, and loss of appetite.
- IV administration should be through a large vein to decrease incidence of extravasation.
- Monitor vital signs and electrocardiogram (EKG) during treatment.
- Toxicity of these drugs is usually indicated by an extension or increase of the common adverse effects.
- Because of the short half-life of these medications, discontinuing the drug usually reverses the toxic effects in a fairly short period of time.
- Treatment of toxicity is according to symptoms experienced by the client.

**WHAT DO I NEED TO TEACH MY CLIENT ABOUT
ADRENERGIC AGONIST MEDICATIONS?**

- Explain to the client why they are taking this medication.

- Teach the correct technique for self-administering inhalation or ophthalmic medications.

- Consult physician or pharmacist prior to taking any over-the-counter medications or herbal supplements to ensure there are no adverse drug interactions.

Alpha-adrenergic blockers

HOW DO ALPHA-ADRENERGIC BLOCKERS WORK?

- Inhibit stimulation of the sympathetic nervous system by activating or blocking the alpha-adrenergic, beta-adrenergic, or dopamine receptors.

WHAT ARE ALPHA-ADRENERGIC BLOCKERS USED FOR?

- Used to treat peripheral vascular disease, Raynaud's disease, vascular headaches, adrenergic excess, hypertension, and extravasation of vasopressors.

- Examples of these medications are doxazosin mesylate (Cardura), ergotamine tartrate (Ergostat), and phentolamine (Regitine).

**AS A BRAND NEW NURSE, WHAT DO I NEED TO KNOW
ABOUT ALPHA-ADRENERGIC BLOCKERS?**

- Contraindicated in clients with a history of myocardial infarction, coronary insufficiency, peptic ulcer, and coronary artery disease.

- Adverse effects to monitor for are nasal congestion, orthostatic hypotension, weakness, GI irritation, arrhythmias, tachycardia, and dizziness.

- Use cautiously in clients taking antihypertensive medications.

- Monitor blood pressure and observe for orthostatic hypotension.

- Administer medication with food or milk.

- Monitor client for numbness, tingling, or weakness in the extremities.

- Toxicity of this drug is treated with syrup of ipecac or gastric lavage. Activated charcoal should be given with a cathartic or laxative to facilitate immediate removal of the drug from the body. Other treatments should be provided according to symptoms client is experiencing.

**WHAT DO I NEED TO TEACH MY CLIENT ABOUT
ALPHA-ADRENERGIC BLOCKERS?**

- Slowly change positions to reduce risk of orthostatic hypotension.

- Take medication with food or milk to decrease gastric irritation.

- Consult with physician or pharmacist prior to taking over-the-counter medications while taking these drugs.

Neuromuscular blockers

HOW DO NEUROMUSCULAR BLOCKERS WORK?

- Inhibit nerve transmission in skeletal muscles, causing paralysis.

WHAT ARE NEUROMUSCULAR BLOCKERS USED FOR?

- Used with anesthetics during surgery to maintain muscle relaxation or it can be used in clients with insufficient ventilation, caused by them fighting an endotracheal tube.
- Examples of these medications are pancuronium (Pavulon), vecuronium (Norcuron), and doxacurium chloride (Nuromax).

AS A BRAND NEW NURSE, WHAT DO I NEED TO KNOW ABOUT NEUROMUSCULAR BLOCKERS?

- Be mindful of potential adverse reactions such as apnea, hypotension, skin reactions, bronchospasms, excessive bronchial or salivary secretions.
- Antidotes for toxicity of neuromuscular blockers are anticholinesterase drugs such as neostigmine, pyridostigmine, and edrophonium.
- Monitor closely for potential interactions with other medications.
- Have emergency equipment available in case respiratory support is needed.
- Monitor respirations, ventilation support, and suction as needed.

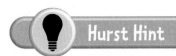

Remember when a client in on the ventilator, and the respiratory muscles have been paralyzed, they are very scared. Be sure to offer *plenty* of emotional support.

Central nervous system (CNS) stimulants

HOW DO CNS STIMULANTS WORK?

- Increase the level of neurotransmitters in the central nervous system causing respiratory stimulation, increased motor activity, mental alertness, dilated pupils, and reduced sense of fatigue.

WHAT ARE CNS STIMULANTS USED FOR?

- These drugs are used in the treatment of attention deficit hyperactivity disorder, narcolepsy, hyperactivity in children, suppressing appetite, and migraines.
- Examples of these medications are dextroamphetamine (Dexedrine), methylphenidate hydrochloride (Concerta), and dexmethylphenidate (Focalin).

AS A BRAND NEW NURSE, WHAT DO I NEED TO KNOW ABOUT CNS STIMULANTS?

- Contraindicated in clients with known anxiety, tic disorders, Tourette's syndrome, glaucoma, and severe cardiovascular disease.
- Use cautiously in elderly or debilitated clients.

- Adverse reactions are increased heart rate, restlessness, tremors, arrhythmias, palpitations, angina, insomnia, anxiety, dry mouth, hypotension, and irritability.
- Monitor client's behavior during drug therapy and assess vital signs prior to medication administration.

WHAT DO I NEED TO TEACH MY CLIENT ABOUT CNS STIMULANTS?

- Take medication at least 6 hours before bedtime to prevent insomnia.
- Avoid caffeine sources and alcohol while taking this medication.
- Ice, hard candy, or gum may assist with symptoms of dry mouth.

Anticonvulsants

HOW DO ANTICONVULSANT MEDICATIONS WORK?

- Depresses abnormal neuronal discharges and stimulations in the CNS that can result in seizures.

WHAT ARE ANTICONVULSANTS USED FOR?

- These medications are used to decrease the occurrence and severity of seizures.
- Other uses of these medications are treatment of arrhythmias and trigeminal neuralgia.
- Examples of anticonvulsants are phenytoin (Dilantin), clonazepam (Klonopin), and diazepam (Valium).

AS A BRAND NEW NURSE, WHAT DO I NEED TO KNOW ABOUT ANTICONVULSANTS?

- Contraindicated in clients with sinus bradycardia, sinoatrial block, heart blocks, and Adam–Stokes syndrome.
- Adverse reactions to anticonvulsants are diplopia, ataxia, drowsiness, gingival hyperplasia, slurred speech, nystagmus, tremors, nausea, vomiting, and dizziness.
- Observe for the following signs and symptoms of anticonvulsant toxicity: ataxia, nystagmus, dysarthria, hypotension, coma, and unresponsive pupils.
- Assess seizure activity.
- Administer medication around the clock to maintain therapeutic drug level.
- When caring for the client receiving oral tube feedings, the feedings need to be scheduled 1 hour before or 2 hours after administering anticonvulsant medications in order for the client to receive maximal absorption of the medication.

WHAT DO I NEED TO TEACH MY CLIENT ABOUT ANTICONVULSANTS?

- It should be taken at the same time everyday to prevent a seizure that could result in a drop of therapeutic blood flow.
- Avoid alcohol and self-medicating with over-the-counter drugs.

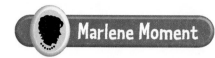

Marlene Moment

You'll have the symptoms associated with CNS stimulants prior to taking the NCLEX®, except you will have hypertension instead of hypotension.

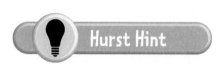

Hurst Hint

When giving Dilantin or Valium IV, you must flush the line with normal saline before and after administration as it will crystallize in other solutions. Dilantin also burns with administration.

- There may be some urine discoloration.
- Provide instruction on proper oral care. (Dilantin can cause gingival hyperplasia.)
- Until the medication's effects are known, use caution with activities requiring alertness.
- Teach the client signs and symptoms of drug toxicity.

Antiparkinson medications

HOW DO ANTIPARKINSON MEDICATIONS WORK?

- Parkinson's disease is caused by an imbalance of the neurotransmitters, ACh, and dopamine in the CNS.
- Antiparkinson medications correct this imbalance by either increasing the dopamine level (dopaminergic agonists) or decreasing the ACh levels (anticholinergics).

WHAT ARE ANTIPARKINSON MEDICATIONS USED FOR?

- Used primarily to treat Parkinson's disease.
- Examples of antiparkinson medications are amantadine (Symmetrel), bromocriptine (Parlodel), and benztropine mesylate (Cogentin).

AS A BRAND NEW NURSE, WHAT DO I NEED TO KNOW ABOUT ANTIPARKINSON MEDICATIONS?

- Contraindicated in clients with angle-closure glaucoma, pyloric or duodenal obstruction, myasthenia gravis, megacolon, and enlarged prostate.
- Adverse reactions are dizziness, confusion, mood changes, involuntary body movements, orthostatic hypotension, hallucinations, tremors, nausea, blurred vision, constipation, urine retention, dry mouth, and vomiting.
- Assess client for parkinsonian symptoms, monitor blood pressure often, and administer medication with food.

WHAT DO I NEED TO TEACH MY CLIENT ABOUT ANTIPARKINSON MEDICATIONS?

- Consult with physician or pharmacist prior to taking other medications.
- Take with food to minimize GI irritation; move slowly or change positions slowly to decrease risk of orthostatic hypotension; do not stop medication abruptly; avoid vitamin B_6 supplements if taking levodopa; use caution if participating in activities that require alertness.

✚ Drugs used for psychiatric disorders

Let's review the three common types of psychotropic medications: antipsychotics, antidepressants, and antimanics.

Antipsychotic medications

HOW DO ANTIPSYCHOTIC MEDICATIONS WORK?

- Block the dopamine receptors, which are where the antipsychotic impulses are transmitted.

WHAT ARE ANTIPSYCHOTIC MEDICATIONS USED FOR?

- Used in the treatment of psychosis, schizophrenia, and schizoaffective disorder.
- Other uses are for nausea, vomiting, and intractable hiccups.
- Examples of antipsychotic medications are chlorpromazine (Thorazine), prochlorperazine (Compazine), and haloperidol (Haldol).

AS A BRAND NEW NURSE, WHAT DO I NEED TO KNOW ABOUT ANTIPSYCHOTIC MEDICATIONS?

- Contraindicated in clients with angle-closure glaucoma, CNS depression, or risk of suicide.
- Adverse reactions are orthostatic hypotension, tardive dyskinesia, neuroleptic malignant syndrome, sedation, blurred vision, dry mouth, constipation, and photosensitivity reaction.
- The biggest concern of antipsychotic medications is extrapyramidal symptoms, which are abnormal, involuntary movements that stop only during sleep.
- Client needs to be informed that the urine may be discolored while taking this medication.
- Needs to call the physician before taking any other medications.
- Assess client's mental status before and throughout therapy.
- Monitor vital signs and observe client when taking medication to ensure it has been swallowed.

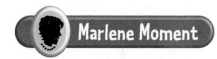

Marlene Moment

Psychiatric clients will try to cheek their drugs (hold the med in their cheek and spit out when you are gone.) Let me clarify: that would be their "mouth" cheek.

WHAT DO I NEED TO TEACH MY CLIENT ABOUT ANTIPSYCHOTIC MEDICATIONS?

- Medication must be taken on a regular basis and cannot be stopped abruptly.
- Avoid alcohol and other CNS depressants while taking this medication.
- Use caution when participating in an activity that requires alertness.
- Sunscreen should be used when outdoors to prevent photosensitivity reactions.
- Provide instruction on preventing dry mouth.
- Instruct client to call physician or pharmacist before using over-the-counter medications or herbal supplements.
- Client should change positions slowly to avoid orthostatic hypotension.

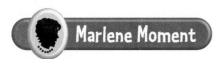

My favorite preacher, Joyce Meyer says that PMS stands for Pretty Mean Sister.

Antidepressant medications

HOW DO ANTIDEPRESSANT MEDICATIONS WORK?

- Depression is a mood disorder usually caused by an inadequate level of serotonin.
- Antidepressants work by blocking the reuptake of serotonin, which keeps the levels increased.

WHAT ARE ANTIDEPRESSANTS USED FOR?

- Used as treatment for depression, anxiety, enuresis, chronic pain syndromes, bulimia, premenstrual dysphoric disorder, obsessive-compulsive disorder, and smoking cessation.
- Examples of antidepressants are citalopram (Celexa), fluoxetine hydrochloride (Prozac), and venlafaxine hydrochloride (Effexor).
- Antidepressants, specifically the SSRIs, block the reuptake and so on.

AS A BRAND NEW NURSE, WHAT DO I NEED TO KNOW ABOUT ANTIDEPRESSANTS?

- Serotonin-selective reuptake inhibitors (SSRIs), second-generation, and third-generation (tricyclic) antidepressants are the newer medications and are replacing the use of monoamine oxidase (MAO) inhibitors.

Let's talk about SSRIs and the second- and third-generation antidepressants first.

- They are contraindicated in clients with angle-closure glaucoma and should be used cautiously in elderly clients or those with cardiovascular disease.
- These medications should not be used concurrently with MAO inhibitors or in clients with active liver disease.
- Discontinuing these drugs should take place gradually.
- Adverse reactions may be orthostatic hypotension, tachycardia, blurred vision, dry mouth, constipation, insomnia, nausea, drowsiness, fatigue, tremors, and sexual disturbances.
- It may be several weeks before desired results of drug therapy are present.
- Antidepressant overdoses are treated by multiple doses of activated charcoal in an attempt to decrease drug absorption.

Now let's talk about MAO inhibitors.

- Contraindicated in clients with heart failure, liver disease, abnormal liver function studies, renal impairment, cerebrovascular accident, cardiovascular disease, and hypertension.
- This medication should not be administered to the client who is also taking other MAO inhibitors, tricyclic antidepressants, anesthetics, CNS depressants, antihypertensives, caffeine, or food with high tyramine content.
- Tyramine containing foods: Beer, wine, aged cheese, sardines, some fruits, sauerkraut, chocolate, nuts, canned meat, bouillon, yeast, pickled or smoked foods, soy products, pepperoni, bologna, salami, summer sausage, liver, avocados.

- The most serious adverse effect to be watching for is hypertensive crisis.
- It may be several weeks before desired results are seen.
- Antidepressant overdoses are treated by multiple doses of activated charcoal to decrease drug absorption.
- It takes about 12 hours before MAO inhibitor toxicity presents itself. The main goal for treatment is removing the toxin and protecting the brain and the heart. Treatments usually involve gastric lavage and hemodialysis.

WHAT DO I NEED TO TEACH MY CLIENT ABOUT SSRIs AND SECOND- AND THIRD-GENERATION ANTIDEPRESSANTS?

- Take medication at the same time every day.
- If discontinuing the medication, do so gradually.
- Avoid alcohol and over-the-counter medications.
- Inform the client that desired effects may not appear for weeks after beginning medication.

WHAT DO I NEED TO TEACH MY CLIENT ABOUT MAO INHIBITORS?

- Avoid alcohol and foods that contain tyramine.
- Teach client the signs and symptoms of hypertensive crisis.
- Other health care providers need to be aware that client is taking MAO inhibitor therapy.

Antimanic medications

HOW DO ANTIMANIC MEDICATIONS WORK?

- Slow down the release of dopamine and norepinephrine and it also work by shifting sodium transfer in nerve and muscle cells.

WHAT ARE ANTIMANIC MEDICATIONS USED FOR?

- Bipolar disorder and mania.
- Examples of these medications are lithium carbonate (Lithane, Lithotabs, Eskalith) and lithium citrate (Cibalith-S).

AS A BRAND NEW NURSE, WHAT DO I NEED TO KNOW ABOUT ANTIMANIC MEDICATIONS?

- Lithium is contraindicated in clients with renal or cardiovascular disease, severe dehydration, and severe sodium depletion.
- Use cautiously in clients that are elderly, debilitated, or have thyroid disease.
- Adverse reactions can indicate lithium toxicity and are seen as hand tremors, muscle weakness, tinnitus, ataxia, confusion, diarrhea, abdominal pain, polyuria, polydipsia, nausea, vomiting, nephrogenic diabetes insipidus, and hypothyroidism.
- Lithium levels need to be monitored carefully.
- Lithium toxicity is managed with osmotic diuretics, as these will pull fluid into the bloodstream and dilute the serum sodium.

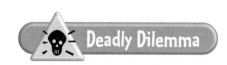

Deadly Dilemma

Clients on lithium must avoid dehydration. Dehydration makes the serum sodium go up, which will cause lithium toxicity.

WHAT DO I NEED TO TEACH MY CLIENT ABOUT ANTIMANIC MEDICATIONS?

- Instruct client to drink 2 to 3 liters of water a day, monitor sodium intake, and avoid excessive amounts of caffeine.
- Consult physician or pharmacist prior to taking over-the-counter medications.
- Teach your client signs and symptoms of lithium toxicity.
- Client should avoid activities requiring alertness until effects of medication are known.

✛ Musculoskeletal system drugs
Antiarthritic medications
HOW DO ANTIARTHRITIC MEDICATIONS WORK?

- Also called gold salts, these medications suppress inflammation by inhibiting prostaglandin synthesis.

WHAT ARE ANTIARTHRITIC MEDICATIONS USED FOR?

- Used to treat rheumatoid arthritis, Crohn's disease, psoriasis, and acute lymphocytic leukemia.
- Examples of these drugs are auranofin (Ridaura), gold sodium thiomalate (Myochrysine), and methotrexate (Rheumatrex).

AS A BRAND NEW NURSE, WHAT DO I NEED TO KNOW ABOUT ANTIARTHRITIC MEDICATIONS?

- Contraindicated in clients with heart failure, systemic lupus erythematosus, severe renal or hepatic dysfunction, diabetes mellitus, and those that have had recent radiation.
- Adverse reactions are dizziness, gold toxicity, hypertension, nausea, vomiting, bone marrow suppression, diarrhea, abdominal pain, respiratory infection, and headache.
- Signs and symptoms of gold toxicity are rash, pruritus, metallic taste, stomatitis, and diarrhea.
- Medication should be administered on an empty stomach to facilitate drug absorption.
- Therapeutic results will not appear in the client for 3 to 6 weeks after therapy is started.

WHAT DO I NEED TO TEACH MY CLIENT ABOUT ANTIARTHRITIC MEDICATIONS?

- Teach your client the signs and symptoms of gold toxicity and to seek immediate health care assistance if they are present.
- Instruct them on good oral hygiene and to wear protective clothing and sunscreen when going outdoors.

Skeletal muscle relaxants

HOW DO SKELETAL MUSCLE RELAXANTS WORK?

- These medications act either centrally on the central nervous system or directly at the neuromuscular junction.
- Nerve-impulse transmission is blocked when the centrally acting medications are used.
- Direct-acting medications interrupt muscle contraction by interfering with calcium release in the muscle fibers.

WHAT ARE SKELETAL MUSCLE RELAXANTS USED FOR?

- Used to treat spasticity or as an adjunctive treatment of acute, painful musculoskeletal conditions. Examples of these medications are baclofen (Lioresal), methocarbamol (Robaxin), and cyclobenzaprine hydrochloride (Flexeril).

AS A BRAND NEW NURSE, WHAT DO I NEED TO KNOW ABOUT SKELETAL MUSCLE RELAXANTS?

- Contraindicated in clients whose posture and balance are maintained by spasticity. They also should not be given to clients with arrhythmias, heart block, recent myocardial infarction, hepatic disease, or within 14 days of MAO inhibitor treatment.
- Adverse reactions are transient dizziness, ataxia, drowsiness, dry mouth, nausea, and GI irritation.
- Give medication with meals.
- Assess pain and mobility levels.

WHAT DO I NEED TO TEACH MY CLIENT ABOUT SKELETAL MUSCLE RELAXANTS?

- Avoid alcohol and other CNS depressants while taking this medication.
- Take with meals.
- Do not stop taking medication abruptly.
- Use caution when participating in activities requiring alertness until effects of medication are known.

✦ Endocrine system drugs

Antidiabetic medications

HOW DO ANTIDIABETIC MEDICATIONS WORK?

- Diabetes occurs when the pancreas does not produce enough of the hormone insulin (or the pancreas may not be making any insulin at all) to maintain a normal glucose level (60–110 mg/dL). Diabetes can also occur if the pancreas produces insulin that doesn't work well.
- Antidiabetics can correct this one of two ways. Insulin can be given to decrease glucose levels by increasing the transport of glucose into cells and facilitating the conversion of glucose into glycogen. The other form of antidiabetic medication is oral hypoglycemics. These drugs decrease the blood glucose level by stimulating the pancreas to secrete more insulin.

- Keep in mind—the client must have a functioning pancreas for the oral hypoglycemics to work.

WHAT ARE ANTIDIABETIC MEDICATIONS USED FOR?

- Insulin may be used in the treatment of type I or type II diabetes mellitus. It comes in rapid-acting, intermediate-acting, and long-acting forms.
- Examples of rapid-acting insulins are regular insulin (Humulin R, Novolin R, and Regular Iletin II), lispro insulins (Humalog), and insulin aspart (NovoLog). Intermediate-acting insulin are isophane insulins suspension (NPH), Humulin N, and Novolin N; and insulin zinc suspension (lente), Humulin L, and Lente Iletin II. Long-acting insulins are insulin glargine (Lantus) and extended insulin zinc suspension (Humulin U).
- Oral hypoglycemic medications are used in the treatment of type II diabetes mellitus that cannot be controlled with diet and exercise.
- Examples of these medications are acarbose (Precose), metformin (Glucophage), glyburide/metformin hydrochloride (Glucovance), tolbutamide (Orinase), meglitinides (Prandin), and rosiglitazone maleate (Avandia).

AS A BRAND NEW NURSE, WHAT DO I NEED TO KNOW ABOUT INSULIN?

- Observe for signs and symptoms of hypoglycemia after administration.
- Do not shake insulin; instead, roll the vial between your hands.
- When mixing insulins, draw up the regular insulin (clear) first, and then the long-acting (cloudy) one.
- Use insulin syringes only and rotate injection sites.
- Regular insulin is the ONLY insulin that can be administered IV and is usually given in acute situations only.
- Monitor client's blood glucose level.
- Know the peak action times of insulin you are administering and coincide this with the client's snacks. Depending on the type used, the peak action times of rapid-acting insulins range from 30 minutes to 3 hours; intermediate-acting insulins range from 4 to 15 hours; and long-acting insulins range from 5 to 30 hours.
- Sugar sources such as hard candy, orange juice, honey, or glucose tablets are used to treat mild to moderate hypoglycemia.
- The treatment for severe hypoglycemia is IV glucose or glucagon (IM).

AS A BRAND NEW NURSE, WHAT DO I NEED TO KNOW ABOUT ORAL HYPOGLYCEMIC MEDICATIONS?

- These medications are contraindicated in clients with type I diabetes mellitus, severe kidney or liver disease, and thyroid or other endocrine dysfunctions.
- Adverse reactions are hypoglycemia, nausea, vomiting, dizziness, drowsiness, diarrhea, heartburn, upper respiratory infections, edema, heart failure, photosensitivity, and headache.
- Be aware of other medications the client is taking that can increase hypoglycemic effects.

- Alpha-glucoside inhibitors need to be taken with the first bite of food.
- Meglitinides need to be taken with 30 minutes of each meal.
- Stressors, internal (illness) or external (work), and the use of certain medications can increase insulin needs, creating the possibility of changing an oral hypoglycemic agent to insulin for a period of time.
- The treatment for hypoglycemia in the client taking oral hypoglycemics is the same as the treatment for the client taking insulin.

WHAT DO I NEED TO TEACH MY CLIENT ABOUT TAKING ANTIDIABETIC MEDICATIONS?

- Teach your client the signs and symptoms of hypoglycemia and what to do if they recognize them (orange juice, hard candy, sugar, milk).
- Explain that this treatment is a lifelong commitment—there is no cure.
- Demonstrate how to check blood glucose levels.
- Instruct in proper technique and care of equipment with self-administration of insulin.
- Encourage prescribed diet, exercise, and avoidance of alcohol consumption.
- Call the physician if ill, unable to eat, or unable to get blood glucose levels under control.

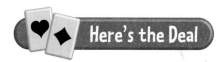

Here's the Deal

Any stress (such as illness) can make the blood glucose go up. The client may need to increase their routine dose of insulin to control the blood glucose and prevent diabetic ketoacidosis.

> Something groovy to know: Hyperkalemia (emergency treatment)
>
> Administer IV insulin, bicarb, glucose, and calcium gluconate
>
> Insulin will "grab" glucose and potassium and bring it into the cell, thereby decreasing potassium levels.
>
> Bicarbonate causes an alkalosis. The body attempts to fix the alkalosis by driving potassium into the cell and hydrogen out of cell.
>
> Potassium and calcium gluconate in the presence of each other inactivate each other.

Thyroid hormones

HOW DO THYROID HORMONE MEDICATIONS WORK?

- These medications correct the hormonal imbalance of thyroid deficiency by providing the same physiological effects as natural hormones.

WHAT ARE THYROID HORMONE MEDICATIONS USED FOR?

- Thyroid hormones are used in the treatment of primary or secondary hypothyroidism, goiters, and some thyroid cancers.
- Examples of these medications are levothyroxine sodium T4 (Levoxine, Synthroid), liothyronine sodium T3 (Triostat), liotrix (Thyrolar), and thyroid USP (desiccated Armour Thyroid).

AS A BRAND NEW NURSE, WHAT DO I NEED TO KNOW ABOUT THYROID HORMONE MEDICATIONS?

- Contraindicated in clients with a recent history of myocardial infarction, adrenal insufficiency, Addison's disease or hyperthyroidism.
- Use cautiously in clients with cardiovascular disease, diabetes mellitus, or diabetes insipidus, and in the elderly.

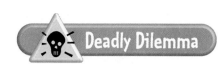

Deadly Dilemma

Be careful when giving "heart" clients thyroid hormones. Thyroid hormones increase energy levels, which will increase work on the heart.

- Adverse reactions are hyperthyroidism, arrhythmias, palpitations, nervousness, sweating, weight loss, hair loss, and insomnia.
- Be aware of drug interactions if client is also taking anticoagulants, beta-blockers, theophylline, adrenergics, insulin, or estrogen.
- Medication should be administered in the morning for prevention of insomnia.
- For maximum drug absorption, medication should be taken on an empty stomach.
- Medication brands differ in potency.

WHAT DO I NEED TO TEACH MY CLIENT ABOUT THYROID HORMONE MEDICATIONS?

- Instruct your client to contact his health care provider if he starts experiencing any of the adverse reactions previously stated.
- Instruct the client to take medication in the morning, on an empty stomach, and to not change medication brands.

Antithyroid medications

HOW DO ANTITHYROID MEDICATIONS WORK?

- Work by slowing down the formation of thyroid hormones.

WHAT ARE ANTITHYROID MEDICATIONS USED FOR?

- Used in the treatment of hyperthyroidism (Graves' disease), thyroid cancer, as a radiation protectant of the thyroid, and as preparation for thyroidectomy.
- Examples of these medications are iodine (Strong Iodine Solution, USP), methimazole (Tapazole), PTU, and sodium iodide I^{131} (Iodotope, Sodium Iodide I^{131} Therapeutic).

AS A BRAND NEW NURSE, WHAT DO I NEED TO KNOW ABOUT ANTITHYROID MEDICATIONS?

- Adverse reactions are diarrhea, hypothyroidism, nausea, vomiting, tachycardia, chest pains, sore throat, and hair loss.
- Iodism is also a potential adverse reaction and can be recognized by vomiting, abdominal pain, metallic taste, rash, and sore salivary glands.
- Administer medication around the same time each day.
- Monitor thyroid function studies.

WHAT DO I NEED TO TEACH MY CLIENT ABOUT ANTITHYROID MEDICATIONS?

- Teach the client to recognize the signs and symptoms of hypothyroidism.
- Assist in identifying iodine sources and practice avoiding or restricting these products from diet.
- Do not discontinue medication without a physician's prescription.
- Take in the morning to prevent insomnia.

Parathyroid medications

HOW DO PARATHYROID MEDICATIONS WORK?

- Increase calcium levels in the body by pulling calcium from the bones and placing it in the blood.

WHAT ARE PARATHYROID MEDICATIONS USED FOR?

- Used to treat clients with hypocalcemia, hypoparathyroidism, and osteoporosis.
- Examples of these medications are calcitriol (Calcijex), calcium carbonate (Os-Cal), calcium citrate, calcium gluconate, and calcium lactate.

AS A BRAND NEW NURSE, WHAT DO I NEED TO KNOW ABOUT PARATHYROID MEDICATIONS?

- Contraindicated in clients with hypercalcemia, vitamin D toxicity, renal calculi, and ventricular fibrillation.
- Use cautiously in clients taking digitalis glycosides (digoxin, lanoxin) and those with renal or cardiac disease, as fluctuating calcium levels can exacerbate arrhythmias.
- Adverse reaction is hypercalcemia.
- Monitor electrolyte levels.

WHAT DO I NEED TO TEACH MY CLIENT ABOUT PARATHYROID MEDICATIONS?

- Avoid use of magnesium-containing antacids.
- Teach the client to limit intake of spinach, whole grains, and rhubarb because they may decrease the absorption of calcium.

✛ Immune system

Corticosteroids

HOW DO CORTICOSTEROIDS WORK?

- Corticosteroids are hormones produced naturally by the adrenal cortex, which are broken down into glucocorticoids and mineralocorticoids.
- Corticosteroids alter the normal immune response and suppress inflammation.

WHAT ARE CORTICOSTEROIDS USED FOR?

- Used to treat many disorders and come in different forms (systemic, topical, inhaled, and nasal).
- Indicated uses for corticosteroids are treatment of clients with adreno-cortical insufficiency, autoimmune response, neoplastic diseases, cerebral edema, and inflammation of the joints, respiratory tract, GI tract, or skin.
- Examples of corticosteroids are betamethasone (Celestone), dexamethasone (Decadron), hydrocortisone (Cortef), and methylprednisolone (Solu-Medrol).

AS A BRAND NEW NURSE, WHAT DO I NEED TO KNOW ABOUT CORTICOSTEROIDS?

- Contraindicated in clients with serious infections as they suppress the immune system.
- Adverse effects are edema, hypertension, convulsions, headaches, vertigo, insomnia, nervousness, Cushing's syndrome, hyperglycemia, peptic ulcers, pancreatitis, muscle weakness, and weight gain.
- Assess client for fluid retention by weighing daily, auscultating breath sounds, and checking for peripheral edema.
- Medication cannot be stopped abruptly or the client could go into an Addisonian crisis (think shock!).
- Administer dosage in the morning if it is prescribed daily as steroids can cause insomnia.

WHAT DO I NEED TO TEACH MY CLIENT ABOUT CORTICOSTEROIDS?

- Take medication exactly as prescribed—do not abruptly discontinue.
- Because of a suppressed immune system, the client should be instructed to avoid contact with people who have contagious illnesses and report any fever, lethargy, weakness, or sore throat to her physician.
- Client should also consult a physician prior to receiving any vaccinations.
- Client needs to be instructed to monitor weight while on this medication and report any significant weight gains, (2–3 pounds or more).
- Take with food; can cause gastric irritation (ulcers).

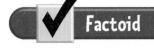

Factoid

Steroids make blood glucose go up. Watch glucose levels closely as the client may need insulin while on these medications.

Immunosuppressants

HOW DO IMMUNOSUPPRESSANTS WORK?

- Suppress the immune response and alter antibody formations.

WHAT ARE IMMUNOSUPPRESSANT MEDICATIONS USED FOR?

- Used in the treatment of clients with rheumatoid arthritis, multiple sclerosis, and organ transplants.
- Examples of these medications are azathioprine (Imuran), prednisone (Deltasone), and tacrolimus (Prograf).

AS A BRAND NEW NURSE, WHAT DO I NEED TO KNOW ABOUT IMMUNOSUPPRESSANTS?

- Contraindicated in clients with GI disorders, infection, bone marrow depression, cancer, impaired liver or kidney function, and hyperlipidemia.
- Adverse effects are leukopenia, thrombocytopenia, nephrotoxicity, chest pain, dyspnea, wheezing, fluid retention, vomiting, nausea, and diarrhea.
- Practice isolation precautions to protect client from infection.
- Monitor vital signs, intake, and output.
- Assess for signs and symptoms of infection which can be fatal.

**WHAT DO I NEED TO TEACH MY CLIENT
ABOUT IMMUNOSUPPRESSANTS?**

- Encourage client to avoid crowds and to report any signs or symptoms of infection.

- Instruct client to use contraception while on immunosuppressant therapy.

- Flowers, plants, fresh fruit, and raw vegetables should be discouraged because of infection risk.

- Emphasize importance of medication compliance.

Antibiotic medications

HOW DO ANTIBIOTIC MEDICATIONS WORK?

- Depending on the type, antibiotics generally work by being bactericidal (killing the bacteria) or bacteriostatic (inhibiting bacterial growth).

- Some medications may do a little of both.

WHAT ARE ANTIBIOTIC MEDICATIONS USED FOR?

- Used to treat infections.

- The type or kind of antibiotic is determined by the bacteria causing the infection.

- Some antibiotics are considered broad-spectrum antibiotics because they can treat a wide range of gram-negative and gram-positive organisms.

- Broad-spectrum antibiotics are often used until the source of the infection is identified and then it is either continued or the medication is switched to a bacteria-specific antibiotic.

- Examples are penicillins (Amoxil, Timentin), cephalosporins (Keflex, Cefzil), aminoglycosides (Garamycin, Nebcin), tetracyclines (Vibramycin, Terramycin), fluoroquinolones (Cipro, Levaquin), and miscellaneous antibiotics (Zithromax, Biaxin).

**AS A BRAND NEW NURSE, WHAT DO I NEED TO KNOW
ABOUT ANTIBIOTIC MEDICATIONS?**

- These medications do not work for illnesses caused by viruses or fungi.

- Prolonged use of antibiotics can increase the client's risk of superinfections, or secondary infections.

- Specimen cultures should be obtained prior to antibiotic therapy; first dose may be given while results are pending.

- Medication should be given around the clock to maintain a therapeutic blood level.

- Penicillins and cephalosporins may inactivate aminoglycosides and should be given separately.

- Monitor kidney and liver function studies, because the kidneys and liver are where most antibiotics are metabolized.

- Peak and trough levels should be monitored on the client receiving aminoglycosides.

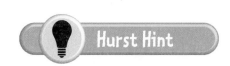

With "mycin" drugs, think ototoxicity and nephrotoxicity.

- The most common adverse reactions of antibiotics are nausea, vomiting, and diarrhea.

WHAT DO I NEED TO TEACH MY CLIENTS ABOUT ANTIBIOTIC MEDICATIONS?

- Take this medication consistently and until it is all gone, even if you are feeling better.
- Women who are taking oral contraceptives should use an alternate method of contraception (especially while taking any of the penicillin or tetracycline drugs.)
- Including yogurt in the diet can alleviate diarrhea caused by antibiotics.
- Avoid alcohol consumption during antibiotic therapy.

Antifungal medications

HOW DO ANTIFUNGAL MEDICATIONS WORK?

- Work by altering permeability of fungal cell membranes and either killing the cell or inhibiting growth by preventing reproduction of the cell.

WHAT ARE ANTIFUNGAL MEDICATIONS USED FOR?

- Used in the treatment of systemic or topical fungal infections, such as ringworm and Candida infections.
- As with antibiotics, the medication used is specific to the type of fungus present.
- Examples of antifungal medications are amphotericin B (Amphocin, Fungizone), clotrimazole (Gyne-Lotrimin, Mycelex), fluconazole (Diflucan), and nystatin (Mycostatin).

AS A BRAND NEW NURSE, WHAT DO I NEED TO KNOW ABOUT ANTIFUNGAL MEDICATIONS?

- Specimens for culture and sensitivity need to be obtained prior to starting antifungal therapy.
- Administer medication around the clock to achieve therapeutic level.
- Monitor renal and *liver* function studies with systemic antifungal medications due to the risk of toxicity.
- Amphotericin B should be infused via infusion pump and with close monitoring of the client.

WHAT DO I NEED TO TEACH MY CLIENT ABOUT ANTIFUNGAL MEDICATIONS?

- Take this medication for the prescribed time even if you are feeling better or symptoms have disappeared.
- Teach the client proper technique for medication administration.
- Women who are being treated for vaginal infections should abstain from sexual intercourse until infection is completely resolved.
- Do not cover infected area with an occlusive dressing.

Antiviral medications

HOW DO ANTIVIRAL MEDICATIONS WORK?

- Viruses are microorganisms that can only reproduce inside a host cell.

- Antiviral medications work by interfering with this reproduction.

- By halting reproduction, the concentration of the virus becomes small enough that the client's immune system can eliminate it from the body.

WHAT ARE ANTIVIRAL MEDICATIONS USED FOR?

- Antiviral medications are used to treat viral disorders such as herpes simplex, shingles, chickenpox (varicella), influenza A and B, cytomegalovirus, and HIV.

- Examples of these medications are acyclovir (Zovirax), amantadine (Symmetrel), and zidovudine (AZT Retrovir).

AS A BRAND NEW NURSE, WHAT DO I NEED TO KNOW ABOUT ANTIVIRAL MEDICATIONS?

- Administer IV mixtures by infusion pump.

- Monitor renal and liver function studies for possible nephrotoxicity and hepatoxicity.

- If treating lesions, assess daily for resolution.

- Maintain adequate fluid intake.

- Antiviral medications do not prevent the transmission of the viruses so universal precautions should be practiced.

WHAT DO I NEED TO TEACH MY CLIENT ABOUT ANTIVIRAL MEDICATIONS?

- Take medication around the clock for the prescribed length of time, even if you are feeling better or symptoms are no longer present.

- Teach proper medication administration technique.

- If being treated for genital lesions, practice abstinence or condom use until lesions are healed.

- Teach client infection control methods to prevent the transmission of the virus to others.

Antituberculotic medications

HOW DO ANTITUBERCULOTIC MEDICATIONS WORK?

- Work by either killing or inhibiting the growth of mycobacterium that cause tuberculosis (TB).

WHAT ARE ANTITUBERCULOTIC MEDICATIONS USED FOR?

- Used in the treatment of tuberculosis.

- Examples of these medications are rifampin (Rifadin, Rimactane), isoniazid (INH, Nydrazid), and capreomycin (Capastat).

AS A BRAND NEW NURSE, WHAT DO I NEED TO KNOW ABOUT ANTITUBERCULOTIC MEDICATIONS?

- Obtain specimens for culture and sensitivity prior to beginning drug therapy.
- Monitor renal and liver function studies.
- Assess breath sounds and sputum prior to and throughout drug therapy.
- Give medication around the clock to maintain therapeutic level.
- Use universal precautions when caring for the client with TB.

WHAT DO I NEED TO TEACH MY CLIENT ABOUT ANTITUBERCULOTIC MEDICATIONS?

- Avoid alcohol consumption while taking this medication.
- Take for the prescribed length of time, even if you are feeling better.
- Teach client methods of preventing the transmission of TB to others.

✚ Gastrointestinal system drugs
Antiulcerative medications

HOW DO ANTIULCERATIVE MEDICATIONS WORK?

- Work by altering the gastric acid content in the GI tract.
- They can reduce production of gastric acid (histamine$_2$-receptors, proton-pump inhibitors), neutralize the acid, and/or protect the mucosal membrane (antacids).

WHAT ARE ANTIULCERATIVE MEDICATIONS USED FOR?

- Used in the treatment and/or prevention of gastric ulcers.
- Cimetidine (Tagamet) and ranitidine (Zantac) are examples of histamine$_2$-receptors, and esomeprazole (Nexium) and lansoprazole (Prevacid) are proton-pump inhibitors.
- Used to treat indigestion and reflux esophagitis.
- Examples of these medications are aluminum hydroxide (Amphojel) and magnesium hydroxide (Milk of Magnesia).

AS A BRAND NEW NURSE, WHAT DO I NEED TO KNOW ABOUT ANTIULCERATIVE MEDICATIONS?

- Do not administer magnesium-based antacids to clients with renal failure, as they may not be able to excrete the excess.
- Antacids can cause enteric-coated tablets to dissolve too quickly.
- Monitor the client for abdominal pain and gastric bleeding.

WHAT DO I NEED TO TEACH MY CLIENT ABOUT ANTIULCERATIVE MEDICATIONS?

- Take medication at prescribed times (prior to meals and at bedtime).
- Avoid alcohol, cigarettes, aspirin products, and other gastric irritants.

- Teach client to read labels to identify sodium and magnesium content if on dietary restrictions.

Antiemetic medications

HOW DO ANTIEMETIC MEDICATIONS WORK?

- Work by acting on the central nervous system to prevent nausea and vomiting, stopping impulses from the inner ear to the vestibular system, or by emptying gastric contents quicker and improving the gastroesophageal sphincter tone.

WHAT ARE ANTIEMETIC MEDICATIONS USED FOR?

- Used in the treatment of nausea and vomiting.
- Examples of these medications are promethazine (Phenergan), dimenhydrinate (Dramamine), metoclopramide (Reglan), and prochlorperazine (Compazine).
- Used in the prevention of nausea and vomiting for preoperative and postoperative clients and for those receiving chemotherapy.

AS A BRAND NEW NURSE WHAT DO I NEED TO KNOW ABOUT ANTIEMETIC MEDICATIONS?

- Assess hydration, bowel sounds, nausea, and vomiting prior to and during treatment with these medications.
- Actions of central nervous system depressants are enhanced when given with antiemetics.

WHAT DO I NEED TO TEACH MY CLIENT ABOUT ANTIEMETIC MEDICATIONS?

- Avoid activities requiring alertness when taking these drugs.
- Teach the appropriate administration and timing of antiemetic medications.

✚ Cancer drugs

Antineoplastic medications

HOW DO ANTINEOPLASTIC MEDICATIONS WORK?

- Work by interfering with cancer cell replication, changing the hormonal setting, or a combination of both.
- The different kinds of antineoplastic medications are alkylating drugs, antitumor antibiotics, antimetabolites, hormonal drugs, and vinca alkaloid drugs.

WHAT ARE ANTINEOPLASTIC MEDICATIONS USED FOR?

- Used primarily in the treatment of cancer.
- Some antineoplastics are used to treat autoimmune disorders.
- Examples of antineoplastic medications are cisplatin (Platinol), doxorubicin (Adriamycin), methotrexate (Folex), megestrol acetate (Megace), and paclitaxel (Taxol).

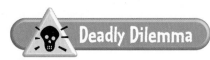

Deadly Dilemma

Never give chemotherapeutic agents if the client's WBC count is below 3000. You do not want to decrease the white count even more, which these drugs will do. Doing so could be fatal.

AS A BRAND NEW NURSE, WHAT DO I NEED TO KNOW ABOUT ANTINEOPLASTIC MEDICATIONS?

- These medications kill healthy cells as well as the cancerous ones, placing the client in an immunocompromised state.
- Almost all of these medications have adverse side effects with nausea, vomiting, alpecia, stomatitis, bone marrow depression, and anorexia being the most common.
- Monitor lab work including platelet count, CBC, renal and liver function studies.
- These medications can be ototoxic, nephrotoxic, and/or hepatotoxic.
- Peripheral IV sites should be monitored frequently during administration of these drugs because of the risk of tissue necrosis caused by extravastion of an IV infiltration.
- Monitor vital signs throughout treatment.
- Administer antiemetic medications before, during, and after treatment with antineoplastics.

WHAT DO I NEED TO TEACH MY CLIENT ABOUT ANTINEOPLASTIC MEDICATIONS?

- The client needs to recognize and report any signs or symptoms of GI bleeding.
- They also need to report tinnitus, dizziness, or hearing loss.
- Teach the client infection-control measures (washing hands, staying away from crowds, etc.).
- Female clients should use a barrier method of contraception during treatment.
- Mouth should be inspected daily for redness or ulcerations and a soft toothbrush used when doing oral care.

✚ Cardiovascuclar medications

You need to remember that with any heart client we do everything we can to decrease workload on the heart. You would never want to increase workload on the heart with heart clients. This is a very important concept. The pathophysiology involved in heart failure tells us why we do not want to increase workload on the heart. When you increase workload on the heart, compensatory mechanisms kick in. The renin angiotensin aldosterone system (RAAS) kicks in. Epinephrine (epi) and norepinephrine (norepi) are released. The RAAS system, through release of aldosterone, causes sodium and water retention and vasoconstriction from conversion of angiotensin I to angiotensin II. Epi causes the heart to contract more strongly (positive inotropic effect) and causes vasoconstriction. Norepi causes peripheral vasoconstriction. These stressors damage heart myofibrils (muscle fibers). Once damaged, myofibrils attempt to repair themselves. The term given to this repair process is remodeling. Remodeling results in bizarre-shaped, poorly functioning myofibrils. More damage results in more remodeling and worsening of the heart failure. So you see "why" it is so important to decrease workload on the heart?

I want to make one more point before we move on. Ischemia can lead to arrhythmias. Drugs that increase oxygen supply or decrease oxygen demand (workload) can prevent ischemic arrhythmias.

Two final concepts will assist you in understanding cardiac medications. These are preload and afterload.

Define time

Afterload is defined as the pressure in the aorta and peripheral arteries the heart has to work against to get blood out. This pressure is referred to as resistance or systemic vascular resistance (SVR), which is the resistance the left ventricle has to overcome to get the blood out of the ventricle and out to the body. A high blood pressure indicates a high SVR. A low blood pressure indicates a low SVR. A low afterload decreases workload on the heart and is preferable for your heart clients.

Define time

Preload is defined as the amount of blood returning to the right side of the heart. To remember preload, think volume; you can have too much or not enough volume. Normal volume (euvolemia) or a little less than normal is okay, because this decreases workload on heart. Two events decrease preload. One is diuresis and the other is vasodilation. When the vascular system vasodilates, blood pools in the extremities so less blood returns to the right side of the heart (less preload). Therefore, the heart doesn't have to work as hard to pump extra blood. When diuresis occurs, there is actually less volume in the cardiovascular system for the heart to have to pump. So once again, preload decreases.

Now let's start checking out the different types of cardiovascular drugs.

Nitroglycerin (sublingual)

HOW DOES NITROGLYCERIN SL WORK?

- Relaxes vascular smooth muscle, causing vasodilation of both the arterial and venous system. This decreases preload (blood pools in extremities with vasodilation) and afterload (decreased pressure in aorta).
- Nitroglycerin also dilates coronary arteries. This effect allows more oxygenated blood to go into the actual heart muscle.

WHAT IS NITROGLYCERIN SL USED FOR?

- Treatment of acute angina or prevention of angina before a stressful event (e.g., stair climbing.).

AS A BRAND NEW NURSE WHAT DO I NEED TO KNOW ABOUT NITROGLYCERIN?

- See Table 11-2.

Table 11-2. Examples of Nitroglycerin

Generic name	Brand name
SL nitroglycerin	Nitro-bid
SL nitroglycerin	Tridil

Table 11-3. Actions of Nitroglycerin Derivatives

Standard monitoring	What do you need to "worry" about?
For relief of acute anginal attacks. Dilates coronary arteries to increase blood supply (oxygen delivery) to heart muscle.	Nitroglycerin decreases blood pressure. On NCLEX® after you give NTG stay with the client. This client is considered unstable. There is a chance blood pressure could drop out the bottom. On NCLEX® never, EVER leave an unstable client. This answer will always be wrong.
Vasodilation of veins and arteries. This decreases preload and afterload. Yeah! This decreases workload on heart.	The client will get a headache. Should you call the doctor? NO! Don't call the doctor about that. We expect that to occur. That's not life threatening.
Take one every 5 minutes to a maximum of 3 doses. The key is a maximum of 3 doses. If chest pain (CP) is unrelieved, call the physician.	

- How do I remember this medication? Whenever the generic has the word "nitrate," it is a nitroglycerin derivative (Table 11-3).
- What vitals signs are most important? Monitor your client's blood pressure. If your client's blood pressure (BP) is less than 90 mm Hg, hold the med and call the doctor.
- Antidote: For drops in blood pressure consider IV fluids to build volume and elevate legs to increase venous return. This is usually transient, as NTG has a short half-life.

WHAT DO I NEED TO TEACH MY CLIENTS ABOUT NITROGLYCERIN?

- Do not swallow this medicine. It is taken under the tongue.
- NTG should be kept in a dark, glass bottle.
- Keep it cool, keep it dry.
- If it burns or fizzes under the tongue, this means it is fresh.
- NTG is to be renewed every 6 months.
- Monitor BP. Hold medicine for BP less than 90 mm Hg.
- For persistent chest pain, call the physician.

Beta-blockers

HOW DO BETA-BLOCKERS WORK?

- Beta-blockers block the effects of epinephrine (adrenergic) and norepinephrine (alpha-1), which decreases afterload (BP) and contractility. This decreases workload on heart. They also slow A-V node conduction, which makes them useful in preventing fast arrhythmias like atrial fibrillation or even ventricular tachycardia.

WHAT ARE BETA-BLOCKERS USED FOR?

- Hypertension and/or fast arrhythmias

Table 11-4. Examples of Beta-Blockers

Generic name	Brand name	Uses
Metoprolol	Lopressor, Toprol XL (extended release)	Control hypertension and slow fast arrhythmias
Propanolol	Inderal	Control hypertension and slow fast arrhythmias
Atenolol	Tenormin	Control hypertension
Labetolol	Trandate	Control hypertension
Carvedilol	Coreg	Control hypertension

AS A BRAND NEW NURSE, WHAT DO I NEED TO KNOW ABOUT BETA-BLOCKERS?

- See Table 11-4.
- How do I remember this medication? Each of these medications has something in common. They all end in "lol" (Table 11-5).

Table 11-5. Actions of Beta-Blockers

Standard monitoring	What do you need to "worry" about?
Adjunctive therapy for clients experiencing an MI. Helps to decrease workload on heart, thereby decrease the size of the infarction.	Beta-blockers decrease contractility. This is O.K. to a point, but it could drop the cardiac output out the bottom. So you had better watch for it! (e.g., decreased LOC, HR, BP, cold and clammy.)
The standard of care is for CHF clients to be discharged on a beta-blocker, ACE inhibitor, or both. Research shows improved long-term outcome when clients are on these medications.	Use caution with diabetic clients. Beta-blockers may "mask" normal tachycardiac events caused by hypoglycemia. The hypoglycemia may go unrecognized. The client may become unresponsive and you can't figure out why. That would be bad.
	Use with caution in asthmatics. Beta-1 cells are in your heart. Beta-2 cells are in the lungs. There is a risk beta-blockers will block the beta cells in the lungs. This is bad for an asthmatic. This could send your asthmatic client into status asthmaticus.
	Beta-blockers slow heart rates and drop BP. Be careful they don't drop the HR and BP out the bottom. That's what I am "scared of." Your client could have a sudden atrioventricular block (slow HR) and their BP can drop out the bottom.
	NEVER stop beta-blockers abruptly. If the client were to stop taking beta-blockers he is at risk for developing a sudden rapid HR. Now workload on heart has really increased. The client could start complaining of chest pain, or, even worse, might just go ahead and have an MI.

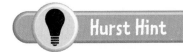

Hurst Hint

Diabetics should never take beta-blockers, as these drugs mask the signs of hypoglycemia. A client needs to know when she is becoming hypoglycemic!

- What vital signs are most important? Check HR and BP. If your client's HR is less than 60 or BP less than 90 mm Hg, hold the med and call the doctor.
- Antidote: For slow rhythms with drop in CO and BP give adenosine or with a drop in the cardiac output (CO) epinephrine. Dopamine is recommended for drops in BP.

WHAT DO I NEED TO TEACH MY CLIENTS ABOUT BETA-BLOCKERS?

- NEVER stop your medicine abruptly.

ACE (angiotensin-converting enzyme) inhibitors

HOW DO ACE INHIBITORS WORK?

- ACE inhibitors block angiotensin-converting enzyme from converting angiotensin I to angiotensin II (a potent vasoconstrictor). This decreases preload and afterload, ultimately decreasing workload on heart.

AS A BRAND NEW NURSE, WHAT DO I NEED TO KNOW ABOUT ACE INHIBITORS?

- Uses: Hypertension (Table 11-6).
- How do I remember this medication? If it ends in "pril" it is probably an ACE inhibitor (Table 11-7).
- What vital signs are most important? Monitor your client's blood pressure. If your client's BP is less than 90 mm Hg, hold the med and call the doctor.

WHAT DO I NEED TO TEACH MY CLIENTS ABOUT ACE INHIBITORS?

- Monitor BP. Hold medicine for BP less than 90 mm Hg.
- Antidote: For drops in blood pressure consider IV fluids. If HR is normal dopamine may be initiated.

Angiotensin II receptor blockers (ARBs)

HOW DO ARBs WORK?

- ARBs block angiotensin I from converting to angiotensin II (a potent vasoconstrictor).

Table 11-6. Examples of ACE Inhibitors

Generic name	Brand name
Enalapril	Vasotec
Fosinopril	Monopril
Lisinopril	Zestril
Captopril	Capoten

Table 11-7. Actions of ACE Inhibitors

Standard monitoring	What do you need to "worry" about?
The standard of care is for CHF clients to be discharged on a beta-blocker, ACE inhibitor, or both. Research shows improved long-term outcome when clients are on these medications.	I am happy to decrease workload on heart by decreasing preload and afterload. I am "worried" my client's blood pressure could drop out the bottom.
A decreased afterload decreases the resistance the heart has to work against to eject blood out of left ventricle. There is an improvement in CO without increasing the demand.	One unusual side effect is a big fat tongue (angioedema). So you had better watch for it. This could occlude their airway!
	Watch for elevated liver enzymes, because a rare syndrome that damages liver may occur and cause liver necrosis and death.
	May cause renal problems, so watch BUN and creatinine.
	ACE inhibitors lower aldosterone levels. Drops in aldosterone levels cause your client to lose sodium and water. This is okay to a certain point. If the client is losing sodium, he will retain potassium. (Sodium and potassium have an inverse relationship.) Your client can become hyperkalemic. Hyperkalemia can cause lethal arrhythmias. That's what you need to "worry" about.

WHAT ARE ARBs USED FOR?

- Hypertension and for clients who do not tolerate ACE inhibitors.

AS A BRAND NEW NURSE, WHAT DO I NEED TO KNOW ABOUT ARBs?

- Examples of ARBs (Table 11-8).

Table 11-8. Examples of ARBs

Generic name	Brand name
Valsartan	Diovan
Losartan	Cozaar
Irbesartan	Avapro
Candesartan	Atacand

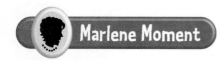

- How do I remember this medication? If the generic ends in "sartan," it is probably an ARB.

> Refer to ACE inhibitors for standard monitoring and things you need to "worry" about.

- Please note: ARBs are newer than a lot of other cardiac medications. Research into their effectiveness is in progress.

Calcium-channel blockers

HOW DO CALCIUM-CHANNEL BLOCKERS WORK?

- The strength of a cardiac contraction, in part, is related to the influx of calcium into the cell during depolarization. When calcium channels are blocked, contractility is decreased. This decreases workload on the heart.
- Calcium-channel blockers also block influx of calcium in vascular smooth muscle cells, thereby causing vasodilation and a drop in blood pressure.
- Calcium-channel blockers are unique in that they also cause coronary artery vasodilation.
- Finally, calcium-channel blockers decrease A-V node conduction and prolong the refractory period, so are useful in treating and preventing fast, narrow-complex tachycardias.

WHAT ARE CALCIUM-CHANNEL BLOCKERS USED FOR?

- Hypertension; control of fast rhythms and prevention of angina.

AS A BRAND NEW NURSE, WHAT DO I NEED TO KNOW ABOUT CALCIUM-CHANNEL BLOCKERS?

- See Table 11-9.
- How do I remember this medication? Nifedipine and amlodipine end in "pine." The others will need to be memorized. Yuk! (Table 11-10).
- What vital signs are most important? Check HR and BP. If your client's HR is less than 60 or BP less than 90 mm Hg, hold the med and call the doctor.
- Antidote: Calcium chloride can reverse life-threatening effects of calcium-channel blockers.

WHAT DO I NEED TO TEACH MY CLIENTS ABOUT CALCIUM-CHANNEL BLOCKERS?

- Monitor HR and BP. Hold medicine if your HR is less than 60 or BP less than 90 mm Hg.

Hydralazine

HOW DOES HYDRALAZINE WORK?

- Can be given PO or IV. Causes direct relaxation of the smooth muscles of arteries.

Table 11-9. Actions of Calcium-Channel Blockers

Standard monitoring	What do you need to "worry" about?
Used to treat clients with angina because they dilate the coronary arteries.	We want the blood pressure and HR to come down, but be careful they don't drop out the bottom.
May be selected over beta-blockers for diabetic clients.	Calcium-channel blockers decrease contractility. This is okay to a point, but, it could drop cardiac output out the bottom. So you had better watch for it! (e.g., decreased LOC, HR, BP, cold and clammy.)
	May cause heart block (slowed HR).
	Watch for orthostatic hypotension and/or syncope.
	Nifedipine (Procardia) is no longer given sub-lingual. Clients who where given SL Procardia were found to have rebound hypertension. Procardia XL (extended release) PO is acceptable.
	Norvasc is only given PO and should not be given with grapefruit juice, as this can increase the drug level and adverse side effects.

WHAT IS HYDRALAZINE USED FOR?

- Major implication is to watch BP carefully. Your client may develop chest pain. Discontinue the medication STAT and call the physician if your pt. c/o chest pain.

AS A BRAND NEW NURSE, WHAT DO I NEED TO KNOW ABOUT HYDRALAZINE?

- Monitor BP. Hold medicine if BP is less than 90 mm Hg and call the physician.

Diuretics

HOW DO DIURETICS WORK?

- Diuretics act on the proximal, distal, or loop of Henle in the renal tubules to promote the excretion of sodium and water. There are two types of diuretics K⁺ sparing K⁺ losing.

Table 11-10. Examples of Calcium-Channel Blockers

Generic name	Brand name
Nifedipine	Procardia
Amlodipine	Norvasc
Diltiazem	Cardizem
Verapamil	Calan or Isoptin

WHAT ARE DIURETICS USED FOR?

- Diuretic effects lower blood pressure.(Whenever you have less volume in the vascular space you will have less pressure.)
- Decrease edema in CHF and clients with renal disease.
- May be used in clients with ascites.

Hurst Hint

To prevent degradation, IV Lasix is protected from light. (Usually it is covered with a little brown bag.)

AS A BRAND NEW NURSE WHAT DO I NEED TO KNOW ABOUT DIURETICS?

- See Table 11-11.
- How do I remember this medication? Except for metolazone (Zaroxolyn) the generics tend to end in "ide." The most common diuretic, of course, is furosemide.
- What vital signs are most important? Check BP. If your client's BP is less than 90 mm Hg, hold the med and call the doctor.
- Antidote: If BP drops too low, the physician may order IV fluids. In this case, isotonic fluids will be ordered. Isotonic fluids go into the vascular space and build up therefore making the BP go up. Remember . . . more volume, more pressure.

WHAT DO I NEED TO TEACH MY CLIENTS ABOUT DIURETICS?

- See Table 11-12.
- Take in the morning so you are not up all night going to the bathroom.
- Monitor BP. Hold medicine if BP is less than 90 mm Hg.
- Your doctor will be monitoring your lab values periodically.
- Report any involuntary finger contractions immediately (sign of hypocalcemia).
- Weigh yourself daily (teach proper method for weighing a client).
- Hold the medicine and call the doctor if you lose more than 2–3 pounds overnight.
- It is okay to eat foods high in potassium such as fresh produce.
- Advise client to stand slowly to prevent orthostatic hypotension.
- Hold the medicine and call the doctor if any ringing in the ears or hearing problems occur.

Table 11-11. Examples of Diuretics

Generic name	Brand name
HCTZ- hydrochlorthiazide	hydroDiuril
Furosemide	Lasix
Bumetanide	Bumex
Torsemide	Demadex
Metolazone	Zaroxolyn

Table 11-12. Actions of Diuretics

Standard monitoring	What do you need to "worry" about?
CHF: Assess your client for decreasing signs and symptoms of CHF. For instance, client reports she can breathe better, has decreased bibasilian crackles and increased oxygen saturation. Client exhibits decreased work of breathing. All of these indicate the medicine is working.	Diuretics, in general, make you lose sodium and water. That's O.K., but, they also make you lose lots of other electrolytes. That's what you "worry" about. The electrolyte you worry about the most is potassium. Hypokalemia can cause life-threatening arrhythmias. DO NOT administer without checking this electrolyte.
Monitor for decreased peripheral edema.	Calcium is lost with many diuretics. You need to assess your patient for hypocalcemia (tetany, Trousseau's sign, Chvostek's sign, twitching). Low calcium levels can cause life-threatening arrhythmias, but doesn't occur as often as low potassium.
Weigh clients daily. Weight losses of greater than 2–3 pounds overnight are of concern.	When client loses more than 2–3 pounds overnight, you "worry" they may be hypotensive or worse, they could go into shock.
Monitor I and O. On ANY client receiving a diuretic we monitor I and O. A good response would be increased UOP.	Use cautiously in clients with impaired kidney or liver function because these meds can worsen the problem. Monitor BUN, creatinine, and liver function tests (LFTs).
For clients with ascites measure the abdominal girth.	
	ALWAYS check for allergies. Use cautiously in clients who are allergic to sulfa drugs. (Diuretics are sulfonamide derivatives.) Ototoxicity is the number one toxicity to "worry" about. If your client complains of hearing loss or any weird ear complaint, hold the med and call the doctor.

Potassium-sparing diuretics

HOW DO POTASSIUM-SPARING DIURETICS WORK?

- Antagonize aldosterone in the distal tubule in the kidneys, thus promoting excretion of sodium and water and retention of potassium. (Sodium and potassium have an inverse relationship.)

WHAT ARE POTASSIUM-SPARING DIURETICS USED FOR?

- Hypertension, hyperaldosteronism, edema, diuretic-induced hypokalemia; also reduce ascites.

AS A BRAND NEW NURSE, WHAT DO I NEED TO KNOW ABOUT POTASSIUM-SPARING DIURETICS?

- See Table 11-13.

Table 11-13. Example of Potassium-Sparing Diuretics

Generic name	Brand name
Spironolactone	Aldactone

- How do I remember this medication? Aldactone acts on aldosterone . . . therefore the client will lose sodium and water and retain potassium.
- The most important thing to remember is to monitor your client for hyperkalemia. This could cause a lethal arrhythmia.
- Other than the hyperkalemia, follow the other recommendations listed above when giving diuretics.
- Antidote: If BP drops too low the physician may order IV fluids. In this case, isotonic fluids will be ordered. Remember how isotonic solutions work?

WHAT DO I NEED TO TEACH MY CLIENTS ABOUT POTASSIUM-SPARING DIURETICS?

- Avoid foods high in potassium like fresh produce.
- Be careful with salt substitutes because they have a lot of potassium.
- Except for the above listed items see other teaching under diuretics.

Brain natriuretic peptide (BNP) (Natrecor)

HOW DOES BNP WORK?

- BNP was assigned this name because it was originally discovered in the brain. Body makes BNP and Natrecor is a synthetic form of BNP.
- BNP is mainly produced by the ventricle in the heart in response to stretching of the myocardium
- BNP causes relaxation of the heart and vascular smooth muscle. This results in ventricular, venous, and arterial relaxation. In this way, preload and afterload are reduced.
- Natrecor provides a diuretic effect by inhibiting sodium resorption in the glomeruli filtrate.

WHAT IS NATRECOR USED FOR?

- Uses: Treatment for decompensated CHF (Table 11-14).

AS A BRAND NEW NURSE, WHAT DO I NEED TO KNOW ABOUT NATRECOR?

- How do I remember this medication? BNP is normally released in the body in response to stretching of the left ventricle. This is a good

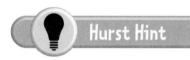

Hurst Hint

Natrecor must be stopped 2 hours before a serum BNP is drawn or the results will be falsely elevated.

Table 11-14. Example of Treatment for Decompensated CHF

Generic name	Brand name
Nesiritide	Natrecor (infusion; short-term therapy; not to be given for more then 48 hours)

Table 11-15. Actions of Serum BNP

Standard monitoring	What do you need to "worry" about?
I and O . . . anytime your client is receiving a diuretic, monitor I and O.	Vasodilation may drop your client's blood pressure out the bottom. The half-life is longer than NTG. (Hypotension may last for hours.)
Monitor EKG	Electrolyte disturbances can lead to EKG changes.
Daily weights	Notify MD of weight losses greater than 2–3 pounds overnight.

thing, because when secreted into the blood it causes diuresis which will decrease preload and afterload. This is what your client needs.

- A serum BNP can be drawn and indicates the level of heart failure your client is in. The higher the number, the worse the heart failure (Table 11-15).

- What vital signs are most important? BP, BP, BP . . . < 90 mm Hg, call the doctor.

- Antidote: If BP drops really low, place the client in Trendelenberg position. Call the physician. If your client is severely hypotensive and symptomatic, initiate ACLS (advanced cardiac life support) or call the Rapid Response Team.

WHAT DO I NEED TO TEACH MY CLIENTS ABOUT NATRECOR?

- Tell your client what to expect with a Natrecor infusion.
- Tell your client you are measuring I and O.

Positive inotropes

- Inotropic medications increase the strength of a contraction.
- The major positive inotrope we will discuss is digitalis ("Dig").

HOW DOES DIGITALIS WORK?

- This medicine is derived from a plant called digitalis lanata. Dig inhibits the sodium-potassium activated ATP_a pump. This allows calcium to move from outside to inside the myocytes. Additional calcium makes a contraction stronger. Which will help push more blood out ($\uparrow CO$).

- Dig also increases vagal tone. Increased vagal tone slows the heart rate, which allows the ventricles more time to fill with blood. Therefore, cardiac output increases when Dig begins working within 5 to 30 minutes. Its effects can last up to 24 hours.

CASE IN POINT The client's heart rate has been slowed. This allows more time for the ventricles to fill up. Now, the ventricles are squeezing down harder on more volume. Cardiac output just went up! Yeah! Now more volume is moving forward. If your client is in CHF they need more forward flow of blood (if the blood goes backward, it will go into the lungs). The bad part of all this is that workload on the heart just went up. You could stress a client's heart too much on this medicine and worsen the heart failure. This is why digoxin is not as popular as it used to be.

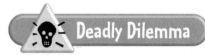

Deadly Dilemma

Your client is on a diuretic. Don't forget to give them a urinal or provide a bedside commode. It is a safety thing. Assess your client. Can they tolerate getting up and down frequently? Ask them to call for help as needed. Be sure to have the call light with in the clients reach.

Table 11-16. Example of Positive Ionotropes

Generic name	Brand name
Digoxin	Lanoxin

WHAT IS DIGITALIS USED FOR?

- Controls rate or converts atrial fibrillation and supraventricular tachycardias.
- Treatment for CHF.

AS A BRAND NEW NURSE, WHAT DO I NEED TO KNOW ABOUT DIG?

- It's the BIG cardiac glycoside to "worry" about (Tables 11-16 and 11-17).

Table 11-17. Actions of Positive Ionotropes

Standard monitoring	What do you need to "worry" about?
If your client's HR is really fast, their ventricles don't have time to fill up with blood. Digoxin slows fast heart rates. That's a good thing. You slow the HR so the ventricles have more time to fill. You must check your client's apical HR. It must be at least 60 bpm or the med should not be given.	Hold the digoxin if the HR is less than 60 bpm. Digoxin could drop the HR so much the CO will drop. When CO drops, your client may become short of breath. They may have a change in LOC, feel cold and clammy, and might start having chest pain.
Monitor potassium levels. All electrolytes are important, but potassium is the one to monitor closely.	Here's our formula: Dig + hypokalemia = toxicity.
Monitor for therapeutic levels, between 0.5 and 2.0 ng/mL.	Anything more than 2.0 ng/mL, consider your client to be toxic.
The MD will order a "digitalizing dose" or loading dose. This is a larger initial dose and one or two lesser dosages 4 to 6 hours later. She is trying to get the digoxin level therapeutic.	
	Monitor the client for s/s of toxicity. Early signs are visual changes like yellow halos or nausea and vomiting. Late changes are arrhythmias like A-V blocks or really, really slow heart rates. This can drop their CO out the bottom.
	Clients with hypothyroidism are extremely sensitive to this medication. Use with caution.
	Use caution in giving digoxin. If your client already has any degree of heart block, digoxin could make the block worse.

- What vital signs are most important? Heart rate must be above 60. Hold the medication for a HR of 60 bpm or below.

WHAT DO I NEED TO TEACH MY CLIENTS ABOUT DIGITALIS?

- Inform your client the doctor will be monitoring their digoxin and electrolyte levels.

- Tell your client to report ANY vision changes and/or nausea and vomiting.

- Tell client to inform MD if they are taking any of these OTCs: herbs such as oleander, St. John's wort, ginseng, and licorice, as these can alter Dig levels.

- Teach your client how to take her pulse and hold her medicine when HR drops below 60 bpm and call her physician.

- Antidote: Digibind or DigiFab is a medicine that binds to digoxin and can reverse life-threatening arrhythmias.

Inotropic medications

- The major IV Inotropic medications we will review are dopamine and dobutamine.

HOW DO IV INOTROPIC MEDICATIONS WORK?

- Inotropic medications increase myocardial contractility. They do this by stimulating the beta-adrenergic receptor cells in the heart.

- Dopamine, in addition to stimulating beta-1 receptor cells, acts on alpha (peripheral) receptors in the body. The final result is an increase in cardiac output and increased workload on the heart.

- Dobutamine tends to stimulate the beta-1 (heart) cells selectively, whereas dopamine affects beta and alpha cells (especially in higher dosages). This means dopamine causes more peripheral vasoconstriction (increases BP).

WHAT ARE DOPAMINE AND DOBUTAMINE USED FOR?

- Dobutamine is used for uncompensated CHF. For IV use only in decompensated CHF. Dopamine is the drug of choice for shock syndromes (septic shock, cardiac shock) due to its vasoconstricting effects.

AS A BRAND NEW NURSE, WHAT DO I NEED TO KNOW ABOUT DOPAMINE AND DOBUTAMINE?

- See Table 11-18.

Table 11-18. Examples of IV Inotropic Medications

Generic name	Brand name
Dobutamine	Dobutrex
Dopamine hydrochloride	Intropin

- How do you remember this medication? Dobutrex and dopamine sound similar. Dopamine is used for hypotension; Dobutrex is used for decompensated CHF. Both increase cardiac output, but dopamine increases workload on heart more than dobutamine (Table 11-19).
- What vital signs are most important? Monitor all the vital signs very closely. Monitor for s/s of decrease in CO (change in LOC, restlessness, complaints of shortness of breath, chest pain, cold clammy skin, and decrease in urine output).

WHAT DO I NEED TO TEACH MY CLIENTS ABOUT DOPAMINE AND DOBUTAMINE?

- Clients on these medications are really sick. You as the nurse need to offer the client and family emotional support.

Let's review some miscellaneous information regarding cardiovascular drugs

DIRECT VASODILATING INOTROPIC MEDICATIONS

- This is the most recent class of inotropic medications (Table 11-20).
- If you even get a question on NCLEX® on this medication just remember it is used in decompensated CHF. It improves CO by decreasing afterload and preload.

Table 11-19. Actions of IV Inotropic Medications

Standard monitoring	What do you need to "worry" about?
The client receiving low-dose dopamine or dobutamine needs to be on the telemetry unit to be monitored. High doses (>5 μg/kg/min is the standard) require ICU monitoring.	These medicines stimulate the sympathetic nervous system. This is the "fight or flight" response. They increase HR (chronotropic effect) and cardiac output. Guess what? They also have a dromotrophic (increased myocardial conduction). These medications can cause too much stimulation. The client can have lethal arrhythmias.
	These meds also increase workload on heart. This can cause ischemia and subsequent arrhythmias. People in the medical field worry about the side effects of these medications. These meds are reserved for clients who have poor COs or dangerously low BP.
	Call the MD if your client is having arrhythmias.
Monitor for changes in cardiac output	Assess LOC, respirations, c/o chest pain, skin, and UOP frequently.
Monitor I and O, daily weights, electrolytes	Clients on these medicines are critically ill. They need careful monitoring.
	Dopamine at high dosages can create so much vasoconstriction that your patient may lose peripheral pulses. You had better be checking for this often.
	Both meds should be given in a central line. Dopamine can cause tissue necrosis if extravasation occurs. If extravasation occurs, regitine is the antidote. (It will cause a localized vasodilation to the area to hopefully restore circulation.)

Table 11-20. Example of Direct Vasodilating Inotropic
Medications (for IV Use Only)

Generic name	Brand name
Milrinone	Primacor

NOW LET'S TALK ABOUT THE WORST-CASE SCENARIO IN CHF

- Your client develops pulmonary edema. Some or all of the medications may be given to save the client's life.

- Lasix (decreases preload through diuresis and vasodilation); 40-mg IV push given over 1 to 2 minutes.

- What do you worry about? Hypotension and ototoxicity.

- Bumex can be given IV push or as continuous IV to provide rapid fluid removal; 1- to 2-mg IV push given over 1 to 2 minutes. What do you "worry" about? Hypotension.

- Nitroglycerin IV vasodilation; decreases afterload. What do you "worry" about? Hypotension.

- Digoxin (some still use this to get the blood moving forward); remember it increases workload on heart, so it is not always used.

- Morphine sulfate 2-mg IV push for vasodilation to decrease preload and afterload. Now your client doesn't care that they can't breathe! What do you "worry" about? Respiratory depression.

- Natrecor (infusion; short-term therapy; not to be given more then 48 hours). Vasodilates veins and arteries.

- Primacor (infusion; short-term therapy); vasodilates veins and arteries. What do you "worry" about? Hypotension.

- Dobutamine (increases cardiac output, so more blood is moving forward instead of backward into lungs). What do you "worry" about? Arrhythmias, and the increased workload on heart.

LET'S TALK ABOUT THE CLIENT EXPERIENCING
A MYOCARDIAL INFARCTION (MI)

- Fibrinolytics are given to clients experiencing an acute myocardial infarction and who are more than 60 minutes from a hospital that can perform a percutaneous coronary intervention (PCI). PCIs are the gold standard when the door to cath lab time is < 90 minutes. These medications dissolve the clot that has formed in the coronary artery.

- Examples of fibrinolytics:

  TPA (tissue plasminogen activator)

  TNKase

  Retavase

  Streptokinase

- Things to remember for NCLEX®:

  The fibrinolytic your client is most likely to have an allergic response to is streptokinase.

The med must be given to your client within the first 12 hours from the onset of the MI.

Major complication to remember is BLEEDING! Your client is placed on bleeding precautions like: Watch for bleeding gums, watch for hematuria, watch for black stools, use an electric razor, use a soft toothbrush.

No IMs (intramusculars).

There are four absolute contraindications for administering this drug to your client: (1) known intracranial neoplasm; (2) hemorrhagic stroke at any time, other stroke within one year; (3) active internal bleeding; and (4) suspected aortic dissection.

- How can you remember the four absolute contraindications? Remember two in the head and two in the belly. Two in the head meaning an intracerebral bleed or stroke within last year or a tumor in your client's head. Two in the belly meaning internal bleeding or suspected aortic dissection.

- If your client had any of these and you gave them a fibrinolytic what would happen? Your client would bleed to death.

PREVENTING PLATELET AGGREGATION

- Medications to prevent clotting by inhibiting platelet aggregation include ASA (recommended for prevention of MIs) and Plavix (platelet aggregate inhibitor).

- Reopro and Integrilin are given by IV infusion. They are given to very unstable MI clients at risk for re-occluding. They too prevent clotting but, are more potent than ASA or Plavix.

TREATING VENTRICULAR TACHYCARDIA OR VENTRICULAR FIBRILLATION

- The most common arrhythmia for your patient during a MI is ventricular fibrillation (V-fib).

- If your client has an episode of V-fib, the first thing you do is "defib" (defibrillate) V-fib. Once they return with a perfusing rhythm, the doctor may place them on one of the antiarrhythmics listed in Table 11-21.

- Major complication to remember with amiodarone is hypotension.

- The major toxic effects with lidocaine are CNS changes. You may think your client has had a stroke because they are having neurourological changes. If they are on lidocaine they may be toxic.

LET'S FINISH WITH A COMMON CARDIOVASCULAR PROBLEM

- First on the list is DVT (deep vein thrombosis).

Table 11-21. Examples of Antiarrhythmics

Generic name	Brand name
Amiodarone	Cordarone
Lidocaine	Lidocaine hydrochloride

Table 11-22. Labs to Monitor and Antidote to Medications if Client Has DVT or Is at Risk for Developing DVT

Medication	Lab	Antidote
Heparin	aPTT	Protamine sulfate
Fibrinolytics	PT, fibrinogen level, aPTT, HCT	Amicar
Coumadin	INR, PT	Vitamin K
Plavix	No labs required	N/A
Aspirin	No labs required	N/A
Lovenox	No labs required	Protamine sulfate
Persantine	No labs required	N/A

- If the client has a DVT or is at risk for developing a DVT, he may be placed on medications listed in Table 11-22.
- NCLEX® may try to trick you into choosing lab to monitor for Lovenox effectiveness. Don't let them fool you! There are no labs required. Leave the air bubble in the Lovenox syringe. Expelling the air could result in loss of medication and incorrect dosing.

✚ Immunizations

One more group of medications to review is immunizations. These medications work by producing antibodies to specific infectious diseases, providing immunity to them. Active or acquired immunity occurs when the body produces its own antibodies by being exposed to an infectious disease or receiving a vaccination. Passive immunity involves the transference of antibodies from another person or by vaccination, so the body does not have to produce its own antibodies to a particular disease. Immunizations are contraindicated in clients who are allergic to egg products and those who are immunocompromised. Common adverse effects of immunizations are local reactions to injection sites and fever. Nursing interventions would be to place warm compresses at the site of inflammation and administer acetaminophen as prescribed (Table 11-23).

Table 11-23. Recommended Immunization Schedule

Vaccine	Age given
Hepatitis B	Birth; 2, 4, and 6 months
Hepatitis A	After first birthday and 6 months later
Rotavirus	3 doses total at 2, 4, and 6 months (must be given prior to 32 weeks of age)
DtaP	2, 4, 6, 12 months; age 4 or before school
Haemophilus influenzae Type B	2 months, 4 months, and another dose after 1st birthday

(Continued)

Table 11-23. Recommended Immunization Schedule (*Continued*)

Vaccine	Age given
Pneumoccal	2, 4, 6, 12 months
Inactivated poliovirus	2 months, 4 months, 6 months or 12 months, and a fourth dose at age 4
Influenza	After 6 months and yearly thereafter
Measles, mumps, rubella	After age 1; age 4
Varicella	12 months; age 4
Meningococcal	24 months through age 18 (not given routinely . . . usually requested before college as client will be living in a dormitory setting)
Human papillomavirus (HPV)	9 to 26 years of age; 3 doses total; give first dose; 2 months later give second dose; 6 months later give third dose

Adapted from CDC website **www.cdc.gov/nip/acip.**

CONCLUSION

I know what you are thinking. The name of this chapter is "Pharmacology in a Nutshell." That must have been a nut on anabolic steroids, because that was a lot of content! You do not have to memorize everything in this chapter. A general understanding will be fine, because you are a brand new nurse whose major focus is client safety. Yes, it's a lot to remember, but there are at least 60,000 drugs in the United States. I know you would rather review this chapter than every single drug out there!

Bibliography

Centers for Disease Control: **www.cdc.gov/nip/acip.**

Hurst Review Services: **www.hurstreview.com.**

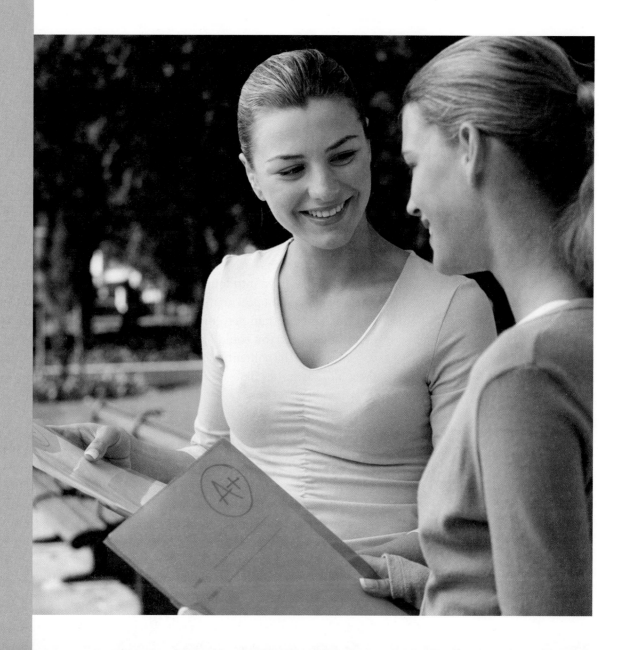

12 Potential Test Question Topics According to the PN Test Plan

EVERYTHING YOU WANTED TO KNOW ABOUT THE TEST PLAN BUT WERE AFRAID TO ASK

The purpose of this chapter is to get a better understanding of the NCLEX-PN® test plan. This plan was developed by the National Council of State Boards of Nursing and is updated every 3 years. The purpose of this document is to provide detailed information on the content areas that are tested on the NCLEX-PN® exam. Extensive research is performed to ensure the test plan accurately reflects what a new nurse will be faced with in a client care setting. This test plan is the guide question writers (item writers) use when writing questions for your test. The test plan is broken down into four major categories called Client Needs. Each category has certain potential test question topics. From each category you will have a certain percentage of questions. There is no way to know every single topic you could have on your exam. This chapter will give you an idea of the content that could be tested per category. Let's look at the major categories first.

CONTENT CATEGORIES AND PERCENTAGES OF QUESTIONS/CATEGORY

Table 12-1 outlines the different categories the test plan is broken into. The percentages tell you how much of your test will come from each category.

Let's take a look at each category separately.

Table 12-1. Subdivision of Categories in the NCLEX-PN® Test Plan

Client needs categories	Percentage of questions in each category
Safe and effective care environment	
Coordinated care	11–17%
Safety and infection control	8–14%
Health promotion and maintenance	7–13%
Psychosocial integrity	8–14%
Physiological integrity	
Basic care and comfort	11–17%
Pharmacological therapies	9–15%
Reduction of risk potential	10–16%
Physiological adaptation	12–18%

Information from National Council of State Boards of Nursing. *2005 NCLEX-PN® Detailed Test Plan, NCLEX® Examinations.*

REVIEWING THE CATEGORIES

Now we are going to breakdown each category even more! We will now review, in general, the types of question topics that fall into each area.

✛ Safe and effective care environment

As you can see from Table 12-1, this category has two subheadings, which are Coordinated Care and Safety and Infection Control. A total of 19% to 31% of your test will come from this overall category. Safe and Effective Care Environment refers to the nurse's ability to provide nursing care to a specific client. This category also includes the nurse assisting with the protection of other health care personnel. Let's look at the topics you could be tested on under each of these subheadings.

Coordinated care

Coordinated Care is the nurse's ability to work with other members of the health care team to promote effective client care. 11% to 17% of your test questions will come from this subheading. Let's look at some of the potential test question topics that fall under this category.

- *Advance Directives:* Living wills, health care proxy, Durable Power of Attorney. Does your client have a living will? If not, can you explain what each of these items are correctly?

- *Advocacy:* Acting as a client advocate. Promoting self-advocacy.

- *Assignments:* Correctly assigning care to appropriate personnel while making sure the person you are assigning care to has the ability to carry out the task safely. Recognizing when an assignment needs to be altered due to a change in the client's health status. Recognizing when you or another heath care team member is not prepared to accept a task or assignment.

- *Client Rights:* Do you and the client understand the "rights" of a client? Can you recognize when a client's rights have been violated and do you know what to do? Understanding of confidentiality and informed consent. Do you know what to do when a client refuses treatment (notification of physician or charge nurse, proper documentation)? Includes client in decision making regarding care.

- *Management and Supervision:* Conflict resolution. Uses appropriate chain of command. Understands what other health care team members do. Recognizes and intervenes in unsafe situations. Participates in staff education seminars. Assists in evaluating other staff members. Knows when to supervise care given by other personnel. Knows the staff's skills, abilities, and knowledge level. Time management. Assists with orientation of a new employee.

- *Confidentiality:* Recognizes situations that could affect client confidentiality (inappropriate staff looking at client's records; discussing client situations in inappropriate places). Maintains and respects client's privacy (during procedures, when interviewing a client).

- *Consulting with Other Members of the Health Care Team:* Knows when to consult with others and participates accordingly.

- *Continuity of Care:* Admission histories. Transferring clients. Discharging clients/ following up after discharge. Revising plan of care as needed (especially if client's condition changes). Participates in interdisciplinary conferences. Shift report. Documents transfers/ discharges/referrals appropriately. Uses care plans to guide client's care.

- *Priority Setting:* Knows what actions take priority. Which client do I see first? Recognizes and reports a change in client's health status. When caring for multiple clients, can you determine what takes priority/what do I do first?

- *Ethics:* Can you identify ethical issues that could affect the staff or client and share this information appropriately? Do you know when to intervene to promote ethical practice?

- *Informed Consent:* Do you understand informed consent requirements? If client is unable to give informed consent, can you identify the appropriate person to do so?

- *Legalities:* Documentation. Reports client problems such as child abuse, a communicable disease, or gunshot wounds. Reports errors appropriately. Obtains verbal, telephone, and written prescriptions appropriately. Transcribes physician's orders appropriately. Cares for client's valuables appropriately. How to deal with a physician prescription that is confusing or illegible. Do you know your scope of practice? Do you know when to report unsafe practice of another staff member (improper care, substance abuse)?

- *Quality Assurance:* Participates in facility quality-assurance activities (collecting data or serving on a quality-improvement committee). Reports client care issues to appropriate personnel.

- *Referring:* Identifies and utilizes community resources (hospice, social services, shelters, support groups). Identifies the client's need for further assistance (physical therapy, home health care).

- *Resource Management:* Uses equipment appropriately (oxygen, suction machine). Are you cost-effective when providing care?

Safety issues and infection control

Safety Issues and Infection Control refers to the nurse's ability to protect clients and other members of the health care team from any type of hazard (health or environmental). Eight to fourteen percent of your test questions will come from this subheading. Let's take a look at some potential test question topics.

- *Error and Injury Prevention (including accidents):* Is aware of client's and health care team members' knowledge of safety procedures/issues and how to prevent them. Correct use of infant seats. Being able to identify factors that could increase accidents or injuries (age, confused clients). Identification of allergies and reporting/documenting appropriately.

All content related to fire safety. Insuring client has a way to call staff members if needed. Utilization of client protection mechanisms (bed alarms, ID bracelet, allergy bracelets). Recognizing, reporting, and intervening if environmental hazard is identified (spills on floor, frayed electrical cord, malfunctioning call light). Ensures proper identification of client.

- *Hazardous and Infectious Materials:* Understands protocols for handling infectious products and hazardous chemicals (chemotherapy, radioactive substances, cleaning fluids, flammable substances). Utilizes appropriate methods to prevent infection. Identifies and reports hazardous working conditions (chemical spills, blood spills, smoking by client or other health care team member). Is able to locate the Material Safety Data Sheets.

- *Safety in the Home:* Do you know how to adapt a client's home environment to improve safety (lighting, clearing floor of throw rugs, use of handrails)? Identification of fire or environmental hazards in the home (frayed electrical cords, wearing socks on slick floors). Providing client information to improve home safety (proper disposal of syringes, kitchen safety). Fall prevention.

- *Internal and External Disasters:* Do you understand evacuation protocols? Triage. Knowing who is responsible for what during a disaster. Participating in disaster drills.

- *Asepsis (medical and surgical):* Assesses the client's environment for potential infectious sources. Set up a sterile field and use proper supplies and equipment to maintain an aseptic environment (gloves or mask). Use of sterile technique. Proper use of methods to control or eliminate infectious substances (proper use of cleaning solutions, proper hand-washing technique).

- *Incident/Event/Irregular Occurrence/Variance:* Can you complete the proper reports if a variance occurs? Do you know the proper time to complete a report (medication errors, client falls)?

- *Using Equipment Safely:* Can you check equipment to ensure its safe functioning or identify any safety hazards (frayed electrical cords, loose parts, safe administration of oxygen, safe use of canes, crutches and walkers, safe use of continuous passive motion machine)? Do you know what to do with malfunctioning equipment and who should be notified?

- *Security:* Do you know the agency security plan and is it effective? Triage. Evacuation of clients.

- *Standard/Transmission Precautions:* Infection control principles (isolation, sterile technique, standard precautions). Teaching clients infection control procedures (proper disposal of sputum in tuberculosis client). Knowing which diseases are communicable and how the organism is transmitted (airborne, droplet). Utilizes equipment to prevent the spread of infectious diseases (placing tuberculosis client in properly ventilated room, keeping door closed). Identifying immunocompromised clients and preventing exposure to infection. Hand-washing.

- *Restraints/Safety Devices:* Proper application of restraints/bed alarms. Utilizes least restrictive restraint devices. Continuously monitors client for the need of restraints or safety devices. Proper documentation of restraints/safety devices. Documents client's response to use of restraints or safety devices. Recognizes the need for monitoring and proper documentation of a client in seclusion. Follows agency protocols for timed client monitoring (suicide precautions, restraint/seclusion check or any safety checks).

✚ Health promotion/maintenance

Health Promotion and Maintenance refers to the nurse's knowledge and utilization of growth and development and early detection of health problems. Seven to thirteen percent of the questions will come from this category. Now let's look at some potential test question topics.

- *The Aging Process:* Do you consider the client's age and adapt care accordingly? What is the client's attitude on aging? Expected changes related to aging. Developmental tasks. Developmental stages. Expected physiological changes associated with aging, especially in clients over 65 years of age. Provides resources for end-of-life needs.

- *Ante/Intra/Postpartum Care and Care of the Newborn:* Stages of labor. Relaxation techniques during labor. Non–stress-test. Postpartum complications. Assessing client's ability to care for a newborn infant. Normal pregnancy. Postpartum care (perineal care, assisting with feeding of infant). Supports client's labor coach. Care of newborn (cord care, maintaining proper temperature). Teaching infant care skills (bathing, positioning, and circumcision care). Identifies emotional needs during pregnancy. Fetal heart monitoring. Is able to monitor a client in labor or one who is postpartum.

- *Data Collection:* Can you complete an admission and health history properly? Physical examination. Reporting and documenting physical exam findings. Is able to identify barriers to communication. Is able to identify barriers to learning.

- *Developmental Stages/Transitions:* Selection of age-appropriate activities. Assists with activities that specifically relate to client's developmental stage (attachment to newborn, parenting, puberty, aging issues such as retirement). Identifies normal developmental tasks and behavioral characteristics specific to a certain age (when does separation anxiety occur). Explains nursing care/procedures according to client's age and developmental stage. Recognizes when client is not at appropriate developmental stage for age.

- *Prevention of Disease:* Provides information on disease prevention (yearly Pap tests, mammograms). Recognizes risks for disease (family history, lifestyle, precancerous skin change). Identifies disease risk factors (age, ethnicity, family history). Recognizes actions that prevent disease (smoking cessation, exercise, healthy diet).

- *Body Image Changes:* Identifies and determines client's acceptance of expected body image changes (aging, pregnancy, menopause).

Determines how expected body image changes impacts client (temperament).

- *Family Interaction:* Assists family with introduction of new infant into present family structure. Identifies present family structure and roles of each family member. Identifies stressors that could affect family functioning.

- *Family Planning:* Reviews client's preferred contraceptive. Can identify factors that could influence the outcome of the contraceptive method (smoking with oral contraceptives). Genetic counseling. Infertility assessment.

- *Promoting Health/Screening Programs:* Can you accurately check results of client's screening test (Pap test, hemoccult tests)? Can you select the appropriate teaching strategy for health programs (return demonstration, pamphlets, showing videos)? Complimentary and alternative medicine (yoga, journaling, meditation). Identifies and encourages client's participation in health-seeking programs (breast exams, testicular exams, blood pressure screenings, stress prevention, health fairs). Helps client to understand health promotion activities. Emphasizes teaching in regard to health risks. Emphasizes teaching in regard to health promotion.

- *High-Risk Behaviors:* Helps client identify high-risk behaviors and the expected outcome of these behaviors (use of tanning beds, not exercising regularly, needle sharing, unprotected sex). Can you teach about high-risk behaviors?

- *Human Sexuality:* Can you identify the client's perspective on human sexuality? Do you respect the client's sexual orientation? Is able to discuss issues such as family planning, menopause, or erectile dysfunction.

- *Administering Immunizations:* Immunization schedule. Checking immunization status. Recognizing contraindications for immunizations. Identifying abnormal responses to immunizations.

- *Lifestyle Choices:* Identifies lifestyle choices that may result in illness (smoking). Does client use alternative health practices? Identifies other lifestyle choices (choosing to not have children, choosing to home school). Can you teach about healthy lifestyle choices (exercising regularly, stopping smoking)?

- *Self-Care:* Identifies whether client can meet her own self-care needs or not (feeding, dressing, hygiene).

✛ Psychosocial integrity

Psychosocial Integrity refers to the nurse's ability to assist and provide care for promotion of the emotional, mental, and social well-being of clients. A total of 8% to 14% of the exam will come from this category. Now let's review some potential test question topics.

- *Abuse/Neglect:* Does the client possess risk factors that make them more apt to abuse or neglect others? Can identify signs and symptoms of abuse or neglect (client losing weight, poor hygiene of client). Provides a safe environment, emotional care, and physical care for the abused/

neglected client. Is able to identify the abused/neglected client's response to care. Identify client at high risk for being abused/neglected. Reinforces teaching on coping strategies associated with preventing abuse/neglect.

- *Behavioral Intervention/Management:* Assists client in using behavioral techniques in an effort to decrease anxiety. Assists client with mental illness to participate in therapy. Encourages client to use suggested interventions to correct inappropriate behavior. Identifies stressors in the client's life that could interfere with behavioral intervention. Is able to identify inappropriate/abnormal behaviors and compare them to the norm. Checks clients response to behavioral management strategies. Checks for changes in appearance, mood, and psychomotor behavior. Appropriately orients the client to reality. Participates in behavioral management programs for client. Promotes independence, especially in those with impaired cognition (Alzheimer's disease). Identifies/documents response to behavioral management interventions. Reinforces participation in group/family therapy. Reinforces education of family/caregivers on specific behavioral management interventions. Sets limits on inappropriate behavior (especially dangerous behavior). Uses behavioral strategies to help clients in controlling behavior (contract or behavioral modification techniques). Assists client in understanding her own behavior.

- *Coping Mechanisms:* Collects data on effective and ineffective coping mechanisms. Discusses ways to help client cope with illness. Identifies emotional response to present illness (hopefulness or anger). Does client use any support systems for coping? What is the family's emotional reaction to illness?

- *Crisis Intervention:* Identifies orientation to reality. Can identify a client in crisis. Provides time to express feelings about crisis. Reinforces resources to assist in recovery from crisis. Reports developing crises to supervisor. Appropriately utilizes crises intervention techniques.

- *Cultural Awareness:* Considers/respects culture of client when providing nursing care, especially to a client who has died or is dying. Documents language needs are being met. When reinforcing teaching, provides sensitivity to client's cultural practices. Recognizes cultural practices that could affect interventions (using direct eye contact during care). Recognizes cultural differences that could potentiate complications (use of folk remedies, refusing blood transfusions). Recognizes cultural differences in regard to having children and raising children (disciplinary techniques, toilet training techniques). Recognizes that different cultures perceive and respond to pain differently. Recognizes cultural differences that could affect the understanding of a psychiatric diagnoses. Recognizes that different cultures go through the grieving process differently. Recognizes when client does not understand English. Respects different cultural backgrounds and practices. Uses interpreters appropriately.

- *End-of-Life Issues:* Helps client understand end-of-life interventions and their purpose. Helps in resolution of end-of- life issues.

Recognizes end-of-life needs (fear, changes in role, loss of control, financial concerns). Is able to perform postmortem care. Appropriately provides end-of- life interventions.

- *Grief/Loss:* Assists with resolution of grief and loss (loss of a child, loss of a limb). Helps to refer clients to appropriate grief and loss resources (use of a pastor, support group). Is able to collect data on reactions to loss. Recognizes the ability to understand grief/loss. Encourages reminiscing. What are client's fears related to grief/loss? Reinforces teaching on expected reactions to grief/loss (denial, fear, anger). Provides support during anticipatory grieving.

- *Mental Health Issues:* Assists in promoting independence and a sense of hope. Discusses refusal to follow treatment plan. Establishes trust in the nurse–client relationship. What are the barriers to compliance with treatment? Recognizes when there are differences between the client's and health care providers' feelings/views. Promotes increased self-esteem. Recognizes when relapse may be occurring. Recognizes defense mechanisms used by the client. Supports client's involvement in making decisions about his health care when appropriate.

- *Mental Illness Issues:* Assists family in planning care for clients with impaired cognition, dementia or Alzheimer's disease. Assists in teaching regarding diagnoses. Is able to recognize changes in mental status. Can client follow a treatment plan? Is able to recognize abnormal mood, judgment, cognition, or reasoning. What is the client's reaction to the mental illness diagnoses (anxiety, depression)? Recognizes signs of mental illness (schizophrenia, bipolar disorder). Recognizes the signs of impaired cognition (loss of memory, decreased hygiene). Validates that client is adhering to treatment plan (is the client taking her medicine?).

- *Religious or Spiritual Influences:* Helps clients meet religious/spiritual needs (getting their pastor involved). Does client feel conflict between the treatment that has been recommended and their beliefs? Recognizes different religious/spiritual beliefs can affect the plan of care. Always respects different beliefs.

- *Sensory/Perceptual Alterations:* Assists client when compensating for impairment of sensory or perceptual type (hearing loss, vision loss). Recognizes communication problems (hearing loss; cannot speak English; is the client intubated? does the client have expressive aphasia?). Provides other methods of communication when needed (translator, sign board). Ensures client has the ability to communicate needs effectively.

- *Situational Role Changes:* Helps client adjust to temporary role changes. Identifies scenarios that could change the role of the client or impact the client's recovery (death of a parent or spouse with a long-term illness). Does the client have the ability to adapt to temporary/permanent role changes? Can you recognize successful adaptation to a situational role change?

- *Stress Management:* Recognizes client stressors. Has the client's stress level changed? What is the client's response to stress-management interventions? Does the client use any stress-management techniques? What kinds of things are stressful to the client (a noisy environment, uncertainty, lack of knowledge)? Reinforces teaching on stress-management interventions (relaxation exercises, physical activities, meditation).

- *Substance Disorders:* Assists in dealing with signs and symptoms of substance abuse. Encourages use of support groups such as Alcoholics Anonymous or Narcotics Anonymous. Encourages counseling for drug/alcohol dependency. What is the client's reaction to a chemical dependency diagnosis? What are the signs and symptoms of intoxication/dependency of a substance or withdrawal from a particular substance? Recognizes unhealthy behaviors that could reinforce chemical dependency (stressors, family dynamics). What is the client's response to the substance-related treatment plan? Provide care in non–substance-related dependencies (gambling, pornography). Provide care for those going through alcohol or drug withdrawal.

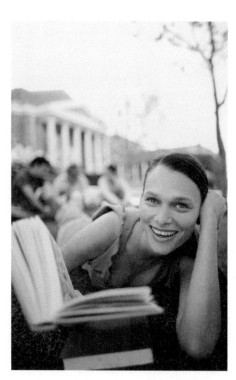

- *Suicide or Violence:* What is the client's potential for suicide or violence? What is the client's risk for self-injury or violence?

- *Support Systems:* Does the family or do significant others have the ability to provide appropriate support to the client? What are the client's support systems or resources? What are the family dynamics? What is the family's response to the present illness? Provides emotional support.

- *Therapeutic Communication:* Helps client to communicate their needs to other health care team members. Always communicates respect to the client. Promotes and maintains a therapeutic relationship. Encourages appropriate verbal/nonverbal communications. Encourages the client to verbalize feelings. Identifies dynamics of client/family and reports changes accordingly. Listens effectively. Provides emotional support as needed. Utilizes active listening skills.

- *Therapeutic Environment:* Maintains a safe/supportive environment. Actively participates in community meetings as needed. What is the client response to the therapeutic environment?

- *Unexpected Body Image Changes:* Helps client keep an appropriate level of independence, especially after unexpected body image changes (mastectomy). Monitors progress in achieving an improved body image (Is the client accepting the loss? Are they using effective coping skills?). Monitors reactions to body image changes that could affect the recovery (loss of sight or paralysis).

✚ Physiological integrity

Physiological Integrity refers to the nurse's ability to provide care and comfort to promote physical health and well-being. This also includes decreasing the client's risk potential and assisting the client with management of health issues. If we add all of the percentages from the subcategories that fall under Physiological Integrity, we can see that 42% to 66% of your test will come from this content. I would say this is a very important category! Here are some potential test question topics.

Basic care/comfort

Basic care/comfort refers to the nurse's ability to provide comfort and assistance with activities of daily living. A total of 11% to 17% of your exam will come from this subheading. Let's look at a few potential test topics.

- *Assistive Devices:* Assists with ambulation using a gait belt, lift, crutches, walker, or cane. Assists in care of clients who use assistive devices or prosthesis (crutches, dentures, artificial limbs, or telecommunication devices). Is the client using the assistive device appropriately? Reviews the correct use of assistive devices with other members of the health care team and client. Uses appropriate transfer devices (mechanical lift, T-belt).

- *Elimination:* Assists with developing a bowel/bladder retraining program. Assists in teaching ostomy care. Is able to discontinue a urinary catheter. Is able to insert a urinary catheter. Is able to provide interventions for altered bowel elimination (removes impactions, administers enema). Is able to irrigate urinary catheter. Measures output. Provides ostomy care. Is able to care for incontinent client. Recognizes issues that could interfere with elimination (medications or fluid restrictions). Is able to record output from nasogastric tube, vomitus, or urine. Reinforces teaching on ways to prevent constipation and or incontinence. Uses alternative methods to assist client with voiding (turns on water faucet).

- *Mobility/Immobility:* Is able to apply and remove mobilization equipment (brace or splint). Considering mobility level, assists in teaching client to change positions frequently. Checks mobility, strength, gait, and motor skills. Is able to maintain correct body alignment. Monitors improvements from the hazards of immobility (improvement of skin breakdown areas or contractures). What is the client's response to immobility? Prevents complications of immobility (performs range of motion, uses equipment to prevent contractures). Reinforces teaching and requests return demonstration on exercises that increase and maintain mobility (range of motion, isometric exercises). Uses correct body mechanics at all times. Protects and maintains skin integrity (turns client at regular intervals, utilizes alternating pressure mattresses).

- *Nonpharmacological Interventions for Comfort:* Is able to apply heat/cold treatments appropriately. Monitors for nonverbal signs of discomfort (grimacing). Monitors response after pain-relief interventions (utilizes a pain rating scale). Has the client verbally report on effectiveness of interventions and notes nonverbal behaviors as well. Incorporates complementary/alternative therapies into care (massage or music relaxation therapy). Utilizes nonpharmacological interventions to decrease or relieve pain (repositioning or distraction therapy). Recognizes initial discomfort and pain level. Is nonjudgmental of client's rating of pain or response to interventions.

- *Nutrition/Oral Hydration:* Checks for proper feeding tube placement. Collects data regarding diet history. Considers food preferences. Reinforces teaching in regard to diet restrictions (low-sodium diet, low-fat diet). Determines nutritional status (skin turgor check, review of diet history). Can determine hydration status (I & O, signs of dehydration, presence of edema). Monitors ability to chew or swallow. Recognizes food/medication interactions. Monitors for side effects associated with tube feedings and intervenes appropriately (is the client having any gastrointestinal symptoms such as diarrhea?). Does the client have signs of dehydration? Monitors weight. How does the client's disease affect the nutritional status? Initiates/cares for/discontinues tube feedings (nasogastric tube, gastrostomy tube). Is able to perform calorie counts. Assists client to be independent while eating (proper placement of food on meal tray, proper client positioning). Provides nutritional substances as appropriate (high-protein beverages). Provides special diets based on diagnosis and specific nutritional needs (low-sodium diet, high-protein diet, calorie-restrictive diet). Reinforces teaching on specific foods and diet changes needed as related to a specific health problem (low-sodium diet is needed for congestive heart failure clients). Utilizes ways to improve intake (administers small feedings, administers tube feedings, feeds the client if needed). Is able to weigh client accurately.

- *Palliative/Comfort Care:* Is able to identify the need for palliative/comfort care and monitors response to interventions accordingly. Is able to monitor symptoms related to palliative/comfort care (Is the client fatigued? Are they having breathing difficulty?). Notes response to care after palliative/comfort care interventions.

- *Personal Hygiene:* Assists with basic hygiene as needed. Determines ability to perform activities of daily living. Reinforces understanding of equipment used for personal hygiene (use of shower, use of a chair in shower, or use of handrails).

- *Rest and Sleep:* Identifies usual rest/sleep patterns (What time does the client usually go to bed? Does he have any bedtime rituals?). Helps plan interventions to improve clients rest/sleep. Schedules activities to promote proper rest and sleep.

Since I know you are dying for more topics you could be tested on, I've included a few more: proper body mechanics; acupressure; administering feedings through a nasogastric tube; feeding through gastrointestinal tube/jejunal tube; flushing after a tube feeding; administering a tube-feeding bolus; caring for a continuous feeding; changing the feeding bag appropriately; checking residuals; checking for placement of tubes; use of nonpharmacological measures for pain relief (imagery, massage, or repositioning); discontinuing or removing an intravenous line/nasogastric tube/urinary catheter; performing irrigation of a urinary catheter/bladder/ear/wound/nose/eye; providing care for a client in traction.

Pharmacological therapy

Pharmacological therapy refers to the nurse's ability to provide appropriate care in relation to the administration of medication. This also includes monitoring the client who is receiving parenteral therapy. A total of 9% to 15% of your test will come from this subheading. Potential test question topics are as follows.

- *Adverse Effects:* Appropriately documents adverse effects to medication/parenteral therapy. Follows the proper procedure to counteract adverse effects of medication (this includes identifying and documenting the client's response). Is able to recognize symptoms of an adverse medication effect (allergic reaction). Constantly monitors for adverse effects of medications (whether the medication is prescribed or an herbal supplement). Notifies the primary health care provider in regard to adverse effects of medications/parenteral therapy. Reinforces teaching on possible adverse medication side effects. Reviews common side effects with the client and reinforces when the client is to notify their primary health care provider. Knows when to withhold a medication dose (if client is experiencing an adverse reaction to medication).

- *Expected Effects:* Is able to identify the expected response of the medication. Reinforces teaching on expected effects of medication. Is the client improving with new prescription or over-the-counter medication?

- *Medication Administration:* Is able to administer eye, ear, and nose drops. Is able to administer oral, intradermal, subcutaneous, intramuscular, topical, or internal medications. Prepares the client for insertion of a central line. Properly calculates the client's medication dose. Can discontinue an IV line. Disposes of unused medications according to agency policy. Documents medication administration properly. Identifies the need for PRN medications. Provides information regarding the actions and therapeutic effects of medications. Appropriately maintains medication administration schedule and record. Maintains controlled substances according to legal guidelines and agency policy. Is able to mix medications from two vials. Is able to monitor client's condition during blood transfusions or during intravenous administration of drugs. Monitors IV site and flow rate. Is able to phone a prescription into the pharmacy. Reinforces teaching on self-administration of medications. Frequently checks chart for medication prescription changes. Always uses the five "rights" when administering medications.

- *Pharmacological Actions and Agents:* Identifies incompatibilities of medications. Identifies contraindications to over-the-counter medications. Is able to recognize and report appropriately the client's response to pharmacological agents and over-the-counter drugs. Knows when to use resources in seeking further information and uses them appropriately in regard to pharmacological agents. Reinforces teaching on the actions of medications and the therapeutic effects of medications.

- *Side Effects:* Documents appropriately side effects to medications/parenteral therapy. Monitors response to the management of side effects. Knows when to notify the primary health care provider about side effects. Reviews ways to manage side effects.

Here are some more goodies you may be interested in: administers rectal and vaginal medications, performs narcotic count/controlled substance count.

Reduction of risk potential

Reduction of Risk Potential refers to the nurse's ability to decrease the potential for clients to develop complications/health problems as it relates to their treatments/procedures/existing conditions. 10–16% of your exam will come from this subheading. Here are some potential test question topics.

- *Diagnostic Tests:* Determines if the client is prepared for the test. Monitors test results (blood glucose, pulse oximetry). Monitors client during/after test. Performs tests appropriately. Prepares the client for the test. Recognizes if the client understands purpose of test. Reinforces any teaching about test. Is able to review pacemaker function.

- *Lab Values:* Collects lab specimens. Compares client's lab values to normal lab values. Is able to explain the proper procedure for specimen collection. Monitors for abnormal lab values. Knows when to notify the primary health care provider about lab tests. Reinforces any teaching regarding the purpose of lab tests.

- *Potential for Alterations in the Systems of the Body:* Collects specimens (urine, stool, or sputum). Compares present clinical data to baseline data. Knows symptoms of diseases. Identifies clients at risk for poor circulation (postsurgical clients, diabetic clients). Is able to identify a client at risk for aspiration (clients with a feeding tube, sedated clients, or clients with swallowing problems). Identifies clients at risk for skin breakdown (immobile clients, poorly nourished clients, or incontinent clients). Identifies factors that could interfere with wound healing (poor circulation). Identifies appropriate interventions that could prevent complications associated with the present health problem (foot care for the diabetic client). Identifies signs of potential prenatal complications (bleeding, contractions, high blood pressure). Monitors for peripheral edema. Monitors for hypoglycemia. Monitors for hyperglycemia. Monitors for bowel sounds. Monitors output and recognizes changes from baseline. Monitors peripheral pulses. Is able to perform a bladder scan. Performs neurological checks. Recognizes changes in neurological status (level of consciousness, muscle strength). Reinforces teaching on ways to prevent complications associated with present health problems and a decreased activity level (ways to prevent contractures, ways to prevent problems with the feet in a diabetic client).

- *Potential for Complications Related to Diagnostic Tests/Treatments/Procedures/Surgery:* Identifies response to diagnostic tests/treatments/procedures/surgery. Identifies signs of aspiration and is able to intervene to prevent aspiration (checks feeding tube placement, knows proper positioning of client when administering a tube feeding). Identifies signs of neurological complications (foot drop, numbness/tingling). Identifies signs of poor venous return and utilizes interventions to improve venous return (utilizes elastic stockings or sequential compression devices). Identifies signs of circulatory complications and utilizes interventions to manage circulatory complications (hemorrhage, embolus, shock). Intervenes to control symptoms of hypoglycemia/hyperglycemia.

Maintains tube placement (gastric tubes, chest tubes, tracheostomy tubes). Is able to monitor client recovering from conscious sedation. Monitors for signs of bleeding. Monitors wounds for signs of infection. Notifies health care provider in the presence of complications or potential complications (fever, limb pain, thrombus formation, low blood pressure, poor circulation of casted extremity). Provides care for clients receiving electroconvulsive therapy. Recognizes the client's response to interventions that check for or prevent complications (checks breath sounds, checks pulse oximeter, checks bowel sounds, checks mobility). Reinforces teaching that can prevent complications (the importance of coughing and deep breathing postoperatively, the use of elastic stockings to prevent blood clots). Recognizes responses to interventions (decreased fever after administration of Tylenol, normal vital signs).

- *Therapeutic Procedures:* Is able to determine if client is prepared properly for procedures/surgery. Identifies client's response to procedures/surgery. Documents appropriately. Is able to monitor client before, during, and after procedure/surgery. Monitors proper functioning of therapeutic devices (chest tubes, drainage tubes, continuous bladder irrigation). Is able to perform an EKG. Prepares client for procedure/surgery (maintains NPO status before surgery). Provides intraoperative/perioperative care (positioning of client, maintaining a sterile field). Observes accurately during a procedure and documents response appropriately. Recognizes proper recovery from local/regional/general anesthesia. Recognizes appropriate understanding of procedure/surgery.

- *Vital Signs:* Is able to compare present vital signs to baseline vital signs and documents appropriately. Reinforces teaching regarding normal/abnormal vital signs. Accurately obtains vital signs.

You want some more? O.K., here it is: performs risk assessment (potential for falls); follows up appropriately post-incidents such as a fall, elopement of client, or a medication error; monitors continuous/intermittent suction of a nasogastric tube; insertion of a nasogastric tube; monitors O_2 saturation.

Physiological adaptation

Physiological Adaptation refers to the nurse's ability to participate in providing care for clients with acute/chronic/life-threatening physical health conditions. A total of 12% to 18% of your exam will come from this subheading. Here are some potential test question topics to review.

- *Alterations in Body Systems/Basic Pathophysiology:* Understands general principles of disease processes (injury/repair of tissue, immunity). Appropriately documents response to interventions (pacemaker, chest tubes). Is able to identify signs of infection. Intervenes as appropriate to improve respiratory status (teaches turning, coughing, and deep breathing; suctions when needed). Is able to care for clients with alterations in skin integrity. Is able to care for clients in traction (external fixation devices, halo traction, skeletal traction). Maintains appropriate body temperature (use of hypothermia units, cold packs, or blankets).

Is able to monitor a closed wound drainage system (documents amount and characteristics of drainage). Knows when to notify the primary health care provider if a client's health status has changed. Promotion of wound healing (application of dressing, proper nutrition, irrigation of wound). Provides care of the client experiencing complications of pregnancy/labor/delivery (eclampsia, precipitous labor, hemorrhage). Is able to provide care for the client with increased intracranial pressure. Provides care for the client with a drainage device (chest tubes, wound drains). Provides care when a vascular access for hemodialysis is present (atrioventricular shunt, fistula). Provides care for physiological problems (hypoglycemia or hyperglycemia). Provides care for the client who has had a seizure. Provides care for someone on a ventilator. Is able to provide care that will correct an alteration in a body system (administers phototherapy to newborns). Provides care for a client receiving peritoneal dialysis according to agency protocol. Provides wound care. Reinforces teaching on management of health issues (chronic illnesses such as autoimmune deficiency syndrome and diabetes). Reinforces the client's understanding of care needs with impaired tissue perfusion (care of the client with a decubitis ulcer/incision/skin graft).

- *Fluid and Electrolyte Balance:* Monitors response to interventions that will correct fluid and electrolyte imbalances. Provides interventions to re-establish fluid and electrolyte balance (encourages fluids appropriately). Recognizes signs of a fluid and electrolyte imbalance (dehydration).

- *Medical Emergencies:* Is able to explain emergency interventions. Understands and implements cardiopulmonary resuscitation appropriately. Recognizes and intervenes in life-threatening situations (CPR/Heimlich maneuver, intervenes during fetal distress, intervenes if a pacemaker malfunctions). Notifies health care provider in emergency situations. Is able to provide care for wound complications (evisceration, dehiscence). Follows up appropriately after a medical emergency. Recognizes signs of a medical emergency (increasing intracranial pressure or hemorrhage).

- *Radiation Therapy:* Documents client's response to radiation therapy (documents condition of skin post-radiation therapy). Is able to provide appropriate interventions if client is having side effects of radiation therapy (teaches client to avoid the sun, small frequent meals for nausea). Recognizes side effects or adverse side effects of radiation therapy.

- *Unexpected Response to Therapies:* Documents appropriately unexpected responses. Identifies unexpected negative responses to therapy (increased intracranial pressure or hemorrhage). Intervenes appropriately when unexpected negative responses to therapy occur (bleeding). Promotes recovery from unexpected negative responses to therapy.

We have a few more fun topics to include here: removes drains (hemovac, Jackson–Pratt, or penrose); improves respiratory status by administering a breathing treatment/suctioning/repositioning; provides care of a tracheostomy; recognizes when an intravenous line has infiltrated; is able to remove sutures or staples; recognizes abnormalities on the EKG.

LET'S WRAP IT UP

Let me make you feel better. You do not have to know everything in this chapter to pass! If you see something you've never heard of, go ahead and review that topic to decrease your anxiety. Don't forget . . . the NCLEX® Lady thinks of you as a new nurse with 2 weeks of vast nursing knowledge. Therefore, you are expected to have a *basic* understanding of these topics, because the NCLEX® Lady knows you're not an expert yet!

Bibliography

Hurst Review Services. **www.hurstreviewservices.com** National Council of State Boards of Nursing. *2005 NCLEX-PN® Detailed Test Plan, NCLEX® Examinations.*

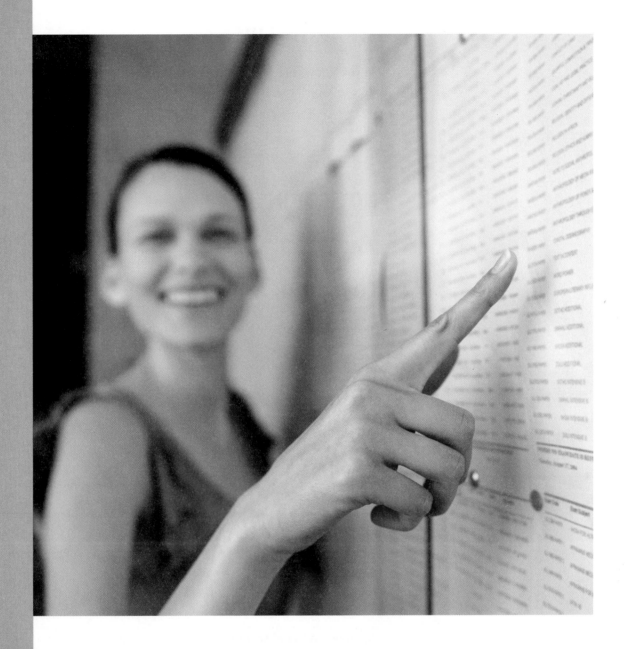

13 Cool Charts You Just Have to Know

LET'S GET THE NORMAL STUFF STRAIGHT FIRST

As you know there are so many numbers, skills, and little gems of knowledge to keep straight in nursing. I've compiled everything right here in easy-to-read charts with helpful drawings and photos. What do you think of the sexy blond in the photos? Not bad for an ol' Southern nurse author, huh?

NOT AGAIN . . .

Yes, here it is again . . . the nursing process. Just read over it one last time.

COMMUNICATION

As nurses, our job isn't to yak all the time, but to communicate effectively. These charts will remind you how to communicate therapeutically with clients and family.

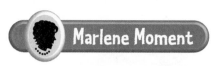

Marlene Moment

I hope your client doesn't hold up a sign that says, "I want another nurse!"

Table 13-1. The Nursing Process

Assessment	• Collecting and organizing data • Recording of subjective/objective data
Forming a Diagnosis	• Analyzing data • Identifying specific client needs • Establishing a nursing diagnosis
Planning and Goal Setting	• Prioritizing how to solve client problems • Identifying goals or client outcomes to measure the effectiveness of nursing actions • Selecting nursing interventions • Writing nursing orders
Implementation	• Reassessing the client • Implementing the nursing orders • Delegating and supervising • Documenting nursing actions
Evaluation	• Collecting data related to outcomes • Comparing data with outcomes • Drawing conclusions • Continuing, modifying, or terminating client's plan of care

Table 13-2. How to Communicate with the Nonverbal Patient

Ask the client to point to the appropriate word, or if that is not possible, ask the client to blink when you call out the appropriate word.

I am too: COLD HOT	Close: BLINDS DOOR
I am: HUNGRY THIRSTY	
YES NO THANK YOU PLEASE OK	I need: GLASSES BATH SHOWER
Pain: 0 1 2 3 4 5 6 7 8 9 10	
Please turn on/off: LIGHT TV	I am: NAUSEATED FRUSTRATED CONFUSED
Please help me: TURN OVER SIT UP GET UP	
Please call: SPOUSE FRIEND CHILD DOCTOR	

Table 13-3. Therapeutic Communication Barriers

Giving advice	Judging
Stereotyping	Being defensive
Appearing distracted or uninterested	Agreeing or disagreeing
Not being a good listener	Appearing biased
Excessive probing	

FOOD!
....

We can't live without it, and when ill, we require special dietary considerations. Nutritional deficits can have severe consequences.

Table 13-4. Nutrients

What nutrient?	Why is it needed?	Where does it come from?
Water	Water carries nutrients, lubricates joints, and regulates body function and processes	Water, other beverages/liquids, fruits, vegetables
Carbohydrates	Regulates body temperature, brain function, and energy	Sugars, fruits, grains, nuts, potatoes, breads, milk, fruit
Protein	Tissue repair and growth	Nuts, beans, milk, fish, eggs, poultry, meat
Fat	Carries vitamins A and D, energy	Nuts, milk, fish, animal fat

** The food list above includes examples of food sources but is not an exhaustive list**

Figure 13-1
Figure 13-2

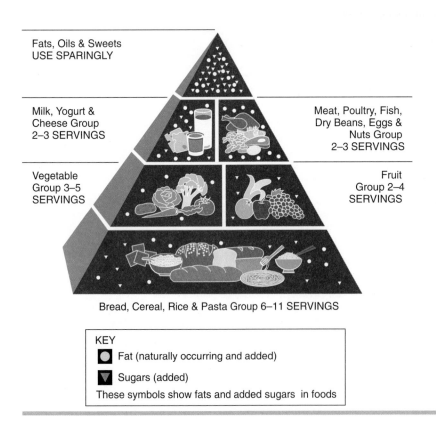

Fats, Oils & Sweets
USE SPARINGLY

Milk, Yogurt &
Cheese Group
2–3 SERVINGS

Meat, Poultry, Fish,
Dry Beans, Eggs &
Nuts Group
2–3 SERVINGS

Vegetable
Group 3–5
SERVINGS

Fruit
Group 2–4
SERVINGS

Bread, Cereal, Rice & Pasta Group 6–11 SERVINGS

KEY
◯ Fat (naturally occurring and added)
▼ Sugars (added)
These symbols show fats and added sugars in foods

Nutrition Facts

Serving Size 1/2 cup (114 g)
Servings Per Container 4

Amount Per Serving	
Calories 90	Calories from Fat 30

	% Daily value*
Total Fat 3 g	5%
Saturated Fat 0 g	0%
Cholesterol 0 mg	0%
Sodium 300 mg	13%
Total Carbohydrate 13 g	4%
Dietary Fiber 3 g	12%
Sugars 3 g	
Protein 3 g	

Vitamin A	80%	•	Vitamin C	60%
Calcium	4%	•	Iron	4%

* Percent Daily Values are based on a 2000 calorie diet. Your daily values may be higher or lower depending on your calorie needs;

	Calories	2000	2000
Total Fat	Less than	66 g	80 g
Sat Fat	Less than	20 g	25 g
Cholesterol	Less than	300 mg	300 mg
Sodium	Less than	2400 mg	2400 mg
Total Carbohydrate		300 g	375 g
Fiber		25 g	30 g

Calories per gram:
Fat 9 • Carbohydrate 4 • Protein 4

Table 13-5. Special Dietary Considerations

Pancreatitis	• Avoid alcohol • Bland foods • Small, frequent meals • Decrease fat
Cholecystitis	• Decrease fat • Small, frequent meals
Hepatitis	• NPO initially • Low fat • High protein/carbohydrates
Cirrhosis	• Small, frequent meals • Low sodium/protein
Diaphragmatic Hernia	• Decrease portion sizes • Decrease fat • Increase frequency of meals • Increase protein
Dumping Syndrome	• Increase fat/protein/fiber • Increase frequency of meals • Decrease portion sizes/fluids with meals • Decrease carbohydrate intake
Diverticulosis	• NPO initially • Increase fluids • Bland/soft foods • High-fiber foods, but avoid foods that are difficult to digest such as corn, seeds, and nuts
Ulcerative Colitis	• AVOID coarse, high-fiber, raw fruits/veggies, cold beverages • Increase bland foods • Increase protein • Increase calories
Celiac Disease	• No gluten • Increase calories • Increase protein
Renal Failure (Acute)	• Increase carbohydrates • Limit protein (good rule of thumb for anyone with kidney failure until otherwise specified by physician) • Decrease sodium • Fluid restriction
Renal Failure (Chronic)	• Avoid high potassium foods • Low sodium • High iron • High calcium, vitamins B, C, D

(Continued)

Table 13-5. Special Dietary Considerations (*Continued*)

Cushing's Syndrome	• Increase protein • Increase potassium • Decrease sodium • Decrease calories
Addison's Disease	• Increase sodium • Low potassium
Ménière's Disease	• No alcohol • Low sodium
Heart Failure	• Low sodium • Low fat • Fluid restriction in some patients

✛ Eating disorders

Table 13-6. Characteristics Eating Disorders

Anorexia nervosa (self-induced starvation)	Bulimia (binge-and-purge)
• 10–25 years old (average 13) • Denies eating pattern is abnormal • Increase physical activity • Intense fear of becoming obese • Slow eating • Preoccupation with food • Body image disturbances • Low caloric intake (usually 400–800 calories) • Hair loss • Amenorrhea (absence of menstruation) • Loss of 20–40% of usual body weight	• Older, college age • Recognize that the eating pattern is abnormal • Keeps weight within normal range • Unable to control food intake • Binging is the consumption of 5000–25,000 calories/day • Purging is the intentional elimination of food from the body by vomiting, enemas, diuretics, laxatives (used alone or in combination)

✚ Fluid

Fluid leaves the body each day by several different routes. This is important to remember when assessing, evaluating, and recording fluid loss.

Table 13-7. Fluid Escape

Skin	Lungs	GI tract	Kidneys
	● Diffusion (Skin): 400 mL		
	● Perspiration (Skin): 100 mL		
	● Lungs: 325–350 mL		
	● Feces (GI tract): 120–150 mL		
	● Kidneys: 1200–1500 mL		

✚ Conversions

You need to know basic conversions for those pesky NCLEX® questions on drug dosing and client intake.

Table 13-8. Basic Volume/Weight Conversions

Volume	Weight
1 tsp = 5 mL	1 mg = 1000 µg
1 tbsp = 15 mL	1 g = 1000 mg
1 oz = 30 mL	1 gr = 60 mg
1 cup (8 oz) = 240 mL	1 kg = 2.2 lb
1 soda (12 oz) = 360 mL	1 L of water = 1 kg
1 pint = 480 mL	
1 quart = 960 mL	

STRIKE A POSE

Body positioning is very important for:
- Maintaining body alignment.
- Preventing friction and sheer on the tissue, thus helping maintain skin integrity.
- Preventing injury and limiting deformity.
- Promoting comfort.
- Promoting optimal lung expansion.

Table 13-9. Body Positioning

Position	Purpose	Description
Fowler's Figure 13-3A 	• Prevents aspiration • Promotes comfort • Improves breathing capacity	• HOB 30–90 degrees • Knees slightly flexed • Semi-sitting position
Supine Figure 13-3B 	• Position of choice after certain procedures	• Flat on back • Body in alignment
Prone Figure 13-3C 	• Positioning alternative for bedridden client • Rotating position for low-limb amputees to promote extension of the stump	• Flat on the abdomen • Knees slightly flexed • Feet over the end of the mattress to support normal flexion
Lateral (side-lying) Figure 13-3D 	• Positioning alternative • Used for some procedures	• Lying on the side with the upper leg flexed at the hip and knee • Top arm flexed

Table 13-9. Body Positioning (*Continued*)

Position	Purpose	Description
Sims Figure 13-3E 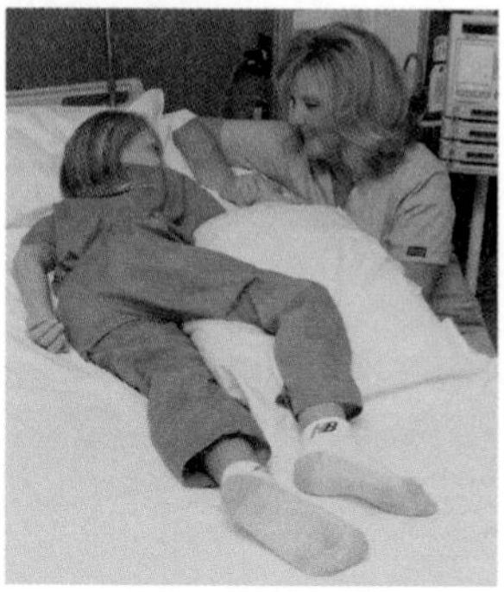	• Positioning alternative • Used for some procedures	• Positioned between prone and side-lying • Knees slightly flexed • Upper arm flexed • Lower arm behind back
Lithotomy Figure 13-3F 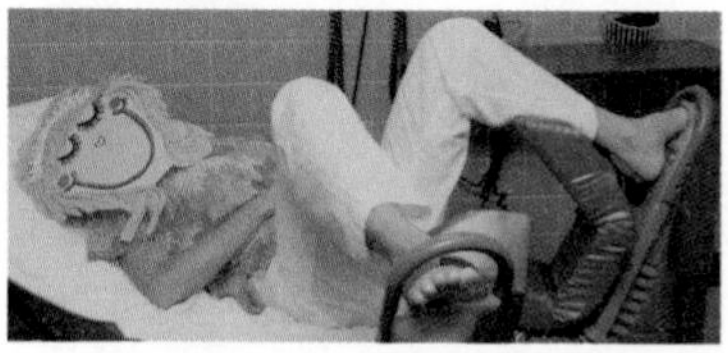	• Position for anal/rectal or vaginal exams	• Client supine with legs flexed at 90 degrees • Feet in stirrups
Modified Trendelenburg Figure 13-3G 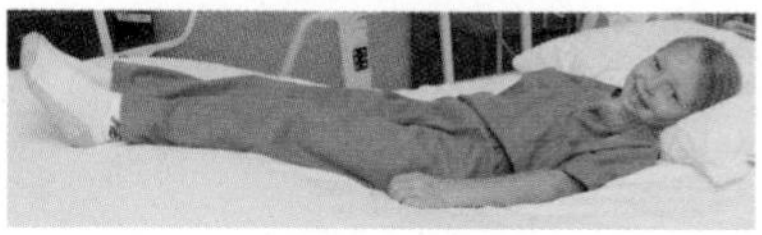	• "Shock" position • Increases blood flow to the heart and brain	• Supine • Legs straight and elevated at the hips • Head slightly raised

VITAL SIGNS ARE KEY!

Taking and monitoring vital signs are a critical nursing skill. You must be aware of the normal and abnormal vital signs of the different age populations. It is important to remember that vital signs will vary across the lifespan.

✚ Vital signs at a glance

Table 13-10. Vital Signs

Age	Temperature (°F)	Pulse rate (beats/min)	Respiratory rate (breaths/min)	Blood pressure (mm Hg)
Neonate	98.6–99.8	110–160	30–50	70–73/45–48
1 month–3 years	98.5–99.5	80–130	20–30	90–100/55–63
6–10 years	97.5–98.6	75–115	17–25	96–110/57–72
16 years	97.6–98.6	55–100	15–20	120–123/76–80
Adult	96.8–98.6	50–95	15–20	120/80
Elderly >70	96.5–97.5	55–95	15–20	120/80

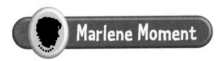

Marlene Moment

Your BP and pulse are going to be very high, and you will be diaphoretic when you take the NCLEX®. That's because your adrenals will kick in!

Table 13-11. Blood Pressure Monitoring

To obtain an accurate BP reading be aware of the following:

- Make sure the patient does not smoke or consume caffeine within 30 minutes prior to measurement.
- Place the arm at the level of the heart in a straight position (if the arm is below the heart level, the BP reading will be elevated; if it is above the heart, the BP reading will be decreased).
- Determine the size cuff that will be needed and apply it to the patient's arm. Make sure that the bladder of the cuff encircles at least $2/3$ of the arm and the width of the cuff covers $1/2$ to $2/3$ of the upper arm.
- Inflate the cuff 30 mm Hg higher than the expected systolic reading.
- Record your finding.
- Always wait at least 1 minute before taking the BP in the same arm again.
- If the cuff is too small, you will get a false high reading; if the cuff is too big, you will get a false low reading.

PROTECT YOURSELF AND YOUR CLIENTS

Wearing gloves and washing your hands before and after every client contact will protect you and your clients from transferring microbes.

Table 13-12. Universal Precautions

- ALWAYS wear gloves
- Wash hands before and after patient contact
- Do not recap or bend needles
- Wear eye shields when there is a potential for splash
- Wear mask when the patient is coughing or sneezing
- Wear gowns when warranted
- Get appropriate vaccinations

✛ It's sterile . . . be careful

Table 13-13. Sterile Field

- Do not turn your back on the sterile field
- Do not talk or laugh
- Do not place sterile objects below your waist
- Keep all sterile objects within view
- Open all sterile packages away from the sterile field
- Avoid moisture on the sterile field
- Do not reach across the sterile field

Table 13-14. Latex Allergy

Interventions	Products to be aware of
<ul><li>Use nonlatex gloves</li><li>Use latex-free/safe supplies</li><li>Use a barrier between the BP cuff and the client's skin</li><li>Keep the latex-free/safe supplies in a designated place that is easily accessible</li><li>Label the chart clearly indicating patient's allergy</li><li>Make sure the patient has an armband with the allergy listed and that signs are posted in the room</li></ul>	<ul><li>Ambu bag</li><li>Catheters</li><li>ACE bandages</li><li>Blood pressure cuff/tubing/bladder</li><li>Elastic pressure stockings</li><li>EKG pads</li><li>Gloves</li><li>IV catheters</li><li>Pads for crutches</li><li>Prepackaged enema kits</li><li>Syringes</li><li>Tourniquets</li><li>Stethoscopes</li></ul>

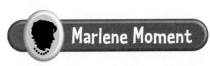

Marlene Moment

For you latex condom users, you might want to swap up a little every now and then and use something different, or you may develop a latex allergy. Just a little advice from Aunt Marlene . . . .

SKIN

The skin is our largest organ and can give us so much information about what is going on with our clients.

Table 13-15. Skin Assessment

Color	• Pallor
	• Redness
	• Cyanosis
	• Jaundice
Moisture	• Dry
	• Excessively moist (diaphoresis)
Temperature	• Cool
	• Warm
Turgor	• Poor
	• Good
Swelling/Edema	• Bilateral
	• Unilateral
Lesions	• Presence and type of skin lesion

✚ Skin turgor

Table 13-16. The Pinch Test

Pinch the skin of the forearm or sternum. The skin normally will resume its shape within a few seconds. If it does not and remains wrinkled for >20 seconds, the skin turgor is poor. Poor skin turgor may indicate recent weight loss or dehydration. It may, however, be a normal variant of aging.

Figure 13-4

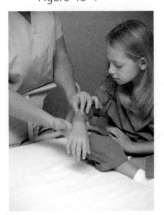

Table 13-17. Skin Breakdown

Stages	Description
I	• Intact skin • Nonblanching erythema
II	• Epidermis interrupted • Dermis may be interrupted • Abrasion or blister
III	• Full thickness • Damage and/or necrosis down to the fascia
IV	• Full thickness • Penetrates the fascia • Involves muscle, tendon, and/or bone

Table 13-18. Skin Lesions

Lesion	Description	Example
Macule	Flat, nonpalpable, <1 cm	Freckle
Papule	Palpable, elevated, <1 cm	Wart or mole
Nodule	Elevated, firm with circumscribed borders, 1–2 cm	Lipomas
Pustule	Elevated, serous/pus filled vesicle, vary in size, <1 cm	Impetigo, acne
Wheal	Elevated, erythematous with irregular borders that contain fluid in the tissue	Insect bite, hives
Vesicle	Elevated, fluid filled <1 cm	Herpes zoster (shingles)
Bulla	Elevated, fluid filled >1 cm	Varicella (chickenpox), small burns, herpes lesions
Cyst	Elevated, firm	Sebaceous

Table 13-19. Skin Cancer Lesions

• Irregular shape
• Color variation with hues of tan, black, brown, or blue
• Red, nodular lesion
• Bleeding lesion
• Crusting lesion
• Waxy nodule
• Mole, freckle, or birthmark that changes in appearance, texture, or size

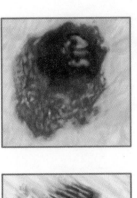
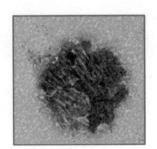
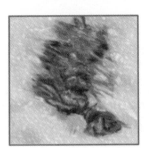
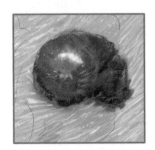
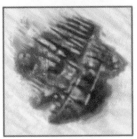

Figure 13-5 ▶

Table 13-20. Causes of Burns

Thermal	Excessive heat from a fire, flames, hot liquids, hot objects, steam, or heating pad
Electrical	Lightning, electrical current
Chemical	Acids, bases, or caustics
Light	Sunlight, ultraviolet light
Radiation	Ultraviolet light, nuclear radiation

Table 13-21. Burn Classification

First-Degree Burn (Superficial thickness)	Limited to the epidermis Painful Skin will appear red Requires local wound care (Example: sunburn)
Second-Degree Burn (Partial thickness)	Extends beyond the epidermis into the dermis Painful Skin will appear red, swollen, and blisters will appear
Third-Degree Burn (Full thickness)	Extends through the dermis leaving only the subcutaneous tissue Painless Skin will be dry and have a leathery appearance
Fourth-Degree Burn	Rare and usually fatal Extends through the subcutaneous tissue into the muscles, fascia, and bone

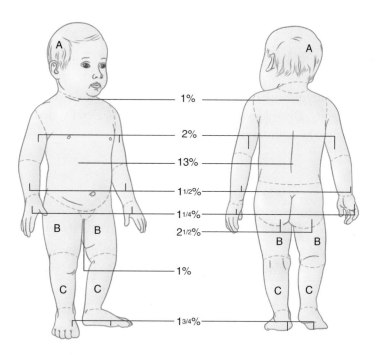

◀ Figure 13-6. Lund and Browder classification.

▶ Figure 13-7. Rule of nines.

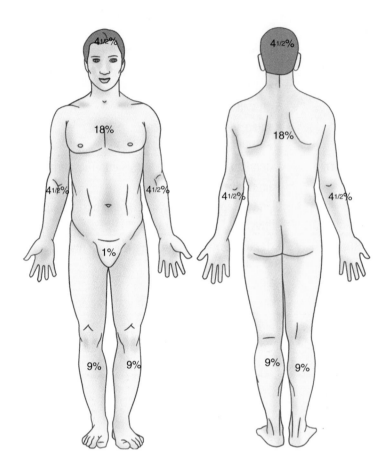

MUSCULOSKELETAL SYSTEM

The musculoskeletal assessment is important for detecting injury and disability. Disorders that affect the musculoskeletal system may also involve the neurologic system.

Table 13-22. Muscle Strength

5/5 Normal	The patient has full ROM against gravity and full resistance
4/5 Good	The patient has full ROM against gravity and moderate resistance
3/5 Fair	The patient has full ROM against gravity ONLY
2/5 Poor	The patient has only passive ROM
1/5 Trace	The patient has muscle contraction that is palpable but no joint movement is noted
0/5 Absent	The patient has NO evidence of muscle contraction

Table 13-23. Traction

- Ensure that all ropes, weights, and pulleys are hanging freely
- Keep all lines off of the traction ropes
- Do not lift the weights for any reason
- Avoid jarring the bed or equipment
- Provide frequent neuron checks
- Provide frequent circulatory checks including: color, temperature, pulses, and capillary refill
- Perform periodic skin assessments
- Keep the body in proper alignment
- Monitor for infection (fever, localized warmth, redness, swelling, odor, or increasing pain)
- Do not massage the calves
- Increase fluid and fiber intake (unless medically contraindicated)
- Encourage coughing and deep breathing
- Encourage use of the overhead trapeze bar
- Provide diversional activities

Table 13-24. Compartment Syndrome

Occurs when swelling or bleeding increases within the muscle compartment to the point that it interferes with circulation. It is life threatening to the limb and requires immediate attention. Most common sites include forearm, hand, lower leg, and foot.

Signs and symptoms	Immediate nursing actions
- Recent injury - Intense deep, throbbing pain that does not improve with pain medications - The pain is often out of proportion to the injury - Pulses may be weak or absent - Sensation and strength may be decreased - May have numbness and tingling	- Monitor vital signs for low blood pressure and tachycardia - Remove dressings, cast, rings, etc. from the area (relieve the pressure . . . restore the circulation) - Elevate the extremity above the level of the heart - Provide frequent neuro/circulatory checks - Prepare for probable procedures - Administer pain medications as ordered - Administer IV fluids as ordered - Call physician at once

NEUROLOGICAL SYSTEM

The great thing about performing a neurological assessment is using that hammer to tap away on people. I just love that!

Table 13-25. Deep Tendon Reflexes

Reflexes

0 = Absent

+ = Hypoactive

+ + = Normal

+ + + = Increased (brisk)

+ + + + = Hyperactive

Figure 13-8

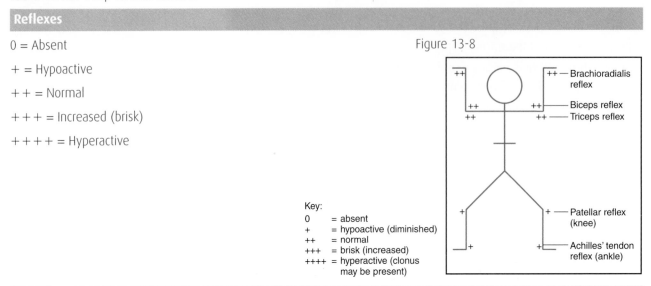

Key:
0	= absent
+	= hypoactive (diminished)
++	= normal
+++	= brisk (increased)
++++	= hyperactive (clonus may be present)

✚ The Frenchman and the German

Table 13-26. Cranial Nerve Function

On **O**ld **O**lympus **T**owing **T**ops **A** **F**renchman **A**nd **G**erman **V**iewed **S**ome **H**ops	
CN I **O**lfactory	Smell
CN II **O**ptic	Vision
CN III **O**cculomotor	Upper eyelid elevation, pupillary constriction, extraocular movement
CN IV **T**rochlear	Downward and inward eye movement
CN V **T**rigeminal	Corneal reflex, chewing, face and scalp sensations
CN VI **A**bducens	Lateral eye movement
CN VII **F**acial	Taste, expressions in the forehead, eye, and mouth
CN VIII **A**coustic	Hearing and balance
CN IX **G**lossopharyngeal	Taste, swallowing, and salivation
CN X **V**agus	Gag reflex, swallowing, talking, sensations of the throat and larynx
CN XI **S**pinal accessory	Head rotation, shoulder shrug (movement)
CN XII **H**ypoglossal	Tongue movement

Table 13-27. Pupil Assessment

1. Equal or unequal
2. Reactive or nonreactive
3. Brisk or sluggish
4. Size

Pupil gauge

Figure 13-9

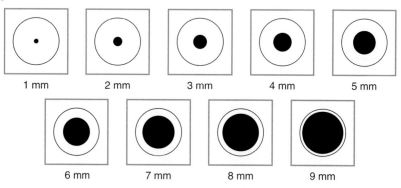

| 1 mm | 2 mm | 3 mm | 4 mm | 5 mm |

| 6 mm | 7 mm | 8 mm | 9 mm |

Table 13-28. Beware of the Following Findings

Battle Sign	Ecchymoses over the mastoid process in basilar skull fractures. This sign usually occurs 48 hours after the event
Diplopia	Double vision
Nystagmus	Constant, involuntary movement of the eyeball
Ptosis	Drooping
Hippus	Rhythmical and rapid dilation and constriction of the pupil

Table 13-29 Signs and Symptoms of the Neurologicaly Injured Patient

- Doll's eyes
- Absence of the oculocephalic reflex
- Extraocular range of motion—abnormal EOROM
- Babinski—upper motor sign that indicates dysfunction (Fig. 13-10)
- Decerebrate posturing (Fig. 13-11A)
- Decorticate posturing (Fig. 13-11B)
- Flexion withdrawal
- Localization

▶ Figure 13-10A Notice the toes are curled toward the top of the foot. This is a negative response. You want to see the toes curl toward the sole of the foot in client greater than 1 year of age.

▶ Figure 13-10B Notice how the toes fan out when the sole of the foot is stroked. This is a positive response. You do not want a positive Babinski in clients over the age of 1.

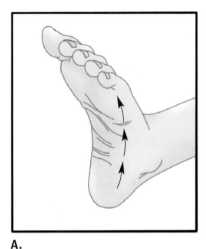
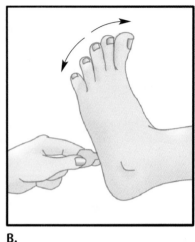

A.   **B.**

▶ Figure 13-11A Decerebrate posturing.

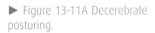

▶ Figure 13-11B Decorticate posturing.

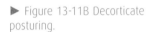

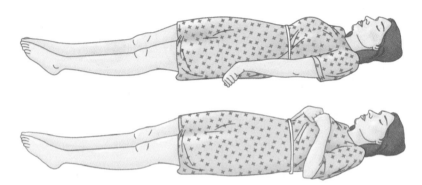

Table 13-30. Seizure

What is it? A seizure is an abnormal electrical discharge that interrupts the brain's nerve conduction. It can be localized or widespread. It is manifested through motor, sensory, or behavioral changes and can occur with or without loss of consciousness.

Generalized	Partial
Absence—brief of consciousness or posture	*Simple*—Focal seizures without loss of consciousness. An aura often precedes the seizure
Myoclonic—repetitive muscle contractions, brief jerking	*Complex*—focal seizure with alteration on level of consciousness. There may be lip smacking, picking at bed clothes, or rocking back and forth
Tonic-clonic—Stiffness followed by loss of consciousness and rhythmic contractions of all four extremities	**Do Not Forget** *Febrile seizures*—Fever is the cause of the seizure

Status Epilepticus

This is a **CONTINUOUS** seizure that **MUST** be interrupted by **emergency** measures

It is **ALWAYS** an **EMERGENCY** because it is often accompanied by respiratory distress

It is usually managed with diazepam (Valium), phenytoin (Dilantin), or phenobarbitol (Luminal). If the condition is related to hypoglycemia (low blood glucose), D50 is used

ABDOMEN

Remember that when performing an abdominal assessment, your assessment order is not in order. Keep this in mind: the abdominal assessment order is atypical!

Table 13-31. Abdominal Assessment

Inspect	• Skin
	• Scars
	• Distention
	• Hernias
Auscultate	• Bowel sounds
	1. Normal = every 15–20 seconds
	2. Hypoactive = every minute
	3. Hyperactive = every 3 seconds
Percuss	• Dullness
	• Tympany
	• Resonance
	• Flatness
Palpate	• Masses
	• Tenderness
	• Pulsations

Table 13-32. Percussion Sounds

Sounds	Pitch	Example
Flat	High	Sternum
Dull	Medium	Kidney, liver
Resonance	Low	Normal lung
Hyperresonance	Lower	Lungs with emphysemic changes
Tympanic	High	stomach

Table 13-33. Referred Pain

Organ involved	Pain referred to . . .
• Appendix	• Right lower quad, right inguinal region
• Abdominal aneurism	• Severe burning back pain
• Bladder	• Suprapubic, posterior gluteus/thigh
• Biliary tract	• Right side of the scapula
• Gallbladder	• Umbilical region, chest, shoulder and scapula
• Liver	• Right shoulder, right side
• Pancreas	• Left upper quad, left hypochondriac region
• Spleen	• Left shoulder, right back
• Renal colic	• Groin and external genitalia, back
• Ruptured peptic ulcer	• Back
• Heart	• Left arm, jaw, shoulder, chest

Table 13-34. Ileostomy versus Colostomy

Type	Purpose	Nursing considerations
Ileostomy	Curative for ulcerative colitis	• One stoma at the terminal ileum • Drains gastric juices • Very irritating and destructive to the skin
Colostomy (loop colostomy)	Relieves obstruction distal to the colostomy site. Usually temporary	• Two openings • Proximal and distal stomas • Proximal stoma drainage is very irritating and destructive to the tissue
Colostomy (end colostomy)	Curative for rectal and colon cancer	• One small stoma • Limit gas-forming foods • Limit high-residue foods • Client may be taught to irrigate the stoma

Table 13-35. GERD (Gastroesophageal Reflux Disease)

Signs and symptoms include sore throat, cough, dyspepsia, heartburn, nausea, and abdominal pain (usually mid-epigastric)

Factors that lessen sphincter tone and increase symptoms:

- Alcohol
- Bending/stooping
- Caffeine
- Chocolate
- Calcium-channel blockers
- Diazepam
- Fatty foods
- Hital hernia
- High levels of estrogen/progesterone (pregnancy)
- Peppermint
- Smoking
- Tight/binding clothes
- Decongestants

Avoid or decrease intake of the above when possible!

HEART

O.K., the heart can get kinda tricky. We know that. These charts help simplify some of the more difficult concepts.

✛ Define time

Table 13-36. Cardiac Terms to Know

Cardiac output	• Volume of blood ejected by the heart in one minute
	• Cardiac output = heart rate × stroke volume
Heart rate	• Influenced by many things, and normal rates vary greatly depending on age
Stroke volume	• The amount of blood ejected by the heart in any one contraction
Preload	• The volume of blood returning to the heart of the circulating blood volume
Afterload	• The resistance against which the ventricles must pump when ejecting blood

Table 13-37. Cardiac Cycle

1. Atria contract (systole) and eject blood into relaxed (diastole) ventricles (ventricles can fill with blood when relaxed)
2. When the atria have completely ejected, atrial relaxation (diastole) occurs. When relaxed, the atria are able to accept blood (as #3 occurs) from the systemic and pulmonary veins.
3. Ventricles begin to contract and eject blood into the pulmonary artery and aorta; atria begin to refill as well.

+ Chambers and valves

Table 13-38. Normal Heart and Blood Flow

Chambers and valves (One-way valves to direct blood flow)
Blood enters right atrium → goes through tricuspid valve → enters right ventricle → goes through pulmonic valve into lungs → leaves lungs through pulmonary veins → enters left atrium → goes through mitral valve (bicuspid) → enters left ventricle → goes through aortic valve out to the systemic circulation
The chambers on the right side of the heart receive blood from the veins ("blue" blood). The chambers on the left side pump oxygenated ("red" blood) out of the heart to the rest of the body
A wall (septum) divides the right and left sides of the heart

Table 13-39. Heart Sounds

	Valve	Location to listen
LISTEN (Auscultate)	Aortic valve (AV)	Right second intercostal space
	Pulmonic valve (PV)	Left second intercostal space
	Tricuspid valve (TV)	Left third and fourth intercostal space
	Mitral valve (MV)	Left mid-clavicular line
Normal Heart Sounds	S1 (apex)	Closure of the tricuspid and mitral valves (SYSTOLE) "Lub"
	S2 (base)	Closure of the pulmonic and aortic valves (Diastole) "Dub"
Abnormal Heart Sounds	S3 (apex)	Ventricles rapidly filling "Ken-tuck-y"
	S4 (tricuspid/mitral)	Increased resistance to ventricular filling "Ten-nes-see"
	Pericardial friction rub (left sternal border)	Pericardial inflammation "Grating"
	Other heart sounds	Clicks, snaps, and murmurs

Table 13-40. Cardiovascular Markers

Capillary refill	Jugular vein distention	Grading pulses	Edema scale
Normal <3 seconds	*Normal:* <4 cm in diameter	0 = absent	0—None
Abnormal >3 seconds	**Abnormal** >4 cm in diameter	+1 = weak	+1—Minimal (<2 mm)
		+2 = *NORMAL*	+2—Depression (2–4 mm)
		+3 = Increased	+3—Depression (5–8 mm)
		+4 = bounding	+4—Depression (>8) PITTING

Table 13-41. Cardiac Enzymes

Enzyme	Normal	Onset	Peak	Duration
Troponin-I	0–0.1 ng/mL	3–6 hr	12–24 hr	4–7 days
Troponin-T	0–0.2 ng/mL	3–4 hr	10–24 hr	10–14 days
CK	♂38–174 ♀96–140	4–6 hr	12–24 hr	3–4 days
CK-MB	0–5 ng/mL	4–6 hr	14–20 hr	2–3 days
Myoglobin	<55 ng/mL	1–3 hr	6–10 hr	12–24 hr

✛ Rhythm strips? Yikes!

Table 13-42. How Do I Read an EKG Rhythm Strip? Questions to Ask

- What is the rhythm?
- What is the rate?
- What does the P-wave look like?
- What does the QRS measure?
- What is the duration of the QRS?
- What do the T-waves look like?
- What is the measurement of the QT interval?
- Are there any abnormal beats or FLTs (funny-looking things)?

Table 13-43. Heart Rhythms You Just Have to Know

EKG Strip Facts
• Each little box is 0.04
• Normal PR interval is 0.08–0.20
• Normal QRS interval is 0.06–0.10
• Normal QT interval is 0.20–0.40

Rhythm	Strip	Facts
Normal sinus rhythm	Figure 13-12	• Normal PQRST • Rhythm—regular • Normal heart rate • P-wave for every QRS • Regular intervals between complexes

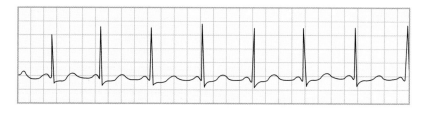

Atrial fibrillation	Figure 13-13	• No recognizable P-waves • Irregular intervals between QRS complexes • Narrow QRS • Chaotic waves between QRS complexes

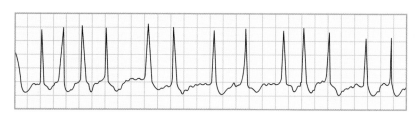

Atrial flutter	Figure 13-14	• Flutter waves • No P-waves • Narrow QRS complexes

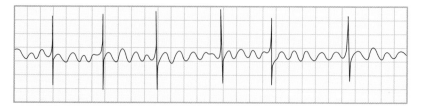

Table 13-43. Heart Rhythms You Just Have to Know (*Continued*)

Rhythm	Strip	Facts
Supraventricular tachycardia	Figure 13-15	• No recognizable P-wave • Regular intervals between QRS complexes • Narrow QRS complex • Heart rate—rapid (usually >150 bpm)

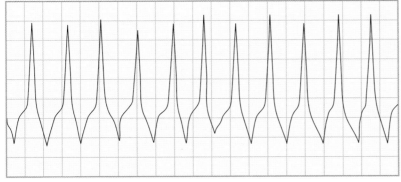

First-degree AV block	Figure 13-16	• Prolonged PR interval (>0.20)

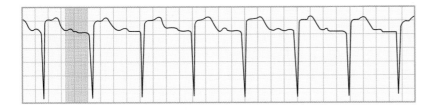

Second-degree AV block (type I) (Wenckebach)	Figure 13-17	• Prolonged PR interval with each QRS until it will drop a QRS • Often intermittent

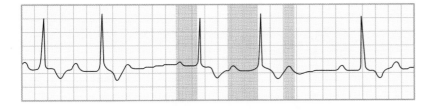

Second-degree AV block (type II)	Figure 13-18	• PR intervals are not prolonged, they remain consistent • QRS complexes will drop randomly or consistently

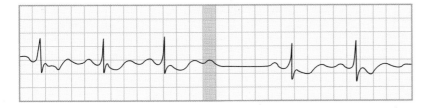

(Continued)

Table 13-43. Heart Rhythms You Just Have to Know (*Continued*)

Rhythm	Strip	Facts
Third-degree AV block	Figure 13-19	• P-waves and QRS complexes are regular • Disassociation between the atria and ventricles • QRS complexes are wide • Heart rate is slow

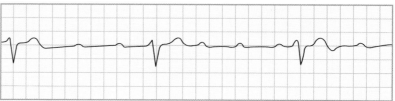

Ventricular tachycardia	Figure 13-20	• No P-waves • Wide, deformed QRS complexes • Usually caused by a PVC (premature ventricular contraction)

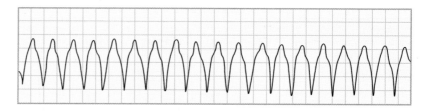

Ventricular fibrillation	Figure 13-21	• Erratic ventricular activity • No QRS complexes

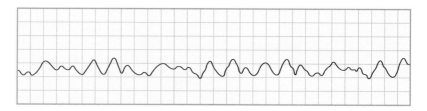

Asystole	Figure 13-22	• No activity

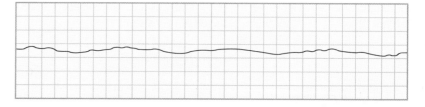

Table 13-44. Grading Heart Murmurs

Grade I	Barely audible
Grade II	Quiet and soft
Grade III	Moderately loud, no thrill
Grade IV	Loud with a thrill
Grade V	Very loud, with a palpable thrill
Grade VI	Extremely loud, can be heard without a stethoscope, with a palpable thrill
When documenting a murmur . . .	Use Roman numerals and always place your finding over VI . (Example: "grade II/VI")

✚ Failing hearts

Table 13-45. Heart Failure

Right-sided heart failure	Left-sided heart failure
• Jugular-vein distention	• Anxiety
• Edema (peripheral)	• Cyanosis
• Liver/spleen enlargement	• Pulmonary crackles
• Bounding pulses	• Wheezes
• Decreased or absent urinary output	• ↑ Respiratory rate
	• S3/S4 gallop
	• Apical murmurs
	• ↓ BP/peripheral pulses

✚ Heart medications

Table 13-46. Antihypertensives: What You Need to Know!

Antihypertensive drugs act on the vascular, cardiac, renal, and sympathetic nervous systems

They also do the following:
- Lower blood pressure
- Lower cardiac output
- Decrease peripheral vascular resistance

Class	Action	Nursing Implications
ACE inhibitors (-"pril")	• Block the conversion of angiotensin I to angiotensin II, which is a potent vasoconstrictor • Vasodilitation occurs • Peripheral resistance decreased • BP decreases • Aldosterone is blocked • There is a decrease in water and sodium retention	• Teach to rise slowly from a sitting position • Ask if client has history of renal disease • Give on an empty stomach to enhance absorption • Teach client to never stop taking medication abruptly • Teach client to never double up if missed dose
Beta-blockers (-"olol")	• Acts primarily on the heart • Beta$_2$ also blocks receptors in the lungs that may cause bronchospasm • Decreases heart rate • Decreases force of contraction • Delays impulse conduction	• Teach client to report dizziness, weakness, headache • Always hold medication if the systolic BP is <90 mm Hg • Teach client to never stop taking the medication abruptly • Teach the client to never double-up if missed dose
Calcium-channel blockers	• Block calcium access to the cells • Decrease the force of myocardial contractility • Decrease conductivity • Decrease oxygen demand • Decrease heart rate and PVR	• Watch for decreased BP • Weigh and report weight gain • Teach client to rise slowly from sitting to standing position • Give before meals • Report dry cough • Teach client to never stop taking the medication abrubtly

LUNGS

O.K., we all know why we need lungs. I'll huff, and I'll puff, and I'll blow Newt over!

Table 13-47. Common Causes of Respiratory Disorders

- Allergies
- Crowded living conditions
- Recurrent respiratory infections
- Smoking
- Surgery
- Travel to foreign countries
- Family history of infectious/respiratory diseases
- Chemical exposure
- Exposure to environmental pollutants
- Noncompliance with respiratory medications/hygiene

Table 13-48. Respiratory Assessment

Inspection	Chest symmetry, tracheal position, skin condition, accessory muscle use, nasal flaring, respiratory rate, respiratory pattern, cyanosis, clubbing
Palpation	Chest wall symmetry, chest wall expansion, scars, lumps, lesions, pain, tactile fremitus, crepitus
Percussion	Resonance (NORMAL), hyper-resonance, dullness, tympany
Auscultation	The breath sounds over normal lung fields are: tracheal, bronchial, bronchovesicular, and vesicular

Table 13-49. Breath Sounds

	Where (location)	What (description)
Normal	Bronchial (trachea)	• Loud • High pitched • Harsh • Expiration > inspiration
	Vesicular (peripheral lung tissue)	• Soft • Swishing • Low pitched • May sound like a breeze • Inspiration > expiration
	Bronchovesicular (mainstem bronchi)	• Soft • Blowing • Inspiration = expiration
	Wheezes (can be heard anywhere)	• High pitched • Musical • Whistling sound • May be heard on inspiration and expiration
Abnormal	Rhonchi (central airways)	• Course • Rumbling • Low pitched • Snoring sound • May be heard with inspiration and expiration
	Pleural friction rub (lateral lung field)	• Grating or squeaking • May sound like pieces of sandpaper being rubbed together • Heard on inspiration and expiration
	Rales (can be heard anywhere)	• Soft crackling • Bubbling
	Stridor (louder in the neck)	• High pitched • Crowing sound

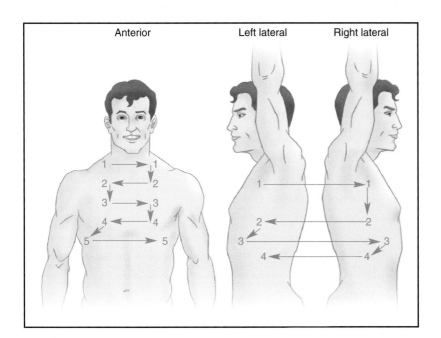

◀ Figure 13-23

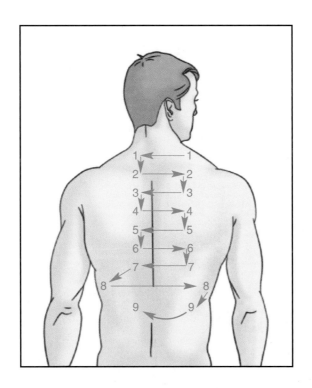

◀ Figure 13-24

✚ What's the incentive?

Table 13-50. Incentive Spirometry

WHAT?	• Encourages maximal inspirations • Mimics yawning or sighing • Promotes lung expansion
WHY?	• Prevents atelectasis • Increases ventilation to the lung bases • Mobilizes secretions • Decreases risk of pneumonia secondary to inability/unwillingness to take deep cleansing breaths (example: pain secondary to rib fractures)
HOW?	• Sitting position • Place mouth tightly around the mouthpiece • Inhale slowly (maintain 500–900 marks) • Hold breath for 5 seconds • Exhale through pursed lips • Repeat 5–10 times each hour

CAUTION: <u>DO NOT USE</u> if the patient is hypoxic with interruption of O_2, or if the patient is resistant to instructions of proper usage.

Figure 13-25

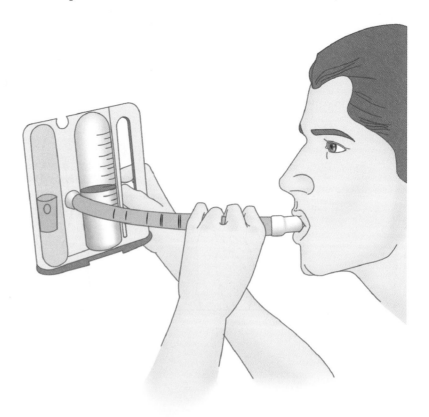

Table 13-51. Pulse Oximetry

Ranges	Treatment
Normal: 95–99%	
Mild hypoxia: 91–94%	Give O_2
Moderate hypoxia: 86–90%	Give 100% O_2
Severe hypoxia: <85%	Give 100% O_2, prepare to ventilate
False high (may be caused from anemia or carbon monoxide poisoning)	False low (may be caused from cool extremities, hypothermia, hypovolemia)

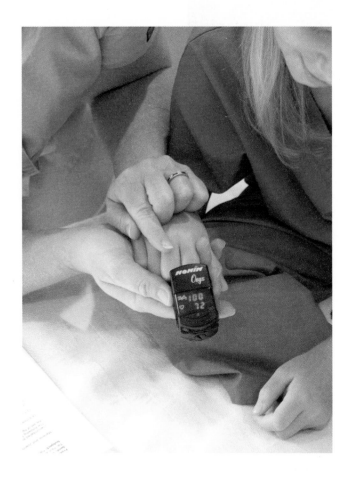

◀ Figure 13-26

+ Oh delivery boy . . .

Table 13-52. Oxygen Delivery Equipment

O₂	Percent of O₂	O₂ flow rate
Room air	21%	
Nasal cannula REMEMBER: Should be humidified if used for an extended period of time Figure 13-27	24–44%	1–6 L/min

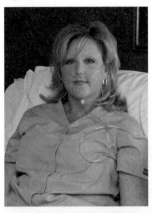

Simple face mask Figure 13-28	30–60%	6–10 L/min

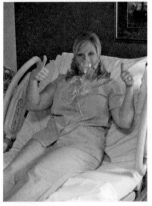

Venturi mask	24–50%	3–15 L/min
Nonrebreather mask	50–100%	6–15 L/min
Bag-valve mask (Ambu bag)	100% with reservoir	15 L/min
Trach collar	28–100%	
Ventilator	Mechanical breathing device	
CPAP	Variable oxygen concentration	
Aerosols	Variable; high-humidity oxygen	

Table 13-53. Suctioning

WHY? Maintains the airway for breathing assistance and promotes the clearance of secretions.

1. Check the order
2. Explain the procedure to the patient (even if they are unresponsive)
3. Wash your hands
4. Determine the length of the catheter

   Nasal tracheal: Measure the distance from the tip of the nose to the earlobe and along the side of the neck to the Adam's apple

   Oral tracheal: Measure from the mouth to the midsternum
5. Position the patient on the side or back with the HOB elevated
6. Hyper-oxygenate the patient using the Ambu bag
7. Lubricate the catheter with sterile water
8. DO NOT APPLY SUCTION while inserting the catheter
9. Insert the catheter until resistance is met or until the cough reflex is stimulated
10. Apply suction intermittently for 10 seconds
11. Rotate the catheter and withdraw
12. Hyper-oxygenate the patient

✛ "Postural" not "pastural" drainage

Table 13-54. Postural Drainage Positions

Lung segment	Position of the patient
Upper lung lobes (*anterior right/left apical*) Have the patient sit upright in a bed or chair	Figure 13-29A 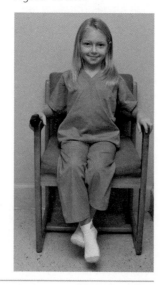

(Continued)

Table 13-54. Postural Drainage Positions (*Continued*)

Lung segment	Position of the patient
Upper lung lobes (*posterior right/left apical*) Have the patient lean forward in the sitting position	Figure 13-29B 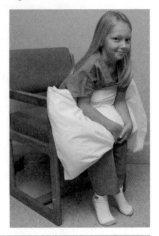
Middle lobe (*middle anterior lobe*) Have the patient supine, tilted to the left side in Trendelenburg's position	Figure 13-29C 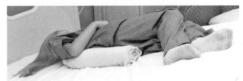
Middle lobe (*middle posterior lobe*) Have the patient prone, tilted to the left side with the hips elevated	Figure 13-29D 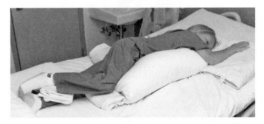
Lower lobes (*anterior lower lobes*) Have the patient supine in Trendelenburg's position	Figure 13-29E 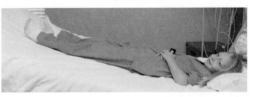
Lower lobes (*posterior lower lobes*) Have the patient prone in Trendelenburg's position	Figure 13-29F 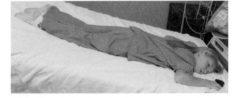

Table 13-54. Postural Drainage Positions (*Continued*)

Lung segment	Position of the patient
Lower lobes (*lateral lower lobes*) Have the patient on right or left side in Trendelenburg's position	Figure 13-29G

Table 13-55. Respiratory Isolation

- Private room
- Keep the door closed
- Wash hands before and after attending to client
- Use precaution when handling secretions
- Patient MUST wear a mask when being transported outside the room
- Mask must be located outside the room for visitor and staff usage

ALWAYS check your hospital policy for specific guidelines.

ENDOCRINE SYSTEM

Diabetes is the major disorder that affects the endocrine system. You will encounter clients with diabetes for as long as you remain in patient care. Therefore, you can be sure that you will be asked questions about the disease on NCLEX®.

+ The showdown

Table 13-56. HYPERglycemia Versus HYPOglycemia

"DKA or ketoacidosis"	"Insulin shock"
• Blood sugar—HIGH >180 mg%	• Blood Sugar—LOW
• Gradual onset	• Sudden onset
• Warm dry skin	• Cool, moist skin
• Rapid weak pulse	• Normal to slightly ↑ pulse
• "Sweet" acetone breath	• Normal breath
• Urine output ↑	• Seizures are common
• Weak	• Urine output is normal
• Give IV fluids and insulin	• Disoriented, coma
• Slow steady recovery	• Give glucose IV (PO only if the airway is not compromised)
• Monitor EKG	• Rapid recovery
	CAUTION
	Hypoglycemia can mimic a stroke or alcohol intoxication.

Pour some sugar on me . . .

Table 13-57. How Do I Treat Hypoglycemia?

Treat ONLY if the patient is conscious and does not have swallowing difficulty:
- Glucose tablets/gel
- 1 TBS of honey
- 1 TBS of sugar
- $\frac{1}{2}$ cup of fruit juice or regular soda
- 3 graham crackers

ALWAYS follow with a protein such as peanut butter, cheese, or $\frac{1}{2}$ meat sandwich

✚ These boots were made for walking

Foot care is vitally important in diabetics and other patients who have lost protective sensation in their feet.

Table 13-58. Foot Care

- Inspect the feet daily and monitor for redness, swelling, or breaks in skin integrity
- Notify the physician if redness, swelling, or breaks in the skin occur
- Instruct the patient to avoid using heating pads, hot water bottles, or hot water soaks
- Do NOT soak feet
- Dry feet completely, especially between the toes
- Do not treat calluses, ingrown nails, or blisters
- May use moisturizing lotions but avoid placing between the toes
- Wear clean, white, cotton socks
- Do not wear open-toed shoes, shoes with a strap, or flip-flops
- Check shoes for foreign objects before putting them on
- Cut nails straight across or allow someone else to assist with nail care
- File nails with an emery board to avoid snagging nail that can cause injury

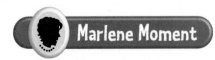
Marlene Moment

I had a client one time who had really long toenails that he did not want trimmed. He said he used them to climb trees!

SEE NO EVIL, HEAR NO EVIL, SPEAK NO EVIL

This section reviews eye illnesses and proper care of hearing aids and dentures.

✛ My, what big eyes you have!

Table 13-59. Special Eye Considerations

Artificial Eye Care

1. Don gloves

2. Exert pressure below the lower eyelid (this will make the eye prosthesis "pop" out)

3. Cleanse carefully with normal saline and gauze

4. Cleanse from the inner to the outer canthus

5. Wash the prosthesis in warm normal saline

6. To reinsert, pull down on the patient's lower lid and slip the prosthesis gently into the socket

7. Release the lids

Eye Medications	
My**D**riatic—**D**ialate pupils	Mioti**C**—**C**onstricted pupils

Glaucoma

Acute closed angle	Chronic open angle
• Severe pain	• Loss of peripheral vision
• Headache	• Eye fatigue
• Nausea/vomiting	• Vision changes
• Blurring of vision	
• Halos around the lights	
• **MEDICAL EMERGENCY!!**	

Retinal Detachment

• Sudden onset of blurred vision	• Bed rest
• Blank spots in visual field	• Cover eyes
• Flashes of light	• Decrease anxiety
• Floating particles	• Flat or low Fowler's position
• Surgery required	• No stooping or bending
	• No prone position

Trauma

Major/minor	Treatments
• Chemical injury	• (Especially alkali exposure)—profuse irrigation with normal saline
• Ruptured globe	• No drops or ointments
• Blunt trauma	• Decrease anxiety, wait for ophthalmology consult

Cataracts

• Blurred vision	• Surgery often required
• Distortion	• Avoid straining, vomiting, coughing, brushing teeth, stooping, lifting, rubbing eye (these increase IOP)
• Photophobia	

✚ Ear care

Table 13-60. Care of a Hearing Aid

- Clean the ear as often as needed
- May use warm water and soap
- Keep the hearing aid dry
- Do NOT shower with the aid in
- Turn the aid off when not in use
- Store it away from animals and small children
- Store it in the same place every time

✚ What do I do with these teeth?

Table 13-61. Care of Dentures

- Don gloves
- Allow the patient to remove their own dentures
- If the patient needs assistance, grasp the upper plate at the front teeth and move them up and down to release the suction
- Lift the lower plate up on one side at a time
- Use warm water to clean . . . do not use hot water!
- Avoid soaking for long periods of time
- Beware of sharp edges
- Check the oral cavity
- Replace the dentures in the patient's mouth
- If the dentures are to be stored away, be sure to label properly

✚ Swallowing issues

Table 13-62. Swallowing Problems

Stage 1 (pureed)	Stage 2 (minced/ground)	Stage 3 (soft)	Stage 4 (slightly modified)
Minimize Complications by:			

- Position client prior to eating (sitting upright when possible)
- Provide a pleasant, relaxed eating environment
- Make sure the patient has cleared the throat with each bite
- Do not use liquids
- Encourage the patient to feed self when possible
- Thickeners may be ordered (dried apple flakes, baby rice cereal, mashed potatoes, or commercial thickeners)

MATERNAL–NEWBORN

Table 13-63. Signs and Symptoms of Pregnancy

Presumptive	Probable	Positive
• Amenorrhea • Nausea • Vomiting • Fatigue • Breast tenderness • Breast enlargement • Frequent urination • Stretch marks (striae) • Quickening	• Positive urine/serum pregnancy • Heger's sign (lower uterine softening) • Ballottement • Braxton–Hicks contractions • Chadwick's sign (bluish coloration of the vagina) • Goodell's sign (cervix softening)	• Fetal heartbeat per Doppler ultrasound • Sonogram of the fetus • Fetal movement felt by the health care provider

+ Off to the doctor . . . again

Table 13-64 is for patients who do not have special needs that require a change in the normal visit schedule.

Table 13-64. Schedule of Prenatal Visits

28–32 Weeks	Visits are made every 4 weeks
32–36 Weeks	Visits are made every 2 weeks
36–40 Weeks	Visits are made every week

+ Honey, I need more pickles and ice cream

Table 13-65. Special Nutritional Needs and Weight Gain During Pregnancy

Normal Weight Gain	Approximately 25 lbs (total)
↑ Caloric Needs	Additional 300 cal/day (total 2500 calories)
Protein	75–80 g/day
Carbohydrates	Limited in certain patients
Folic Acid	400 μg every day
Sodium	≤2400 mg/day
Iron	30 mg/day
Calcium	1200 mg/day
Other Dietary Considerations	• No alcohol • Limit fish intake to 6 oz/week (cooked). No shark, swordfish, tuna due to mercury concerns • No feta, brie, or Mexican-style cheeses (to prevent listeriosis) • Leftovers should be cooked to at least 165°F

✛ Are you smarter than a fifth-grader?

Table 13-66. Pregnancy Facts

G—*Gravida* = the number of pregnancies the patient has had including the present one

T—*Term* = the total number of infants born >37 weeks

P—*Preterm* = the total number of infants born <37 weeks

A—*Abortions* = total number of spontaneous or induced deaths

L—*Living* = total number of children still living

Nägele's rule: First day of the last menstrual period, minus 3 months, plus 7 days.

Example: First day of the last menstrual period = October 5

Subtract 3 months = July 5

Add 7 days = July 12

Estimated date of delivery = July 12

True labor	False labor
• Regular contractions	• Irregular contractions
• Back pain followed by abdominal pain	• Pain localized to the abdomen
• Progressive cervical dilation and effacement	• No change in the cervix
• Progressive effacement	• No change in intervals between the contractions or quality of the contractions
• Shorter intervals between contractions with increased intensity	• May be relieved with ambulation

DANGER signs of pregnancy

- Unusual or severe abdominal cramping
- Severe vomiting
- Fluid discharge or bleeding from the vagina
- Vision changes
- Swelling of the fingers, face
- Change in fetal movement or absence of movement
- Severe headaches
- Seizure activity
- Progressive contraction in duration and consistency

Table 13-67. OB/GYN Emergencies

What is the problem?	What happens?	When does it happen?	What will I see?	What do I dD?
Abruptio placentae (Fig. 13-30)	Separation of the placenta from the uterine wall	Usually >20 weeks gestation	**PAINful** dark red vaginal bleeding, BP↓, Pulse↑, ↓fetal heart tones, ↑fundal height, pale, diaphoretic skin	O₂, IV, prepare for an emergency C-section
Placenta previa (Fig. 13-31)	The placenta covers the cervical os	This can occur during the 2nd & 3rd trimester	**PainLESS,** bright red vaginal bleeding, BP↓, pulse↑	O₂, IV, bedrest, ultrasound. If the bleeding is heavy, prepare for C-section
Preeclampsia/PIH (Fig. 13-32)	Pregnancy-induced hypertension	Anytime during the pregnancy	BP↑; headache; proteinuria; swelling of the hands, feet, and face, weight gain; ↓ UOP; visual disturbances; hyperreflexia; possible seizures; ↓FHT	Place the patient in a quiet room, supportive care, seizure precautions. The HTN may be treated with magnesium sulfate

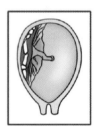
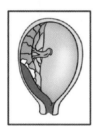
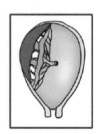

◄ Figure 13-30   Abruptio placentae

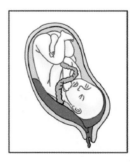
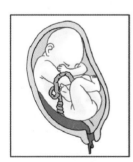
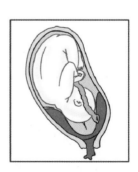

◄ Figure 13-31   Placenta previa

▶ Figure 13-32   Fetal positions

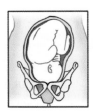

Right occiput
anterior
(ROA)

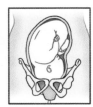

Right occiput
transverse
(ROT)

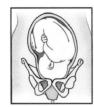

Left occiput
anterior
(LOA)

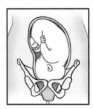

Right occiput
transverse
(LOT)

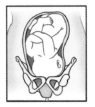

Right
mentum
anterior
(RMA)

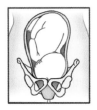

Right
mentum
posterior
(RMP)

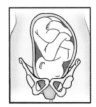

Left mentum
anterior
(LMA)

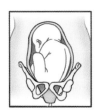

Left sacrum
anterior
(LSaA)

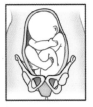

Left sacrum
posterior
(LSaP)

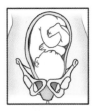

Right occiput
posterior
(ROP)

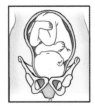

Left occiput
posterior
(LOP)

▶ Figure 13-33   Assessing fetal
engagement.

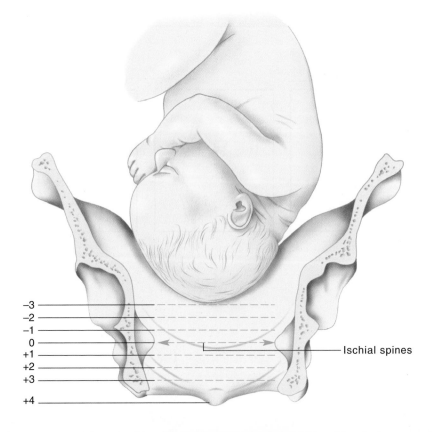

−3
−2
−1
0
+1
+2
+3

+4

Ischial spines

Table 13-68. Postpartum Checks

Lochia	• **Days 1–3:** rubra (red) • **Days 3–7:** serosa (pink to brown) • **Days 10–14:** alba (creamy white to clear)
Fundal Height and Consistency	• **After delivery:** At the umbilicus and about the size of a grapefruit • **Day 1:** One finger-breadth above the umbilicas • **Days 2–10:** Descends one finger-breadth daily • **Day 10:** Nonpalpable, located behind the symphysis pubis Figure 13-34 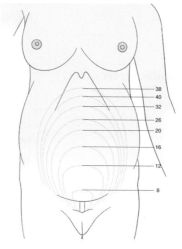
Uterine Involution	Figure 13-35
Nipple Checks and Care	• Good hand-washing • Nurse on each breast (alternate "beginning" breast) • Make sure the whole areola is in the infant's mouth • Break the suction before removing the infant from the breast • Allow nipples to air-dry • May apply lanolin (avoid creams, lotions, or ointments)

✚ Something's not right with the baby . . .

Infants may be born with illnesses or defects that are inherited or caused by the uterine environment.

Congenital heart defects

Table 13-69. Acyanotic Defect

Left-to-right shunt—increased pulmonary blood flow; blood is oxygenated

Defect	Description
Red blood = oxygenated blood	Blue blood = deoxygenated blood
Atrial septal defect (ASD)	• There is a hole between the top two chambers (atria) of the heart • The hole allows the blue blood and red blood to mix • Repair: The hole is closed with stitches or a patch of pericardium
Atrioventricular septal defect	• There is a hole between the top two defect (AVSD) chambers (atria) and the bottom two chambers (ventricles) • There is only one (AV) valve rather than two separate valves • The blue blood and red blood mix together freely • The right side of the heart and the lungs receive too much blood • The body receives less oxygenated blood than it needs • Repair: Top two chambers are separated; bottom two chambers are separated; two valves are made from the one large valve
Coartation of the aorta	• There is a narrowing of the major artery from the heart (aorta) to the body • The narrowing decreases blood flow to the body • The heart has to pump harder • Repair: Cutting out the narrow part and connecting the two ends together using a blood vessel (subclavian) to widen the narrowed area
Patent ductus arteriosus (PDA)	• There is an open connection between the aorta and the pulmonary artery • Essential at birth, but usually closes shortly after birth • If a large amount of blood flowing through it, can lead to CHF • This blood vessel increases the risks of endocarditis (infection of the heart) • Repair: The connection from the aorta to the pulmonary artery is tied off and/or cut

Table 13-70. Cyanotic Defect

Right-to-left shunt—blood shunted from the right side of the heart (pulmonary) to the left (systemic) side. Pulmonary circulation is bypassed

Defect	Description
Red blood = oxygenated blood	Blue blood = deoxygenated blood
Tetralogy of Fallot (TOF)	• A hole between the bottom two chambers of the heart (VSD)
	• A narrowing under or at the pulmonary valve (pulmonary stenosis)
	• An enlargement of the bottom of the right side of the heart
	• Aorta is lined up just over the hole between the bottom two chambers
	• Mixing of the red and blue blood through the VSD
	• Blood to the lungs is restricted by the narrowing of the pulmonary valve
	• Repair: VSD closed, narrowing relieved
Transposition of the great arteries (TGA)	• The pulmonary artery and the aorta are in opposite position of where they should be
	• There may also be a VSD
	• When the vessels are switched, the body receives blue blood instead of red blood. The lungs receive red blood rather than normal blue blood. If there is a VSD, there is mixing of red and blue blood
	• Repair: Pulmonary artery and aorta are moved to their proper position, the hole is closed, and the coronary vessels are moved
Truncus arteriosus (TA)	• One large blood vessel (truncus) with a single valve leaves the heart
	• It has branches that go to the lungs, body, and coronary arteries
	• There is always a large hole between the bottom two chambers (VSD)
	• Repair: VSD repair, connection is made between the bottom right heart chamber and the branch pulmonary arteries going to the lungs, and the areas of the truncal vessel where the branch pulmonary arteries have been removed are patched closed

Congenital heart disease in infants

Table 13-71. Signs and Symptoms of Congenital Heart Disease in Infants

Dyspnea with crying or eating	Cyanosis with crying or eating
Pallor	Fatigue
Poor feeding	No weight gain
Sweating	Irritable
Murmur	

PEDIATRICS

There are so many things that can go wrong with those little bodies. These charts will help you focus on the core content of caring for little ones.

Table 13-72. Pediatric Developmental Markers

Age	Actions
1 month	Stares at faces, blinks at loud noises or bright lights, lifts head briefly when prone (lying on stomach)
2 months	Smiles, coos, follows objects with eyes, more control over the head
3 months	Recognizes faces, smiles and giggles, holds head steady when upright, kicks legs and flings arms
4 months	Responds with cooing when talked to, tries to hold weight on both legs when held upright
5 months	Notices objects when they are placed in front of the face, rolls over, reaches for objects
6 months	Mimics sounds and facial expressions, sits up with minimal support, rolls freely from back to stomach and stomach to back
7 months	Goes after toys, begins to feed self finger foods, sits freely
8 months	Begins forming words out of previous sounds ("mama"), crawls, responds to name, chews on objects
9–10 months	Pulls up, looks for objects that are dropped, very attached to the primary caregiver, walks while holding onto furniture
11–12 months	Plays ball; begins to associate the word "No"; lets you know wants and dislikes; fear of strangers; removes shoes, socks, hats
13–14 months	Takes a few steps, puts two words together, puts objects into a container, dumps all toys on the floor

Table 13-72. Pediatric Developmental Markers (*Continued*)

Age	Actions
15–16 months	Toddles, vocabulary increases to 5–10 words, laughs, likes video and books, loves to play, attaches to a stuffed animal or blanket.
18–20 months	Feeds self with eating utensil, runs, colors (scribbles), undresses self
24 months	Forms 3- to 4-word sentences, counts to 5, understandable much of the time

✛ Erikson's like the music group *Aerosmith*: He's withstood the test of time

Table 13-73. Erikson's Theory of Development (Psychosocial)

Trust vs. mistrust	• Develops trust as the needs are met by the primary caregiver • Develops mistrust if the needs are not adequately met
Autonomy vs. shame and doubt	• Becomes increasingly independent • Learns to control bodily functions
Initiative vs. guilt	• Develops conscience • Learns about the world through play
Industry vs. inferiority	• Learns to socialize • Learns to follow the rules • Enjoys playing with others
Identity vs. role confusion	• Tries to establish own identity while attempting to meet the expectations of peers • Consumed with looks and view point of others

Table 13-74. Measuring Head Circumference

• Use a paper measuring tape to avoid stretching
• Place the tape just above the infant's eyebrows and around the occipital prominence at the back of the head to measure the largest diameter of the head

Figure 13-36

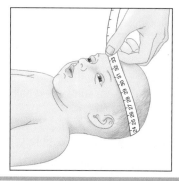

✛ Checking reflexes without the fun hammer

Table 13-75. Normal Infant Reflexes

Reflex	Description	Age reflex disappears
Babinski	When the sole of the foot on the side of the little toe is stroked, the neonate's toes fan upward. This is a positive reflex.	1 year old
Moro (startle)	When there is a loud noise, or when lifted above the crib and lowered quickly, there is symmetrical abduction and extension of the arms with the fingers extended to form a "C"	4–6 months
Palmer grasp	When a finger is placed in the neonate's palm, the fingers grasps tightly	3–4 months
Stepping	When held in an upright position with the feet in contact with a hard surface, the neonate will alternately raise feet as if stepping or dancing	Varies
Rooting	With stimulation (stroking) the cheek, the neonate turns toward the stimulus	3–4 months
Sucking	Immediate sucking when something placed in the mouth	6 months
Tonic neck (fencing)	When the head is turned to one side, the arm and leg on that side extend and the opposite arm and leg flex	2–3 months

Table 13-76. Signs and Symptoms of Dehydration in Infants and Children

- **Skin:** poor skin turgor, cool to touch, pale/gray
- **Mucous membranes:** dry, pasty
- **Weight loss:** 5–15%
- **Fontanel** (anterior): sunken in infants
- **Eyes:** absence of tears when crying, sunken eyeballs
- **Urine:** decreased or absent urinary output
- **Level of consciousness:** irritable, coma, possible seizures
- **Shock:** ↑↑ pulse and respirations, ↓ blood pressure

✛ Poisoning

Infants and children are at high risk for poisoning. It is imperative that you know what to do in this emergency situation.

When not to hurl

Table 13-77. Ingestions and Poisonings: When NOT to Induce Vomiting

- Child with decreased level of consciousness or comatose
- Child is having seizures
- Child has a decreased or absent gag reflex
- Child ingested a corrosive substance
- Child is in shock

Acetaminophen poisoning

Acetaminophen (Tylenol) is the most common substance for drug poisoning in children. Poisoning occurs from acute ingestion. Acetaminophen is metabolized by the liver, so hepatic damage may occur. Most children recover if treated promptly!

Table 13-78. Acetaminophen Poisoning

Stages	Time since ingestion	Characteristics
I	0.5–24 hours	Nausea, vomiting, malaise, pallor, diaphoresis, decreased appetite
II	24–48 hours	Upper abdominal pain, tenderness with palpation; elevated liver enzymes, bilirubin, and prothrombin time
III	72–96 hours	Peak liver function abnormalities; nausea, vomiting, and malaise may reappear
IV	4–14 days	Resolution of symptoms, normalization of liver functions (resolution of hepatic dysfunction)
Nursing Care		
• Empty stomach—lavage or induced vomiting • Mucomyst is the antidote (may be placed in carbonated beverage)	• Active charcoal absorbs acetaminophen • Monitor VS, lab, and I & O • Be very supportive!	

Lead poisoning (plumbism)

Lead poisoning results when a child repeatedly ingests or absorbs substances containing lead (e.g., paint, auto exhaust, foods, water). Lead poisonings are more common in the summer months.

Table 13-79. Lead Poisoning Symptoms

Mild	Moderate	Severe
• Irritability	• Headache	• Severe, intermittent abdominal cramps
• Mild fatigue	• Abdominal pain	• Paralysis
• Myalgias	• Weight loss	• Lead line (blue-black) on the gingival tissue
• Paresthesias	• Constipation	• Seizure
• Mild abdominal pain or discomfort	• Vomiting	• Decreased LOC
	• Fatigue	• Coma
	• Arthralgia	• Death

✚ Choking hazards

There are hundreds of deaths each year related to asphyxiation in infants and children. It is strongly advised that the following foods be avoided. Small children should always be supervised while eating.

Table 13-80. Choking Hazards

Infants	Children
• Biscuits	• Hot dogs
• Hot dogs	• Corn
• Cookies	• Nuts
• Apples	• Gum
	• Hard candy
	• Grapes
	• Popcorn
	• Raw vegetables
	• Celery

Toys that don't cause choking

Table 13-81. Safe Toddler Play

- Building blocks
- Pot's, pans, play food
- Play dough
- Toy telephones
- Wooden puzzles
- Cloth books
- Tricycle
- Coloring books and large crayons
- Musical instruments
- Trucks/trains/cars that roll
- Balls (medium to large)
- Stuffed animals without buttons (choking hazard)

✚ Acute illnesses

Following are several acute illnesses that young children may experience. The NCLEX® Lady may test your knowledge on these topics during the exam, but don't let that terrible Newt distract you! Keep telling yourself: I love peds! I love peds! I love peds!

Increased intracranial pressure

Table 13-82. Symptoms of Increased ICP in Children

- Irritable/fussy
- Vomiting
- Altered or decreased level of consciousness
- Seizure activity
- ↑ BP
- ↓ Pulse and respirations

Sudden infant death syndrome

Table 13-83. SIDS (Sudden Infant Death Syndrome)

- The sudden death of a previously healthy infant for which a routine autopsy fails to identify the cause
- Most common cause of death between 1 month and 1 year (peak 2–4 months)
- More common in low-birthweight babies, boys, families with crowded living conditions, and in the winter months
- SIDS has decreased by more than 40% since the initiative to position babies on their backs during sleep

Prevention	• Sleep infants on their backs • No smoking • Keep the infant warm while sleeping • Remove all pillows and toys from the infant's sleeping area • Do not cover the infant's head while sleeping • Use a firm mattress • Make sure bed linens fit properly • Do not sleep the infant in the bed with parents or other children • Do not allow pets to sleep with or in the same room as the infant • Apnea monitors are available if needed

A CHILD'S GRIEF

Children experience the emotion of grief, although they express it differently than adults. The child's age influences the grief process and response.

Table 13-84. Children and Grief

Age	Process
<1 year	• Infants may react to the loss of the mother or primary caregiver • Infants have no concept of death
12–24 months	• Child may become irritable, disinterested, withdrawn; may exhibit temper tantrums or irrational behavior • Response expected ONLY if the loss is someone of significance in the child's life • Child may see death as reversible
2–4 years	• Aggressive behavior or regression • Withdrawal from normal activities • The child may be overly concerned about who will care for them • Child may see death as reversible
4–9 years	• Child may assume responsibility for the death • May have difficulty with tasks and school; performance secondary to inability to concentrate • Child may begin to see death as permanent
9–Adolescence	• There will likely be a strong emotional reaction • Regression and rebellion are common • Outbursts of anger and questioning • See death as permanent

Table 13-85. Grief Response

Shock/Disbelief	• Denial • Extremes of emotional expression • Difficulty concentrating or making decisions
Loss Experience	• Anger or guilt • Depression may occur at this stage • Isolation/withdrawal are common
Reintegration	• Begin to reorganize life • Adaptation to life without loved one • Acceptance of the loss

CHILD ABUSE

Child abuse is an unfortunate occurrence and one that nurses are responsible to report by law. Therefore, nurses should be aware of the signs and symptoms of possible child abuse. Much of the time, children will exhibit several signs and symptoms in combination.

Table 13-86. Signs and Symptoms of Child Abuse

- Unexplained broken bones, bruises, burns, or facial contusions
- Begs or steals
- Cries when time to go home
- Neglect of medical/dental needs
- Dirty or inappropriately dressed
- Reports nightmares or bedwetting
- Pain with walking or sitting
- Extremes in behavior
- Overly demanding, withdrawn, or aggressive

Reactions from Parents (When to Be Concerned)

- Show little concern for the child
- Deny responsibility or blame the child for injuries or problems
- View the child as burdensome
- Demand unrealistic performance by the child
- Open admittance that they do not like the child
- Rarely look at the child
- Minimize the situation no matter how serious

Table 13-87. Family Violence and Neglect

Physical Neglect	Failure to provide health care for the treatment or prevention of illness or injury
Emotional Violence	Inflicting mental anguish
Developmental Neglect	Failure to provide appropriate stimulation (cognitive) that is needed to prevent developmental delays or deficits
Sexual Violence	Sexual contact (of any kind) without consent
Educational Neglect	Failure to provide the child with appropriate educational opportunities
Physical Violence	Inflicting physical pain or bodily harm

✚ Bruises

Bruises in dark-skinned children will vary according to the degree of skin pigmentation. Bruises may occur with bleeding disorders or liver dysfunction, but in the absence of disease suspect trauma or abuse.

Table 13-88. Bruises—What They Can Tell You

Color	Time
Red, blue, or purple (light-skinned person) Dark, deep blue (dark-skinned person)	Immediate to 24 hours
Purple	1–5 days
Green	5–7 days
Yellow	7–10 days
Brown/resolving	10–14 days

PSYCHIATRIC NURSING

This is an area of nursing you will use in your career more than you think! Be prepared to recognize the signs and symptoms of psychiatric disorders, communicate effectively with your clients, and make appropriate referrals.

Table 13-89. Signs and Symptoms of Client with Suicidal Thoughts

- Crying, sadness, weight loss/gain, loss of interest, inability to concentrate, inability to perform daily activities/tasks
- Withdrawal
- Getting personal things in order
- Making unusual statements such as "Everyone would be better off without me."
- Isolation from family and friends

Nursing Actions

- Provide a safe environment
- Remove all dangerous objects such as belts, razors, clippers, knives, glass, and cords
- Observe the patient at all times
- Communicate clearly the plan and restrictions for the client

Table 13-90. Alcohol Withdrawal

Early (Stage I)	Advanced (Stage II and III)
(No alcohol intake for 2–12 hours)	(24–36 hours later)
• Memory impairment	• Profound confusion
• Poor judgment	• Delusions
• Insomnia	• Hallucinations
• Irritable/anxious/agitated	• Tremors
• Cramps/abdominal pain	• Profuse sweating
• Weakness	• Fever >102°F
• Diarrhea	• Severe agitation
• Bloating	• ↑↑ Pulse
• ↑ BP, pulse	• Grand mal seizures
• Sweating	• Death can occur
• ↑↑ Startle response	

Table 13-91. Incompetent Clients

- Under the influence of drugs or alcohol
- Unconscious
- Chronic dementia/Alzheimer's
- Other psychological or mental deficiency
- Declared incompetent

USE CAUTION IN CANCER

As a nurse, it is imperative that you know the warning signs of cancer. The NCLEX® Lady will surely expect you to know these and the preventative measures for the various cancers.

Table 13-92. The Warning Signs of Cancer

C : Change in bladder or bowel function
A : A sore that will not heal
U : Unusual bleeding or discharge
T : Thickening or lump in the tissue
I : Indigestion or unusual GI disturbances
O : Obvious change in a wart or mole
N : Nagging hoarseness, or cough

LABORATORY VALUES

If you haven't learned them yet, here's your last chance to commit them to memory. You will **definitely** be asked questions about laboratory values on NCLEX®.

Table 13-93. Common Hematology Lab Values

RBC	(♂) 4.2–5.6 ; (♀) 3.6–5.0 M/μL
Hgb	(♂) 14–18; (♀) 12–16 g/dL
Hct	(♂) 42–52%; (♀) 36–48%
MCH	26–34 pg
MCHC	31–37%
MCV	78–98 fL
WBC	4–10 K/mm³
Neutrophils	54–75%
Monocytes	2–8%
Lymphocytes	25–40%
Eosinophils	1–5%
Basophils	0–1%
Bands	0–5%
Platelets	140,000–400,000

✦ Is it positive or negative?

The following substances can cause false results in common hematology lab values.

Table 13-94. Common Substances Causing False Results

False positive	False negative
• Red meat	• Vitamin C
• Fish	• Turnips
• Oral iron supplements	• Horseradish
• Iodine	• Beets
• Boric acid	• Melons
• ASA	
• NSAIDs	
• Corticosteroids	

Table 13-95. Metabolic Panel

	Test	Conventional units
	Albumin	3.5–5.0 g/dL
	Alkaline phosphatase	32–115 U/L
	Urinalysis	
Color	Straw to yellow	
Specific gravity	1.003–1.040	
pH	5–8	
Glucose	Negative	
Sodium	10–40 mEq/L	
Potassium	<8 mEq/L	
Chloride	<8 mEq/L	
Protein	Negative	
Osmolality	80–1300 mOsm/L	
ALT		♂10–40 units/L; ♀7–35 units/L
AST		11–39 U/L
Bilirubin (total)		0.2–1.1 mg/dL
BUN		6–23 mg/dL
Calcium		8.2–10.9 mg/dL
Carbon dioxide		22–31 mmol/L
Chloride		98–108 mEq/L
Creatinine		0.6–1.3 mg/dL
Glucose		70–100 mg/dL
Potassium		3.5–5 mEq/L
Protein (total)		6.3–8 g/dL
Sodium		135–145 mEq/L

ACID–BASE IMBALANCES
....

Acid–base balance is very important to your nursing practice, because many diseases and disorders include a malfunction of acid–base homeostasis.

Table 13-96. Normal Blood Gases

pH	7.35–7.45 pH units
P_{O_2}	80–100 mmHg
P_{CO_2}	35–45 mmHg
HCO_3	22–26 mmol/L
CO_2	19–24 mmol/L
Sa_{O_2}	>95%

Table 13-97. Acid–Base Imbalances

State	pH	Hco₃	Pco₂	Compensation
Metabolic acidosis	↓	↓	↓ or normal	Lungs blow off CO_2 and hold on to HCO_3
Metabolic alkalosis	↑	↑	↑	Lungs hold on to CO_2, the kidneys hold on to H^+ and get rid of HCO_3
Respiratory acidosis	↓	↑ or normal	↑	Kidneys hold on to HCO_3 and get rid of H^+
Respiratory alkalosis	↑	↓ or normal	↓	Kidneys get rid of HCO_3 and hold on to H^+

Table 13-98. Causes of Acid–Base Imbalances

State	Cause	Signs/symptoms
Metabolic acidosis **pH < 7.35**	Aspirin overdose, renal failure, diarrhea, sepsis, diabetic ketoacidosis	Drowsiness, confusion, ↑ respiratory rate, N/V, headache
Metabolic alkalosis **pH > 7.45**	Vomiting, excessive antacids, GI suctioning, ↓ K^+, ↑ Ca^+	Stiff muscles, tingling in extremities, dizziness
Respiratory acidosis **pH < 7.35**	CNS depression, hypoventilation, airway obstruction, chest trauma, pneumonia, aspiration, drug overdose, pulmonary edema, respiratory depression	↑ BP/pulse/respiratory rate, dysrhythmias, restless, confused, weakness
Respiratory alkalosis **pH > 7.45**	Anxiety, hyperventilation, pulmonary embolism, hypoxia	Light-headedness, inability to concentrate, confusion, numbness/tingling

FLUIDS AND ELECTROLYTES

Nursing practice requires diligent monitoring and in-depth understanding of fluids and electrolytes. First, you must understand how these fluids and electrolytes work.

Table 13-99. Osmolarity

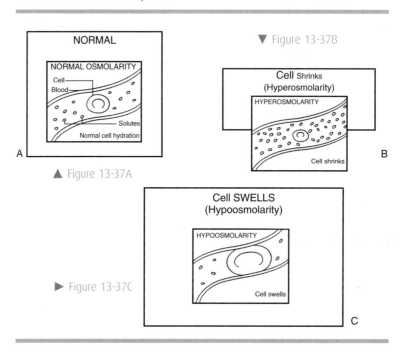

▲ Figure 13-37A

▼ Figure 13-37B

▶ Figure 13-37C

Table 13-100. Hormones that Balance Sodium and Water

ADH (hypothalamus)	Antidiuretic hormone is released and acts on the kidneys (distal renal tubules and collecting duct) to reabsorb or excrete water
Aldosterone (adrenal gland)	Volume receptors stimulate the release of aldosterone to reabsorb or excrete sodium

Table 13-101. Sodium and Potassium Imbalance

	Hypernatremia >145 mEq/L	Hyponatremia <135 mEq/L
Sodium	• Thirst • Flushed skin • Restlessness • Decreased LOC • Tremors • Weakness Foods high in sodium include cheese, pork, sardines, dried fruits, ketchup, mustard, pickles, snack foods, soy sauce, and packaged foods	• Lethargic • Decreased LOC • Inability to concentrate • Twitching • Nausea/vomiting • Seizures
	Hyperkalemia >5.5 mEq/L	**Hypokalemia <3.5 mEq/L**
Potassium	• Anxious • Diarrhea/cramps • Paresthesia • Leg weakness • EKG changes: peak T-wave, wide QRS, irregular pulse, low BP, dysrhythmias Foods high in potassium include apricots, avocado, banana, dates, chocolate, dried peas and beans, oranges, potatoes, spinach, sweet potatoes, tomatoes	• Malaise/fatigue • Nausea/vomiting • Increased urine output • Cramps, numbness, ↓DTRs • Flat T-, U-wave, low BP, dysrhythmias, irregular/weak pulse

Table 13-102. Calcium and Magnesium Imbalance

	Hypercalcemia >11 mg/dL	Hypocalcemia <8 mg/dL
Calcium	• Fatigue • Bone pain • Itching • Nausea/vomiting • Constipation • Renal dysfunction • Poor coordination/unsteady gait • ↓ ST/QT; increased PR interval • Ventricular dysrhythmias Foods high in calcium include cheese, milk chocolate, seafood, tofu, yogurt, oat flakes, molasses, meat, cereal, and beans	• Anxious, irritable • Seizures • Confusion • Diarrhea • Stridor • Hyperreflexia • Tremors • +Trousseau's/Chvostek's sign • Muscle cramps • Ventricular dysrhythmias • Torsades • Heart block • ST/QT ↑
	Hypermagnesemia >2.5 mg/dL	**Hypomagnesemia <1.5 mg/dL**
Magnesium	• Flushing • Drowsiness • Nausea/vomiting • Weakness • ↓ HR/BP • Wide QRS, tall T-wave • Hyporeflexia Foods high in magnesium include chocolate, legumes, seafood, soy, bananas, coconuts, green leafy veggies, oranges	• Hallucinations • Anorexia • Confusion • Tetany/hyperreflexia • Leg cramps • ↑ BP/HR/QT • Dysrhythmias

Table 13-103. Trousseau's and Chvostek's Signs in Hypocalcemia

Hypocalcemia causes nerve fiber membranes to become partially charged, causing muscular irritability. You will see carpopedal spasms, cramps, and muscle twitching/spasms in your clients

Trousseau's sign: Place a blood pressure cuff on the patient's arm, pump it up, and occlude the arterial blood flow. You will see a carpopedal spasm. The thumb will adduct and the phalangeal joints will extend. This indicates tetany.

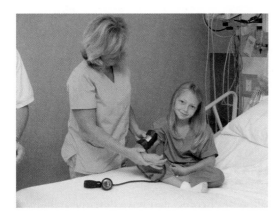

Figure 13-38

Chvostek's sign: Tap the side of the patient's face (facial nerve) adjacent to the patient's ear. You will see a brief contraction of the nose, upper lip, or side of the face. This is a positive sign.

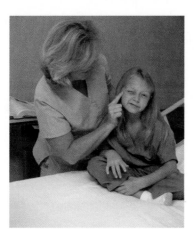

Figure 13-39

Table 13-104. Phosphorus Imbalance

	Hyperphosphatemia >4.8 mg/dL	Hypophosphatemia <2.2 mg/dL
Phosphorus	• Nausea/vomiting • Hyperreflexia • Spasms • Muscle cramps • Paresthesias • ↑ HR • Oliguria Foods high in phosphorus include eggs, nuts, milk, cheese, organ meats, fish, beans, and dried peas	• Malaise/lethargy • Bleeding • Infection • Confusion/memory loss • Decreased GI motility • Weakness • Paresthesias • Hypoxia

PAIN, PAIN GO AWAY . . .

Pain, whether acute or chronic, can have detrimental effects on the client. Remember: pain is whatever the client says it is, whenever the client says it is. It is not up to nurses to judge a client's pain. The client is the expert on her pain.

✚ Harmful effects of pain

The client should be given PRN pain medications for acute pain with no fear of addiction or long-term problems.

Table 13-105. Harmful Effects of Pain

Acute	Chronic
• Sleep disturbance	• Fatigue/exhaustion
• Decreased appetite	• Weight gain/loss
• Nausea/vomiting	• Inability to concentrate
• Decreased fluid intake	• Job loss
• Agitation/anxiety	• Marital strain
	• Depression
	• Loss of interest

Table 13-106. The ABCs of Pain Management

Assess	Assess the pain level by asking the patient to rate it
Believe	Believe what the patient tells you
Choices	Choices are important to the patient, tell them what they are
Do	Do what you say you will do
Ensure	Ensure that the patient has control over his pain

Table 13-107. PQRST of Pain Assessment

P	• **P**oint to where you feel the pain
Q	• What is the **Q**uality of the pain? Is it sharp, dull, throbbing, aching?
R	• Does it **R**adiate? • Where does it radiate? • What makes the pain better/worse?
S	• What is the **S**everity of your pain? • Use appropriate pain rating scale.
T	• What **T**ime did the pain start? • Did anything help the pain? • How long did the pain last?

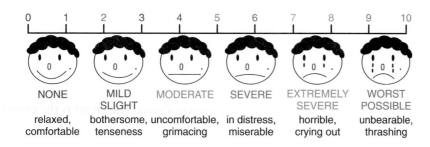

◀ Figure 13-40

MEDICATION ADMINISTRATION

Administering medications is one of the tasks you will perform most as a nurse. It is crucial that you understand the basics of medication administration listed in the following charts.

Table 13-108. Medication Administration

The "SIX RIGHTS"
RIGHT patient
RIGHT drug
RIGHT dose
RIGHT time
RIGHT route
RIGHT documentation

The "Five CHECKS"
• **WHEN** the medication is removed from storage
• **WHEN** the dose is removed from the container just prior to administration
• **WITH** the MAR and the doctor's order
• **WHEN** administering (just before)
• **WHEN** the medication is returned to storage

Table 13-109. Routes of Medication Administration

Topical	Applied to the skin
Sublingual	Administered under the tongue
PO	Given by mouth
Intradermal	Injected under the skin
Subcutaneous	Injected into the fatty tissue (45-degree angle using $\frac{1}{2}$- to 1-inch needle)
Intramuscular	Injected into the muscle (90-degree angle using $\frac{5}{8}$- to 3-inch needle) **The needle MUST be long enough to pass through the fatty tissue and into the muscle**
Intravenous	Given into a vein
Rectal	Inserted into the rectum
Vaginal	Inserted into the vagina
Intranasal	Into the nasal cavities
Opthalmic	Instilled into the eyes
Otic	Instilled into the ears

Table 13-110. Routes of Administration and Absorption Rates of Medications

Topical (Skin)	The absorption rate depends on the medication and the delivery system. It can take hours to days
Sublingual (under the tongue)	3–5 minutes
PO (by mouth)	Usually within 30–90 minutes
Inhalation	3 minutes
Subcutaneous (into fatty tissue)	Usually within 3–20 minutes (45-degree angle using $\frac{1}{2}$- to 1-inch needle)
Intramuscular (into muscle)	Usually within 3–20 minutes (90-degree angle with $\frac{5}{8}$- to 3-inch needle) REMEMBER: The needle must be long enough to pass through the fatty tissue into the muscle
Intravenous (into the vein)	Usually within 30–60 seconds
Rectal (into the rectum)	5–30 minutes (very unpredictable)
Endotracheal	3 minutes

Table 13-111. Medication Administration Special Reminder

- **Always** confirm that the MAR is up to date
- **Always** triple check (label/MAR/recheck)
- **Always** check for allergies
- **Always** confirm compatibility
- **Always** use a straw when administering PO iron to prevent staining the patient's teeth
- **DO NOT** crush time-release tablets
- **DO NOT** crush enteric-coated tablets
- **DO NOT** aspirate when administering SQ heparin or insulin

Table 13-112. Abbreviations You Have to Know

Abbreviation	Meaning	Abbreviation	Meaning
mL/kg	Milliliters per kilogram	q	Every
mm/hr	Millimeters per hour	qhs	Every night, bedtime
μg/mL	Micrograms per milliliter	qid	Four times a day
units/L	Units per liter	qs	Sufficient amount
mEq/L	Milliequivalents per liter	Rx	Prescription
mg/dL	Milligrams per deciliter	SC	Subcutaneous
μg/dL	Micrograms per deciliter	sup	Suspension
g/dL	Grams per deciliter	tid	Three times a day
AC	Before meals	bid	Two times a day
ad lib	As desired	g	Gram
mg	Milligrams	gr	Grain
mL	Milliliter	gtt	Drops
OD	Right eye	h	An hour
OS	Left eye	hs	At bedtime
OU	Both eyes	IM	Intramuscular
PC	After meals	IV	Intravenous
PO	By mouth	PRN	When needed

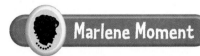

Marlene Moment

You are a mean nurse if you let the eye drop fall directly on the pupil!

Table 13-113. Administration of Eye Drops

Figure 13-41

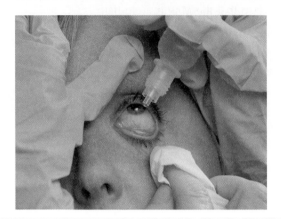

- Gently retract the lower lid
- Ask the patient to look up. WHY? This will diminish the corneal reflex
- Instill the drop into the inner corner of the eye (conjunctival sac)
- Gently release the lid

Table 13-114. Administration of Ear Drops

Infant or child (<3 years old)	Child (>3 years old) and adults
Down and Back	**Up and Back**
Position the child on the unaffected ear. Pull the pinna ↓ ← (down and back)	Position on the unaffected ear. Pull the pinna ↑ ←
Instill the drops and release the pinna	Up and back
	Direct the drops toward the ear canal. WHY? To avoid hitting the tympanic membrane. OUCH!
	The patient should remain in the position for 5–10 minutes
Figure 13-42A	Figure 13-42B

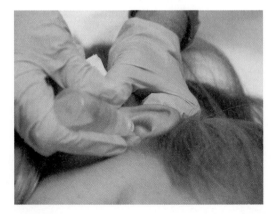

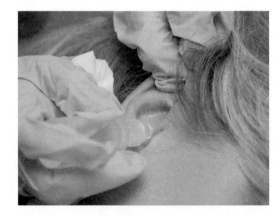

Table 13-115. Administration of a Rectal Suppository

- Position the patient on the side
- Remove the suppository from the wrapping
- Apply water-soluble lubricant
- Insert the suppository into the rectum (approx. 1 inch)
- Don't forget your gloves!

Figure 13-43

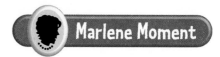

Please use A LOT of water-soluble lubricant!

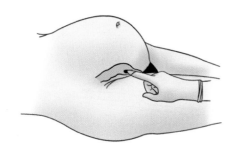

Table 13-116. Enema Volume Administration

Age	Amount of solution	Tube insertion
Infant	100 mL	1 inch
2–4 years old	200 mL	2 inches
4–10 years old	200–400 mL	3 inches
>10 years old	500 mL	3 inches
Remember: The enema position is on the left side!		

Table 13-117. Administration of Vaginal Medication

- Insert the applicator into the vagina up to the hub
- Push the plunger to deposit the medication

Figure 13-44

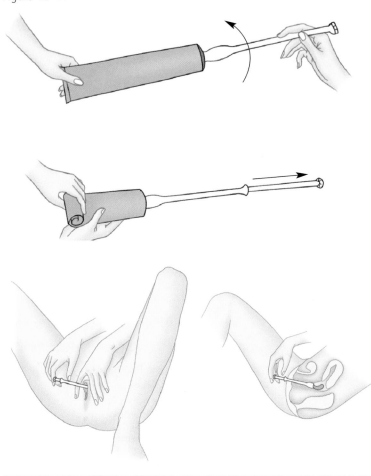

Table 13-118. Administration of Metered Dose Inhaler

- Have the patient take a deep breath and blow out all of the air
- Open the mouth and place the inhaler's mouthpiece in the mouth
- Instruct the patient to close the lips tightly around the mouthpiece
- As the patient begins to take the next breath, have her squeeze the canister
- If another inhalation is needed, repeat the process

Figure 13-45

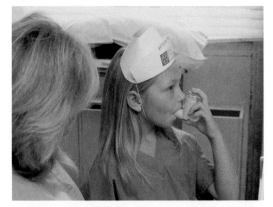

Table 13-119. Preparing Medication from an Ampule

- Wash hands
- Gather equipment
- Check the label of the medication "6 Rights"
- Calculate the dosage if needed
- Hold the ampule and gently tap the top of the ampule or make a complete circle by rotating your wrist
- Place alcohol swab or gauze pad around the neck of the ampule
- Hold the ampule with your dominant hand
- Grip firmly the base with your nondominant hand
- Snap! Break the ampule away from you and others
- Place the top on a safe surface or immediately discard
- Remove the needle cap
- Push the plunger all the way down
- Do not aspirate air into the syringe
- Place the needle in the ampule
- Withdraw the appropriate amount of solution
- Discard the ampule immediately

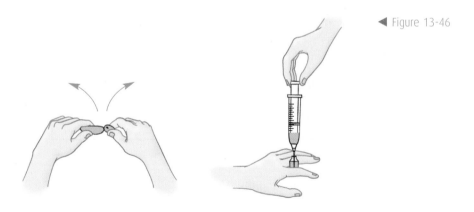

◀ Figure 13-46

Table 13-120. Injections

Type	Site	Angle	Gauge and length of the needle		Volume
Intradermal (ID) (skin)	Inner forearm, back, or chest	10–15 degrees	25–27 g	$\frac{1}{4}$–$\frac{3}{8}$″	0.1 mL
Subcutaneous (SQ) (fatty tissue underlying the skin)	Abdomen, outer upper arm, or anterior thigh	90 degrees *If less than an inch can be pinched between the fingers, inject at a 45–degree angle*	27–28 g	$\frac{3}{8}$–$\frac{5}{8}$″	0.5–1 mL
Subcutaneous Heparin	Abdomen, posterior upper arm, low back, thigh, or upper back	90 degrees *If less than an inch can be pinched between the fingers, inject at a 45–degree angle*	25–26 g	$\frac{3}{8}$″	**DO NOT ASPIRATE OR MASSAGE THE SITE!**
Intramuscular (IM)	Deltoid (DO NOT use if volume > 2 mL)	90 degrees	23–25 g	$\frac{5}{8}$–1.0″	0.5–2.0 mL
	Ventrogluteal (preferred site for adults)	90 degrees	20–23 g	$\frac{5}{8}$–1.5–3″	Up to 3 mL
	Dorsogluteal (WATCH out for the sciatic nerve)	90 degrees	23 g × $\frac{5}{8}$–1.5–3″		Up to 4 mL
	Vastus lateralis Figure 13-47	90 degrees	23 g × $\frac{5}{8}$–1.5″		Up to 3 mL

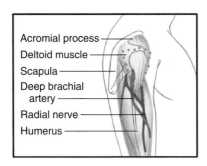

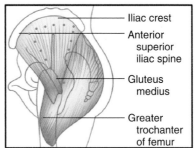

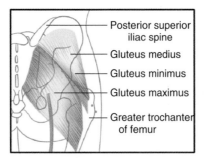

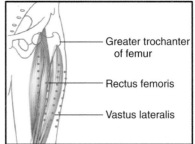

Center of red dots shows safe place to administer injections.

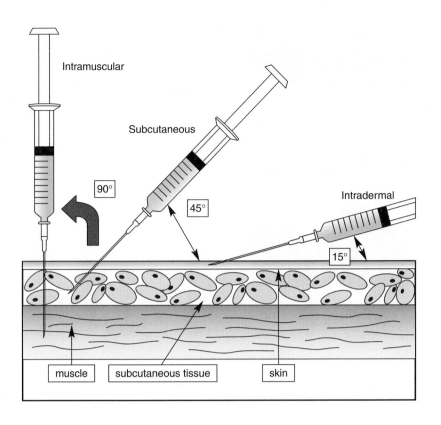

◄ Figure 13-48

Table 13-121. Administering Medication Through a Nasogastric Tube

1. Wash your hands
2. Prepare the medication "6 RIGHTS"
3. Explain the procedure to the patient
4. Tell the client WHAT drug you are giving and WHY
5. Verify allergies
6. Prepare the medication
7. Semi-Fowler's position
8. Gloves
9. Place a pad or towel over the client's chest
10. Disconnect the tube feeding or unclamp the tube
11. DO NOT FORGET TO CHECK TUBE PLACEMENT
    - Attach the syringe to the tube
    - Place the stethoscope on the left upper/outer quadrant of the abdomen
    - JUST below the sternum
    - Instill 20 mL of air
    - LISTEN for the "swishing" sound
    - Aspirate
    - Flush the tube with 30–60 mL of water (may be order specific)
    - Attach the syringe that contains the medication
    - GENTLY push the medication through the tube
    - Flush the tube with 30–60 mL of water
    - Clamp the tube for 30–60 minutes
    - Document

Figure 13-49 ▶

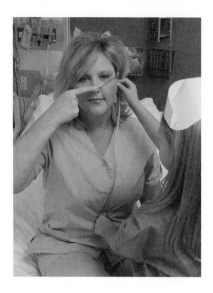

Table 13-122. Angles of Injections

Intradermal	Subcutaneous	Intramuscular
5–15 degrees	45–90 degrees	90 degrees

Table 13-123. Adapting IM Injections for Children
The age, weight, and muscular development MUST be considered!

Goal	Principles
• Minimize trauma	• Be honest with the child
• Minimize discomfort	• Give simple, age-appropriate explanation
• Provide safe, efficient administration of the medication	• Praise the child/never shame
	• Give the child a bandage

Site	Age	Needle size/length	Amount	Remember!
Vastus lateralis	Infants Toddlers	**<4 months** 23–25 g, ⅝-inch needle **>4 months** 22–25 g, 1-inch needle	**Infants:** 1 mL or less **Toddlers:** 2 mL or less	This muscle is large and well developed. It does not have a lot of major nerves or blood vessels so it is a safe site for IM injections
Ventrogluteal	All ages Infants Toddlers Pre/school age Adolescents	**<4 months** 23–25 g, ⅝-inch needle **>4 months** 22–25 g, 1-inch needle	**Infants:** 1 mL or less **Toddlers:** 2 mL or less **Pre/school age:** 3 mL or less **Adolescents:** 5 mL or less	This site does not have a lot of major nerves or blood vessels so it is a safe site for IM injections This site may be less painful than the vastus lateralis
Dorsogluteal	>2 years old	20–25 g, ½- to 1.5-inch needle	**Age 2–6:** 1.5 mL or less **Age > 6:** 2 mL	**Careful:** the sciatic nerve is near!!! Not recommended for children who have been walking <1 year
Deltoid	Toddlers Pre/school age Adolescents	22–25 g, ⅝- to 1-inch needle	**Age < 12:** 1 mL **Age > 12:** 1–1.5 mL	Drug absorption is faster in the deltoid These sites tend to be less painful than the vastus lateralis

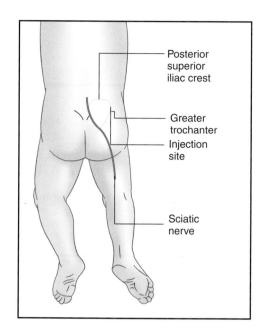

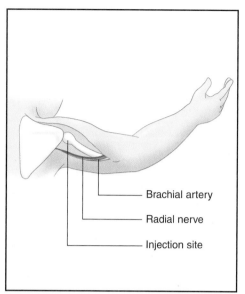

◀ Figure 13-50A—D
Injection sites for children

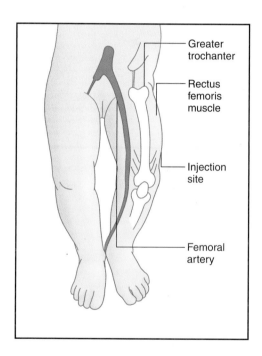

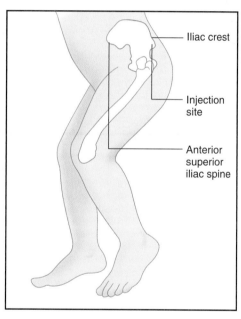

Table 13-124. Z-Track Technique

What Is It?

It is an intramuscular injection

How Do I Do It?

The skin is pulled laterally, then the injection administered. After the needle is withdrawn, remove the needle

Why Do I Use This?

This will help decrease discomfort and prevent the medication from leaking out

Figure 13-51

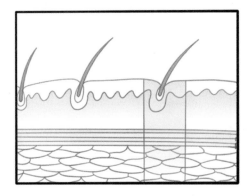
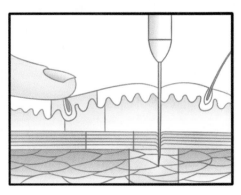
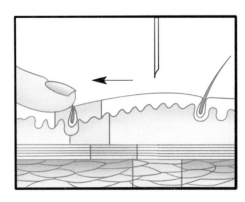
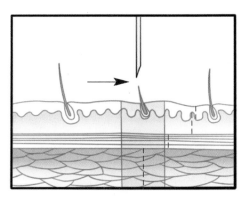

PHARMACOLOGY

If you need to know medication administration, then you can bet your boots that you need to have a good handle on pharmacology. This section will help!

Table 13-125. Drugs and Antidotes

Drug	Antidote
Acetaminophen	Mucomyst (N-acetylcysteine)
Anticoagulants	Protamine/vitamin K
Anticholinergics	Physostigmine (Antilirium)
Benzodiazepines	Flumazenil (Romazicon)
Calcium-channel blockers	Calcium chloride
Digoxin	Digoxin immune Fab (Digibind)
Ethylene glycol	Ethanol
Heparin	Protamine sulfate
Insulin-induced hypoglycemia	Glucagon
Iron	Deferoxamine (Desferal)
Lead	Edetate calcium disodium (Calcium EDTA)
Naphthalene (mothballs)	Methylene blue
Opiates	Methylene blue
Organophosphate	Naloxone (Narcan) Atropine and pralidoxime (Protopam)

Table 13-126. What Can Drug Name Endings Tell You?

If they end in this	They belong to this
-caine	Local anesthetics
-cillin	Antibiotics
-done	Opiod analgesics
-mycin	Antibiotics
-olol	Beta-blockers
-pril	ACE inhibitors
-sone	Steroids
-statin	Antihyperlipidemics
-zide	Diuretics

Table 13-127. Peak and Trough Values of Antibiotics

	Peak	Trough
Gentamycin	5–12 μg/mL	<2 μg/mL
Vancomycin	20–40 μg/mL	5–10 μg/mL
Tobramycin	5–12 μg/mL	<2 μg/mL

Table 13-128. Toxic Drug Levels to Know

Drug	Normal	Toxic level	Signs and symptoms of toxicity
Lithium	<1.5 mEq/L	>2.0 mEq/L	**Mild:** fine hand tremors, polyuria, thirst, nausea **Moderate:** vomiting, diarrhea, confusion, muscle irritability **Severe:** seizures, severe hypotension, coma, death
Digoxin	<2.0 ng/mL	>2.0 ng/mL	**Mild:** GI—anorexia, nausea/vomiting **Moderate:** CNS—headache, confusion, weakness, fatigue **Severe:** cardiac—dysrhythmias, bradycardia, irregular pulse
Theophylline	<20 µg/mL	>20 µg/mL	**Mild/Moderate:** infused rapidly—hypotension, hyperventilation, tachycardia **Severe:** seizures, severe dysrhythmias, cardiovascular collapse

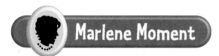 **Marlene Moment**

No sardines and pickled pigs' feet when on MAO inhibitors. Shucks!

Table 13-129. Don't Forget about . . . the MAO Inhibitors

- Used for clinical depression, manic-depression, and psychosis
- Used in patients who have severe depression that has failed other treatments
- Nardil, Marplan, Parnate

Side Effects: Constipation, dizziness, orthostatic hypotension

Remember!!

The patient MUST be warned of the medications and food items that could cause a hypertensive crisis!
- Over-the-counter cold medications
- Foods containing tyramines, such as aged, fermented, or dried, foods; beer, wine

Table 13-130. Insulin

Course	Insulin type	Onset	Peak	Duration
Rapid acting	Insulin aspart	5–10 min	1–3 hr	3–5 hr
	Insulin lispro	15–30 min	30–90 min	4–6 hr
	Regular	30–60 min	2–3 hr	3–6 hr
	Regular IV	10–30 min	15–30 min	30–60 min
	Only insulin that can be given IV			
Fast acting	NPH/regular	30 min	4–8 hr	24 hr
Intermediate acting	NPH	2–4 hr	4–10 hr	10–16 hr
Long acting	Ultralente	6–10 hr	—	18–20 hr

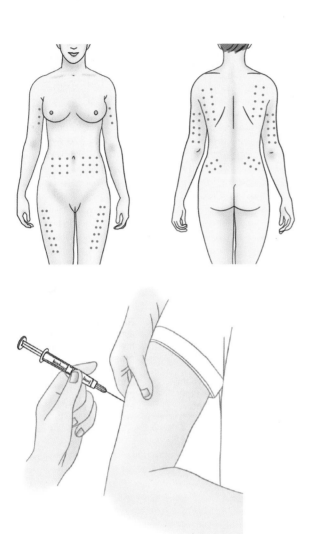

◀ Figure 13-52A,B,C.

Table 13-131. Mixing Insulin

Clear then cloudy

- Use the proper size syringe
- Draw up enough air to equal the TOTAL amount of both insulins being used
- Wipe the runner top with alcohol
- Gently roll the cloudy insulin between your palms
- Inject the amount of air to equal the amount of cloudy insulin that you want into the cloudy vial. Be careful not to inject into the solution
- Inject the remaining air into the clear vial and draw up the clear insulin
- Reinsert the needle into the cloudy vial and withdraw the desired amount

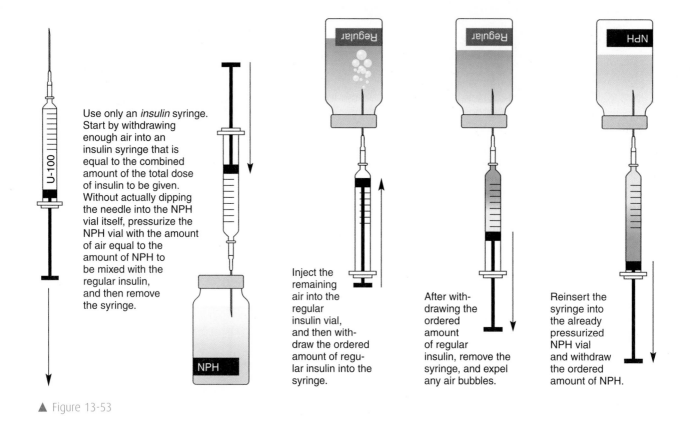

Use only an *insulin* syringe. Start by withdrawing enough air into an insulin syringe that is equal to the combined amount of the total dose of insulin to be given. Without actually dipping the needle into the NPH vial itself, pressurize the NPH vial with the amount of air equal to the amount of NPH to be mixed with the regular insulin, and then remove the syringe.

Inject the remaining air into the regular insulin vial, and then withdraw the ordered amount of regular insulin into the syringe.

After withdrawing the ordered amount of regular insulin, remove the syringe, and expel any air bubbles.

Reinsert the syringe into the already pressurized NPH vial and withdraw the ordered amount of NPH.

▲ Figure 13-53

Table 13-132. Storing Insulin

- Avoid exposure to temperature extremes
- Do NOT freeze
- Do NOT expose to direct sunlight
- Should be at room temperature before injection
- Store at room temperature if the vial will be used within 30 days. If not, store in the refrigerator

Table 13-133. Drugs that Can Cause Confusion in the Elderly

- Antipsychotics
- Antihistamines
- Anticholinergics
- Antiemetics
- Antihypertensives

- Antiarrhythmics
- Diuretics
- Histamine blockers
- Opioid analgesics
- Tranquilizers

Table 13-134. Oral Anticoagulants

Warfarin (Coumadin) is a drug that interferes with the use of vitamin K. This in turn affects the liver's ability to manufacture several clotting factors. Vitamin K intake through foods must be limited and in some cases restricted. Remember:

- Avoid drastic dietary changes
- Eat the same amount of food and green leafy vegetables each day

Avoid	Limit to 1 serving/day	Be careful
• Parsley	• Broccoli	• Green tea
• Kale	• Turnip greens	• Green vegetables
	• Spinach	• Liver
	• Brussels sprouts	• Soybeans
		• Lentils
		• Garbanzo beans

Table 13-135. Street Drugs

Drug	AKA	Toxic side effects	Treatment	WARNING
Cocaine (stimulant/anesthetic)	Coke, crack, snow	Headache, N/V, chest pain, euphoria, ↑ temp, pulse, acute MI, dilated pupils	O_2, IV, set up for intubation, control HTN, cool patient, minimize stimulation	Patient may be violent!
Ecstasy (stimulant/hallucinogen)	Love drug, XTC, MDMA, empathy	Euphoria, hallucinations, agitation, nausea, sweating, ↑ temp, dilated pupils, seizures, electrolyte imbalance	O_2, IV, vitals, EKG, cool the patient, prepare to intubate, benzodiazepines for seizures	Do not give beta-blockers!
Hallucinogens (alter perception)	LSD, mushrooms	Hallucinations, panic, N/V, disoriented, anxious	Calm and reassure the patient	Watch for violent and unexpected behavior!
PCP (tranquilizer)	Angel dust, horse tranquilizer	Hallucinations, HTN, nystagmus, stupor, mania, dilated pupils	O_2, vitals, IV, EKG	Watch for violent behavior!
GHB (depressant)	G, easy lay, liquid x, cherry meth	Dizziness, euphoria, sedation, N/V, headache, apnea, ↓ pulse	ABCs, manage airway, prepare to ventilate if needed	Common "date rape" drug

BLOOD PRODUCT ADMINISTRATION

Administering blood products can be life threatening if the client experiences an adverse reaction. Be sure to constantly monitor your clients as they receive blood products.

Table 13-136. Blood Transfusion Compatibility

Blood type	Compatible donors	Incompatible
O− (O− is the universal donor)	O−	O+, A−, A+, B−, B+, AB−, and AB+
O+	O− and O+	A−, A+, B−, B+, AB−, and AB+
A−	O− and A−	O+, A+, B−, B+, AB−, and AB+
A+	O−, O+, A−, and A+	B−, B+, AB−, and AB+
B−	O− and B−	O+, A−, A+, B+, AB−, and AB+
B+	O−, O+, B−, and B+	A−, A+, AB−, and AB+
AB−	O−, B−, A−, and AB−	O+, A+, B+, AB+
AB+ (Universal recipient)	O−, O+, A−, A+, B−, B+, AB−, and AB+	NONE
Rh factor	Do a Coomb's test to evaluate the Rh status	In a person previously sensitized to Rh-positive blood, another exposure to Rh-positive blood will cause a severe hemolytic reaction

Table 13-137. Blood Product Infusion

STOP the Infusion If the Following Occur

- Pain in the area
- Burning or stinging at the entry site
- Rash
- Flushing
- Warm sensation
- Itching
- Chills
- Fever
- Marked change in vital signs
- Stay with the patient and have someone notify the physician!

IV ADMINISTRATION

Table 13-138. Tonicity of IV Fluids

Isotonic	Hypotonic	Hypertonic
• 0.9% saline • D5W • LR	• ½ NS • ¼ NS	• D5LR • D5 ½ NS • D5 NS • D10W
• Isotonic solutions go where you put them and they stay there • They expand the intravascular space • Monitor for fluid overload	• Less salt and more water • Water pulled from the intravascular space into the cell • The cell will swell! • Monitor for cardiovascular collapse	• They greatly expand the intravascular space and draw fluid from intravascular areas • The cell will shrink! • Monitor for fluid overload

Table 13-139. IV Catheter Gauge Selection

Remember: Always use the shortest length and smallest diameter needed to get the job done

Gauge	Use	Indications
>16 clients	• Large fluid/volume • Rapid infusions	• Usually in trauma or surgical • Large vein needed
18	• Surgery • Blood products	• Large vein needed
20	• Routine IV access	• Very common selection
22	• Good for most infusions that are running slowly • Good for small, fragile veins	• Difficult to insert through tough skin • Easier to insert into small, fragile veins
24, 26	• Pediatric and elderly • Slow-flow infusions	• Easier to insert into small, fragile veins

Table 13-140. Intravenous Administration

The ABCs of IVs

- Prepare and gather the equipment (gloves, tubing, sharps container, catheter, tape, tourniquet, and antiseptic wipe)
- Apply the tourniquet
- Select a vein
- Cleanse the site
- Don gloves
- Lightly press the skin with the thumb of your nondominant hand
- Bevel up, 15–30 degrees
- Insert the needle bevel up through the skin and into the vein
- Observe for flashback
- Lower the catheter so that it is parallel to the skin and then insert it an additional 1–2 mm to ensure the catheter tip is in the vein
- Advance the catheter
- Release the tourniquet. Apply pressure just above the end of the catheter tip while stabilizing the hub of the catheter
- Remove or retract the needle and discard into approved sharps container
- Connect the IV tubing, watch for free flow
- Secure the IV with supplies according to the facility's policy
- Document, document, document!

Table 13-141. IV Site Complications

Assessment	Infiltration	Phlebitis
Color	Pale	Red
Temperature	Cool	Warm
Swelling	Puffy	Cord-like
Pain	Yes	Yes
Flow	Slowed or stopped	No change or slowed
Actions:	<ul><li>Lower the bag</li><li>Discontinue the IV</li><li>Get an order for warm (phlebitis), cool (infiltration) compresses</li><li>Elevate the extremity</li></ul>	<ul><li>Stop the infusion</li><li>Discontinue the IV</li><li>Elevate the extremity</li><li>Get an order for warm compresses</li></ul>

Table 13-142. High-Risk IV Infusions

Insulin	• Regular insulin is the ***ONLY*** insulin that can be given IV
	• **ALWAYS** use an infusion pump
	• Label well
Heparin	• Look closely at the concentration of the solution
	• **ALWAYS** use an infusion pump
	• Label well

VENOUS AND ARTERIAL PUNCTURES

Table 13-143. Allen's Test

Purpose	• This is a test that **MUST** be preformed prior to using the radial artery for obtaining a blood specimen
Location	• Apply direct pressure over the radial and ulnar arteries
	• While applying pressure, ask the patient to open and close his hand repeatedly
Result	• The hand should blanch
	• Release pressure from the ulnar artery while maintaining pressure over the radial artery
	• Assess the color of the distal extremity
	• If the extremity fails to pink up within 6 seconds, the ulnar artery is insufficient. Do not use the radial artery!
	• Remember to document!

Table 13-144. Venipuncture Technique

Check Your Institution's Policy

1. Don gloves
2. Select a site (vein)
3. Apply the tourniquet
4. Palpate the vein
5. Cleanse the skin
6. Bevel up
7. Syringe at 45 degrees
8. Insert the needle through the skin and into the vein
9. Slowly reduce the angle of your syringe
10. When you see blood . . .
11. Withdraw blood with syringe or connect the collection device
12. Remove the tourniquet when collection complete
13. Remove the needle and dispose in a proper container
14. Place a dressing
15. Label container and dressing with time, date, and person performing the VP
    Figure 13-54A,B

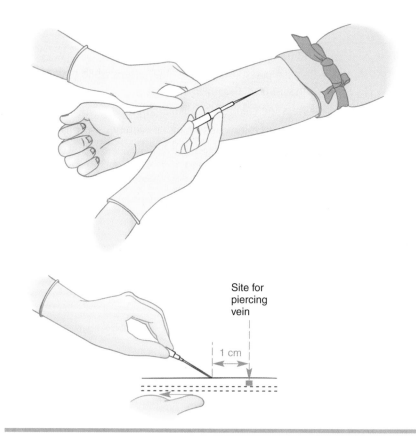

SIGNS AND SYMPTOMS THAT MEAN SOMETHING

Table 13-145. Signs and Symptoms that Mean Something

Rebound tenderness

Indicates peritoneal inflammation or peritonitis

To elicit rebound tenderness, place the patient in a supine position, then push your fingers deeply into the abdomen. Quickly release the pressure and assess for pain. The pain that is produced is called rebound tenderness

Frequent cause: Appendicitis

Figure 13-55

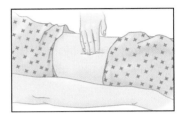

Carpopedal spasm

Violent, painful spasm of the muscles in the hands and feet. It is an important sign of tetany, a potentially life-threatening condition

In the hand, carpopedal spasm involves adduction of the thumb over the palm, followed by flexion of the metacarpophalangeal joints, flexion of the wrist and elbows

Frequent cause: Hypocalcemia and tetanus

Figure 13-56A and B

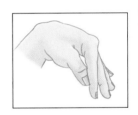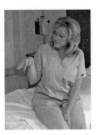

Pitting edema

Pitting edema is noted when the tissue fails to return to normal when the fluid is displaced by pressure application

To check for pitting edema, apply pressure with your finger to the swollen area for 5 seconds, and then quickly remove your finger. With pitting the indentation is slow to fill. To determine the severity of the pitting edema, estimate the depth of the indentation in millimeters.

$$+1 = 2 \text{ mm}$$
$$+2 = 4 \text{ mm}$$
$$+3 = 6 \text{ mm}$$
$$+4 = 8 \text{ mm}$$

Frequent cause: Congestive heart failure (CHF)

Figure 13-57

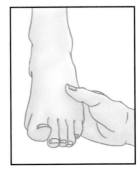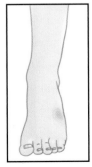

Testing for pitting edema | Pitting edema

Angioedema

Swelling of the lips, tongue, and/or eyelids.

It is characterized by rapid onset of painless, nonpitting, subcutaneous swelling. It usually resolves in 1–2 days

Careful! The airway (laryngeal edema) may occur, which could cause a life-threatening airway obstruction

Frequent causes: Allergic reaction, ACE inhibitors, or hereditary angioedema

Figure 13-58

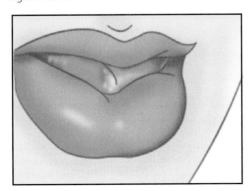

(Continued)

Table 13-145. Signs and Symptoms that Mean Something (*Continued*)

Homan's sign	Jugular vein distention
Deep calf pain with flexion	Normally, jugular veins only distend if the patient is lying flat
To elicit Homan's sign, support the patient's thigh with one hand and his foot with the other, bend his leg slightly at the knee, then abruptly dorsiflex the ankle. Pain = + Homan's sign	To measure JVD:
Frequent causes: Deep vein thrombosis (DVT), deep vein thrombophlebitis, or cellulitis	1. Elevate the head of the bed @ 45–90 degrees
	2. Locate the angle of Louis (sternal notch)
Even though you were probably still taught about the Homan's sign, it is a Killer Assessment. Why? Because you can dislodge the clot and possibly kill your patient. It is no longer acceptable to perform the Homan's sign, but the NCLEX® Lady may still ask you about it!	3. Find the internal jugular vein
	4. Shine a light across the neck to create shadows that highlight the venous pulse
	5. Locate the highest point of the vein where pulsations are seen
	6. Using a centimeter ruler, measure the distance between that high point and the sternal notch
	7. A finding > 3–4 cm above the sternal notch with the HOB @ 45 degrees indicates JVD

Figure 13-59

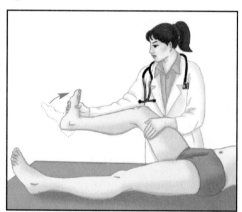

Frequent causes: Cardiac tamponade, heart failure, hypervolemia, pericarditis, superior vena cava obstruction

Figure 13-60

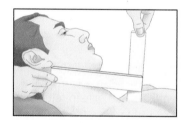

Retractions

When observing retractions in infants and children, it is important that you observe the exact location. This will provide an important clue to the cause of the respiratory distress

Locations of retractions include:

- Subcostal: lower respiratory tract disorder
- Substernal: lower respiratory tract disorder
- Suprasternal: upper respiratory tract disorder
- Intercostal: alone may be normal, but if accompanied by any of the other sites, may indicate moderate respiratory distress

Frequent causes: Asthma, croup, bronchiolitis, epiglottiditis, pneumonia, heart failure, laryngotracheobronchitis, respiratory distress syndrome

Figure 13-61

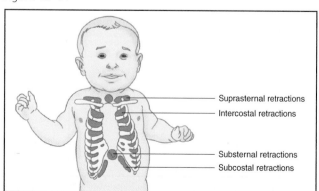

MISCELLANEOUS MED-SURG

Table 13-146. SHOCK: What Does it Look Like & What Do I DO?

Type	Physical findings	Action/treatment
Anaphylactic	Cool, pale skin, BP↓↓, rash, swelling, HR↑, respiratory distress, anxious	O_2, IV fluids, epinephrine, antihistamines, steroids
Hypovolemic	Cool, clammy skin, BP↓↓, rapid, thready pulse, rapid shallow respirations, LOC↓	Fast and furious fluid and volume replacement, + inotropics (e.g., dopamine)
Cardiogenic	Cool, clammy skin, LOC↓, rapid, thready pulse, rapid shallow respirations, BP↓↓↓ (usually < 60), gallop, distant heart sounds	O_2, analgesics/sedatives, osmotic diuretics, vasopressors, vasoconstrictors, inotropics, A-line for BP monitoring
Neurogenic	Pale, warm, dry skin, BP↓, pulse↓, bounding pulse, LOC may be altered	O_2, IV fluids, place the patient SUPINE, vasopressors
Septic	**Initially:** Flushed skin; BP normal to slightly elevated; rapid, full, bounding pulse; rapid, shallow respirations **Progressed/Late:** Pale, cyanotic skin; BP↓; rapid, weak, thready pulse; rapid, shallow respiratons	O_2, antimicrobials (Abx), diuretics, IV fluid (colloids/crystalloids), vasopressors

✛ Who invited all these hormones?

Table 13-147. Hormone Overview

Gland	Hormones secreted
Pituitary	ADH, ACTH, LH, FSH, prolactin, TSH
Thyroid/parathyroid	T3, T4, calcitonin, PTH
Adrenal	Aldosterone, cortisol, catecholamines
Stomach	Gastrin
Pancreas	Insulin
Ovary	Estrogen, progesterone
Placenta	HCG, HPL
Testis	Males: testosterone

✚ Common tube types and function

Table 13-148. Common Tubes

Type	Description	Function
Levin Tube (suctioning or feeding)	• **Nasogastric** • Single lumen tube with a solid tip • May be inserted into the stomach via the nose or the mouth	• Used to drain fluid and gas from the stomach • Continuous irrigation is NOT possible with this tube • MUST be connected to suction to low suction to prevent gastric irritation
Lavacuator Tube (suctioning)	• **Nasogastric** • Large suction lumen • Smaller lavage/vent lumen that provides continuous suction • Irrigation solution enters the lavage lumen while stomach contents are removed via the suction lumen	• Used to remove toxic substances from the stomach
Miller–Abbot Tube (suctioning)	• **Small to large intestine** • Long double-lumen tube • One lumen is filled with mercury once in the stomach • The second lumen is used for irrigation and drainage	• Used to decompress the small intestine
Salem Sump Tube (suctioning or feeding)	• **Nasogastric** • Short double-lumen tube • Small vent tube within a large suction tube	• Used to decompress the stomach • Maintains suction @ 25 mm Hg without damaging mucosal tissue
Jejunostomy (feeding)	• **Jejunum**	• Feedings may be intermittent or continuous with an infusion pump
Dobhoff (feeding)	• **Jejunum** • Has a mercury tip for x-ray visualization and to assist with passage	• CAUTION: Use a 50-mL syringe with 20 mL of water to irrigate. (Small syringes may cause tube rupture from excessive pressure.) ALWAYS use an infusion pump! (40 psi)
Sengstaken–Blakemore Tube (compression of esophageal varices)	• **Esophagus and stomach** • Three lumen tube • Two ports inflate balloons (gastric and esophageal) • The third port is used for nasogastric suction	• Used when tamponade is needed • Does not provide esophageal suctioning • An NG tube may be placed in the opposite nare or the mouth to rest on top of the esophageal balloon. This will help prevent aspiration
Hemovac	• Rigid drain tube • Closed wound drainage system that is connected to suction • Often used for mastectomy, total knee/hip replacement	• Used to drain large amounts of fluid from under incisions

Table 13-148. Common Tubes (*Continued*)

Type	Description	Function
Jackson–Pratt	• Closed wound suction drainage system • Often used for neurosurgery, neck surgery, abdominal surgery, urologic problems	• Indicated when tissue trauma may occur with a rigid drain tube (i.e. Hemovac)
T-tube	• Used post-cholecystectomy	• Used to drain bile from the common bile duct until the edema has subsided
Penrose	• Soft collapsible latex rubber drain • Used in bowel resections	• Drains serosanguineous fluid from surgical site

DEATH AND DYING

Table 13-149. Dying "Fears" of Clients

Pain	• Fear that pain may occur or become increasingly worse • Feel very anxious about the uncertainties of the dying process • **REMEMBER**: Do not withhold or delay pain relief measures to a terminally ill patient
Abandonment	• The family/friends should be allowed to stay with the patient • Listening to, touching, and providing support as needed by the patient • Assuring them that someone will remain with them
Meaningless	• Focus on the positive aspects of the patients life • Encourage them to talk about the past • They may feel powerless and that there is no hope • **REMEMBER:** Do not bring up things that will cause the patient undue anxiety or fear

✚ Impending death: what to do?

Table 13-150. Impending Death

Signs and symptoms	Nursing interventions
• Decreased appetite • Weakness • Fatigue • Decreased fluid intake • Cool hands and feet secondary to decreased circulation • Urine output will decrease • Level of consciousness will change • Respiratory rate and rhythm will change • Coughing may increase secondary to the client decreased ability to swallow adequately • May become restless	• Assist the client with needs as her energy level will be low • Keep the mucous membranes moist • Keep the client clean and dry • Give pain medications as ordered to ensure that the patient is not in pain • Encourage the family to talk about the impending death • Support the family when they feel as if the patient "is giving up" • Provide dignity, comfort, guidance, and education • Respect and assist the family as needed

PSYCHOSOCIAL

Table 13-151. Expressions of Sexuality

Heterosexuality	Sexual relationship solely between a male and female
Homosexuality	Sexual attraction and/or relationship with a member of the same sex
Bisexuality	Sexual attraction and/or relationship with both sexes
Transvestism	Wearing clothes and pretending to be a member of the opposite sex

REPORTING

What information to give and to whom in certain situations is listed in the following tables.

Table 13-152. Reportable Situations

Report WHAT	To WHOM
• Assaults	• Law enforcement
• Animal bites	• Law enforcement/animal control
• Abuse of elderly	• Adult protective services
• Child abuse	• Child protective services
• Communicable diseases	• States specific(most states are reportable to the health department)
• Deaths	• Coroner
• Suicide	• Law enforcement/coroner

+ Elder abuse report

If you suspect abuse, make sure the patient is safe and report the possible abuse to law enforcement. Do not confront the alleged abuser! If sexual abuse is suspected, do not allow the patient to bathe or shower until the police arrive.

Table 13-153. Signs and Symptoms of Elder Abuse

- Fractures and/or bruises in various stages of healing
- Unexplained cigarette burns on the torso or extremities
- Unexplained malnourishment/dehydration/listlessness
- Mental status or neurological changes
- Poor hygiene (urine or feces on the clothing)
- Strange or unusual interaction between the client and the caregiver

+ Shift report

The shift report is VERY important for the ongoing care of the patient and their family.

Table 13-154. Shift Report

- Patient identification information
- Patient present status and any special circumstances (language barrier, cultural concern, safety needs, etc.)
- Nursing diagnosis (priority)
- Assessment information
- Interventions including treatments, monitoring, teaching
- Evaluation
- New orders
- Test results
- Infusions
- Drains/tubes if applicable
- Pending treatments
- Family knowledge and concerns

ENVIRONMENTAL SAFETY

Use the following tables to keep you and your clients safe!

Table 13-155. Incidents

- Falls/Injuries
- Needle-sticks
- Medication administration errors
- Accidental omission of an order
- Equipment-related accidents
- Procedure-related accidents

Do not ignore the above incidents if they occur. Follow the policy in your institution for reporting and follow-up

Table 13-156. Fire

1. Keep the environment free of clutter
2. Make sure the fire exits are clearly marked
3. Know the location of fire alarms, exits, and extinguishers
4. Know the number to call to report a fire
5. Know the evacuation plan
6. NEVER use the elevator in the event of a fire
7. Turn off all oxygen in the area of the fire
8. Be prepared to offer respiratory support to ventilator patients (Ambu bag)
9. Move all clients to a safe area as quickly as possible

Priority Actions

1. **R**—Rescue: Remove all clients from the vicinity of the fire
2. **A**—Alarm: Activate the fire alarm
3. **C**—Confine: Close all doors and windows
4. **E**—Extinguish: Extinguish the fire by using the appropriate fire extinguisher

PASS (Use of a Fire Extinguisher)

P   Pull the pin

A   Aim at the base of the fire

S   Squeeze the handle

S   Sweep the fire from side to side

Table 13-157. Radiation Source

- Private room with private bath
- Place a caution sign on the door
- Minimize exposure to the patient
- Rotate nursing assignments so that no one is overexposed
- Wear a lead shield to reduce transmission of radiation
- Limit exposure time to 30 minutes
- Wear a radiation badge to measure exposure
- Do not allow a pregnant nurse to care for the client
- Do not allow a pregnant person or a child to visit the client
- Limit visitors to 30 minutes
- Do not allow visitors any closer than 6 feet to the client
- Dispose of linens and supplies per hospital policy

Management of Dislodged Radiation Source

- Do not touch with bare hands
- Use long-handled forceps to place the source in the lead container. Make sure that there is a lead container in the room at all times
- Call the physician
- If you cannot locate the dislodged source, DO NOT allow visitors
- Reassure the client

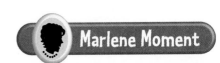 **Marlene Moment**

If the radiation source falls out of the client and you see it glowing in the bed, please do not take it out to the nurses' station to show everybody what you found.

DELEGATION AND LEADERSHIP

These topics are HUGE on NCLEX®. But if you've been paying attention to me all along, you'll do just great!

Table 13-158. Delegation: "The Four Rights"

Right person	Who is the right person to carry out the task?
Right task	Can the task be delegated?
Right communication	Can I communicate what I need to the person who is assigned the task?
Right response	Was the right person selected for the right task, and was the need communicated so that the task was accomplished?

Table 13-159. Leadership Styles

Style	Strengths	Limitations
Democratic	• Everyone participates in the decision making • Group consensus reached • High productivity • Preferred management style	• Limited personal growth
Authoritarian	• Immediate task is completed quickly • Organization during times of crisis remains • Structure/order	• Limited growth of members • No attention to the growth process
Facilitative	• Maximizes personal growth • Personal commitment high	• Limited when immediate action is needed to maintain safety
Laissez-faire	• No limit on members • Minimal direction or control	• No structure • No commitment to the group • No cohesiveness

LAW AND ORDER

The remaining tables demonstrate the different legal and ethical content you may encounter on NCLEX®.

Table 13-160. Consents

Admission	• Identify the health care facility's responsibility to the client • Obtain at the time of admission
Blood transfusion	• Indicate that the client was informed about the risks and benefits of the transfusion • Some clients refuse blood products because of religious beliefs even in the event of life-threatening illnesses or injury
Research	• Indicates the client's willingness to participate in a research study • The client is informed regarding risks, consequences, and the benefits of the research
Surgical	• This consent is obtained for all surgical procedures, invasive procedures, or invasive diagnostic test • The risks, benefits, alternative options (if applicable) are explained to the client by the surgeon, physician, or anesthesiologist
Special	• There are some special cases where consent is required. They include the following: organ recovery after death, photographs, use of restraints, disposal of body parts, and autopsy

Table 13-161. Invasion of Privacy

• Allowing others to observe a procedure without the client's consent
• Assessing medical records when you have not been authorized to do so
• Leaving the door or curtain open while performing a procedure or treatment
• Interviewing a patient in a room with only the curtain between clients, or where the conversation can be overheard
• Taking photographs of the client without the client's consent
• Releasing information without the client's consent
• Using the client's name or picture for the sole purpose of the institution's sole advantage
• Public disclosure of private information
• Leaving a confused client in the hallway
• Discussing patient information with unauthorized persons

Table 13-162. Maintaining Confidentiality

- Do not discuss client issues with other clients
- Do not discuss client issues with staff who are not involved in caring for that client
- Do not share client information with family or friends without the client's consent
- Do not share client information in a public place where the information can be overheard
- Do not allow anyone to read the medical record who is not authorized to do so

Table 13-163. Ethical Principles

Ethics: The distinction between right and wrong based not on opinion but rather on a body of knowledge

Autonomy	• Respect for an individual's right to self-determination
Beneficence	• To do good • To implement actions that benefit the client and their support persons
Nonmaleficence	• The duty to do no harm
Veracity	• Telling the truth
Justice	• Often referred to as fairness
Fidelity	• To be faithful to agreement and promises

Table 13-164. EMTALA (Emergency Medical Treatment and Active Labor Act)

This act was passed by Congress in 1988 and states the following:

1. Any patient presenting to the emergency department requesting examination and treatment must be provided an appropriate medical screening to determine if they have an emergency medical condition.
2. If the patient does have an emergency medical condition, the hospital must either treat the patient until stable or transfer the patient to another hospital in conformance with the statute's directives.
3. If the patient does not have an emergency medical condition, EMTALA imposes no further obligation on the hospital.
4. Hospitals must have an updated list of on-call physicians who are available to provide emergency stabilization of the patient.
5. The hospital cannot admit a patient with no intention to treat him and then inappropriately transfer or discharge the patient.
6. The hospital cannot delay screening or treatment to obtain information about payment method.

Table 13-165. Liability: Action = Responsibility

Individual Liability

- Every person is liable for her own actions and conduct
- May be shared by another person or group
- Cannot be removed by the statements or actions of another

Vicarious Liability

Does not lessen individual liability even though shared

1. **Respondeat superior:** Employer can be held liable for the actions of an employee
2. **Supervisory negligence:** Supervisors may share liability if
   - Assignments are not within the nurse's capabilities
   - Assignments are not appropriate for the educational training of the nurse
   - Assignments are outside of the legal limitations of the nurse
3. **Physicians:** They may share liability but cannot assume or alter the personal liability of the nurse

Table 13-166. Your License: Protect It or You Will Lose It!

- Do not let anyone borrow your license
- If you loose it, report it immediately to the Board of Nursing
- Be sure to notify the Board of Nursing of any address or telephone number changes
- Never practice outside of your scope of practice as set by the Board of Nursing
- Know the rules and stick by them!
- Never take chances!

SUMMARY

Use these cool charts to help jog your memory on some of the core content. I can promise you that you will use these basics on a regular basis if your career keeps you in patient care.

Bibliography

Hurst M. *A Critical Thinking and Application NCLEX® Review.* Brookhaven, MS: Hurst Review Services; 2006.

McCance K, Huether S. *Pathophysiology: The Biological Basis for Disease in Adults and Children.* 4th ed. St. Louis: Mosby-Year Book; 2002.

Becker D, Franges EZ, Geiter H, et al. *Critical Care Nursing Made Incredibly Easy.* Amble, PA: Lippincott, Williams & Wilkins; 2004.

Hurst Review Services. **www.hurstreview.com.**

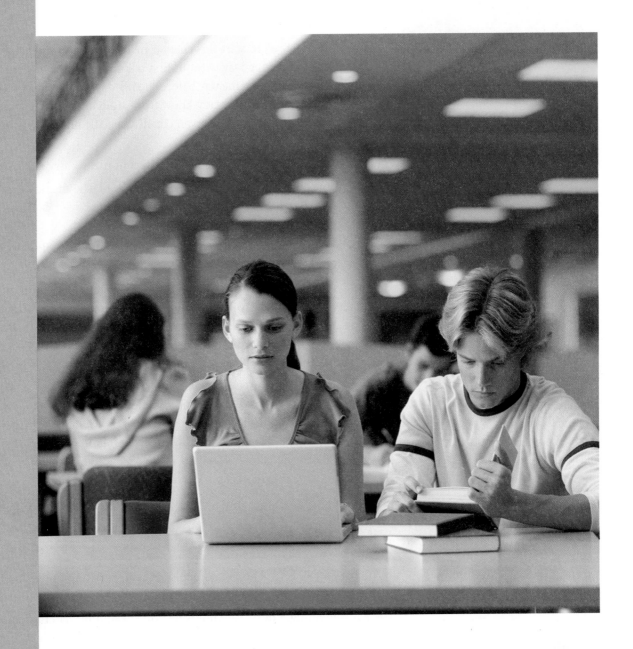

14 A Day in the Life

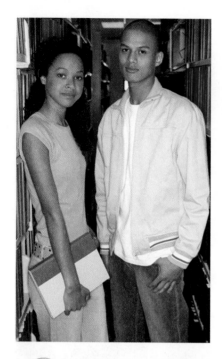

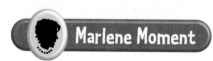
Marlene Moment

The best thing to drink is milk or a protein shake. These types of drinks not only get your blood sugar up, but will sustain your blood sugar longer than a cola.

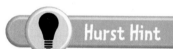
Marlene Moment

Don't forget your valid identification when you head to the testing center.

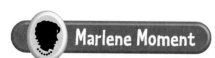
Hurst Hint

Don't worry about not sleeping the night before . . . you will be able to sleep after the exam!

Marlene Moment

If you do not eat properly, you will not have the power required to fight Newt. I can assure you he is waiting for you at the testing center!

THE DAY BEFORE THE BIG DAY

I know I'm supposed to start this chapter by talking about the Big Day, but I can't start with the Big Day without first talking about the day *before* the big day. As you approach the day before the big day, your anxiety level will naturally increase. As you already know from studying psychiatric nursing, anxious people do better when given concise, specific information!

So here goes:

1. Get specific directions to the testing site and make a dry run.

2. Buy some snacks, water, soft drinks, juice, headache medicine, and your anti-diarrheal of choice. Put a little cooler in your car for the drinks and snacks.

3. Place your ATT and forms of identification with your belongings to be taken to the testing center.

4. Study 'til you can't study anymore. I know what you are thinking: "Everybody else says to take the day off prior to the exam." Aunt Marlene says study 'til the bitter end. That last little bit of studying may be what bumps you into the passing zone!

5. Get a good night's rest. That sounds so therapeutic, doesn't it? You can forget it! You are going to wake up every hour on the hour staring at your digital clock just like you did the night before clinical. Please do not take medications to help you sleep unless you take these medications regularly, as they will cloud your thinking on exam day. Don't worry about the "sleep" deal; you will have enough adrenalin running through your veins to keep you going during the exam.

THE DAY OF THE EXAM

The Big Day is here! The old adrenals are really starting to pump out the catecholamines. Here are specific tips about how to approach exam day:

1. Eat something. I don't care if it is just one peanut butter cracker and one half of a glass of milk. Your brain is going to need all the glucose your body can provide. You may feel nauseous prior to the exam and you may feel like you can't eat. Try to eat a little bit at a time on the way to the testing center. However, I do not recommend drinking or eating **too many** sweets such as colas, candy, or donuts. These will shoot your blood sugar up and then it will bottom out. When your blood sugar bottoms out, you will not think as sharply and your mood may change. Your mood will switch from one of confidence to one of insecurity: "I don't know if I should have taken this exam today; I don't recognize anything on this exam; I wonder if they have given me the correct test?"

2. Dress in layers. Who knows what the temperature of the testing center may be. Post-menopausal ladies with raging hormones may run the center resulting in an air-conditioning setting of a frigid 50 degrees!

3. Get your thoughts straight. Test-taking anxiety is natural.

The next section will help lessen the impact of test-taking anxiety.

✛ Test-taking anxiety

A big part of being successful on this test is to keep your emotions under control. Let's get the mental aspect straight. As you drive to the testing center, it is normal to think you are forgetting everything you ever learned about nursing. You're not. This is only anxiety. When taking a test at school, have you ever felt like you needed to write down everything you knew on the back of the test before you forgot the material? The same thing may happen on NCLEX® day, but don't waste your time trying to write down everything you know on the cute little dry-erase board the testing center provides you.

- Prepare yourself to take the entire test. This way, you won't panic if you receive all of the questions. Repeat to yourself the mantra: I am special. I am special. I am special. You are so special that you **know**, without a doubt and without hesitation that the computer is going to give you **all** the test questions. Then you will not get upset if the computer does not stop on the lowest number of available test questions. You WILL tell yourself you are PASSING as you answer each question, even if the exam goes to the bitter end!

- Assure yourself you may need the entire amount of time allotted to take the test. This is perfectly okay! As long as you are there, you are passing! You do not care that your friends finish the exam in 1.5 hours!

- Tell yourself: "I promise not to get hung up trying to figure out if I am getting high-, medium-, or low-level questions." There is no way for you to judge what level of question you are getting, and spending the time figuring it out only wastes valuable brain energy. You may think a question is low level, but in reality, it may be a high-level question. So give this up!

- Think this: "I will not get discouraged during the exam even if I feel as if I know nothing. I know I know SOMETHING! I've come too far to know NOTHING! When I feel as if I know nothing, I will be aware that this is just Newt trying to make me feel inadequate."

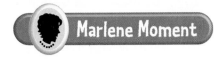

Marlene Moment

Every time you get another test question, you know you are very close to passing.

✛ Let's get organized

Getting organized the day before the test is very important, so that you aren't rattled on exam day. There are a few things that you can do to help alleviate the "jitters."

1. Don't forget your stuff. Make a list of the items you will need to bring with you to the testing center. These may include:

   - Snacks
   - Water
   - Soft drinks, juices, protein drinks
   - Sweater or jacket
   - Medications
   - ATT
   - Identification cards
   - Tissues

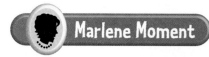

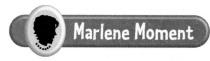

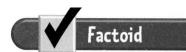

You may want to get these items packed up the night before the test and leave them by your door with your car keys.

2. Plan on getting to the testing center at least 30 minutes ahead of time. You should have already done at least one dry run prior to exam day to figure out directions, travel time, and parking.

3. As you drive to the testing center, you should play the theme music to *Mission Impossible* or whatever music pumps you up or settles you down.

✚ Test center guidelines

The testing center has guidelines you must follow upon your arrival.

● Check in and have a seat in the waiting area. A nice person will call your name to fingerprint and photograph you.[1] No matter how hard you try to look good in this picture, you will have a sudden onset of exophthalamus! You just need to accept this less-than-perfect photo of yourself!

● You need to provide a digital signature verifying your photograph.

● A dry-erase board is provided for calculations. You will turn in your noteboard after testing is completed.

● You can ask for earplugs. The testing center administers other tests than NCLEX®. So you may hear some background noises, such as typing.

● You cannot take anything into the testing area with you. You cannot wear your hat or coat and you cannot carry your purse into the actual testing area either. Don't worry. A safe place for your personal belongings is provided.

● Throughout the entire test, you are monitored by a real person and videotaped for security purposes.[1]

✚ Conquering the computer

The testing center is manned by real people, but the computer is the main focus of your exam day. The following are helpful hints to help you through the computer world if you are not familiar with it already.

1. Computer skills are not necessary to take the actual test. You do not need to know how a computer works, or to have ever touched one, to take this exam.

2. Once you are seated at the computer, a tutorial introduces you to computer testing. This alleviates any fears or insecurities you may have regarding the computer.

3. Next, the real exam begins. Each screen prompts you for the next action you must take in order to progress through the exam.

4. You use a mouse to select answers to the exam questions.

5. You may use the on-screen calculator or your trusty dry-erase board if you have a calculation to make.

6. The "Time Remaining" clock is located in the top right-hand corner of the computer screen.

7. You can change your answer as many times as you wish by clicking another answer. However, once you click NEXT, that question is gone forever. This is true with all questions, no matter what the format.[1]

8. At the end of 2 hours of testing, you will be given an optional 10-minute break. Take it! However, if you need a break prior to this, just raise your hand.

9. You will have to sign in and out each time you take a break. You will be re-fingerprinted every time you re-enter the exam room after taking a break.[1]

10. The computer will offer you another break after another few hours. Make use of your breaks! Go eat and drink something, even if it's only a few bites and a few sips. I insist you do 20 jumping jacks every time you take a break, unless you are incontinent! You will be amazed how this little bit of exercise will increase the blood flow to your brain, thus improving your thinking!

11. Remember, the clock is still ticking while you take breaks.

12. Your test will stop when one of the following occurs:

    * You pass or fail.
    * You take the maximum number of questions allowed.
    * You use up all of the allotted time.

13. When the test ends, the screen will read: "Your test has concluded." You will be asked to complete a survey about your testing experience. You have 2 weeks to contact the NCSBN about specific questions you may have regarding your testing experience.[1]

14. As we all know, computers are not perfect and sometimes experience technical problems. The computers at the testing center are no different. If technical difficulties arise, do not hesitate to report the problem immediately.

15. Your test will be scored twice—once at the testing center and once at Pearson Vue headquarters.[1]

NOW WHAT DO I DO?

Now you have completed your test. If you are like every other nursing student in the country, the worrying process begins. Some students start remembering all kinds of questions they surely missed, and other students can't remember how to get home. Still other students will tell everybody they know that they never heard of any of the information asked on the test, and that there is no way to study for an exam like this. Others will say things like, "My whole test was on pharmacology!" even if in reality they only got one drug question.

You will experience an array of emotions upon leaving the test. Many students are angry and bitter; many are in a zombie-like state; many experience uncontrollable crying; and many are just indifferent. You may cry to your mother and she may say, "Don't worry, I'm sure you did fine, sugar." Then you will say very loudly through bursts of crying, "How do

Hurst Hint

When you click NEXT, forget about the previous question and just focus on the one in front of you! No going back and no sense worrying!

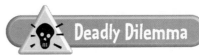

Deadly Dilemma

Taking the stance of "I will not stop until I finish this exam" is a poor way to approach this exam. Your brain needs a break every now and then to rest and continue to process information.

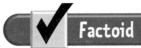

Factoid

Prior to leaving the testing center, you may request a confidential comment sheet if you feel that you need to inform the NCSBN about your testing experience.

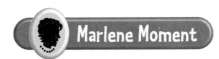

Marlene Moment

Take your candidate bulletin with you to the exam. If technical difficulties arise with your computer, you can find what your options are according to the NCLEX® people!

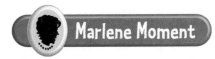

Marlene Moment

Just because the test is graded at the testing center does not mean the people who work at the testing center know your results. So if the testing lady winks at you, this doesn't mean you passed!

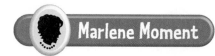

No one ever leaves the testing center skipping and laughing as they make their way to the car.

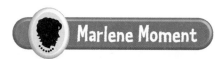

Remember, you will always feel like you were asked more questions in the areas where you feel you have a weakness.

you know? You don't know what I've been through!" Many tell anyone who will listen, "There is no way I passed." This is a common defense mechanism used to begin preparing for the possibility of failing the exam. Some call the Quick Results line repetitively every hour. You must wait at least 2 business days before you even have a chance of getting your results.

If your state is one that only delivers results by mail, this is when you might start making frequent visits or calls to the post office. If you live in a rural area as I do, you may start stalking the postal carrier and chasing his little post-office car or truck with the strobe light on top all over the country roads!

Some students have actually called me from the post office with cell phone in hand as they gazed into the clear post-office box window and said, "Aunt Marlene, I think it's in there." I instructed them to open the mailbox, retrieve the envelope, and call me back. Then they would call me from the car, sitting in the post-office parking lot, and say, "I have the envelope." I would ask, "Well, did you pass?" and they would say, "I don't know, I haven't opened it."

Now that we've been through the common feelings and phases that may occur post-test, let's look at how we can get our results.

HOW DO I GET MY RESULTS?

Do not call the board of nursing, NCLEX® candidate services, or Pearson Vue to try to get your results. Many states allow you to access your "unofficial" results through either the NCLEX® Candidate website or via the NCLEX® Quick Results Line. Here are the steps to take:

1. Log onto **www.ncsbn.org.**

2. On the left side of the screen you will see "NCLEX® Examinations." Click this.

3. Now you will see "NCLEX®" on the left side of the screen. Click this.

4. A drop-down menu will appear. Click on "After the Exam."

5. In the middle of the screen at the top you will see "Quick Results." Click this.

Here you will find the states that allow release of unofficial results within 2 business days after the exam date.

If your state participates in the Quick Results program, here are the steps you follow:

Get your credit card ready because it's going to cost $7.95.[1]

1. Log onto **www.pearsonvue.com/nclex.**

2. Type in your user name and password.

3. Look for "Current Activity."

4. Look under "Recent Appointments."

5. Find the row with your current test.

6. Click on "Status" and then double click on "Quick Results."

7. If your results are available, a payment page will appear so you can type in your credit card information.

8. Click continue.

9. Confirm your order by clicking on the "Confirm Order" only once.

You may also get your results by phone. This costs $9.95. This charge will appear on your phone bill as "NCLEX® Test." Dial 1-900-776-2539. If your results are not available, you will not be charged.[1]

SUMMARY

This is going to be a stressful day. You've done all you can do, so try to keep busy while you are waiting for your results. Odds are, no matter how horrible you feel, you probably passed and can get on with your life!

Reference

1. National Council of State Boards of Nursing. NCLEX Examinations. Available at: **www.ncsbn.org**. Accessed October 25, 2006.

Bibliography

Hurst Review Services. Available at **www.hurstreview.com**.

National Council of State Boards of Nursing. Available at **www.ncsbn.org**.

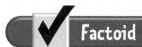

Marlene Moment

If your results are available and you passed, please don't call the number over and over again so that you can hear that you passed repetitively! Why? You are going to run up a huge phone bill!

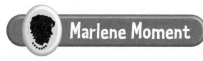

Factoid

Just because you have unofficial results that you passed does not make it legal to practice nursing just yet. You must wait until you get the official results from your state board of nursing.

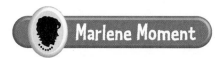

Marlene Moment

If you are unsuccessful, this does not mean you are a horrible nurse and a failure in life. It means you had better call me at once, because you are retaking the exam in 45 days. I'm going to help you pass and we've got work to do!

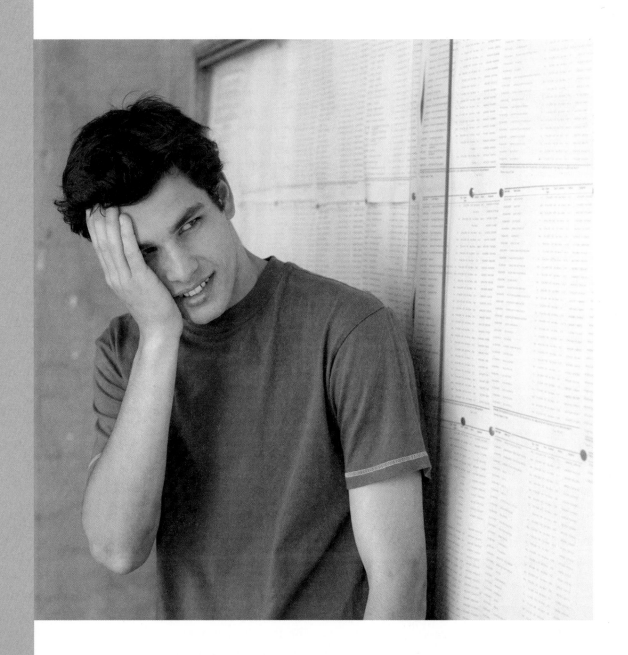

CHAPTER

15

I've Already Failed Once . . . What Do I Do Now?

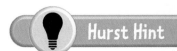

Marlene Moment

You do what Aunt Marlene says to do, and you will pass whether you want to or not!

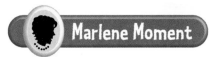

Hurst Hint

Your NCLEX® results do not have any bearing on what kind of nurse you are now or what kind of future you will have in nursing.

Marlene Moment

Get self-centered and do what is best for you!

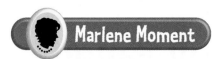

Marlene Moment

I guarantee that somehow this situation will be used in the future to benefit you or someone else. Something positive will come out of this!

KEEPING IT POSITIVE

Okay, we're going to make this short and sweet because I refuse to dwell on the negative. If you did not pass the NCLEX® the first time you took it, most states will allow you to take the test again in 45 days.[1] So there is not much time to waste being negative and wondering what went wrong during your first attempt.

Many things can play a part in not being successful on the NCLEX®. Don't fear! If you want to pass you can, but you have to decide you are willing to do the work and get it done! Don't forget, Hurst Review will be here for you **until you pass.**

ACKNOWLEDGE YOUR FEELINGS AND THEN GET THEM OUT OF THE WAY

Once you discover that you have not been successful the first go-around, there is an array of feelings that may overcome you: defeat, embarrassment, anger, confusion, surprise, and guilt . . . just to name a few. For some reason, when nurses fail their licensure exam, they are abnormally hard on themselves. Other professionals—attorneys and certified public accountants—also must take licensure exams, but when they are unsuccessful they do not go crazy downing themselves. They immediately start planning to retake the exam, but without all of the self-loathing. For some reason, possibly the fact that our nursing school experience emphasized that only perfection was allowed, it's just our nature to be hard on ourselves.

You may feel embarrassed in front of your friends and family during this phase of your life—and remember, it is only a phase. If you only knew how many people in the nursing world took boards more than one time, you would be amazed! These results do not have any bearing on what kind of nurse you are now or what kind of future you will have in nursing. This is only a temporary setback and will not affect your career for the rest of your life. In fact, once you pass, no one will ever ask, "How many times did you take the NCLEX®?"

Maybe you have some people in your life who are being hard on you regarding this issue. It is time for you to focus on yourself and stop listening to those negative words and thoughts. Maybe it was that negative situation you were in to begin with that influenced your exam results.

Many students become upset because they feel like they were the only ones in their class who failed. They really become defeated when they learn that someone who struggled in school (you know . . . the dumb girl who could never get anything right) passed. Maybe you were the president of your class with a 4.0 grade point average. Believe it or not, I have found that many times NCLEX® failure hits the best students from a class.

WHAT DID I DO WRONG?

I guarantee you will hear many theories and opinions regarding what you could have done differently during the exam. Many thoughts will go through your head. Let's look at some things that might have influenced your results, so we can avoid these in the future, for sure.

1. *Major life events.* Getting married, getting divorced, and a death in the family are all examples of major life events that can lend to failure on NCLEX®. If any of these things were going on during the time you prepared for NCLEX®, then there is no way you were as focused as you needed to be. You may have thought you were, but I promise you weren't.

2. *Test anxiety.* This is probably the most common cause of exam failure according to the students. Everyone has test anxiety . . . just differing degrees of it. If you made it through nursing school having test anxiety, you can make it through NCLEX® as well. I know there are people in the world with true test anxiety, but I do not believe it just started with taking NCLEX®.

3. *You only studied the practice questions.* Maybe someone gave you lots of discs with thousands of test questions to practice. You knew every one of those questions like the back of your hand. This is definitely the wrong way to approach studying for NCLEX®. Why? Because no matter how many questions you memorized and studied ahead of time, there will always be thousands more waiting for you at the testing center, which you have never seen.

4. *I just studied too much.* No way! There is no way to study too much for any test. How do you study too much and fail? You may have studied the wrong way, but not "too much!"

5. *I didn't know the core content.* If you do not know the core content of nursing, then there is no way to pass NCLEX®. As the core content is way too much information to read, you can <u>hear</u> me discuss it at **www.hurstreview.com** (if you feel you need to).

6. *False reassurance.* Maybe you thought since your school had such a high pass rate and was certainly the hardest school in the whole entire world, there was no way you could fail. Let's not think like this anymore!

I could go on and on listing things that may have caused you to do poorly. I really do not think you should spend a whole lot of time trying to figure out what you did wrong. Why? Because you have **THIS BOOK** in your hands, which means you are headed in the right direction no matter what detour you may have taken in the past!

WHAT DO I DO WITH MY CANDIDATE PERFORMANCE REPORT?

You received the candidate performance report (CPR) in the mail that outlined your strengths and weaknesses.[1] Students will sometimes look at this and say things like, "Well, I was mainly weak in psychiatric nursing, so

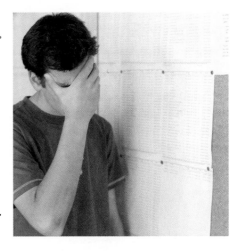

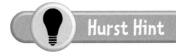
Marlene Moment

The best cure for test anxiety is being prepared the right way!

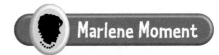
Hurst Hint

If you are retaking NCLEX®, you will not have the exact same questions as you had before. They have been blocked in the computer and will not show up again on your next test.

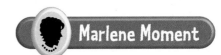
Marlene Moment

I've heard students say, "Well, the reason I failed is because I know that testing center lady didn't like me!"

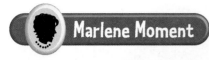

Marlene Moment

You probably felt as if you were going to need the other kind of CPR when you opened your results envelope. You know . . . the kind with the chest compressions!

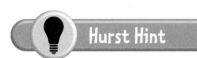

Hurst Hint

If you have taken NCLEX® three times, then you have to study three times as hard as you did the very first time you took the exam. Why? Because as time goes by, the information that was once very fresh on our minds just isn't anymore.

I'm just going to study that for my next test." Bad move. You have to study EVERYTHING again like you have never studied before. Use the CPR to check out your strengths and weaknesses. If there are some specific things you can actually look up and study on the CPR, like immunizations, then do it.

SHOULD I RETAKE THE EXAM?

"Maybe I wasn't meant to be a nurse." "I don't know if I will even take the test again." I don't EVEN want to hear this kind of talk. Yes, you are going to retake the exam, and you are going to pass. You have a degree in nursing! Now let's get busy and pass this test, and stop wasting energy on this kind of thinking. Hey, at least the next time you take it you'll know what to expect!

BUT WHAT DO I DO?

What do I do to pass the NCLEX® the next time I take it? It's easier to pass than it may seem to you right now. Believe it or not, your biggest obstacle is not the content of the exam. Your biggest obstacle is conquering your emotions and finding the energy and motivation to study!

Take this book and study every single chapter. Passing NCLEX®, whether it is your first time or fifth time, is the entire purpose of this book you are reading. Do not pick and choose which chapters you THINK you need to study. If you want additional insurance, then get on my website **www.hurstreview.com** and **listen** to Aunt Marlene talk you through NCLEX® success step-by-step. The only risk you are taking by getting online with me is developing my southern country accent! Don't worry; the accent wears off in approximately 2 weeks!

SUMMARY

I heard a lady minister from Tupelo, Mississippi—Ms. Paula White, another good ol' Mississippi girl—say, "You may feel broke, busted, and disgusted, but there is hope for you!" This is how you may be feeling as well, but there is hope for you! Now start studying the Marlene way!

Reference

1. National Council of State Boards of Nursing. 2006 NCLEX Examination Candidate Bulletin. Available at: **https://www.ncsbn.org/ 2006_Candidate_Bulletin.pdf.** Accessed December 15, 2006.

Bibliography

Hurst Review Services. **www.hurstreview.com.**

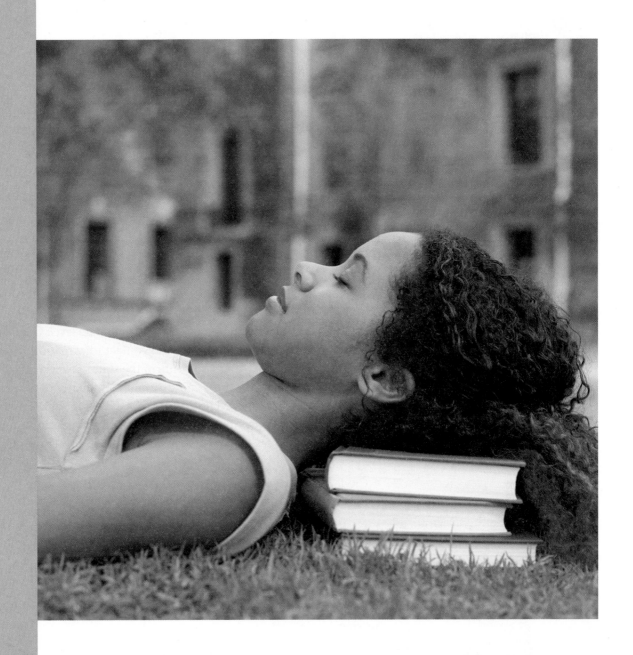

16 Tips for International Students

Hurst Hint

Don't forget that you must meet criteria at the state level for NCLEX® as well as the criteria from the Commission on Graduates of Foreign Nursing Schools (CGFNS)!

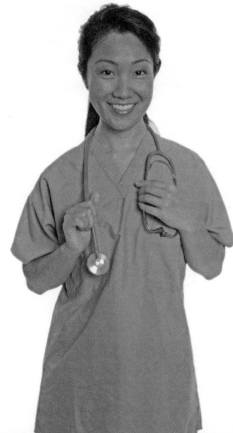

TIPS FOR INTERNATIONAL STUDENTS

This chapter is for those students who completed their nursing education outside the United States and now need to meet the special criteria required to practice nursing in the United States. Remember, my goal is to help you pass the NCLEX® the first time! In this chapter, I will give you the tools needed to maneuver the licensing agencies and meet their criteria.

THE PROCESS YOU MUST GO THROUGH

How many times have you heard the phrase "the process you must go through?" There are many steps to complete prior to taking NCLEX® if you graduated from nursing school in the United States. There are even more steps to take if you completed nursing school outside the United States! Each state has certain criteria that you must meet (see Chapter 2); to do this, you should begin your journey at the state level. Chapter 18 provides the directory of the names and contact information for each state board of nursing. After you confirm the state's criteria, make sure you meet all the steps for the Commission on Graduates of Foreign Nursing Schools (CGFNS). The website for CGFNS is **www.cgfns.org.** The CGFNS is a nonprofit organization that helps you become a successful, trained nurse. The main steps you must go through for CGFNS are listed below.

- Credentials review
- Qualification testing
- English proficiency exam

After you pass the above, you will be awarded a CGFNS certificate, which allows you to take the NCLEX®. I will discuss each of these steps in this chapter to steer you in the right direction. Don't forget that you still have to meet all the criteria at the state level where you will be practicing nursing.

✚ Credentials review

According to CGNFS, there are three questions that must be satisfied to meet the eligibility requirements to continue with the certification testing. These questions are:

- Are you a first-level, general nurse?
- Do you meet the educational requirements?
- Do you have appropriate licensure and registration documents?

First-level, general nurse

The first-level or general nurse is usually a registered nurse. The educational criteria require that you graduate from a government-approved or recognized school of nursing. In some countries, the educational program is specialized and not considered to be a "generalist" curriculum. Those nurses who receive specialized training, such as a midwife or psychiatric nurse, are not considered general nurses unless they complete a general nursing program as well as the specialized program. They are not permitted to take the CGNFS qualifying exam.

Educational requirements

The educational requirements include successful completion of a senior secondary education, successful completion of an approved general nursing program, and clinical and theoretical education regarding nursing care of adult, children, maternity/infant, and psychiatric/mental health clients. Some schools of nursing may not include the clinical and theoretical nursing care of these client populations. The CGNFS determines if your nursing program meets these criteria and provides suggestions if your education does not meet the requirements.

Appropriate licensure and registration documents

The appropriate registration or licensure is simply a current license to practice nursing in your country. The CGNFS will verify that your licensure is valid and up to date.

+ Qualification testing

The CGNFS qualifying exam was originally developed in order to determine if students educated internationally were likely to pass the U.S. registered nurse licensure exam. Now the qualifying exam is necessary prior to taking NCLEX-RN® and becoming a registered nurse in the United States. The qualifying exam is given four times per year using an objective multiple-choice format administered in pen and pencil. The exam tests nursing knowledge based on current nursing practice in the United States.

+ English proficiency exam

The English language proficiency exam determines if you have adequate English language skills. The role of the nurse in the United States requires excellent communication skills and a good command of the English language. CGFNS accepts successful completion of any one of the following as fulfillment of the English proficiency exam criteria.

- Test of English as a Foreign Language (TOEFL), which is administered by the Educational Testing Service (ETS).
- Test of English for International Communication (TOEIC), administered by the ETS.
- International English Language Testing System (IELTS), Academic Module, which is administered by IELTS, Inc.

CGFNS provides excellent resources for preparation for both the qualifying exam and the English-language proficiency exam. Contact information for the specific tests follows.

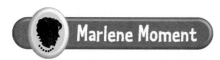

Marlene Moment

Don't forget your "therapeutic communication" (in English, that is)!

TOEFL and *TOEIC*

Educational Testing Service (ETS)

P.O. Box 6151

Princeton, NJ 08541-6151 USA

Telephone (609) 771-7100

www.ets.org

IELTS

IELTS, Inc.

100 East Corson St., Suite 200

Pasadena, CA 91103 USA

Telephone (626) 564-2954

www.ielts.org

SUMMARY

Foreign nurses play an integral role in the care of clients in the United States. Planning a move to the United States and preparing all the necessary steps in order to practice nursing in the United States can be overwhelming. Be very careful in following the state licensure requirements as well as those requirements of the CGFNS. Studying for the NCLEX® the "Marlene" way will help you pass the NCLEX® as well as the CGFNS the first time!

Bibliography

Commission on Graduates of Foreign Nursing Schools. *Characteristics of Foreign Nurse Graduates in the Unites States Workforce 2000–2001.* Philadelphia: CGFNS; 2001.

Commission on Graduates of Foreign Nursing Schools. *Official Study Guide for the CGFNS Qualifying Exam.* 5th ed. Philadelphia: CGFNS; 2006.

Commission on Graduates of Foreign Nursing Schools. **www.cgfns.org.**

Educational Testing Service (ETS). **www.ets.org.**

Hurst Review Services. **www.hurstreview.com.**

International English Language Testing System. **www.ielts.org.**

National Council of State Boards of Nursing. The CGNFS Certification Program (CP) Page. Retrieved from **www.ncsbn.org.** Accessed September 16, 2006.

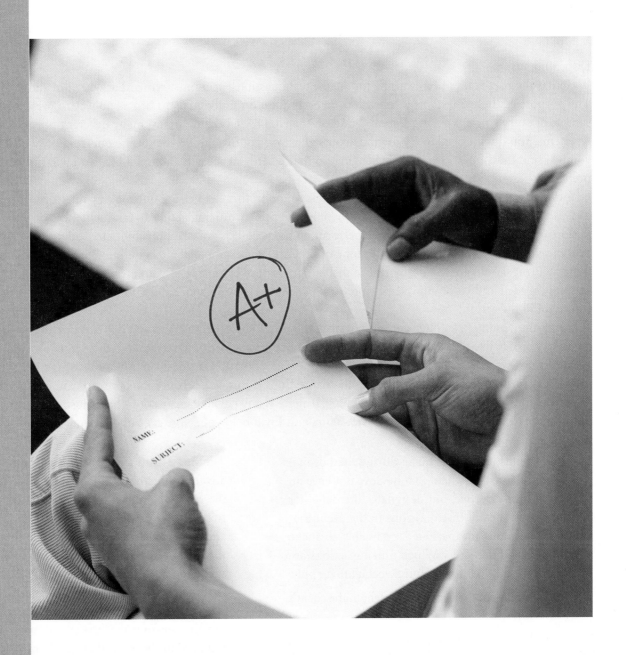

17 Sample Test Questions

INTRODUCTION

Dear Students:

Here is the part you've been waiting for . . . the test questions! You must remember what I'm about to say: The purpose of these questions is to learn from each question individually. There is no way to present to you a sample of every single type of question found on the NCLEX®, because many, many different people write the test items. You do not need to try to grade yourself as you go through these practice questions. My goal is that you will find these questions very challenging, so that when you actually take NCLEX® you will be MORE than prepared!

You may feel like a few of the practice questions found in this chapter are outside of your scope of practice. This is a good thing! Remember, you need to know the proper nursing action to take, whether you are the one performing the task or an RN is the one performing the task. It is your responsibility to understand all nursing actions even if they fall outside of your scope of practice. For example, if a test question states, "Give morphine 2 mg IV," you should automatically realize this nursing action is outside of your scope of practice. But if this action is needed and you cannot legally perform it, then it is your responsibility to locate the appropriate person to fulfill the action!

In addition, many PNs think they do not need to know "RN" material. Yes, you do! Not because you are going to practice like a RN, but because you need to know what actions are required to adequately care for your clients. I've always said the PN has to know the role of the RN in addition to the role of the PN.

Another positive thing about reviewing these questions is this—these questions prepare you for the higher-level questions you will encounter on NCLEX®. If there is any particular question that is just giving you fits, please write to me at marlene2@hurstreview.com, and I will help you. Now get busy!

1. A client informs the nurse during the hospital admission assessment that he does not have an advance directive, but designates the daughter to make health care decisions in the event that he becomes incapacitated or unable to make informed decisions. Which nursing actions are appropriate for this client? Select all that apply.

A. Document the client's statement in the client's own words.

B. Provide information on advance directives to the client.

C. Inform the client that personnel are available to assist with completing an advance directive if the client wishes to do so.

D. The nurse inquiring about a client's advance directive could cause the client anxiety and concern, and should be avoided.

Answer: A, B, & C. The nurse should document the client's statement in the client's own words. The nurse should provide the client with information on advance directives and reassurance that there are hospital personnel to assist with completing the advance directive.

The nurse who avoids inquiry about a client's advance directive is not serving the client's best interests. The nurse should explain to the client that the law requires all clients to be asked about the existence of an advance directive at the time of hospital admission. Inquiring about a client's advance directive does not indicate that the client's health status is deteriorating or is expected to deteriorate. Preparing an advance directive ensures that the client's wishes will be followed in the event that the client is unable to make health care decisions.

TEST-TAKING STRATEGY: Use the process of elimination to disregard incorrect answer choices and focus on the correct answer. In "select all that apply" questions, there may be more than one correct answer.

Note: On the actual licensure test, the answer choices are given as 1, 2, 3 & 4 rather than A, B, C & D.

2. A Durable Power of Attorney for Health Care is an example of (select all that apply):

A. An advance directive.

B. A legal document that identifies a surrogate decision-maker for the client's financial matters in the event that the client becomes incapacitated.

C. A legal document that identifies a surrogate decision-maker in the event the client becomes incapacitated or unable to make informed health care decisions.

D. A legal document that becomes a permanent part of the client's medical record.

Answer: A, D, & C. A Health Care Durable Power of Attorney is one example of an advance directive. Advance directives are documents signed by a competent person giving direction to health care providers about treatment choices in certain circumstances. A Durable Power of Attorney for Health Care is a legal document that identifies a surrogate decision-maker in the event the client becomes incapacitated or unable to make informed health care decisions. The document becomes a permanent part of the client's medical record. A legal document that identifies a client's surrogate for financial matters is incorrect because a Durable Power of Attorney for Health Care identifies a surrogate decision maker for health care decisions only; this document does not designate a surrogate for financial matters.

TEST-TAKING STRATEGY: When answering "Select all that apply" questions, be sure and treat each answer as a true or false statement. There may be one correct answer or more.

3. A client with a Do Not Resuscitate/Do Not Intubate order in the medical record becomes unresponsive and a code blue is called. The code team arrives and the physician is preparing to intubate the client. What action should the nurse take regarding the DNR/DNI order?

A. Prepare the client for immediate intubation. Assist the physician with the intubation procedure as needed.

B. Immediately inform the physician and code team of the client's DNR/DNI order in the medical record.

C. Assist the code team with the code blue per Advanced Care Life Support protocol.

D. Notify the physician and code team of the client's DNR/DNI order in the medical record, but the physician responding to the code blue will make the decision whether or not to intubate the client.

Answer: B. It is the nurse's responsibility to know the client's code status and the treatment wishes of the client when a DNR order is in effect. The nurse must communicate this information to the other health care providers. A DNR order indicates that a client does not want treatment in the event of respiratory or cardiac arrest. Providing treatment to a client who desires no treatment is considered battery. The nurse and health care personnel providing treatment without the client's consent are liable for the treatment provided.

TEST-TAKING STRATEGY: Read the questions twice to ensure that you understand what the question is asking, especially if the question is tricky or confusing. Focus on what the question is asking: what action should the nurse take regarding the DNR/DNI order?

4. A disoriented client is admitted to the med-surg unit with a diagnosis of acute renal failure. The physician orders a hemodialysis line to be placed to facilitate acute hemodialysis. The client's spouse presents the nurse with an advance directive that gives instructions that no hemodialysis treatment be provided if the client becomes incapacitated and unable to make informed health care decisions. What is the appropriate immediate action for the nurse to take at this time?

A. Inform the physician immediately of the advance directive and the client's wishes regarding no hemodialysis treatment. Place a copy of the advance directive in the client's medical record.

B. Obtain consent from the client's spouse for placement of the hemodialysis line and for acute hemodialysis.

C. Inform the physician immediately of the advance directive and the client's wishes regarding no hemodialysis treatment.

D. Tell the client's spouse to speak with the physician in order to make an informed decision on whether or not to proceed with hemodialysis.

Answer: A. The physician should be informed immediately if orders conflict with the client's wishes for treatment. A copy of the advance directive should always be placed in the client's medical record. Obtaining consent from the client's spouse for insertion of a hemodialysis line and acute hemodialysis is incorrect because these orders conflict with the client's treatment wishes. Providing treatment to a client against the client's documented wishes is considered battery. The advance directive is a legally binding document outlining the client's wishes for treatment should the client become incapacitated and unable to make informed health care decisions.

TEST-TAKING STRATEGY: Use the process of elimination to rule out incorrect answer selections to help choose the correct answer.

5. A client presents a Durable Power of Attorney for Health Care designating the client's niece as the person to make health care decisions for the client should the client become incapacitated

and unable to make informed health care decisions. The Durable Power of Attorney identifies the niece as the:

A. Legal next of kin.

B. Health care proxy or surrogate decision-maker for health care issues only.

C. Health care proxy or surrogate decision-maker for health care and financial issues.

D. Person responsible for the client's hospital bill.

Answer: B. A Durable Power of Attorney for Health Care is an advance directive prepared by a competent individual designating a proxy, or surrogate decision-maker, should the client become incapacitated. This document does not address a client's legal next of kin and identifies a surrogate decision-maker for health care issues only. Designating a health care proxy or surrogate decision-maker does not make the surrogate responsible for the client's health care costs.

TEST-TAKING STRATEGY: Use the process of elimination to rule out incorrect answer selections.

6. A nurse is taking a client's medical history in the emergency room. The nurse asks if the client has an advance directive. The client responds by saying, "I have heard of advance directives, but I do not have one. What is an advance directive?" What is the nurse's best response to the client's question?

A. "An advance directive is a document that specifies your wishes regarding your personal effects and finances should you become unable to make decisions."

B. "An advance directive is a document that specifies your wishes regarding health care and your finances should you become incapacitated."

C. "An advance directive is a document similar to a will, and specifies your wishes for burial should you die during hospitalization."

D. "An advance directive is a form of a living will. It specifies your wishes regarding health care and treatment options should you become incapacitated."

Answer: D. An advance directive is a legal document prepared by a competent individual that specifies what treatments, if any, the client desires should the client become incapacitated or unable to make informed health care decisions in the future. The document includes wishes regarding resuscitation measures, withdrawing treatment and life support, and end-of-life care. An advance directive does not address client personal effects, finances, or burial wishes. These might be included in a last will and testament, but are not part of an advance directive.

TEST-TAKING STRATEGY: Questions that ask you to prioritize your nursing actions use terms like *priority, first, best, initial, most important,* and *next.*

7. Which documents are correctly identified as advance directives? Select all that apply.

   A. Durable Power of Attorney for Health Care.

   B. Living Will.

   C. Last Will and Testament.

   D. Client's Bill of Rights.

Answer: A & B. Both the Durable Power of Attorney for Health Care and Living Will are examples of advance directives. Advance directives are documents prepared by a competent individual that specify the client's wishes regarding health care treatments, resuscitation and life-support measures, end-of-life care, and other specific wishes of the client should the client become incapacitated in the future. The Durable Power of Attorney for Health Care identifies a health care proxy or surrogate decision-maker for the client should the client be unable to make informed health care decisions. A Last Will and Testament goes into effect after the client is deceased. The client's Bill of Rights outlines the rights of a client receiving medical treatment and is not an advance directive.

TEST-TAKING STRATEGY: When answering "Select all that apply" questions, be sure and treat each answer as a true or false statement. There may be one correct answer or more.

8. Which statements are true regarding advance directives? Select all that apply.

   A. Advance directives are used as guidelines for client treatment should the client's family deem them necessary.

   B. Advance directives are legally binding documents.

   C. Advance directives should be placed in the client's medical record.

   D. Advance directives specify a client's wishes for health care treatment should the client become incapacitated.

Answer: B, C, & D. Advance directives are legally binding documents, which should be placed in the client's medical record. The document is prepared by the client detailing wishes for treatment should the client become unable to make informed health care decisions. The family's wishes for treatment of the client do not take the place of or negate the client's advance directive.

TEST-TAKING STRATEGY: When answering "Select all that apply" questions, be sure and treat each answer as a true or false statement. There may be one correct answer or more.

9. It is the nurse's responsibility to act as client advocate. What is the definition of client advocacy?

   A. Advocacy is to inform the client to accept medical treatments that conflict with the client's beliefs or health care wishes because the health care team knows what is best for the client.

   B. Advocacy is the act of arguing or negotiating on behalf of a particular issue, idea, or person.

   C. Advocacy is providing assurance to the client that a surgical procedure will be successful and will achieve the desired outcome.

   D. Advocacy is informing the client that the client does not have the right to refuse medical treatment in certain circumstances where doing so is detrimental to the client's health.

Answer: B. Advocacy is the act of arguing or negotiating on behalf of a particular issue, idea, or person. The nurse plays an important role as the client's advocate. Informing a client that they should accept treatment conflicting with the client's beliefs or health care wishes demonstrates lack of advocacy. Assurance about the outcome of a pending surgical procedure makes a false claim to the client; the outcome is not guaranteed. Clients have the right to refuse proposed medical treatment, and to be informed of the medical consequences of their decisions.

TEST-TAKING STRATEGY: Use the process of elimination to rule out incorrect answer selections to help choose the correct answer.

10. An intubated client admitted to the intensive care unit appears anxious and fearful of the equipment in the room. The nurse observes this and takes the time to explain each piece of equipment and its role in providing care to the client. This is an example of the nurse acting as a client advocate by:

   A. Providing information to the client and fostering a sense of security.

   B. Promoting client privacy.

   C. Assuring client safety.

   D. Ensuring the client's wishes for treatment are followed.

Answer: A. The nurse acts as a client advocate by providing information to the client to alleviate fear of the unfamiliar equipment and to foster a sense of security. This question addressing client advocacy is not related to client privacy, safety, or the client's health care treatment wishes.

TEST-TAKING STRATEGY: Read the questions twice to ensure that you understand what the question is asking, especially if the question is tricky or confusing. Focus on what the question is asking: identifying an example of client advocacy.

11. The nurse identifies the new medication noted in a recent medication order to be on the client's list of allergies. In the role of patient advocate, what actions should the nurse take to ensure client safety? Select all that apply.

   A. Document the medication with times and doses to be given, then administer the medication as ordered.

   B. Notify the physician immediately that the medication ordered is on the client's list of medication allergies.

   C. Discontinue the medication on the client's medication administration record.

   D. Check the client's allergy band against the list of client allergies documented in the medical record.

Answer: B, C, & D. Administration of a medication that the client is allergic to could result in harm to the client. The physician should be notified immediately of a medication order that conflicts with the client's list of medication allergies. The medication should be discontinued on the medication administration record, and the client's allergy band checked against the list of allergies documented in the medication record for accuracy.

TEST-TAKING STRATEGY: When answering "Select all that apply" questions, be sure and treat each answer as a true or false statement. There may be one correct answer or more.

12. An elderly client from a long-term care facility arrives in the emergency department by ambulance with altered level of consciousness. The physician instructs the respiratory therapist to prepare for intubation. The nurse discovers a Do Not Resuscitate (DNR) bracelet on the client's wrist during the initial assessment. Which immediate action should the nurse take to appropriately advocate for this client?

   A. Assist the respiratory therapist to prepare the client for immediate intubation.

   B. Attempt to contact the client's family.

   C. Notify the physician immediately of the client's DNR bracelet.

   D. Notify the dietician immediately of the client's DNR bracelet.

Answer: C. The nurse should immediately notify the physician upon discovering the client's DNR bracelet. The DNR bracelet is an indicator that the client or her health care surrogate decision-maker desires the client's wishes be known regarding health care treatment and resuscitation. Ignoring the DNR bracelet and assisting the respiratory therapist to prepare for immediate intubation is incorrect because the client has DNR notification on her person and should not be intubated. Reaching the client's family allows the family to be with the client and to provide additional health history, but this should be done after notifying the physician. Notifying the dietician of the client's DNR bracelet is not appropriate and delays addressing the immediate problem.

TEST-TAKING STRATEGY: Questions that ask you to prioritize your nursing actions use terms like *priority, first, best, initial, most important, immediate,* and *next.*

13. The client's physician orders a blood transfusion for a client whose hemoglobin level is 5.0 mg/dL. The nurse informs the client that blood will be drawn for a type and cross-match prior to the blood transfusion. The client avoids eye contact with the nurse, and then states, "I am a Jehovah's Witness. I thought that was on my chart." The nurse demonstrates the role of client advocate by which response to the client?

   A. "Your hemoglobin is very low. I can notify your physician to discuss with you how important it is for you to receive the blood."

   B. "I will place that information in your medical record. You have the right to refuse treatment that conflicts with your beliefs. Would you like to speak with your physician about other treatment options?"

   C. "Your physician ordered this blood transfusion because your hemoglobin is low. You should do as your physician recommends."

   D. "Why do Jehovah's Witnesses choose not to receive blood transfusions?"

   Answer: B. The nurse as client advocate supports the client's beliefs and treatment wishes. Reaffirming that the client's beliefs and treatment wishes are important to the health care team promotes a sense of security and respect for the individual. The information that the client is a Jehovah's Witness who refuses blood products should be placed prominently in the medical record per the facility's policy to avoid further confusion. Providing reasonable health care treatment choices that do not conflict with the client's beliefs is the responsibility of the multidisciplinary health care team.

TEST-TAKING STRATEGY: Use the process of elimination to rule out incorrect answer selections to help choose the correct answer.

14. The nurse has a duty to act as client advocate. Failure to do so could result in possible (select all that apply):

   A. Life-threatening complications for the client.

   B. Legal action against the nurse and/or health care facility.

   C. Suspension of license or loss of license to practice nursing.

   D. Suspension of license or loss of license to practice medicine.

   Answer: A, B, & C. The role of client advocate is a nurse's responsibility. Failure to act as a client advocate could result in a range of complications for the client, including life-threatening or life-ending complications. Failure to act as client advocate exposes the nurse to liability, potential legal action against the nurse and/or health care facility, and potential suspension or loss of license to practice nursing. Practicing medicine outside the scope of nursing could also result in potentially life-threatening complications for the client, legal action against the nurse and/or health care facility, and potential suspension or loss of license to practice nursing.

TEST-TAKING STRATEGY: When answering "Select all that apply" questions, be sure and treat each answer as a true or false statement. There may be one correct answer or more.

15. A client is scheduled for open heart surgery. The nurse enters the client's room to perform preoperative teaching and finds the client crying. The client states, "I really do not want to go through open heart surgery. I have told my children this, but they still want me to go through with the surgery. I don't know what to do." What is the best response for the nurse as client advocate?

A. "Your children are correct. The open heart surgery is the best thing for your health."

B. "From what you are telling me, you have some genuine concerns about the open heart surgery, and you feel as if your children are not addressing your concerns. You and your family will need to resolve this before you go to surgery."

C. "I can contact your physician so that you can discuss your concerns regarding open heart surgery."

D. "From what you are telling me, you have some genuine concerns about the open heart surgery, and you feel as if your children are not addressing your concerns. It is important to me and to the health care team that we follow your wishes regarding surgery and treatment. Would you feel comfortable telling me more about your concerns and your children's attitudes toward the surgery?"

Answer: D. The nurse has a duty to advocate for the client if there is a discrepancy between the care or proposed care and the client's wishes regarding treatment. It is important to acknowledge the client's feelings, and to demonstrate compassion and a willingness to understand. This presents an opportunity for additional communication to help answer some of the client's questions, or set up a client–family conference with the physician. When the nurse agrees with the client's children, the nurse ignores the client's feelings and does not address the issue of the client's treatment wishes. When the nurse restates the client's comment without investigating the client's concerns, the issue goes unresolved. Offering only to contact the physician is an incomplete solution and hints of the nurse not taking responsibility to investigate the client's concerns. The client may be uncomfortable addressing concerns with the physician before resolving the issue of treatment wishes with family members.

TEST-TAKING STRATEGY: Look for similar answer choices to eliminate the detractors and choose the best response.

16. A client seen in the emergency department for a femur fracture is receiving discharge instructions for cast care, use of crutches, and follow-up care. The client complains of chest heaviness to the nurse. The nurse assures the client that the chest heaviness is probably caused by sore chest muscles from using the crutches, and instructs the client to sign the discharge instructions. The nurse neglects to document the complaints of chest heaviness nor does the nurse notify the physician. The nurse failed to implement which measure to intervene on the client's behalf? Select all that apply.

A. Failure to preserve client privacy.

B. Failure to act as a client advocate.

C. Failure to take appropriate action.

D. Failure to appropriately diagnose.

Answer: B & C. The nurse failed to act as a client advocate by neglecting to take appropriate action regarding the client's symptoms, neglecting to document the symptoms, and failing to report the client's complaints of chest heaviness to the physician for further evaluation. The client's privacy is not an issue in this question. Diagnosing the cause of the chest heaviness is not in the nurse's scope of practice, but notifying the physician of the client's complaints and symptoms is the nurse's responsibility.

TEST-TAKING STRATEGY: Never delay treatment or choose an answer option that ignores client symptoms.

17. The nurse knows that case management is:

A. The process of managing the outcomes of client care by quality-improvement measures and involvement of the interdisciplinary team.

B. The process of client assessment and direct client care by the primary nurse, utilizing the nursing process and nursing diagnoses to guide delivery of care.

C. The process used by the health care facility's legal or risk-management department to evaluate legal claims filed against the facility or employees of the facility.

D. The process of overseeing and organizing client care in collaboration with the client's primary health care provider and consulting physicians.

Answer: D. Case management is the process of overseeing and organizing client care in collaboration with the client's primary care physician or health care provider, consulting physicians, and ancillary care providers. The process of managing client care outcomes by quality-improvement measures is a description of outcomes management. Client assessment and direct client care by the primary nurse is a description of bedside primary nursing. The process used to evaluate legal claims against the facility or its employees is a description of risk management.

TEST-TAKING STRATEGY: Look for similar answer choices and eliminate them.

18. The nurse case manager knows case management is an example of which client care model?

A. The outcomes evaluation model of care.

B. The protocol management model of care.

C. The interdisciplinary care management model.

D. The risk assessment care management model.

Answer: C. Case management is an example of the interdisciplinary care management model. Case management is the process of overseeing and organizing client care in collaboration with the client's primary care physician or health care provider, consulting physicians, and ancillary care providers. The outcomes evaluation model of care, the protocol management model of care, and the risk assessment care management model are fictitious client care models. Outcomes evaluation and risk management are two separate methods of evaluating and ensuring safe delivery of client care, but are not care management models.

TEST-TAKING STRATEGY: Read the question twice to ensure that you understand what the question is asking, especially if the question is tricky or confusing. Focus on what the question is asking: identifying client care model, not care management model.

19. The case management nurse focuses on overseeing and organizing client care. Goals of the case management model of client care include (select all that apply):

A. Providing cost-effective care to the client.

B. Providing appropriate care to the client in a timely manner.

C. Providing high-quality care to the client.

D. Providing health care services to the client at no cost.

Answer: A, B, & C. The primary goals of the case management model of interdisciplinary client care are to provide high-quality, appropriate, and cost-effective care to each client in a timely manner. Providing health care services to the client at no cost is not a case management function. The constitution guarantees every citizen *equal access* to health care services; it does not guarantee free health care, although this is a common misunderstanding.

TEST-TAKING STRATEGY: When answering "Select all that apply" questions, be sure and treat each answer as a true or false statement. There may be one correct answer or more.

20. The nurse knows that the case management model of client care is:

A. Implemented throughout a client's entire hospital stay or episode of illness.

B. Implemented only during a client's acute phase of illness.

C. Implemented if a client is unable to recover from an episode of illness within the expected time frame of the client's specific disease process.

D. Focused on the cost of care delivered to a client.

Answer: A. Case management is implemented throughout a client's entire hospital stay or episode of illness, and focuses on the collaboration of all health care personnel involved in the care of the client. Case management implemented only during a client's acute phase of illness and only if a client is unable to recover from an episode of illness in a timely manner are both incorrect because case management is an ongoing process from a client's admission throughout the entire episode of illness and into recovery. Cost-effective care is only one goal of case management.

TEST-TAKING STRATEGY: Use the process of elimination to rule out incorrect answer selections to help choose the correct answer.

21. The role of a case manager in client care is multifaceted and includes coordination of care among all health care personnel involved in the care of a client during an episode of illness, from admission to recovery. Responsibilities of the case manager include (select all that apply):

A. Facilitating referrals for client care to members of the multidisciplinary health care team.

B. Supervising the client's discharge planning process.

C. Providing direct nursing care to the client by the case management team.

D. Providing the client and the client's family and caregivers with the appropriate information and resources to meet the client's needs after discharge from the health care facility.

Answer: A, B, & D. Case management roles include facilitating referrals to members of the multidisciplinary health care team, supervising the discharge planning process, and providing information and resources to the client and the client's family and caregivers to meet the client's needs after discharge from the health care facility. Direct nursing care to the client by the case management team is incorrect because case managers play a coordination role in client care, but generally do not engage in direct hands-on, day-to-day care of the client.

TEST-TAKING STRATEGY: When answering "Select all that apply" questions, be sure and treat each answer as a true or false statement. There may be one correct answer or more.

22. A client's primary physician writes an order to prepare the client for discharge from the hospital the next day. The client expresses concern to the nurse about the ability to provide self-care and perform daily activities of living after arriving home from the hospital. Which member of the health care team should the nurse contact to provide information and assist the client with resources for an effective discharge plan?

A. The client's primary care physician, who will coordinate care and resources for an effective discharge plan individualized to the client's needs.

B. The client's case manager, who will coordinate care and provide information and resources for an effective discharge plan individualized to the client's needs.

C. The client's physical therapist, who will instruct the client to safely navigate the home environment after discharge.

D. The client's occupational therapist, who will evaluate the client's ability to perform self-care and activities of daily living.

Answer: B. The client's case manager should be contacted regarding the order for pending discharge from the health care facility. The case manager coordinates care and provides the client with information and resources for an individualized discharge plan. The primary care physician does not assume the case management role in the acute care facility setting, and generally does not coordinate the discharge planning process. The physical and occupational therapists are members of the multidisciplinary team, but do not coordinate discharge planning. They might assist in evaluation of the client as part of the discharge plan, but they are not responsible for case management and coordination of overall client care for discharge from the facility.

TEST-TAKING STRATEGY: Use the process of elimination to rule out incorrect answer selections to help choose the correct answer.

23. The responsibilities of a case manager are often performed by a nurse. A case manager may also be a(n) (select all that apply):

   A. Allied health care provider.

   B. Social worker or patient-family services care provider.

   C. Primary care physician.

   D. Primary care provider.

   Answer: A, B, & D. A client's case manager can be a nurse, an allied health care professional, a social worker, or the client's primary care provider. The primary care physician generally does not assume the role of the client's case manager.

   TEST-TAKING STRATEGY: Read the question twice to ensure that you understand what the question is asking, especially if the question is tricky or confusing. Focus on what the question is asking: the individuals who may serve as a client's case manager.

24. Case managers use clinical pathways in the process of evaluating and coordinating client care with the multidisciplinary team. A clinical pathway is:

   A. A decision-making flowchart that uses the "if, then" method to address client responses to treatment.

   B. A set of practice guidelines developed by a professional medical organization such as the American Nurses Association or the American College of Surgeons.

   C. A standardized set of preprinted physician orders for client care, which expedite the order process and can be customized to individual clients.

   D. A set of practice guidelines based on a specific client diagnosis, which provides an overview of the multidisciplinary plan of care.

   Answer: D. A clinical pathway is a set of multidisciplinary client care guidelines for a specific diagnosis or condition. It can be used to guide the plan of care and to identify deviations from the plan of care. A decision-making flowchart that uses the "if, then" method is the definition of an algorithm. A set of practice guidelines developed by professional medical organizations is the definition of a practice guideline. A standardized set of preprinted physician orders is the definition of a physician preprinted order set.

   TEST-TAKING STRATEGY: Look for similar answer choices and eliminate them.

25. The nurse performs an admission assessment on a client who is directly admitted to the hospital from the physician's office. The client is worried and distracted, and explains to the nurse that because of the direct admission from the physician's office there was no preparation to be away from home. The client is concerned about the length of stay, pets that need care, and bills that require payment. Which response from the nurse would be most helpful to this client?

A. "An unexpected hospital admission can be very stressful. I will notify the case manager who specializes in helping clients with situations like yours. There is a telephone here beside your bed so that you can contact your family and friends. Is there anything that I can do for you right now to help you?"

B. "I know how you feel. I will be sure to tell your night nurse in shift report that you will probably need something to help you sleep tonight."

C. "An unexpected hospital admission can be very stressful. Is there anyone who I can call for you? You also have a telephone here at your bedside so that you can contact your family and friends."

D. "I can call your physician for you and ask if you could go home today, then schedule another date for your hospital admission."

Answer: A. The case manager should be involved in coordinating the client's care from the date of admission in order to help the client navigate unexpected situations like a last-minute hospital admission. The ability to make telephone calls to notify family and friends will help to decrease the client's sudden sense of isolation from normal daily life, loss of control, and anxiety. Although sleeping medication may be warranted for this client, the nurse neglects to offer a viable solution to the client's problem. Calling the physician is inappropriate as the client requires hospitalization due to the swift nature of the admission.

TEST-TAKING STRATEGY: Questions that ask you to prioritize your nursing actions use terms like *priority, first, best, initial, most important, immediate,* and *next.*

26. Two health care personnel are talking about a client by name in the facility elevator. The conversation is overheard by visitors in the same elevator. Which client right is violated?

A. The client's right to review their medical records.

B. The client's right to privacy.

C. The client's right to have an advanced directive.

D. The client's right to refuse treatment.

Answer: B. Health care information is privileged. The conversation between the health care personnel in the elevator violates the client's right to privacy and could subject the personnel to liability.

TEST-TAKING STRATEGY: Read the question twice to ensure that you understand what the question is asking, especially if the question is tricky or confusing. Focus on what the question is asking: the client right that is violated.

27. A client asks to view the client's medical records. Which response made by the nurse is most appropriate?

A. "You will need to retain an attorney, then have the attorney contact the medical records department in order to view your medical records."

B. "You may only view your medical records after you have been discharged from the health care facility."

C. "You have the right to view the medical records that pertain to your care, and to have those records explained or interpreted for you if necessary."

D. "Why do you want to view your medical records? Are you planning to file a lawsuit?"

Answer: C. According to the Patient's Bill of Rights, the client has the right to view medical records pertaining to the client's care and to have those records explained if necessary. The client does not need to retain an attorney in order to view the medical records unless there is some circumstance where viewing the records is prohibited by law. The client does not need to wait until after discharge from the facility to view the medical records. Challenging the client's desire to view the medical records is an argumentative, antagonistic, and unprofessional response from the nurse.

TEST-TAKING STRATEGY: Use the process of elimination to rule out incorrect answer selections to help choose the correct answer.

28. A client's surgeon discusses the option of surgery and related benefits and risks with the client and the client's family. Which statement by the client demonstrates that the client understands the right to make decisions regarding treatment and the proposed plan of care?

    A. "The surgeon says that I need this operation, so I guess I had better go ahead and have it."

    B. "I am not so sure that I want to have major surgery, but my family will not even talk about other options."

    C. "I am afraid to tell my surgeon about my hesitation to have this operation. The surgeon will think I am being foolish, so I didn't mention it."

    D. "The surgeon explained the risks and benefits of the operation to me, but the decision to have the surgery or to explore other treatment options is mine."

    Answer: D. A client has the right to make decisions regarding recommended treatment options and the proposed plan of care. Ultimately the decision is the client's to make, not the client's physician or the client's family members. The decision should be made after careful consideration of the risks and benefits.

    TEST-TAKING STRATEGY: The phrase "client understands" tells you to select the answer with accurate information.

29. The nurse notices that a client's bedside privacy curtain has been left partially open during the client's bath. Which is the best action for the nurse to take to ensure the client's right to privacy?

    A. Inform the client that the curtain was left partially open and that the client may have been exposed at some point during the bath.

    B. Close the privacy curtain to protect the client's right to privacy.

    C. No action is necessary. The client did not notice the open privacy curtain.

    D. No action is necessary. There are only a few visitors on the unit during this time of the morning.

    Answer: B. The curtain should be closed as soon as the opening is noticed to protect the client's right to privacy. Informing the client that the curtain was open is an embarrassment to the client, and serves no purpose in the client's healing process. The "No action is necessary" options are incorrect because the client has the right to privacy.

    TEST-TAKING STRATEGY: Determine which action would bring the most harm or help to the client. This helps determine the highest nursing priority.

30. A prison inmate is brought to the emergency department with complaints of chest pressure that radiates up the jaw and down the left arm. The nurse overhears another employee speaking rudely to the inmate client. Acting as the client's advocate, the nurse tells the employee privately that all clients are to be treated with equal respect and dignity. Which client right has the nurse protected?

    A. The right to free speech.

    B. The right to privacy.

    C. The right to considerate and respectful care.

    D. The right to confidentiality.

    Answer: C. Every client has the right to considerate and respectful care. The right to free speech is not violated in this example nor is it included in the Patient's Bill of Rights. The client's privacy and right to confidentiality are not breached in this example.

    TEST-TAKING STRATEGY: Use the process of elimination to rule out incorrect answer selections to help choose the correct answer.

31. The Patient Self-Determination Act of 1990 mandates that all clients must be asked whether or not they have a(n):

A. Organ donation card.

B. Advance directive.

C. Last Will and Testament.

D. Funeral home or method of burial preference.

Answer: B. The Patient Self-Determination Act of 1990 mandates that all clients must be asked whether or not they have an advance directive. Organ donation card, Last Will and Testament, and funeral home or burial preference are not included in the Patient Self-Determination Act.

TEST-TAKING STRATEGY: Use the process of elimination to rule out incorrect answer selections to help choose the correct answer.

32. A client with an executed advance directive specifying "do not resuscitate, do not intubate" in the medical record becomes unresponsive during a bed bath, at which time the nursing assistant activates the hospital code blue system. The client's primary nurse arrives quickly at the bedside to find the nursing assistant performing cardiopulmonary resuscitation as the code team enters the client's room. Which action by the nurse is most important in protecting the client's right to self-determination?

A. Instructing the nursing assistant to stop CPR.

B. Assisting the physician with the intubation process.

C. Assisting the nursing assistant in placing the backboard under the client to facilitate compressions.

D. Instructing the nursing assistant to retrieve the crash cart.

Answer: A. The nurse should immediately inform the nursing assistant and the code team of the client's code status and ask the nursing assistant to stop CPR. Assisting with intubation or CPR violates the client's wishes.

TEST-TAKING STRATEGY: Home in on the key words in the stem like "most important." Then eliminate the incorrect answers while focusing on the answer that provides information or an action that is the most important.

33. A client's physician writes the order to "obtain consent for a bronchoscopy and possible lung biopsy." When the nurse presents the consent form to the client, the client states, "I don't know what a bronchoscopy is." Which is the best action by the nurse?

A. The nurse should explain the bronchoscopy procedure to the client and inform the client of the risks, benefits, and treatment alternatives.

B. The nurse should immediately inform the physician that the client requests additional information related to the bronchoscopy procedure.

C. The nurse should give the client an information pamphlet on the bronchoscopy procedure, and tell the client to sign the consent after reading the pamphlet.

D. The nurse should instruct the client to sign the informed consent form. The physician will answer any additional questions right before the procedure is performed.

Answer: B. The physician performing the procedure should explain the risks and benefits, recovery time, and reasonable alternatives, as well as the consequences of refusing treatment prior to the client signing a consent form. The nurse can explain the bronchoscopy procedure and expectations to the client, but the nurse is not performing the bronchoscopy. Providing an information pamphlet to the client may be beneficial, but this should never be substituted for the physician communicating with the client.

TEST-TAKING STRATEGY: Questions that ask you to prioritize your nursing actions use terms like *priority, first, best, initial, most important, immediate,* and *next.*

34. A new client tells the admissions nurse at a rehabilitation facility, "No one asked me which rehabilitation facility I preferred. I feel as if this entire process took place without my involvement. I was not informed of alternative options." Which client right is being violated?

A. The right to considerate and respectful care.

B. The right to self-determination.

C. The right to participate in the plan of care.

D. The right to review medical records related to care and treatment.

Answer: C. A client has the right to participate in the plan of care and to refuse a recommended treatment to the extent permitted by law and by hospital policy. In the case of care refusal, the client has the right to alternative care and treatment, and the right to be transferred to another health care facility if that is the client's choice. The right to considerate and respectful care has not been violated in this situation. The right to self-determination relates to resuscitation and advance directive issues. The client's right to review medical records is not addressed in this question.

TEST-TAKING STRATEGY: Use the process of elimination to rule out incorrect answer selections to help choose the correct answer.

35. A hospital client with abdominal cancer refuses surgical treatment and chemotherapy and asks about options for hospice home care. Later, the client's daughter asks the case manager to talk the client into agreeing to surgery and chemotherapy treatment. The case manager explains to the daughter that this violates which client right?

    A. The right to self-determination.

    B. The right to decline participation in research studies and experimental treatments.

    C. The right to expect reasonable continuity of care.

    D. The right to make decisions about the plan of care.

Answer: D. The client has the right to participate in the plan of care, to refuse a proposed treatment, and to accept alternative care and treatment. The right to self-determination is incorrect because an advance directive or resuscitation status is not involved in this situation. The right to decline participation in research or experimental studies is incorrect because no research or experimental treatment is proposed

to the client. The right to expect reasonable continuity of care appears to be a possible correct answer, but is incorrect because the client has not been transferred to hospice home care.

TEST-TAKING STRATEGY: Look for similar answer choices and eliminate them.

36. Which scenario is an example of violation of a client's right to freedom from unlawful restraint? Select all that apply.

    A. A disoriented client frequently attempts to pull out the nasogastric tube, the urinary catheter, and the endotracheal tube. Multiple attempts to reorient the client and use of alternative methods to promote client safety have been unsuccessful. The nurse obtains an order for soft wrist restraints from the client's physician and applies the restraints, securing them with a quick-release knot.

    B. A client is intubated with an endotracheal tube and is on a mechanical ventilator for respiratory failure. The client is alert, oriented, calm, and cooperative. The client writes the nurse a note asking, "Do I have to wear the wrist restraints? I know that I need the breathing tube and will not attempt to move it."

    C. A mother brings her 18-year-old daughter to the urgent care clinic for a pregnancy test. The daughter refuses to submit to a pregnancy test, and the mother instructs the physician, "I want you to keep her here until she decides to take the pregnancy test."

    D. A mentally competent client has a set of cardiac studies including an EKG and a treadmill study performed at the cardiologist's office. After the studies are completed, the cardiologist recommends that the client be admitted to the hospital for cardiac catheterization and further evaluation. The client refuses to go directly to the hospital because of prior obligations and responsibilities. The client states acceptance for the risks of returning home against medical advice. The cardiologist has the client sign a waiver and documents the client's response.

Answer: B & C. Wrist restraints may appear to be a reasonable safety precaution for an intubated client, but for the client who is alert, oriented, and cooperative, this is an unreasonable restraint. An 18-year-old client has the right to refuse treatment and is not required to submit to a pregnancy test. Wrist restraints are appropriate to prevent self-harm of a disoriented client exhibiting multiple attempts to remove life-support equipment. The cardiologist has no legal right to compel the mentally competent client to accept treatment, nor may the physician admit the client to the hospital against the client's wishes.

TEST-TAKING STRATEGY: When answering "Select all that apply" questions, be sure and treat each answer as a true or false statement. There may be one correct answer or more.

37. The Health Insurance Portability and Accountability Act (HIPAA) of 1996 is federal legislation that protects the privacy and confidentiality of clients' health information. HIPAA also ensures that (select all that apply):

    A. All medical personnel employed at the facility where a client receives treatment can legally access a client's health information at any time.

    B. Additional health-related information revealed by a client to health care personnel must be kept confidential.

    C. The client has the right to access personal health care records and to obtain copies of those records.

    D. A client's information can only be revealed with the client's permission, or when the health care provider or facility is required by law to do so.

    Answer: B, C, & D. HIPAA is federal legislation enacted to protect client health information and privacy. Any information the client reveals to health care personnel must be kept confidential. Clients have the right to access their personal health care records and to obtain copies of the records. A client's health information can only be revealed with the client's permission, or when a health care provider or facility is required to do so by law. Medical personnel do not have the right to access a client's medical records or health information without treatment necessity.

TEST-TAKING STRATEGY: When answering "Select all that apply" questions, be sure and treat each answer as a true or false statement. There may be one correct answer or more.

38. A violently agitated client is brought to the emergency department by police. A Foley catheter is inserted, and the client's urine is sent for a stat urine drug screen. One of the police officers asks the nurse for a copy of the client's drug screen results, stating he believes the client operates a mobile methamphetamine lab. Which response by the nurse indicates that the nurse understands the Health Insurance Portability and Accountability Act (HIPAA) as it relates to the officer's request?

    A. "I understand you believe that this client manufactures methamphetamine. I will make a copy of the urine drug screen results for you."

    B. "I understand you believe this client manufactures methamphetamine. However, this client is unable to consent to the release of personal medical information right now, and it would be a violation of the client's right to privacy under HIPAA to release a copy of the urine drug screen results to you."

    C. "Yes, the client certainly is behaving like someone high on methamphetamine. Did you find the mobile meth lab? These urine drug screen results will help your case against this client for manufacturing illegal drugs."

    D. "Under HIPAA I am not supposed to release the results of the urine drug screen to you, but if you believe this client is manufacturing methamphetamine, you should have the drug screen results. I will not give you a copy, but I will leave the results here on the counter and walk away. You can choose to take them if you want to."

    Answer: B. Releasing confidential health information to anyone, including law enforcement, without the client's consent is a violation of HIPAA's federal legislation to ensure the privacy and confidentiality of client medical records and health information. Nurses are sometimes placed in difficult situations with regard to client privacy issues, but protection of the client's right to privacy and confidentiality is the priority. Any response by the nurse that indicates willingness to release the confidential information, either by commission or by passively leaving the drug screen results out in plain sight, is a violation of HIPAA. Law enforcement can request a client's medical records through the appropriate legal channels if the information is needed.

TEST-TAKING STRATEGY: Never choose an answer option that violates client rights, a stated policy, or federal legislation like HIPAA.

39. A night shift nurse receives shift report from the day shift nurse when the day nurse states, "I have an appointment and I need to leave. Can you get the rest of the client's information from the medical records?" Which client right is violated by the day nurse?

    A. The client's right to reasonable continuity of care.

    B. The client's right to confidentiality.

    C. The client's right to considerate and respectful care.

    D. The client's right to make decisions about the plan of care and proposed treatment.

    Answer: A. An incomplete or uninformative client report from one health care provider to the next violates the client's right to reasonable continuity of care. The client's right to confidentiality is not violated because both nurses have been assigned to care for the client. Information pertaining to client care is passed between health care providers during care reports to safeguard continuity of care. The right to considerate and respectful care and the right to make decisions about the plan of care are not addressed in this scenario, so these answer options are incorrect.

    TEST-TAKING STRATEGY: Choose the answer selection that is the most life threatening or harmful to the client.

40. A client in the intensive care unit is alert and oriented, but loud and verbally abusive to all health care personnel who enter the client's room. Multiple staff members including the charge nurse have spoken to the client about the inappropriate behavior, but all attempts have been ineffective. The client has lorazepam (Ativan) IV ordered as needed for disorientation and agitation. Which client right would be violated if the nurse were to administer the medication to the client under these circumstances?

    A. The client's right to self-determination.

    B. The client's right to freedom from unreasonable restraint.

    C. No client right is violated in this scenario.

    D. The client's right to considerate and respectful care.

    Answer: B. Administering lorazepam (Ativan), an anxiolytic, to an alert and oriented client because of verbally abusive behavior is an inappropriate use of the medication, thus violating the client's right to freedom from unreasonable restraint. The medication is prescribed as needed in the event the client becomes disoriented or agitated. Administering the medication because the staff does not approve of the client's behavior is not consistent with the prescribed use of the medication for this client. The right to self-determination is incorrect because advance directives and resuscitation issues are not discussed in this scenario. The right to considerate and respectful care is this client's due but it is not the client's right in question, with respect to administration of medication.

    TEST-TAKING STRATEGY: Use the process of elimination to rule out incorrect answer selections to help choose the correct answer.

41. A client undergoes hip replacement surgery and requires assistance to ambulate. The client needs to use the bathroom, but the call light has been left out of reach, rendering the client unable to summon staff for assistance. Which client right is violated?

    A. The right to participate in the plan of care and treatment decisions.

    B. The right to freedom from unreasonable restraint.

    C. The right to privacy.

    D. The right to considerate and respectful care.

Answer: B. A client requiring assistance for any activity of daily living needs access to call for assistance from the health care staff. Denial of access to care by removal of access devices is unreasonable restraint. The right to participate in the plan of care and the right to privacy are not violated in this scenario. The right to considerate and respectful care is an important element of client care, but is not the client right in this scenario.

TEST-TAKING STRATEGY: Read the question twice to ensure that you understand what the question is asking, especially if the question is tricky or confusing. Focus on what the question is asking: the client right that is violated by leaving the call light out of client reach.

42. Studies show that collaboration between the members of a multidisciplinary health care team improves quality of client care, decreases length of stay in health care facilities, and decreases the cost of health care to the client. Which members of the multidisciplinary team are responsible for collaboration in client care?

    A. The primary care physician and the case manager.

    B. The primary nurse and the case manager.

    C. All members of the multidisciplinary health care team.

    D. The primary care physician, all consulting physicians, and the case manager.

    Answer: C. All members of the multidisciplinary health care team are responsible for a collaborative care approach to client care. Multidisciplinary care has significantly improved client outcomes and decreased client length of stay in health care facilities.

    TEST-TAKING STRATEGY: Look for similar answer choices and eliminate them.

43. In the multidisciplinary approach to client care, all members of the health care team have the goal of collaborative client care. Which member of the multidisciplinary team oversees and coordinates the care delivery process and organizes the delivery of health care services to the client?

    A. The clinical nutritionist.

    B. The primary nurse each shift.

    C. The primary care physician.

    D. The case manager.

    Answer: D. An important role of the case manager in the multidisciplinary team care approach is coordination of client care. The case manager oversees the process of health care delivery and organizes and coordinates the delivery of health care services to the client. The clinical nutritionist, the primary nurse each shift, and the client's primary physician are all members of the multidisciplinary team.

    TEST-TAKING STRATEGY: Use the process of elimination to rule out incorrect answer selections to help choose the correct answer.

44. A new graduate nurse is asked to present a brief, concise client history and assessment at the unit's daily multidisciplinary client care rounds. Participants in the daily client care rounds include the unit case manager, the charge nurse, the physician conducting rounds, a clinical pharmacist, the unit dietician, a physical therapist and occupational therapist, a respiratory therapist, and each client's primary care nurse in turn. The daily client care rounds are an example of:

    A. A violation of the client's right to privacy. The graduate nurse should decline to give client information to the interdisciplinary team.

    B. A case management model of client care, designed to coordinate care for the client among all members of the multidisciplinary team to improve individual client outcomes.

    C. Collaboration of care with the multidisciplinary health care team, designed to coordinate care for the client among all members of the health care team to improve individual client outcomes.

    D. A violation of HIPAA. Each member of the multidisciplinary team must sign a HIPAA form before participating in the client care rounds.

Answer: C. The daily client care rounds are an example of collaboration of care among the members of the multidisciplinary health care team. Multidisciplinary client care rounds are designed to promote collaborative care and improve client outcomes. They are not a violation of the client's right to privacy nor do they violate HIPAA. The case manager is a member of the multidisciplinary team who often coordinates care, but the "case management model" of client care is fictitious.

TEST-TAKING STRATEGY: Look for similar answer choices and eliminate them.

45. Multidisciplinary client care rounds are a client care tool used by the health care team. List the client care goals of multidisciplinary rounds: Select all that apply.

   A. Documenting multidisciplinary client care rounds complies with Joint Commission on Accreditation for Healthcare Organizations (JCAHO) and state health care regulatory agency requirements.

   B. Multidisciplinary client care rounds promote collaboration of care among members of the multidisciplinary team.

   C. Multidisciplinary client care rounds are shown to improve client outcomes and decrease length of stay in health care facilities.

   D. Multidisciplinary client care rounds are not shown to have any impact on client outcomes or on the cost of health care to the client.

Answer: B & C. Multidisciplinary client care rounds promote collaboration of care among members of the multidisciplinary team, improve client outcomes, and decrease the cost of health care and length of stay in health care facilities. Documenting multidisciplinary client care rounds is not a client care goal.

TEST-TAKING STRATEGY: When answering "Select all that apply" questions, be sure and treat each answer as a true or false statement. There may be one correct answer or more.

46. A clinical pathway is a client care management tool developed by the multidisciplinary team. Which statement describes the purpose and features of a clinical pathway? Select all that apply.

   A. A clinical pathway is an overview of the multidisciplinary plan of care for a select group of clients.

   B. A clinical pathway is the safe area mapped out for ambulatory clients to walk, so they may be monitored by remote telemetry if needed.

   C. A clinical pathway is developed by the multidisciplinary team to standardize care for a specific client group related by a diagnosis or condition, and based on the latest research and practice information.

   D. A clinical pathway is a set of predetermined orders placed in a client's medical record to streamline the order process and expedite care to the client.

Answer: A & C. A clinical pathway is an overview of the client plan of care developed by the multidisciplinary team for a specific client group that is related by diagnosis or condition. The clinical pathway integrates the latest research and practice information into the plan of care. The clinical pathway is not a physical place for clients to ambulate. A set of predetermined orders is the description of an order set.

TEST-TAKING STRATEGY: When answering "Select all that apply" questions, be sure and treat each answer as a true or false statement. There may be one correct answer or more.

47. An algorithm is a client care tool used by the multidisciplinary team designed to improve client outcomes. Algorithms are utilized by members of the multidisciplinary team as (select all that apply):

   A. An overview of the multidisciplinary plan of care.

   B. A decision-making flowchart that employs the "if, then" decision-making process.

   C. Medication titration and weaning guidelines.

   D. Oxygen and ventilator weaning guidelines.

Answer: B, C, & D. An algorithm is a decision-making flowchart utilized by different members of the multidisciplinary health care team that employs the "if, then" decision-making process. Algorithms address client responses to specific medications or treatments delivered and offer treatment options based on those client responses. The ACLS (Advanced Cardiac Life Support) algorithms for resuscitation are an example. The overview of the multidisciplinary plan of care is a description of a multidisciplinary clinical pathway.

TEST-TAKING STRATEGY: When answering "Select all that apply" questions, be sure and treat each answer as a true or false statement. There may be one correct answer or more.

48. During client care rounds with the multidisciplinary team, the nurse reports that a client coughs frequently after taking anything by mouth. The dietician recommends a swallow evaluation for the client, in which the physician participating in rounds writes the order. This is an example of:

    A. Collaboration of client care with the ancillary care providers.

    B. Collaboration of client care between the physician and the dietary department.

    C. Collaboration of care with the risk management team because of the client's risk for aspiration.

    D. Collaboration of care among members of the multidisciplinary team.

    Answer: D. The nurse reporting assessment findings, the dietician suggesting a swallow evaluation, and the physician ordering the swallow evaluation are an example of collaboration of care among members of the multidisciplinary team. Collaboration of care with the ancillary providers is a partial answer as is collaboration of care between the physician and the dietary department. These health care team members are all part of the multidisciplinary team. Risk management is a formal process through which a health care facility or provider agency tracks client outcomes to identify potential problems and ensure safe delivery of care.

TEST-TAKING STRATEGY: Read each answer selection carefully, then choose the option with the most complete answer. Be alert for partial correct answers when a more complete answer option is present.

49. A client with right-sided weakness prepares for discharge home from the rehabilitation facility where the physical therapist works with the client on independent transfers and safe use of a walker and assistive devices. The client expresses concern about self-care during the first week at home. Which response by the physical therapist demonstrates collaboration with the multidisciplinary care team for the safest client outcome?

    A. "I understand you are nervous about the first few days at home, but you have worked hard at physical therapy. Don't worry, you'll be fine."

    B. "Will you have family at home to help you adjust to caring for yourself?"

    C. "I understand you are nervous about the first few days at home. I will suggest a physical therapy evaluation of your home for safety before you are discharged to your case manager."

    D. "Your case manager can give you a list of referral agencies to contact for home health assistance if you would like to have one. Is there anything else I may do to help you?"

    Answer: C. The physical therapist acknowledges the client's feelings of apprehension about going home and the client's worries about self-care. Telling the client not to worry does not address the problem and invalidates the client's expression of anxiety. Asking if the family will be available is a partial correct answer because it does not address the client's concerns or offer assistance from members of the multidisciplinary team. The case manager simply giving the client a list of home health agencies to contact is inappropriate, as it shows lack of responsiveness to the client's concerns regarding care and safety. This answer option demonstrates only minimal involvement by the multidisciplinary team in the client care and discharge process.

TEST-TAKING STRATEGY: Look for similar answer choices and eliminate them.

50. There are multiple theories of management utilized in nursing. Management theories generally fall under one of two distinctly different and opposing schools of thought with regard to the management of people. What are the two current prevailing theories of modern management?

   A. The scientific theory of management and the human relations-based theory of management

   B. The human relations-based theory of management and the democratic theory of management

   C. The scientific theory of management and the theocratic theory of management

   D. The democratic theory of management and the leadership theory of management

   Answer: A. The two current prevailing theories of management are the scientific theory of management and the human relations-based theory of management. The scientific theory of management is task-oriented and emphasizes time-management, efficiency, eliminating excess staff, and increasing productivity. The human relations-based model emphasizes the employee as an individual, focusing on the interpersonal relationships between manager, staff, and clients. Democracies and theocracies are actually management *styles*. Leadership and management are two different concepts.

   TEST-TAKING STRATEGY: Read each question twice to be certain that you know what the question is asking; then read each answer option with the question.

51. Leadership and management are two different concepts. A leader is one who has the ability to influence, motivate, and enable others to contribute toward the success of an organization. A manager is one who directs and controls a group of people toward accomplishing a goal. Which statements describe a manager? Select all that apply.

   A. A manager has an informal role based on influence, knowledge, and experience in a particular field or area of employment.

   B. A manager has a formally appointed role based on authority.

   C. A manager has a formally appointed role and is usually responsible for staff evaluations, hiring, firing, and department financial matters.

   D. A manager has a defined job description and is responsible for work being performed by others.

   Answer: B, C, & D. A manager has a formally appointed role, based on authority, and is usually responsible for staff evaluation, hiring, firing, department budgets, and financial matters. A manager is responsible for the work produced by others. A person who serves in an informal role is a leader.

   TEST-TAKING STRATEGY: Do not panic or become discouraged if you do not know the answer(s) to a question. Study questions are study tools to help you identify topics that you still need to learn or clarify. Read the subjects to refresh your memory and correct the knowledge deficit.

52. Leadership and management are two different concepts. A leader is one who has the ability to influence, motivate, and enable others to contribute toward the success of an organization. A manager is one who directs and controls a group of people toward accomplishing a goal. Which statements describe a leader? Select all that apply.

   A. A leader has a formally appointed role based on authority.

   B. A leader has an earned role, achieved by knowledge and experience, and the respect of coworkers.

   C. A leader has an informal role based on influence and respect of peers.

   D. Being a leader requires collaborative effort and independent thinking.

Answer: B, C, & D. A leader has an informal role; an earned role based on influence that comes from knowledge, experience, and the respect of peers and coworkers. Being a leader requires collaborative effort and independent thinking. A leader in a formally appointed role is a manager.

TEST-TAKING STRATEGY: "Select all that apply" questions may more than one correct answer. Do not panic or become discouraged if you do not know the answer(s) to a question. Study questions are study tools to help you identify what you need to learn or clarify.

53. An effective manager of people must possess qualities that inspire staff to work in an efficient manner, produce a quality work product, work as a team, and perform the work in a professional and ethical manner. Which qualities would describe an effective manager? Select all that apply.

A. Clinical experience and expertise in the field of work under the manager's supervision.

B. Knowledge of finance and business principles.

C. Good communication skills with multiple personality types.

D. Clinical knowledge above and beyond any other staff member under the manager's supervision.

Answer: A, B, & C. An effective manager of people should possess good communication skills and clinical knowledge and expertise in the field of work. Knowledge of finance and business principles allows a manager to run a financially responsible unit of employment. Clinical knowledge *above and beyond* any other staff member is incorrect because this is not a necessary quality of an effective manager.

TEST-TAKING STRATEGY: Look for similarly worded answer selections to help eliminate the incorrect option. "Select all that apply" questions may have more than one correct answer, but usually will not have two correct similarly worded answer selections.

54. The use of good interpersonal skills is essential for a manager to be effective. Which interpersonal skills would be important for an effective manager to possess? Select all that apply.

A. Clinical expertise.

B. Conflict resolution.

C. Communication skills.

D. Business and financial knowledge.

Answer: B & C. Two of the interpersonal skills essential to an effective manager are conflict resolution and good communication skills. Clinical expertise and business and financial knowledge are not interpersonal skills.

TEST-TAKING STRATEGY: Read each question carefully. Use cues in the question to help rule out incorrect answer options. Information in similar questions on the same subject may hold the answer to later questions.

55. The physician has ordered a central IV line insertion and requested the nurse to prepare the client and set up for the procedure. The nurse has not assisted with a central line insertion before and asks the charge nurse for advice and assistance. Which response by the charge nurse indicates that the charge nurse practices the transitional style of management?

A. "I will assist the physician with the procedure so that you will have time to care for the rest of your clients."

B. "I do not have time to go over the procedure with you right now. Look it up in the unit policy and procedure manual."

C. "You have never assisted with a central line insertion before?"

D. "Let's get the supplies that we will need. I want you to assist the physician, but I will be there with you to talk you through the procedure."

Answer: D. The transitional style of management focuses on promotion of staff education and experience in order to enhance each staff member's knowledge and skills. The answer options that quote the charge nurse offering to perform the procedure for the nurse or offer no help to the nurse are incorrect and reflect a transactional management style.

TEST-TAKING STRATEGY: Read each answer option with the question for continuity of content and context. Read each answer option with the question.

56. A managerial position in the health care setting is a complex position. The manager is responsible to the organization, clients, and employees in the manager's area of supervision. Which activity would demonstrate a manager's responsibility to employees? Select all that apply.

   A. Resolving conflicts between employees, clients, client family members, or other members of the organization

   B. Evaluating employees, offering constructive criticism, and developing staff

   C. Representing employees at organizational committee and management meetings

   D. Acting as clinical expert in the area of health care under the manager's supervision

   Answer: A, B, & C. Managers are responsible for conflict resolution, employee evaluation, and staff development. Managers also represent employees at committee and management meetings. A manager is not required to demonstrate expertise in the clinical area of supervision.

   TEST-TAKING STRATEGY: If you do not know the answer to a question, use common sense and good judgment to rule out the obviously incorrect answer options first. This leaves you with the potentially correct answer options. "Select all that apply" indicates that you will choose more than one correct answer selection to complete the question.

57. A high percentage of employees who resign from positions in health care list difficulties with their manager as the main reason for transferring to another department or terminating employment. Which effect could an ineffective manager have on a health care work environment? Select all that apply.

   A. An increase in employee morale.

   B. A decrease in employee morale.

   C. A decrease in the number of staff members to care for clients due to employee resignation or transfer.

   D. A high rate of staff turnover for the unit, resulting in costly new employee hiring and orientation by the health care organization.

   Answer: B, C, & D. An ineffective manager can have a detrimental and costly effect on unit morale, unit staffing, and overall client care.

   TEST-TAKING STRATEGY: Use cues and information in the question to help identify the incorrect answer selections. Look for similarly worded answer selections as an indicator that one of them is an incorrect option.

58. Health care facility departments with effective, supportive managers share common indicators of employee satisfaction. What are some of the indicators of a department with high employee job satisfaction? Select all that apply.

   A. Low employee turnover rate and high unit morale.

   B. Effective conflict resolution and communication.

   C. Employees functioning as an integral part of the multidisciplinary team.

   D. High employee turnover rate and low unit morale.

   Answer: A, B, & C. Indicators of high employee job satisfaction include low employee turnover, high unit morale, effective conflict resolution and communication, and employees who feel as if they are an integral part of the multidisciplinary team.

   TEST-TAKING STRATEGY: Use cues and information in the question to help identify the incorrect answer selections. Look for similarly worded answer selections as an indicator that one of them is an incorrect option.

59. Ensuring the confidentiality of clients' health information and documentation is the responsibility of (select all that apply):

A. The primary physician and all consulting physicians.

B. The health care personnel involved in direct care of the client.

C. The unit secretary.

D. All members of the multidisciplinary team and employees of a health care facility.

Answer: A, B, C, & D. Ensuring the confidentiality of clients' health information is the responsibility of every employee of a health care organization including its physicians.

TEST-TAKING STRATEGY: "Select all that apply" indicates that there will be multiple correct answer selections. Use cues in the answer selections to rule out the clearly incorrect answer options. In the above answer selections, options B and D cannot both be correct, so this would help to identify one of these options as an incorrect answer selection.

60. The Health Insurance Portability and Accountability Act (HIPAA) is federal legislation enacted in 1996. What are some of the components of HIPAA? Select all that apply.

A. HIPAA gives every person access to free health care.

B. HIPAA provides the public more widespread access to health insurance.

C. HIPAA provides protection and privacy of health information.

D. HIPAA designates a health information surrogate for the client in the event the client becomes unable to receive health information and make informed health care decisions.

Answer: B & C. The HIPAA legislation of 1996 provides, in part, more widespread access to health insurance and the protection and privacy of health information. HIPAA provides that every person is guaranteed *access* to health care but does not provide for free health care. HIPAA does not designate a health information surrogate for a client unable to make informed health care decisions.

TEST-TAKING STRATEGY: Use logic and common sense to separate the correct answer selections from the detractors. If you must guess, use cues in the questions and answer options. As above, the longest answer option is not always a correct one.

61. A nurse caring for clients in an OB/GYN physician's office is asked by one of the physician's clients, "How is that girl who was so sick out in the waiting room last week? She told me she was concerned that the physician might admit her to the hospital?" Which response by the office nurse demonstrates confidentiality of client health information within HIPAA guidelines?

A. "I appreciate your concern for that client. She was admitted to the hospital that afternoon. You should call the hospital's information desk and get them to transfer the call to her room, so that you can speak with her."

B. "I appreciate your concern for that client you met last week. The health information of all clients is protected by law and I cannot give you any additional information. Thank you for your kindness in inquiring, though."

C. "That client became very ill and was taken away to the hospital by ambulance. It was a lot of activity for our physician's office!"

D. "I appreciate your concern for that client you met last week. The health information of all clients is protected by law, but since the client told you herself that she might be admitted to the hospital I can tell you that she did go to the hospital by ambulance that afternoon."

Answer: B. The health information of all clients is confidential and protected by law. This answer informs the concerned client of the confidential nature of the information that she is seeking, but validates her concern for the ill client. Further information cannot be given out without the express written consent of the client.

TEST-TAKING STRATEGY: With confidentiality questions and issues, the answer selections that violate a client's right to confidentiality are incorrect. Read similarly worded answers carefully for content—these are the "trick answers" designed to educate you on the importance of reading each answer option carefully. Practice this habit now while studying for the examination.

62. A client in the critical care unit is intubated, mechanically ventilated, and sedated with propofol (*Diprivan*). The client was admitted 1 week ago with an atypical pneumonia and a high fever. A hepatitis panel and an HIV test were drawn with the client's consent before the client was sedated. The client's wife asks the nurse if the test results are back yet, and what the results of those studies were. The client does not have a health care proxy or Durable Power of Attorney executed at this time. How should the nurse respond in compliance with HIPAA (Health Insurance Portability and Accountability Act) regulations regarding the confidentiality of the sedated client's health information?

A. "I can't give you those results. You should ask his doctor, though, the next time that he comes in to examine your husband."

B. "Those test results are confidential, but since you are his wife I can give them to you. Let me look them up in the computer system."

C. "The health information of all clients is confidential and is protected by law. Those test results and all health information cannot be released without the consent of the client. This also applies to family members, and is designed to protect the client's right to choose who receives health information."

D. "Your husband is only lightly sedated on the propofol IV drip. I can wake him up and ask him if it is all right to release these test results to you."

Answer: C. Each client's health information is confidential and protected by law. The nurse should inform the client's wife of this fact, and explain the rationale for health information confidentiality. Family members are often offended or angry upon learning that health information can not be released to them without the client's consent, but health care employees are bound by law to the confidential nature of health information. A client who has received sedative or narcotic medications cannot give legal consent as these medications alter a client's level of consciousness and impair the ability to make informed decisions.

TEST-TAKING STRATEGY: Read each answer selection in conjunction with the question for continuity of content and concept. If you do not know the correct answer, do not panic. Use common sense and what you know about the question's subject matter to rule out the incorrect answer options and narrow the selections down to the probable correct ones.

63. Nurses from a post-anesthesia care unit (PACU) go out for dinner after their shift is completed. One of the nurses says, "Do you remember that last patient I had, the one with the abdominal surgery? They found a tumor during the operation, and the early pathology reports came back as cancer. I wonder if the physician has told the client yet." How does this statement by the PACU nurse violate client confidentiality and HIPAA regulations regarding health care information? Select all that apply.

A. This statement does not violate client confidentiality or HIPAA regulations. All of the nurses present are employed in the post-anesthesia care unit and have access to that client's health information.

B. This statement violates client confidentiality because health information is accessed on a need-to-know basis. This information was not necessary to the care of the client and is not appropriate as a subject of dinner conversation.

C. This statement violates client confidentiality because it is made in a public place where it could be overheard by members of the public with no right to the client's health information.

D. This statement violates client confidentiality because it is revealed by the nurse to other staff not involved in the client's care, without the client's permission.

Answer: B, C, & D. These statements are inappropriate and violate client confidentiality and HIPAA regulations regarding the confidentiality of health care information. Health information is accessed by members of the multidisciplinary team involved in client care on a need-to-know basis only and should never be discussed in a public setting.

TEST-TAKING STRATEGY: "Select all that apply" indicates that there will be multiple correct answer selections in the options listed. Remember to choose more than one answer option. Unless there is an answer option for "all of the above," all four answer options will not be correct.

64. A client is brought to the emergency department by ambulance in an altered state of consciousness. The client does not answer questions appropriately, is alternately agitated and drowsy, and speaks loudly and incoherently at intervals. The client's significant other arrives in the emergency department and asks the nurse for the results of the client's urine drug screen. The client's significant other states that the client has used illegal drugs in the past. The significant other needs the information for personal safety and the safety of the couple's children. What is the best response by the nurse to the request for the results of the urine drug screen?

   A. "The results of the urine drug screen are positive for illegal substances."

   B. "You are wise to ask for the urine drug screen results for your safety and the children's safety. The drug screen results are positive for the drugs you gave me information about."

   C. "Thank you for the information about the client's history of illegal drug use. Because you live together and have children together, I can give you those results."

   D. "Thank you for the information about the client's history of illegal drug use. A complete health history helps us give better care. The health information of every client is confidential and protected by law and cannot be released without the client's consent. Does the client have a Durable Power of Attorney for Health Care listing you as the surrogate decision-maker?"

Answer: D. The health information of every client is confidential, protected by law, and can only be released with the client's consent. Releasing the urine drug screen results, or any health information, to the significant other without an executed Durable Power of Attorney for health care or the client's consent is a violation of client confidentiality and HIPAA regulations regarding the privacy of health information.

TEST-TAKING STRATEGY: Use logic and common sense to figure out the correct answers to questions like this one. If you do not know the answer, do not panic. Study questions are designed to help to identify the areas that you still need to learn or clarify before taking the examination. There is nothing wrong with not knowing an answer, but the correct response is to read and study that subject matter to correct the knowledge deficit.

65. HIPAA is federal legislation enacted in 1996 to protect the privacy of health information and assure broader access to health insurance. "HIPAA" is an acronym for:

   A. Health Insurance Portability and Accountability Act.

   B. Health Information Privacy and Accountability Act.

   C. Health Information Privacy and Access Act.

   D. Hospital Information Privacy and Accountability Act.

Answer: A. "HIPAA" is an acronym for Health Insurance Portability and Accountability Act.

TEST-TAKING STRATEGY: Decide what you believe the answer to be before reading the answer selections. This decreases the likelihood that you will become confused by the incorrect answer options.

66. The violation of client confidentiality, as defined by HIPAA regulations for the privacy and confidentiality of health information is a violation of:

   A. Hospital policy on the confidentiality of health information.

   B. The state nurse practice act.

   C. Federal legislation enacted to assure the confidentiality of health information.

   D. The nursing code of ethics.

Answer: C. The violation of client confidentiality, as defined by HIPAA regulations for the privacy and confidentiality of health information is a violation of federal legislation that was enacted to assure the confidential nature of health information. Conviction of a breach of confidentiality and HIPAA regulations can bring reprimands and consequences from federal, state board of nursing, and health care organization levels.

TEST-TAKING STRATEGY: Often the longest response is the correct answer selection, but not always. Read each answer option carefully to evaluate for content and continuity of context with the question.

67. The neighbor of a nurse working in an urgent care clinic comes in for treatment. That evening after work, the nurse is out working in the yard when another neighbor walks by and says, "I heard that our neighbor went to the urgent care clinic today. Isn't that where you work? Was everything all right?" What response by the nurse demonstrates compliance with the confidentiality of health information?

A. "Since I am off work and it was only a minor injury I can tell you."

B. "It is nice of you to ask, and I do work at that urgent care clinic. The health information of every client is confidential and protected by law. Only our neighbor can give you that information."

C. "I do work at the urgent care clinic. Our neighbor was fine, only a few minor scrapes and bruises. We have such a close, caring neighborhood."

D. "I can neither confirm nor deny whether that client came to our urgent care clinic or not today."

Answer: B. Acknowledge the neighbor's concern and explain that health information is confidential and protected by law, and can only be revealed by the client or the client's consent.

TEST-TAKING STRATEGY: Decide what you believe the answer is before you read the answer options. This will help to keep you from becoming confused by the incorrect answer options.

68. A nurse is accessing a client's computerized health information history to check the list of home medications that the client takes. The information is accessed appropriately for client care necessity. A call light goes on and the nurse walks away to answer the call light without logging off the computer, leaving the client's health information and home medication history visible on the screen. This is a violation of (select all that apply):

A. Health care facility policy regarding the confidentiality of client health information.

B. Client health information confidentiality as defined by HIPAA.

C. The client's right to confidentiality, as defined by the Patient's Bill of Rights.

D. Client health information confidentiality as defined by state law.

Answer: A, B, & C. Leaving a client's health information visible on a computer monitor is a violation of the health care facility's policy regarding client health information confidentiality, federal HIPAA regulations for health information confidentiality, and the client's right to confidentiality as defined by the Patient's Bill of Rights. HIPAA is federal legislation, not state legislation.

TEST-TAKING STRATEGY: "Select all that apply" indicates that there may be multiple correct answer selections, so choose more than one answer option. Unless there is an answer option for "all of the above," all four answer selections will not be correct.

69. A thin, cachectic-appearing client with dry, tenting skin is admitted from a privately operated board and care facility with a diagnosis of urosepsis and altered level of consciousness. The client has skin breakdown and the diaper the client is wearing is soiled and soaked with urine. After photographing the client's condition, bathing the client, and providing the appropriate care, the nurse calls to report the client's condition at the time of admission. To which agencies should the nurse report the client's condition? Select all that apply.

A. Social Services and the Adult Protective Services.

B. Social Services and Dietary Services.

C. Adult Protective Services and Physical Therapy.

D. Physical Therapy and the State Licensing Board for board and care facilities.

Answer: A. Nurses are legally responsible to report any abuse, neglect, or suspicions of abuse or neglect to the Department of Social Services for follow-up on the client's condition, and to Adult Protective Services for the suspicion of abuse or neglect. The State Licensing Board for board and care facilities is usually contacted by Social Services following a formal investigation.

TEST-TAKING STRATEGY: Read the question carefully. Read it twice if necessary to understand what it is asking. This will help to rule out incorrect answer options.

70. A client with a history of supraventricular tachycardia is admitted to the telemetry unit with complaints of dizziness and fainting spells. The client's heart rate suddenly registers 220 beats per minute on the telemetry monitor screen and the rhythm shows atrial tachycardia. The client is alert but complaining of shortness of breath and dizziness. The nurse asks the nursing assistant to repeat a set of vital signs while the nurse notifies the primary care physician. The primary care physician states that the client needs synchronized cardioversion and asks the nurse to contact the on-call cardiologist stat. This collaborative care by the nurse and primary care physician resulted in the client receiving the appropriate cardioversion from the on-call cardiologist in a timely manner. The actions by the nurse to procure appropriate care for the client were an example of:

A. Case management.

B. Cardioversion.

C. Consultation.

D. Delegation.

Answer: C. The nurse assessed the client, reported the assessment information to the client's primary care physician, and then followed the primary care physician's orders by requesting a stat cardiology *consult* for synchronized cardioversion.

TEST-TAKING STRATEGY: The nurse should notify the physician when there is nothing else that the nurse can do to correct the client's problem. This information will result in either additional orders from the physician or orders for consultation with the appropriate members of the multidisciplinary team.

71. A client is admitted with complaints of general fatigue and episodes of syncope. The client's spouse states that the client snores loudly at night and often stops breathing for prolonged periods. The nurse assesses the sleeping client and documents heavy snoring with periods of apnea lasting up to 30 seconds. The nurse reports these assessment findings in multidisciplinary client care rounds and the physician requests a consultation with a specialist for evaluation of possible severe sleep apnea. The collaborative client care effort by the multidisciplinary team resulted in:

A. A diagnosis of sleep apnea.

B. A consultation for further evaluation.

C. The nurse acting as a client advocate.

D. Delegation.

Answer: B. The collaborative client care effort by the multidisciplinary team resulted in a consultation for further client evaluation and treatment.

TEST-TAKING STRATEGY: Read each answer option carefully, then reread it with the question. Decide what the question is asking. In this scenario, is this a respiratory question, a consultation question, or a client advocacy or delegation question?

72. During an initial morning assessment, a client appears to be hallucinating; complaining about "bugs on the wall" and "the dog that ran under the bed." The nurse reorients the client to person, place, and time and the client demonstrates good recall of the information. After the client receives the morning medications, the hallucinations begin again. The nurse notifies the physician that the client's hallucinations returned shortly after the medications were administered. The physician requests the nurse to call the clinical pharmacist to evaluate the client's medication list for a possible medication source of the hallucinations. The actions of the nurse resulted in:

A. Delegation of responsibility.

B. Medication error prevention.

C. Establishing client care priorities.

D. Consultation to the appropriate multidisciplinary team member for further client evaluation and treatment.

Answer: D. The actions of the nurse resulted in consultation to the appropriate multidisciplinary team member for further client evaluation and treatment.

TEST-TAKING STRATEGY: The longest answer option is often the correct one, but not always. Read each answer option carefully for content.

73. A hemodialysis client presents to the dialysis clinic for a regularly scheduled dialysis session. The nurse assesses the client's dialysis access graft before beginning the treatment. The graft site appears reddened and feels abnormally warm to the touch. The client reports a fever and aching joints for the past 2 days and a headache starting that morning. The client's temperature is 101.5°F. What is the most appropriate immediate action by the nurse to provide the correct treatment for the client?

A. The nurse should begin the client's hemodialysis treatment immediately.

B. The nurse should begin the client's hemodialysis treatment, but monitor the client carefully for any worsening of the complaints or symptoms, or an increase in the client's temperature.

C. The nurse should ask if the client feels well enough for dialysis that day.

D. The nurse should immediately notify the client's nephrologist of the assessment findings and vital signs.

Answer: D. The dialysis nurse should immediately consult with the client's nephrologist regarding the client's assessment findings and vital signs. This care consultation by the nurse gives the physician necessary information to provide additional treatment to the client.

TEST-TAKING STRATEGY: If you do not know the answer to a question, remain calm and use common sense and the process of elimination to first rule out the obviously incorrect answer options, and then select the correct answer.

74. A new graduate nurse identifies an abnormal heart sound while performing a client assessment. The graduate nurse asks the charge nurse to listen to the client's heart sounds. The charge nurse confirms that the client has a systolic heart murmur. This action by the graduate nurse is an example of:

A. Continuity of care.

B. Delegation.

C. Consultation.

D. Supervision.

Answer: C. One medical professional asking the opinion of another medical professional regarding an assessment finding is an example of consultation.

TEST-TAKING STRATEGY: Read the question carefully to determine what it is asking. Decide what you believe the answer is before reading the answer options, and then choose the answer option closest to your own answer.

75. The nurse discovers a new stage II pressure ulcer on a client's coccyx area during the bath. What is the most appropriate action for the nurse to take in order to initiate appropriate care for the client?

A. The nurse should notify the physician immediately of the client's new area of skin breakdown.

B. The nurse should place a nursing consultation to the wound care nurse for evaluation of the client's skin breakdown.

C. The nurse should immediately call a "code skin." The skin care team will come quickly to evaluate the client's skin newly identified skin breakdown.

D. The nurse should notify the client's family members immediately of the client's new area of skin breakdown.

Answer: B. The nurse should place a nursing consult to the facility's wound care nurse upon discovery of a new area of skin breakdown. The wound care nurse will evaluate the client for appropriate bed surface and wound treatment.

TEST-TAKING STRATEGY: Do not panic if you do not know the answer to a question. Use common sense and your best judgment to rule out the obviously incorrect answer options first.

76. Consultation is an integral tool that utilizes the combined knowledge, education, and experience levels of different members of the multidisciplinary health care team to provide quality, comprehensive care to clients. Which statements describe the appropriate use of consultation? Select all that apply.

A. Consultation can occur between one physician and another.

B. Consultation can occur between any members of the multidisciplinary health care team.

C. Consultation can occur from one nurse to another.

D. Consultation is rarely done among nursing peers.

Answer: A, B, & C. Consultation is a tool utilized by the multidisciplinary health care team to provide quality, comprehensive client care.

Consultation can occur physician-to-physician, nurse-to-nurse, and between any members of the multidisciplinary team. Consultation among nurses and their peers is a common practice.

TEST-TAKING STRATEGY: Look for cues in the question. Questions such as the one above contain indicators for the correct answer information if you read them carefully.

77. Effective communication between members of the multidisciplinary health care team ensures which important aspect of a safe client care environment?

A. The confidentiality of health information.

B. Reasonable continuity of care.

C. The right to self-determination.

D. Considerate and respectful care.

Answer: B. Effective communication between members of the multidisciplinary team ensures reasonable continuity of care, improves client outcomes, and helps to create a safe environment of care.

TEST-TAKING STRATEGY: Do not change your original answer unless you have positive information the original answer chosen was incorrect. Historically, your first impression is the correct one. Changing an answer usually produces an incorrect result.

78. The night-shift nurse gives an informative end-of-shift report to the day-shift nurse assuming care of the assigned client group. The shift report is an example of which element of a safe client care environment?

A. The shift report is an example of a JCAHO requirement.

B. The shift report is an example of poor communication between members of the health care team.

C. The shift report is an example of continuity of care.

D. The shift report is a breach of confidentiality.

Answer: C. An informative end-of-shift client report is an example of good continuity of care. Effective communication between members of the health care team is a key component of continuity of care and is essential for a safe environment of care. The specific information relayed during a client care shift report is not regulated by JCAHO.

TEST-TAKING STRATEGY: Use the process of elimination to rule out incorrect answer options and select the correct answer. Look for cues or key words in a question that match an answer option in wording or content.

79. A nurse is performing the admission assessment and documenting the health history information on a newly admitted client. The client reports an allergy to penicillin, but the nurse fails to record this allergy information in the medical record. What is the correct definition of this error of omission by the nurse?

    A. A breach of client confidentiality that could result in harm to the client.

    B. A breach of the client's right to participate in the plan of care.

    C. A failure by the nurse to appropriately diagnose the client.

    D. A breach in continuity of care that could result in harm to the client.

Answer: D. The admitting nurse's failure to document the client's stated allergy is a breach in the continuity of care and could result in harm to the client if the medication is ordered and administered.

TEST-TAKING STRATEGY: Look for similarly worded answer options that help identify the incorrect options.

80. A client is being discharged to a rehabilitation facility. The primary nurse caring for the client on the day of discharge carefully inventories the client's belongings and checks the list against the admission list of belongings for accuracy. The nurse then calls a client report the nurse assuming client care at the receiving rehabilitation facility and answers the receiving

nurse's questions before concluding the report. The nurse has demonstrated which element of a safe client care environment?

A. Continuity of care.

B. Case management.

C. Quality improvement.

D. Courteous and respectful care.

Answer: A. The nurse demonstrated good continuity of care by performing an inventory of the client's belongings, calling a client care report to the nurse assuming care of the client at the receiving facility, and answering any questions before concluding the report.

TEST-TAKING STRATEGY: Keep up a steady pace during the exam. If you do not know the answer to a question, use common sense and your best judgment to select an answer, then move on to the next question.

81. A client is brought to the emergency department by ambulance with a head injury. The emergency department physician calls the nurse to be present while addressing the client's family. The physician informs the client's family that the hospital does not have a neurosurgeon on staff. In order to provide the best possible care to the client, the emergency department will stabilize the client and then make transfer arrangements to a nearby hospital with neurosurgical services. This action decision by the physician member of the multidisciplinary team reflects (select all that apply):

    A. Appropriate consultation.

    B. Appropriate disclosure of client health information.

    C. Appropriate continuity of care.

    D. Poor continuity of care.

Answer: B & C. The physician appropriately disclosed client health information to the client's family for purposes of client care. The physician also provides appropriate continuity of care by arranging for the head-injured client to be stabilized and transferred to a health care facility with the services necessary to give the best care to the client.

TEST-TAKING STRATEGY: When answering "Select all that apply" questions, be sure and treat each answer as a true or false statement. There may be one correct answer or more.

82. An informative client care report is essential for good continuity of care and a safe client care environment. What are the components of an effective client care report? Select all that apply.

   A. The client's medical history.

   B. The client's code status and allergy information.

   C. Information overheard about the client or the client's family.

   D. Pertinent events related to the client's current course of illness.

   Answer: A, B, & D. Components of an effective client care report to the nurse assuming client care include, but are not limited to, the client's medical history, code status, allergy information, and pertinent events related to the current course of illness.

TEST-TAKING STRATEGY: Choose answer options that would benefit the client. The answer options that would be detrimental or have no effect on client care can be ruled out as incorrect answers.

83. Which component of the multidisciplinary health care team has been shown, in multiple studies, to decrease clients' length of stay in health care facilities, decrease the cost of health care to the client, and improve continuity of care?

   A. Outcomes management.

   B. Risk management.

   C. Case management.

   D. Infection control.

   Answer: C. Case management has been shown, in multiple studies, to decrease clients' length of stay in health care facilities, decrease the cost of health care to the client, and improve continuity of care.

TEST-TAKING STRATEGY: If you are not certain of the meaning of terms or phrases in the question or answer options, look for cues in the information for the context of the term.

84. Delegation of responsibility between members of the multidisciplinary health care team is essential to provide quality and timely client care. Which statement best describes delegation?

   A. Delegation is the process of overseeing and organizing client care in collaboration with the multidisciplinary team.

   B. Delegation is the reassigning of responsibility for performance of a job or task from one member of the health care team to another.

   C. Delegation of responsibility can only be done by the charge nurse or nurse manager.

   D. Delegation is the process of prioritizing client care to achieve the best possible client outcome.

   Answer: B. Delegation of responsibility is the reassigning of responsibility for performance of a job or task from one member of the health care team to another.

TEST-TAKING STRATEGY: If you discover a term or a question that you do not know the answer to, do not panic—look up the information and correct your knowledge deficit. The purpose of study questions is to help you identify areas you still need to clarify or learn more about prior to taking the actual exam.

85. Nurses use delegation of responsibility as an essential tool to assist in the delivery of high-quality care to clients in a timely manner. What factors must a nurse consider before choosing to delegate a nursing action or responsibility? Select all that apply.

   A. The stability of the client's condition.

   B. The amount of supervision required after delegation of the action or task to ensure quality of care.

   C. The competence of the team member to perform the delegated action or task.

   D. The number of years that the team member has been employed.

Answer: A, B, & C. Nurses use their critical thinking skills and professional judgment to select an appropriate member of the health care team for delegation of a client care responsibility. The accountability for the work product and end result remains with the nurse who delegates the responsibility. Factors that affect the appropriateness of a delegated work assignment include the condition of the client, the competence of the team member receiving the work assignment, and the amount of supervision required to ensure quality care has been delivered to the client in a timely manner.

TEST-TAKING STRATEGY: "Select all that apply" indicates that there may be multiple correct answers. Generally all four answer options will not be correct unless there is an "all of the above" answer option.

86. The nurse must use critical thinking skills and good judgment to appropriately delegate responsibility for portions of client care to other members of the health care team. What are the "Five Rights" of client care delegation?

A. Right medication, right dose, right time, right route of administration, right client.

B. Right medication, right supervision, right symptoms, right time, and right client.

C. Right task, right circumstances, right personnel, right communication, and right supervision.

D. Right client, right site, right procedure, right personnel, and right consent.

Answer: C. The "Five Rights" of delegation are right task, right circumstances (the client is stable enough for the particular task to be delegated), right personnel to perform the task with the correct training and experience, right communication between the nurse who chose to delegate the responsibility and the personnel accepting the responsibility, and the right supervision of the team member with responsibility to perform the task. Accountability for the task remains with the nurse who chose to delegate the task.

TEST-TAKING STRATEGY: Read each question carefully to determine what is being asked, then use cues in the question to identify the correct answer. Do your best to answer each question from your own knowledge base before reading the answer options. Give your full concentration to each question in turn.

87. A nurse who chooses to delegate selected client care tasks to other members of the health care team must use the nursing process to delegate appropriately and effectively. Which components of the nursing process apply to delegation? Select all that apply.

A. Assessing the client needs and the skill levels of health care team members available to assist.

B. Implementing the plan by assigning client care tasks to the appropriate personnel.

C. Planning by assigning client care tasks to the appropriate personnel.

D. Evaluation to determine whether the assigned client care tasks were completed in a manner that met the client's needs.

Answer: A, B, & D. A nurse who chooses to delegate selected client care tasks must use the nursing process of assessing, planning, implementing, and evaluation to delegate appropriately and effectively. Assessing the needs of the client in comparison with the skill level of the health care team member or members, implementing the plan by assigning selected client care tasks to the appropriate personnel, and evaluating the outcome to make certain that the client's needs were met are examples of the way the nursing process is used to delegate care. Planning by assigning client care tasks is an example of implementation, not of planning.

TEST-TAKING STRATEGY: Use your knowledge of the nursing process and the sequence of the nursing process to answer this and related questions. "Select all that apply" indicates that you may need to select multiple correct answers to complete the question.

88. The nurse asks a nursing assistant to administer a preoperative bath to a client using special soap designed to decrease the bacteria count on the client's skin. The nursing assistant has no experience with this type of preoperative bath and asks the nurse for instructions. The nurse replies, "Just read the directions on the soap bottle. You will figure it out." Which "right" of delegation did the nurse fail to perform while delegating the preoperative bath to the nursing assistant?

A. Right client.

B. Right circumstances.

C. Right person.

D. Right communication.

Answer: D. The nurse failed to communicate the process for the preoperative bath to the certified nursing assistant. It is the nurse's responsibility to communicate expectations effectively and, if necessary, talk the nursing assistant through the correct process or demonstrate so that the nursing assistant will be aware of the correct process the next time.

TEST-TAKING STRATEGY: Attempt to answer the question from your own knowledge base before reading the answer options. Choose the answer option closest to the answer that you chose. Do not change your original answer choice without conclusive information that the original answer choice was incorrect. Changed answers are usually incorrect answers.

89. Nurses use delegation of appropriate client care responsibilities as an essential tool to assist in the delivery of quality care to clients in a timely manner. What are some of the advantages provided by appropriate delegation of client care? Select all that apply.

A. Delegation of appropriate client care responsibilities builds trust within the members of the health care team.

B. Delegation of responsibility can be done for client care tasks outside the scope of practice of the nurse choosing to delegate.

C. Delegation allows each health care team member to improve client care skills.

D. Delegation allows the multidisciplinary team to make better use of time.

Answer: A, C, & D. Delegation of appropriate client care builds trust within the health care team, fosters a spirit of teamwork, allows for improvement of each health care team member's skill level, and allows all members of the multidisciplinary team to make better use of time. However, delegation of any responsibility must be within the scope of practice of both the person delegating and the person accepting the delegated responsibility.

TEST-TAKING STRATEGY: When answering "Select all that apply" questions, be sure and treat each answer as a true or false statement. There may be one correct answer or more.

90. A nurse calls the hospital's lift team to assist with transferring an overweight client from the bed to a chair for the first time after hip surgery. Prior to the transfer, the nurse reports the client's recent surgical procedure, surgical site, and any difficulties that the lift team might expect to encounter while assisting the client out of bed to the chair. The nurse then stays in the client's room and supervises the procedure until the client transfer is complete and the client has the nurse call system within reach. What steps of the nursing process did the nurse use to appropriately delegate the client care in this example?

A. Assessment, planning, implementation, and evaluation.

B. Planning, implementation, delegation, and evaluation.

C. Delegation, assessment, implementation, and evaluation.

D. Delegation, planning, assessment, and implementation.

Answer: A. All components of the nursing process were present in this example of appropriate delegation of client care: *assessment* by the nurse to determine how much assistance would be needed to safely transfer the client from the bed to a chair; *planning* by making the decision to contact the lift team for additional assistance; *implementation* by contacting the lift team and by giving them a brief, targeted client situation report upon their arrival; and *evaluation* by staying in the client's room to supervise the client's first transfer out of bed and ensuring client safety during and after completion of the task.

TEST-TAKING STRATEGY: Read each question carefully and use cues in the question to help identify incorrect answer selections. This question is about the elements of the nursing process, so answer options containing "delegation" would be incorrect.

91. Delegation of responsibility for selected client care tasks is performed by nurses and members of the multidisciplinary health care team to manage time effectively and promote quality client care. What is the correct definition of delegation, as defined by the American Nurses Association (ANA)?

    A. Delegation requires direct supervision of the tasks performed by other members of the health care team.

    B. Delegation is the organization and coordination of care between multiple members of the multidisciplinary health care team.

    C. Delegation is the reassigning of responsibility for the performance of a job from one person to another.

    D. Delegation is the process of one person getting as many other persons to perform an assigned workload for them as possible without being noticed.

    Answer: C. Delegation is the reassigning of responsibility for the performance of a job from one person to another, as defined by the ANA.

    TEST-TAKING STRATEGY: Use common sense to identify the incorrect answer selections and choose the correct answer if you do not know the answer and have to guess. Make a list of the subject areas that you need to re-read or to clarify, and correct your knowledge deficit.

92. A nurse colleague who you work with always appears to be busy and overwhelmed. The nurse leaves late after almost every shift. When you offer assistance, the nurse's reply is invariably, "No, I'm all right. I prefer to do it myself but thank you for asking." This nurse is demonstrating difficulty with what important aspect of multidisciplinary client care?

    A. Delegation.

    B. Establishing priorities.

    C. Resource management.

    D. Advocacy.

    Answer: A. The nurse in the above description is demonstrating difficulty with delegation of client care. The statement, "I prefer to do it myself" indicates that the nurse may be hesitant to delegate care or ask for the help of other staff members.

    TEST-TAKING STRATEGY: Use the process of elimination to rule out incorrect answer options. Re-read the question carefully, and use common sense if you do not know the answer to a question.

93. Learning to establish effective client care priorities is an integral part of delivering quality care in a timely manner. Which statements are true regarding effective priority-setting and client care? Select all that apply.

    A. Establishing effective client care priorities is a learned nursing skill that develops with time and experience.

    B. Establishing effective client care priorities can affect a client's health, length of stay, and ultimate outcome.

    C. A large portion of client care priority setting is done by physicians and is not a nursing function.

    D. Priority setting for client care involves all aspects of the nursing process.

    Answer: A, B, & D. Learning to establish effective client care priorities is a nursing skill that develops with time and experience. Client care priorities set by the nurse can affect a client's health, length of stay, and ultimate outcome either positively or adversely. Nurses are the primary health care team members involved in setting direct client care priorities.

    TEST-TAKING STRATEGY: Read each answer option in context with the question. Answer options that do not match in content or context are likely incorrect answers.

94. A postoperative surgery client has orders to be out of bed to a chair 3 times daily and to perform incentive spirometry 10 times hourly while awake. The client resists incentive spirometry instruction by the respiratory therapist and refuses when the nurse and the lift team arrive to assist the client up to a chair at bedside. Which statement by the nurse shows effective priority setting for this postoperative client? Choose the best answer.

A. "You do not have to get up to the chair if you do not want to. You have the right to refuse treatment."

B. "Using the incentive spirometer and increasing your mobility with activities like getting up to the chair are important for your recovery after surgery. They help to prevent complications like pneumonia. You always have the right to refuse treatment, but I want you to know that you are placing yourself at risk for complications if you do so."

C. "If you choose not to get up to the chair or use your incentive spirometer, your physician will be upset. These treatments are designed to help you avoid complications after surgery."

D. "I would not want to get up, either, if I were you. That must be painful after surgery. Maybe you will feel strong enough to get out of bed tomorrow."

Answer: B. The best statement by the nurse that shows appropriate priority setting for this postoperative client is the answer that informs the client of the rationale for getting out of bed to the chair and for using the incentive spirometer. The nurse gives the client the option to refuse treatment, but also informs the client about the potential consequences of not complying with the treatment.

TEST-TAKING STRATEGY: Instructions to "choose the best answer" indicate that there is more than one acceptable answer option present, but one of them is more appropriate or contains more complete information. Select the answer that addresses the client's immediate problem. Watch out for partial answers, as there will usually be a more complete answer option with additional information.

95. Establishing effective client care priorities involves all aspects of the nursing process. What are some of the components of effective client care priority management? Select all that apply.

A. Assessment skills.

B. Critical thinking.

C. Nursing judgment.

D. Risk management assessment.

Answer: A, B, & C. Establishing effective client care priorities involves the nursing process, critical thinking, and nursing judgment. Risk management is the process of identifying potentially unsafe client care practices and changing policy and procedures to ensure safe delivery of client care.

TEST-TAKING STRATEGY: Use your best judgment and common sense to identify the incorrect answer options. If you have no recall of an answer option being associated with the question's subject, it is likely an incorrect answer. "Select all that apply" indicates that there may be one or more than one correct answers.

96. A nurse working on a telemetry unit receives an end-of-shift client care report from the previous nurse. The oncoming nurse receives a report on (1) two stable post-cardiac catheterization clients, (2) a client with frequent PVCs who is diaphoretic and complaining of indigestion, and (3) a client admitted the previous shift for observation after presenting to the emergency department with atypical chest discomfort and cardiac enzyme levels that have been within normal range for 12 hours. Which client should the oncoming nurse assess first?

A. Either of the two clients who are post-cardiac catheterization. Even though both clients are stable, there are potential risks after any invasive procedure.

B. The client with the frequent PVCs who is diaphoretic and complaining of indigestion.

C. The client admitted from the emergency department the previous shift for observation of atypical chest discomfort and negative cardiac enzymes for 12 hours.

D. The order the nurse chooses is not important. All four clients appear to be of the same acuity from the information received from the previous nurse in the shift report.

Answer: B. The client with frequent PVCs showing on the telemetry monitor, who is diaphoretic and complaining of indigestion, is exhibiting symptoms of a possible myocardial infarction. This client requires immediate assessment and further cardiac evaluation.

TEST-TAKING STRATEGY: Select the answer that addresses the client's immediate concern, or the client with the most life-threatening symptoms. Never delay treatment to a client with unstable vital signs or life-threatening assessment findings.

97. A nurse is charting at the nurses' station when a client uses the call light to ask for assistance to the bathroom. As the nurse answers the call light, a second client uses the call system to say, "I think I need some help! My IV site is bleeding a lot!" What criteria should the nurse use to prioritize these two client calls for assistance?

A. The client who called for assistance first should receive assistance first. The bleeding IV is probably not life threatening.

B. The client who called for assistance to the bathroom should be seen first. This client might attempt to get up alone if no one arrives to help.

C. The client who reported the bleeding IV should be seen first. There is no way to know without examining the IV site if it is a central or peripheral IV, how much blood was lost, or what medications might be infusing through the IV.

D. The nurse could choose to assist either client first. Both are of equal acuity and impact on client safety.

Answer: C. The client who reported the bleeding IV site should be assisted first by the nurse. Client care priorities begin with the ABCs, or airway, breathing, and circulation. The nurse should examine the bleeding IV site, but take responsibility for the client who requested assistance to the bathroom by calling another staff member to assist that client, or informing the client that there will be a brief delay.

TEST-TAKING STRATEGY: Use your common sense to answer questions such as the one above. In questions that ask you to prioritize client care, determine the action that will be most helpful or harmful to the client to identify the client care priorities.

98. A nurse is returning to the intensive care unit from the blood bank with packed red blood cells for a stable client with low hemoglobin. A visitor in the lobby waves the nurse over to a woman sitting on a lobby couch. The woman is pregnant and states that her water has broken and she believes the baby is coming. What action by the nurse demonstrates effective priority setting?

A. The nurse should locate a wheelchair and immediately take the pregnant woman to the emergency department or to the OB department, if OB services are available at the facility. The safety of the pregnant woman and her unborn child are a higher priority than the blood for the stable ICU client.

B. The nurse should give the pregnant woman and her friend directions to the facility's OB department.

C. The nurse should continue transporting the blood to the ICU.

D. The nurse should direct the pregnant woman and her friend to the facility's information desk, then continue transporting the blood to the ICU. The ICU client's need for blood is a higher priority than the pregnant woman who was able to walk into the hospital lobby.

Answer: A. The nurse should locate a wheelchair and immediately take the pregnant woman to either the emergency department or to the OB department, if OB services are available at the facility. The safety of the pregnant woman and her unborn child are a higher priority than the blood for the stable ICU client. Once the pregnant woman approaches the nurse for assistance, the nurse is responsible for the client's safety until she is safely in the care of health care professionals who can render further assistance.

TEST-TAKING STRATEGY: Never delay treatment for a client. Choose the answer that addresses the most unstable client's immediate problem.

99. An unstable client's blood pressure is 64/30. The client has hetastarch (Hespan) 500 mL IV bolus ordered PRN for a systolic blood pressure of ≤ 100. What should be the nurse's first priority for the care of this client?

   A. The nurse should contact the client's physician first, to give an update regarding the client's low blood pressure and receive further orders.

   B. The nurse should first begin the hetastarch IV bolus to treat the client's low blood pressure and ask another staff member to place a call to the client's physician.

   C. The nurse should first read the medication information on hetastarch thoroughly, even though the client has a blood pressure of 64/30 and is unstable.

   D. The nurse should take no intervention at this time, but recheck the client's vital signs in 15 minutes to determine the trend of the blood pressure.

Answer: B. The nurse should first begin the hetastarch (Hespan) IV bolus to treat the client's blood pressure. A blood pressure of 64/30 is dangerously low, with a mean arterial pressure that is not perfusing the client's vital organs. A delay in treatment can worsen the client's condition.

TEST-TAKING STRATEGY: Choose the answer that is most life-saving or beneficial to the client. Questions asking you to prioritize nursing actions may have multiple correct answers, but in care priority questions there will be one answer option that should be performed first.

100. Nurses must have an understanding of ethical principles and professional nursing ethics to use as a guide for nursing actions. Which statements are correct regarding nursing ethics? Select all that apply.

   A. Religious beliefs and cultural values are the framework for ethical principles.

   B. Ethics are concerned with the reason for an action, not whether an action is right or wrong.

   C. Ethical principles for decision-making are based on a set of standards and do not address whether a decision is right or wrong.

   D. Ethical principles are used as general guidelines for professional conduct and direction for professional decision-making.

Answer: B, C, & D. Ethics are concerned with the reason for an action, are a framework for the professional decision-making process, and are based on a set of standards, not on whether a decision is right or wrong. Ethical principles are used as guidelines for professional conduct and direction for professional decision-making. Religious beliefs and cultural values are the framework for morals.

TEST-TAKING STRATEGY: Take your time with each question, but keep up a steady pace during the exam. Concentrate on each question in turn. Do not rush.

101. Moral distress over client care issues has recently been identified as a serious problem for health care professionals, especially for nurses. Moral distress can affect the nurse both professionally and personally. Which statements describe moral distress? Select all that apply.

   A. Moral distress can occur when a nurse is asked to care for a client in a manner contrary to the nurse's personal or professional values.

   B. Moral distress often causes feelings of perceived personal integrity compromise for the nurse.

   C. Moral distress can manifest as both emotional and physical stress for the nurse.

   D. Moral distress is an infrequent cause of nurses terminating employment on a specific unit or health care facility, and seeking employment elsewhere.

Answer: A, B, & C. Moral distress can occur when a nurse is asked to care for a client in such a way that is contrary to the nurse's personal or professional values; often causes feelings of perceived compromise of personal integrity for the nurse; and can manifest as both emotional and physical stress. Moral distress is a factor in professional environment dissatisfaction for nurses and health care personnel and is a common cause of nurses terminating employment and/or seeking employment elsewhere.

TEST-TAKING STRATEGY: Do not panic if you do not know the answer to a question. Read the question carefully, use your best judgment to select the answer you believe is correct, and then move on. Give your full concentration to each question, and do not let your thoughts become distracted.

102. Dilemmas regarding ethical principles are common in health care. Which ethical dilemmas are commonly associated with client care in the health care setting? Select all that apply.

   A. Autonomy: the freedom to make choices for one's self without interference from others.

   B. Moral distress: the health care professional knows the ethically correct action to take, but is either legally or professionally prohibited from acting on that knowledge.

   C. Beneficence: the concept of doing good and preventing harm to clients.

   D. Fidelity: the concept of faithfulness and promise-keeping to clients, including client confidentiality.

   Answer: A, C, & D. The ethical principles commonly associated with health care/client care issues are *autonomy, beneficence, nonmaleficence, veracity, fidelity,* and *justice.* Moral distress is not an ethical principle, but a moral-ethical dilemma.

   TEST-TAKING STRATEGY: Read each answer option carefully with the stem question. Identify the answer or answers that do not match the others in content or context. "Select all that apply" indicates that there may be one or more than one correct answers.

103. In the health care setting, the ethical principle of "justice" refers to which aspect of client care?

   A. Each client's right to access to their own medical records and health information.

   B. Each client's constitutional right to health care.

   C. The most appropriate allocation of scarce health care resources.

   D. The right to equal health care, regardless of the client's condition.

   Answer: C. The ethical principle of "justice," in the health care setting, refers to the appropriate allocation of scarce health care resources with regard to client care. The client's right to access their own health information and medical records is guaranteed under HIPAA, the Health Insurance Portability and Accountability Act of 1996. The constitution does not guarantee the client the right to receive health care but guarantees that *access* to health care be provided to all persons.

   TEST-TAKING STRATEGY: Read the question carefully to determine what the question is asking. Try to decide what you believe the correct answer is before reading the answer options, and then choose the answer option that is closest to your own. Do not change your answers without undisputed proof that the original answer was incorrect.

104. The ethical principles most commonly associated with health care and client care decisions are autonomy, beneficence, nonmaleficence, veracity, fidelity, and justice. Informed consent for invasive procedures involves which of these ethical principles?

   A. Autonomy, beneficence, nonmaleficence, veracity, and fidelity.

   B. Autonomy, beneficence, veracity, fidelity, and justice.

   C. Beneficence, nonmaleficence, veracity, fidelity, and justice.

   D. Autonomy and nonmaleficence only.

   Answer: A. Informed consent for invasive procedures involves the ethical principles of autonomy, beneficence, nonmaleficence, veracity, and fidelity. Justice, as an ethical principle, relates to the ethically appropriate allocation of scarce health care resources and generally does not factor into the informed consent process.

TEST-TAKING STRATEGY: You may find that the question does not offer a distinct correct answer. Use your best judgment and select the most correct answer, using what you know about the subject. If you discover a topic or area that you need to refresh your memory on, do so now and correct the knowledge deficit prior to the exam. Practice exams allow you to identify areas that require additional study.

105. What must be obtained from the client or the client's designated surrogate for heath care decisions prior to an invasive procedure?

    A. A Living Will.

    B. A Durable Power of Attorney for Health Care.

    C. Informed consent.

    D. A 12-lead EKG.

    Answer: C. Informed consent must be obtained either from the client or from the client's designated surrogate for health care decisions prior to an invasive procedure. A Living Will is a legal document outlining a client's wishes for treatment and resuscitation. A Durable Power of Attorney for Health Care is a legal document executed by a competent person designating another to make health and treatment-related decisions in the event the client is unable to make informed decisions. A 12-lead EKG is often ordered prior to an invasive procedure, as part of the preoperative workup, but is not a requirement prior to an invasive procedure.

    TEST-TAKING STRATEGY: Decide what you think the answer should be, and then read all answer options carefully and select the option that is closest to what you decided.

106. What is the definition of informed consent? Choose the best answer.

    A. Informed consent is obtained by the client reading the surgical/invasive procedure consent form.

    B. Informed consent is voluntary consent to an invasive procedure given by the client after careful consideration of all information related to the procedure and the client's condition.

    C. Informed consent can be given by a client who is sedated or mentally not competent to make decisions.

    D. Informed consent must be given by a client prior to an invasive procedure for a life-threatening condition requiring emergent treatment.

    Answer: B. Informed consent is voluntarily obtained from a client prior to an invasive procedure after the risks and benefits of the procedure have been explained and the client has been able to give careful consideration of all the information presented. Informed consent does not have to be obtained prior to invasive procedures for life-threatening conditions or situations requiring emergent treatment.

    TEST-TAKING STRATEGY: Read each answer option with the stem question. Use common sense and good judgment to rule out the incorrect answer options, then choose the correct answer from the probable options left.

107. Implied consent differs from informed consent for an invasive procedure. Which scenario describes implied consent?

    A. The nurse enters a client's room with the consent form for an invasive procedure. The client reads and signs the consent form but does not engage in conversation with the nurse.

    B. A fully alert and oriented patient is intubated and unable to speak, but nods, gestures, and writes notes to communicate. The client reads and signs the consent for a tracheotomy after the physician explains the risks and benefits of the procedure to the client with the family present.

    C. A paraplegic client listens carefully to the physician's explanation of a proposed invasive procedure, the risks and benefits, and then gives consent verbally. The physician and nurse both document this and co-sign the consent form as witnesses.

    D. A client arrives at the emergency department severely short of breath, then collapses unconscious on the floor. The ED staff provides emergent treatment to the client for resuscitation and airway protection. The client's consent to treatment was implied by the client voluntarily coming to the ED for treatment, even though the client is currently unconscious and unable to give informed consent.

Answer: D. The client with severe shortness of breath came voluntarily to the emergency department. The implication is that the client desired treatment for the condition, or would not have traveled to the ED and presented for treatment prior to collapsing. The other answer options are examples of legally obtained informed consent.

TEST-TAKING STRATEGY: Read each question carefully to determine what information the question attempting to elicit from you. Each question is designed to test an area of knowledge. Is the question seeking a negative answer or a positive answer?

108. A legally recognized informed consent must meet specific criteria. Which statements are accurate regarding informed consent? Select all that apply.

A. Informed consent must be given voluntarily by a client.

B. Informed consent can only be given by an individual legally competent to make informed health care decisions.

C. Informed consent can only be given after the risks, benefits, and reasonable alternative treatments of the proposed procedure have been explained as well as the health consequences of declining the procedure.

D. Informed consent can be obtained either from a client or from any member of a client's immediate family.

Answer: A, B, & C. Informed consent must be given voluntarily by an individual legally competent to make informed health care decisions and is obtained only after the procedure has been described, preferably by the medical professional who will be performing the procedure, along with the risks, benefits, reasonable treatment alternatives, and the consequences of

doing nothing. Informed consent can only be obtained from the client or the person designated to make health care decisions in the event that the client is incapacitated.

TEST-TAKING STRATEGY: Often the longest answer option is a correct option, but not always. Read each answer option carefully and use good judgment.

109. Physicians commonly write orders for the nurse to obtain informed consent for proposed invasive procedures. This involves the nurse often writing the procedures on the consent form, instructing the client to read the form, and witnessing the client's signature. Which statements describe the legal responsibility of the nurse obtaining an informed consent? Select all that apply.

A. By obtaining and witnessing the client's signature, the nurse is legally obligated to later testify, if requested, to any knowledge of the consent or information given regarding the proposed procedure and consent.

B. The nurse is legally responsible for the outcome of the procedure.

C. The nurse is legally obligated to explain the risks and benefits of the proposed procedure as well as reasonable treatment alternatives.

D. The nurse is legally obligated to assess the competency of the client to give informed consent, to document the concerns and action taken, and to report any concerns regarding client competence to the physician and nursing supervisor.

Answer: A & D. By obtaining informed consent from a client and witnessing the signature, the nurse becomes legally obligated to assess the client's competency to give informed consent prior to obtaining the consent. If there are concerns, the nurse is obligated to document and report those concerns to the physician ordering the consent and to the nursing supervisor. The nurse is not responsible for the outcome of the invasive procedure. The physician or medical professional who will be performing the procedure is legally responsible for explaining the risks, benefits, and therapy alternatives to the client.

TEST-TAKING STRATEGY: When answering "Select all that apply" questions, be sure and treat each answer as a true or false statement. There may be one correct answer or more.

110. What information must the nurse document when obtaining informed consent for an invasive procedure from a client? Select all that apply.

   A. The client's level of consciousness as alert and oriented.

   B. The client's stated understanding of information regarding the invasive procedure.

   C. The client's vital signs.

   D. The client's voluntary signature of the consent.

   Answer: A, B, & D. The nurse should document that the client is alert and oriented; that the client states understanding of the information regarding the proposed invasive procedure and has no further questions; and that the client consented voluntarily to the procedure. The client's vital signs are usually not a factor in obtaining an informed consent. Exceptions that would merit the documentation of client vital signs would be a low blood pressure, a high fever, a high respiratory rate, or any other assessment finding that might cast doubt on the client's ability to make an informed decision.

   TEST-TAKING STRATEGY: When selecting the answers for a "select all that apply" question. If you have difficulty identifying the incorrect answer selections, use common sense and the process of elimination to help rule out the answer option(s) that do not fit with the answers you know to be correct.

111. Informed consent must be voluntary and can be given by a client legally competent to make informed decisions only after the client has been fully informed of the proposed procedure, the risks, the benefits, and any alternative treatments, including refusal. Which scenario contains the elements of a legally appropriate informed consent?

   A. The physician writes the order to obtain informed consent for an invasive procedure from a client. The client states, "My doctor did mention that procedure to me, but I don't understand what is going to be done."

   B. A client states, "I believe that I am well-informed about my procedure. I understand the risks and the benefits, and my right to decline the procedure. May I have a clipboard to write on so that I can sign the consent?"

   C. A client diagnosed with Alzheimer's is admitted from an extended care facility. The client has lucid moments and is oriented to self, but is generally disoriented regarding place and circumstances. There is an order on the chart to obtain informed consent for placement of a central intravenous line.

   D. A 14-year-old client brought to the emergency department states, "I can sign the consent for my procedure. My parents are at work and will not be here for a while. They won't mind me signing the consent."

   Answer: B. The client states understanding of the proposed procedure as well as acceptance of the risks involved and the right to refuse treatment. The client demonstrates competence to sign the informed consent document by appropriate conversation and asking for a clipboard to write on while signing the consent, further correctly identifying the document and necessary action required. No person with dementia can legally make an informed decision for an invasive procedure, even if the client demonstrates occasional lucid thought and is oriented to self. A minor child cannot legally consent to an invasive procedure unless the child is an emancipated minor.

   TEST-TAKING STRATEGY: If you must guess, do so with good logic and common sense. Look for cues in the answer options to identify the obviously incorrect answers, such as the 14-year-old client and the client with Alzheimer's dementia.

112. Just as clients have a "Patient's Bill of Rights," nurses have legal responsibilities toward clients under their care. A nurse's legal responsibilities to clients include, but are not limited to (select all that apply):

A. Protection and promotion of client health, autonomy, and abilities.

B. Prevention of injury and alleviation of suffering.

C. Advocacy for clients, families, and population groups unable to adequately advocate for themselves.

D. Diagnosis of client conditions in a timely manner.

Answer: A, B, & C. A nurse's legal responsibilities toward clients include, but are not limited to, protecting and promoting client health, autonomy, and abilities; preventing injury and alleviating suffering; and advocating for clients, families, and population groups unable to adequately advocate for themselves. Nurses choosing to diagnose client conditions are generally practicing outside the nursing scope of practice and can face legal action for client issues arising from the failure to diagnose.

TEST-TAKING STRATEGY: When answering "Select all that apply" questions, be sure and treat each answer as a true or false statement. There may be one correct answer or more.

113. Nursing negligence issues arise from failures of the nurse to follow the nursing process with regard to client care. Negligence can be due to assessment failures, planning failures, implementation failures, and/or evaluation failures. Which assessment failures can lead to negligence issues and potential client harm? Select all that apply.

A. Failure to assess and analyze the level of care required by the client.

B. Failure to assess the client's wishes with regard to treatment and self-determination.

C. Failure to assess client condition in a timely manner.

D. Failure to implement client care interventions in a timely manner.

Answer: A, B, & C. Assessment failures that constitute nursing negligence or breach of duty include, but are not limited to, failure to assess and analyze the level of care required by the client; failure to assess the client's wishes with regard to treatment and self-determination; and failure to assess client condition in a timely manner. Failure to implement client interventions in a timely manner is an implementation failure.

TEST-TAKING STRATEGY: Read each answer option carefully for cues to help identify incorrect answers. "Select all that apply" indicates that there may be one or more than one correct answers.

114. When a nurse accepts a client assignment, the nurse also accepts a legal duty to provide care to the client that is consistent with the standard of care. A nurse who abandons a client assignment without first procuring comparable and appropriate care for the client during the period of the nurse's absence is guilty of (choose the best answer):

A. Duty.

B. Breach of duty.

C. Damages.

D. Causation.

Answer: B. The nurse establishes a nurse–client relationship when the nurse accepts a client care assignment. Within this relationship, the nurse accepts the duty to provide care for the client within the established standards of practice. If the nurse can no longer care for the client, the nurse is responsible to provide continuity of care by procuring comparable and appropriate care before relinquishing responsibility for the client. Failure to do so is a breach of duty by client abandonment, and the nurse is liable for this action.

TEST-TAKING STRATEGY: Over-learn material prior to the exam. Use the practice questions and practice exams to identify subjects or areas that require additional study. Discovering that you require additional study is alright. Read the material again and correct the knowledge deficit.

115. Nurses are responsible for assessing the client and implementing nursing interventions in a timely manner after accepting the duty of the client care assignment. Which of these examples of breach of duty describe nursing care implementation failures? Select all that apply.

A. Failure to communicate assessment findings in a timely manner.

B. Failure to appropriately diagnose.

C. Failure to document.

D. Failure to take appropriate action.

Answer: A, C, & D. Failure to communicate assessment findings in a timely manner, failure to document, and failure to take appropriate action are all nursing negligence client care implementation failures. Failure to diagnose is a planning failure of the nursing process. Diagnosis of specific client conditions is a physician responsibility, and nurses choosing to diagnose are generally practicing outside the scope of nursing.

TEST-TAKING STRATEGY: Do not change your answers once you have selected them. If you find, in a later question, irrefutable proof or information that an answer was incorrect, changing the first answer is acceptable. Usually your first impression is the correct one. Historically, changed answers are often incorrect.

116. The nurse establishes a nurse–client relationship and a duty to the client upon accepting the client care assignment. What is the correct definition of "breach of duty?"

A. The relationship established between the nurse and the client when the nurse accepts the client care assignment.

B. The failure to act and provide client care consistent with the applicable standards of care.

C. The damages or alleged damages to the client that arise from the nurse's failure to treat the client within the applicable standards of care.

D. The relationship between the alleged damages and the breach of duty.

Answer: B. A breach of duty is the failure to act and provide client care consistent with the

applicable standards of care. For nursing negligence to occur, the nurse's breach of duty or departure from standards of care must have caused the damages for which the client is seeking compensation. Damages are the client issues that arise from the breach of duty/departure from standard of care. The alleged relationship between the damages and the breach of duty is called "causation."

TEST-TAKING STRATEGY: Use cues in the question and answer options to help identify the obviously incorrect answers.

117. A client admitted with a drug-resistant bacterial infection has been placed on contact precautions. The "Contact Precautions" sign is posted on the door to the client's hospital room and personal protective equipment is available and in plain sight outside the room. The nurse observes the client's physician preparing to enter the room without using any of the personal protective equipment provided. What performance improvement action should the nurse take to ensure the physician's safety, the patient's safety, and the safety of other clients who the physician will examine that day?

A. No action is necessary. The client's physician is a medical professional and it is the physician's responsibility to use appropriate contact precautions.

B. The nurse should say, "Doctor, are you aware that this client is on contact precautions? You are not going to enter that room without personal protective equipment, are you?"

C. Tactfully and in a professional manner, inform the physician that the client has been placed on contact precautions. Emphasize the personal protective equipment provided and explain that it is for the client's safety and the safety of other clients that the physician will examine that day.

D. No action is necessary. The physician might be offended if the nurse points out the contact precautions and personal protective equipment.

Answer: C. Client safety is the responsibility of all health care personnel. The nurse, as client advocate, should tactfully and professionally communicate the necessity of contact precautions to any person or health care personnel coming into contact with the client. By reinforcing the importance of contact precautions the nurse will actively participate in providing a safe environment for the care of all clients, and engage in proactive performance improvement for client care.

TEST-TAKING STRATEGY: Use the process of elimination to rule out incorrect answer selections to help choose the correct answer.

118. Health care facilities must have systems in place to ensure that clients receive quality care and services. Two methods of evaluating quality of care are quality assurance and performance improvement. Which statements accurately describe quality assurance? Select all that apply.

    A. Quality assurance is the method of evaluating the safety and efficiency of client care that has previously been given.

    B. Quality assurance focuses on errors and mistakes in client care that has already been delivered.

    C. Quality assurance monitors client care outcomes by comparing delivered care with standards of practice.

    D. Quality assurance utilizes information from both clients who are currently receiving care and clients already discharged from the facility.

Answer: A & B. Quality assurance is the method of evaluating the safety and efficiency of client care that has been previously given. Quality assurance also focuses on errors and mistakes in client care previously delivered. Performance improvement is the process that monitors client outcomes by comparing delivered care with the standards of care.

TEST-TAKING STRATEGY: If you do not know the answer to a question, do not panic. Read the question and answer options again for any cues that you might have missed. Use common sense and your best judgment in selecting the answer(s). "Select all that apply" indicates that you there may be one or more than one correct answers.

119. Quality assurance or quality control is the traditional method of evaluating the safety and efficiency of client care and services that have been previously rendered. A retrospective-only look at client care has drawbacks. Which statements describe the limitations of the quality-assurance system of evaluating client care? Select all that apply.

    A. Quality assurance is a comprehensive system of client care analysis that evaluates care delivered to clients both currently receiving care and clients who have been discharged from the facility.

    B. Quality assurance focuses on clinical errors.

    C. Quality assurance is a retrospective look at care that has been delivered in the past.

    D. Quality assurance is the periodic review of client care that has been previously given and is not a continuous process.

Answer: B, C, & D. Quality assurance is of limited benefit to clients currently receiving treatment and services because it is retrospective, focuses on clinical errors, and is periodic and not a continuously ongoing process. A comprehensive system of client care analysis that evaluates care for both currently admitted and previously discharged clients is a description of performance improvement.

TEST-TAKING STRATEGY: Read the question twice if necessary to understand what the question is asking. Read each answer option carefully. Answer options may be similarly worded at the beginning.

120. Total Quality Management is a comprehensive system of ongoing client care analysis and is beneficial to clients who are currently receiving treatment. The system monitors client care issues as they develop. Which phrases best describe the principles of Total Quality Management? Select all that apply.

A. Emphasizes error prevention rather than focusing on previous client care errors.

B. Evaluates and measures continuously to improve client care.

C. Emphasizes service excellence in the quality of care and services delivered to clients.

D. Evaluates quality and safety of care after care has already been delivered and outcomes have been documented.

Answer: A, B, & C. Total Quality Management is an approach to client care evaluation that is more beneficial to clients currently admitted, or receiving care, because it emphasizes error prevention, is a continuous process of evaluation and measurement, and emphasizes service excellence in the quality of care and services delivered to clients. Quality Assurance/Quality Control is the system of client care evaluation that evaluates the quality and safety of client care retrospectively.

TEST-TAKING STRATEGY: Do not rush your answer selections, but it is important to keep a steady pace while taking the exam. If you do not know the answer to a question, use your common sense and best judgment to select an answer and move on. Focus your full attention on each question in turn.

121. Performance Improvement is a system used by health care facilities to evaluate client care and client care outcomes. Which statements best describe Performance Improvement? Select all that apply.

A. Performance Improvement is of limited benefit to clients currently admitted or receiving treatment because it focuses on care delivered in the past.

B. Performance Improvement monitors client care outcomes by comparing care to established standards of care.

C. Performance Improvement is an ongoing process that evaluates care for clients currently receiving treatment and clients that have received care in the past.

D. Performance Improvement is the formal process of identifying potentially unsafe client care practices and implementing new organizational policies and procedures to ensure safe client care delivery.

Answer: B & C. Performance Improvement monitors client care outcomes by comparing care to established standards of care and is an ongoing process that evaluates both current and previously delivered client care. Quality Assurance/Quality Control is the client care evaluation system that focuses on care delivered in the past. The formal process of identifying unsafe client care practices and implementing new organizational policies and procedures to ensure safe client care is Risk Management.

TEST-TAKING STRATEGY: Use more than one study source for review. The style or organization of information presented may differ from book to book, and the information may be presented in a way that you personally connect with in different sources and on different topics.

122. Performance Improvement is a system used by health care facilities and providers to evaluate client care and client care outcomes. Methods of Performance Improvement include (select all that apply):

A. Staff observations.

B. Error prevention.

C. Peer review and client care audits.

D. National benchmarking for standards of practice.

Answer: A, B, & D. Methods for Performance Improvement of client care for health care facilities include, but are not limited to, staff observations, peer review and client care audits, and national benchmarking for standards of practice. The system that emphasizes client care error prevention is Total Quality Management.

TEST-TAKING STRATEGY: Use the process of elimination to help identify the incorrect answer options. Look for the answer or answers that do not match the others in content and information. "Select all that apply" indicates that there may be one or more than one correct answers.

123. The Performance Improvement process focuses on the nursing process and the effect of the nursing process on client care outcomes. Which statement best describes the Performance Improvement system of client care evaluation?

    A. Performance Improvement focuses on error prevention by identifying the risk of error in delivery of client care.

    B. Performance Improvement has limited benefit to clients who are currently admitted or are receiving care because it looks at care retrospectively focusing on clinical errors that have occurred in the past.

    C. Performance Improvement recognizes the nursing process as a scientifically based process by which nurses deliver client care and focuses on the effects of the nursing process on client care and client outcomes.

    D. Performance Improvement defines nursing standards of practice.

    Answer: C. Performance Improvement recognizes the nursing process as a scientifically based process by which nurses deliver client care and focuses on the effects of the nursing process on client care and client outcomes. The focus on error prevention is a description of Total Quality Management. Limited benefit to clients currently admitted or receiving treatment is a description of Quality Assurance/Quality Control. State and federal nursing boards and regulatory agencies define the standards of care.

    TEST-TAKING STRATEGY: The longest answer option is not always the correct answer.

124. Consultation and referral are two methods of obtaining additional or specialized care for clients by members of the multidisciplinary health care team. Which statements describe referral? Select all that apply.

    A. Referral is the practice of sending a client to another practitioner, specialty service, or member of the multidisciplinary health care team for consultation.

    B. Referral involves delegation of responsibility of client care to another member of the multidisciplinary health care team.

    C. The health care professional who refers a client for additional care or service is responsible for follow-up with the client to ensure that the information or service met the client's needs.

    D. Referrals can only be done by physicians in the health care setting.

    Answer: A, B, & C. Referral is the practice of sending a client to another health care practitioner, specialty service, or member of the multidisciplinary team for consultation. Referral involves delegation of responsibility for client care, and the health care professional requesting the referral is responsible for follow-up to ensure that the client's needs were met. Referrals can be requested by any qualified member of the multidisciplinary health care team.

    TEST-TAKING STRATEGY: When answering "Select all that apply" questions, be sure and treat each answer as a true or false statement. There may be one correct answer or more.

125. A surgical client's primary care physician has written orders to arrange for the client's discharge to home the next day. The client's daughter approaches the case manager regarding the discharge. What statement by the case manager to the client's daughter demonstrates appropriate referral of the client for additional care and services?

A. "I will set up a home health care evaluation before discharge. The home health agency is wonderful at arranging for home care of clients, dressing changes, and assistance with the medication regimen. The home health case manager will contact you today, and I will follow up with you to be sure everything is arranged before discharge."

B. "I will give you a list of home health care agencies to call for additional assistance after discharge from the facility."

C. "The physical and occupational therapy teams have documented in their evaluations that your parent should be capable of self-care after discharge home from this facility. You are worrying unnecessarily."

D. "Is there any way that you can take some time off from work and help your parent out during the first week or two at home after discharge from the hospital?"

Answer: A. The case manager demonstrates appropriate referral for additional care and services for the client by informing the daughter that a call will be placed to the home health care agency and then followed up to be sure that the client's needs were met. Simply giving the client's daughter a list of home health care agencies is not an act of referral and does not demonstrate any responsibility for the client's welfare after discharge or follow-up after client referral. Stating that the client's daughter is unnecessarily worried does not address the daughter's concern, offer a referral of care, or address follow-up. Suggesting that the daughter take time off from work would be only one of the options for the client's care and does not address the daughter's concern, offer a referral, or show responsibility for follow-up.

TEST-TAKING STRATEGY: Use common sense and your best judgment on questions where you are uncertain of the answer, such as dialog answers. Read each answer option carefully with the question for continuity of theme and content.

126. A client is found unconscious in a public park and is brought to the emergency department by ambulance. The client is treated for mild exposure and dehydration and regains consciousness. The client tells the nurse that "the drug rehabilitation facility threw me out because they found drug paraphernalia in my room." What action by the nurse would be most helpful to the client at this time?

A. The nurse should inform the client to be truthful about any recent drug use.

B. The nurse should place a referral to the social worker assigned to the emergency department. The Social Worker will have information and resources to assist the client with appropriate placement and shelter.

C. The nurse should place a referral to the Social Worker for a possible psychiatric evaluation. The client could be a danger to self or others.

D. The nurse should call the client's previous drug rehabilitation facility and inform them that the drug paraphernalia was not the client's and request that the client be accepted back into the facility.

Answer: B. The action by the nurse that will be most helpful at this time would be to place a referral to the Social Worker, who will have information and resources to assist the client with appropriate placement and shelter.

TEST-TAKING STRATEGY: Use Maslow's hierarchy of needs to determine the correct answer. The question instructs you to choose the "most helpful" action for the client. This indicates that there are multiple correct answer options; choose the answer that meets the client's immediate need.

127. A client in the critical care unit is unresponsive and on a mechanical ventilator. Two of the client's children insist that the client previously expressed the desire not to be placed on any life support. The sibling who is named on the client's durable power of attorney for health care refuses to consider discontinuing the mechanical ventilator. This dilemma is causing discontent among the family and an uncomfortable situation for the nurses caring for the client. Which action by the client's nurse would be most appropriate as an attempt to resolve the situation?

A. The nurse should inform the client's family that visiting will be limited until the client's children can resolve the situation and come to an agreement regarding the client's wishes and code status.

B. The nurse should contact the client's primary care physician with information regarding the behavior of the client's family and the effect on the critical care unit nursing staff caring for the client.

C. The nurse should place a referral to the Client-Family Services department. The Client-Family Services representative is trained to speak with the client's family in an attempt to resolve the issue and can coordinate a client family conference with the physicians and members of the multidisciplinary team to speak with the client's family and provide additional information.

D. The nurse should place a referral to the ethics committee regarding the family's inability to come to a decision about the client's code status.

Answer: C. If family members are disagreeing over a client's level of care and/or treatment of code status, the nurse should place a referral to the Client-Family Services representative for the facility of unit. Client-Family Services are members of the health care team trained to assist clients and families and to facilitate communication between family members.

TEST-TAKING STRATEGY: Terms like *most appropriate* and *most accurately* indicate that an undeniably correct answer option is likely not present. You must select the best answer choice.

128. Consultation and referral are two means of obtaining additional or specialized care for clients by members of the multidisciplinary health care team. Which statements accurately describe consultation and referral? Select all that apply.

A. Referral is sending a client to another health care practitioner or service for consultation or additional services. Consultation is the assessment of the client by the health care professional or service to which the client was referred.

B. Consultation is sending a client to another health care practitioner for consultation or additional services. Referral is the assessment of the client by the health care professional or service to which the client was referred.

C. A member of the multidisciplinary health care team caring for the client places a referral. The practitioner who receives the referral performs the consultation by assessing the client or the client's needs.

D. Referrals and consultations can only be initiated by the client's primary care physician.

Answer: A & C. A referral may be made by any member of the multidisciplinary team caring for the client. A consultation is an assessment of the client or client's needs performed by the health care professional or service to which the client was referred.

TEST-TAKING STRATEGY: Look for similarly worded answer options to identify incorrect answers and eliminate them.

129. A thin, malnourished elderly client is admitted from home with a diagnosis of altered mental status and dehydration. During the admission assessment, the client's spouse informs the nurse that the client's mobility has declined and home care has become increasingly difficult for the spouse as the only caregiver. What response by the nurse demonstrates appropriate use of referral to address the spouse/caregiver's concerns and meet the needs of the client?

A. "I will place a referral to the dietitian so that you can receive information on nutrition and feeding techniques for your spouse."

B. "I should place a referral to the Adult Protective Services agency to evaluate your home care situation before your spouse is discharged."

C. "I will place a referral to the physical therapist to evaluate your spouse for mobility issues."

D. "I will place referrals to the case manager, the dietitian, and client-family services for you. These members of the health care team will evaluate the level of care that your spouse requires and help you with information and resources to provide that care."

Answer: D. To address the spouse's concerns and the client's needs, the nurse informs the client's spouse that referrals will be placed to the unit's case manager, dietitian, and client-family services to provide the spouse/caregiver with additional information and resources to assist in the care of the client. Placing a referral to Adult Protective Services is unnecessary and threatening to the client's spouse, as there is no evidence of client abuse.

TEST-TAKING STRATEGY: Choose the answer option that is most helpful to the client in the client's current state of physical or mental health. Read each answer option carefully to identify for partial answers that would be incorrect. Select the answer that offers the most complete and comprehensive care for the client.

130. Resource management is the concept of:

A. Providing the highest quality of health care possible to the client regardless of the cost.

B. Providing quality client care by methods that reduce the costs of care.

C. Keeping an inventory of all items used in the care of a client during an episode of illness, as well as the cost of those items, to present as a bill to the client's insurance company.

D. Staffing a hospital unit with an absolute minimum number of licensed nurses and support personnel as possible.

Answer: B. Resource management is the concept of providing quality health care to clients by methods that reduce costs of care.

TEST-TAKING STRATEGY: The longest answer option is often the correct one, but not always. Read each answer option carefully before deciding to rule out incorrect answers. Do not develop the habit of automatically assuming that the longest answer option will be the correct one.

131. A nurse is preparing to perform the initial assessment of a client. The nurse selects the correct glove size and puts the gloves on. One of the gloves tears across the palm, so the nurse selects and puts a second glove on that hand. The second glove tears across the tip of the nurse's pointer finger. What is the most appropriate action for the nurse to take to demonstrate effective resource management?

A. The nurse should continue to select gloves from the correct-size box until an intact pair of gloves is found, and then proceed with the client's assessment. Most of the gloves in the box are likely intact and nondefective.

B. The nurse should contact the glove manufacturer by the number listed on the glove box and ask why defective protective equipment was sold to a health care facility.

C. The nurse should remove the box of gloves from the client's room, mark the box as "defective—do not use," and then report the multiple amount of defective gloves found in the box to the unit manager or supervisor for further evaluation.

D. The nurse should make an appointment with the facility's chief purchasing officer, demonstrate the defective gloves, and then inquire why defective protective equipment was purchased for health care personnel.

Answer: C. To demonstrate effective resource management, the nurse should remove the box of gloves from the client's room, mark that box as "defective," and then report and demonstrate the defective gloves to the unit manager or supervisor for further evaluation.

TEST-TAKING STRATEGY: Questions that contain terms like *most appropriate* or *most accurate* often have multiple correct answers, so you must choose the best answer.

132. A client in respiratory distress has just been intubated and placed on a mechanical ventilator. A portable chest x-ray is ordered stat to confirm endotracheal tube placement. The radiologic technician arrives with the portable x-ray machine and is preparing to take the x-ray when the nurse remembers that the client also has a nasogastric tube ordered that will also require chest x-ray confirmation. What action should be taken by the nurse to practice good resource management and give quality care to the client?

   A. The nurse should allow the radiologic technician to perform the portable chest x-ray for endotracheal tube placement. The nasogastric tube can be placed at another time and an additional chest x-ray ordered for placement.

   B. The nurse should allow the radiologic technician to perform the portable chest x-ray for endotracheal tube placement, and then stand by for another chest x-ray after the nasogastric tube has been placed. The costs of both stat portable chest x-rays will be covered by the client's insurance plan.

   C. The nurse should inform the radiologic technician that a nasogastric tube still needs to be placed and to come back at a later time to perform the stat portable chest x-ray.

   D. The nurse should inform the radiologic technician to wait briefly while a nasogastric tube is placed and then perform the stat portable chest x-ray for both endotracheal tube and

nasogastric tube placement confirmation with one chest x-ray study.

Answer: D. The nurse should request the radiologic technician to wait briefly while the nasogastric tube is placed. After placement is confirmed by auscultation, the radiologic technician can perform one chest x-ray to confirm placement of both the endotracheal and nasogastric tubes. This is good resource management practice by the nurse and will save the client unnecessary cost and radiation from a second chest x-ray.

TEST-TAKING STRATEGY: Read each question carefully to determine what the question is asking. Do not read information into a question that is not presented in the body of the question. The author of the question did not have your clients in mind while composing the question.

133. A nurse notices soiled linen in the trash receptacle instead of in the soiled linen receptacle in a client's room. The nurse first puts on gloves and then carefully separates the soiled linen from the trash and places it in the soiled linen receptacle to be cleaned by the facility's laundry. This action by the nurse is an example of which principle of client care management?

   A. Resource management.

   B. Case management.

   C. Time management.

   D. Priorities management.

Answer: A. The nurse's action of taking responsibility for the soiled linen found in the trash receptacle, even though another health care team member had placed the linen there, is an example of good resource management. Soiled linen thrown out in the trash is an additional cost to the health care facility and ultimately increases the cost of health care delivery to clients.

TEST-TAKING STRATEGY: If you do not know the answer to a question, do not panic. Read the question again carefully for cues to the correct answer option. Use common sense and your own knowledge base to identify the obviously incorrect answer options and then select from the probable answer options.

134. The practice of good resource management is essential to reducing the costs of client care and to the successful operation of health care facilities in the modern health care environment. Which members of the multidisciplinary health care team are responsible for implementing good resource management practices? Select all that apply.

A. The facility's purchasing department.

B. The facility's billing department.

C. The facility's nurses only.

D. All members of the health care team.

Answer: A, B, & D. All members of the multi-disciplinary health care team are responsible for practicing good resource management—both clinical and nonclinical support staff.

TEST-TAKING STRATEGY: Do not automatically select the longest answer option as correct. Read each answer option carefully. "Select all that apply" indicates that you may need to choose multiple correct answer options to complete the question.

135. The nurse places an overweight client on a bed-pan and notices that the plastic bedpan does not retain its shape under the client's weight. The bedpan flattens, spilling the contents into the client's bed and necessitating an additional bed bath for the client. The nurse must place three bedpans together in order for the bedpan to be used effectively by the overweight client. What action by the nurse would demonstrate good resource management practice?

A. The nurse should pass on in shift report that the bedpans currently purchased by the facility do not hold their shape under heavier clients and that multiple bedpans must be used together for the bedpans to retain their shape and be used correctly.

B. The nurse should notify the unit supervisor or manager of the problem with the bed-pans not supporting the weight of the clients and that multiple bedpans must be stacked together in order for the bedpans to be used effectively.

C. The nurse should call the facility's distribution department and report the defective or weak bedpan issue.

D. The nurse should remember to stack three bedpans together before placing them under a client to increase the strength and retain the shape of the bedpans while in use.

Answer: B. The nurse should notify the unit supervisor or manager of the problem with the weak or defective bedpans. This demonstrates good resource management practice by the nurse. Often managers and supervisors are not aware of issues with poor client care product quality unless nurses and direct client care staff inform them of the problem.

TEST-TAKING STRATEGY: Read each question carefully. Formulate what you believe the answer should be before reading the answer options, and then select the answer that is closest to what you decided was correct before viewing the answer options.

136. The practice of good resource management is the responsibility of every member of the multidisciplinary health care team. Which strategies demonstrate good resource management practices? Select all that apply.

A. Delegation of appropriate client care tasks to manage time and staff resources effectively.

B. Performing quality client care in a timely manner.

C. Charging a client for as many tests and supplies as possible to increase the client's bill for that episode of illness.

D. Notifying the supervisor or manager immediately if client care supplies or equipment are defective so that the appropriate chain of command can be followed to resolve the issue.

Answer: A, B, & D. Delegation of client care tasks maximizes time management and staff resources and allows for performance of quality client care in a timely manner. Notifying the appropriate supervisor or manager immediately of defective or poorly functioning client care supplies and equipment are examples of good resource management practices by nurses.

TEST-TAKING STRATEGY: Use common sense and the process of elimination to identify the incorrect answer options. "Select all that apply" indicates that there may be one or more than one correct answers. All four of the answer options will not be correct unless there is an "all of the above" option among the answers choices.

137. Attracting nursing staff to a facility, hiring, and orienting new nursing staff is a costly process. Implementing programs that result in retention of nursing staff is cost-effective for health care facilities. Programs that result in nursing job satisfaction and nursing staff retention are examples of which client care management principle?

A. Case management.

B. Delegation.

C. Collaboration with the multidisciplinary health care team.

D. Resource management.

Answer: D. Programs that result in increased nursing job satisfaction and nursing staff retention are examples of good resource management practices by the hospital upper-level management team. Retention of currently employed nurses is an effective method of resource management.

TEST-TAKING STRATEGY: Do not panic if you do not know the answer to a question. Use your best judgment and common sense to select an answer and then move on to the next question. Give your full attention to each question.

138. Staff education and development are important components of professional nursing development. Which statements are accurate regarding staff education and development? Select all that apply.

A. Staff education is the responsibility of the unit educator or facility's continuing education department.

B. Every nurse is responsible for continuing professional education and development.

C. Staff education is the responsibility of the manager, charge nurses, and shift supervisors.

D. Staff education and development is an ongoing process of professional learning and development that continues for the entire career of the professional nurse.

Answer: B & D. Every nurse is responsible for continuing professional education and development. Staff education and development is an ongoing process of professional learning and development that continues for the entire career of the professional nurse.

TEST-TAKING STRATEGY: Use the process of elimination to rule out incorrect answer selections. "Select all that apply" indicates that there may be one or more than one correct answers.

139. A physician is preparing to perform a chest tube placement on a client with a pneumothorax. The client's nurse informs a recently hired nurse on the unit that the chest tube placement is about to begin and gives the new-hire nurse the opportunity to observe and assist with the procedure. The client's nurse has just engaged in which form of staff education?

A. Informal staff education and development.

B. Formal staff education and development.

C. Delegation of client care.

D. Quality improvement.

Answer: A. The client's nurse has just engaged in informal staff education and development by providing an opportunity for a recently hired nurse on the unit to obtain needed experience in assisting with chest tube placement.

TEST-TAKING STRATEGY: Look for similarly worded answer options to help identify the incorrect answers. If there are two similarly worded answer options, one will be incorrect in a multiple-choice question with only one correct answer.

140. Staff education and development can be formal or informal. Which statements describe informal staff education? Select all that apply.

A. The unit manager schedules a mandatory staff meeting to inform all staff of new medication administration guidelines.

B. A nurse asks a nurse co-worker about the administration of a medication. The co-worker takes time to explain the correct way to administer the medication and then verifies the information by utilizing the medication administration book on the unit.

C. A new graduate nurse expresses interest in an unfamiliar piece of medical equipment. The nurse caring for the client demonstrates the use of the equipment to the new nurse.

D. The clinical supervisor of an outpatient clinic schedules all members of the clinic staff for a CPR renewal class.

Answer: B & C. Informal staff education and development is an informal exchange of knowledge and experience that takes place daily in a nurturing work environment. Members of the multidisciplinary health care team share knowledge and experience that elevates the overall knowledge and skill level of a unit or facility. The mandatory staff meeting and the scheduled CPR class are examples of formal staff education and development.

TEST-TAKING STRATEGY: Read each question carefully for cues and instructions to help identify the correct answer(s). For example, in this question the word "informal" is a key cue. "Select all that apply" indicates that there may be one or more than one correct answers.

141. Staff education and development is a continuous process designed to improve staff knowledge and skill levels. Which statements are correct regarding effective staff education and development? Select all that apply.

A. Active participation by learners increases learning potential.

B. Critical thinking skills become stronger with continued use and experience.

C. Relevant staff learning experiences enhance clinical experience.

D. Mild learning-related anxiety is detrimental to the learner.

Answer: A, B, & C. Key components of effective staff education and development include, but are not limited to, active participation, critical thinking, and relevant staff learning. Mild learning-related anxiety is actually beneficial to the learner and may increase learning potential.

TEST-TAKING STRATEGY: If there is no clear wrong answer, re-read the answer options carefully. The qualifier "mild learning-related anxiety" is a cue that this is an incorrect answer. "Select all that apply" indicates that there may be one or more than one correct answers.

142. A group of nurses are discussing the benefits of specialized certifications in specific areas of nursing. One of the nurses states, "I believe that the additional knowledge that I acquired by studying for my specialty certification was worth the time and money that I spent. It enhances my client care and benefits my clients every day." Several nurses in the group decide to study for their certifications based on the certified nurse's positive experience. This is an example of which type of staff education and development?

A. Formal staff education and development.

B. Mandatory staff education.

C. Informal staff education and development.

D. Compliance training.

Answer: C. This is an example of informal staff education and development by positive peer influence.

TEST-TAKING STRATEGY: Do not become discouraged or panic if you do not know the answer to a question. The exam is timed and it is important to use your best judgment to answer a question and then be able to move on and concentrate on the next question.

143. The continuous process of both formal and informal staff education benefits a unit or health care facility by increasing the knowledge and skill levels of all staff. Staff education also impacts client care. What are some of the direct benefits of staff education and development to client care? Select all that apply.

A. The overall quality of client care increases.

B. Clients are in danger while client care staff members attend education and development sessions.

C. Mutual goal setting and learning promotes a nurturing work environment and teamwork among staff members.

D. Learning increases both personal and group staff member motivation to deliver service excellence.

Answer: A, C, & D. Some of the direct benefits to client care produced by staff education and development are promotion of teamwork among staff, increased staff motivation to deliver service excellence, and an overall improvement in the quality of client care.

TEST-TAKING STRATEGY: Do not allow your mind to wander. Stay focused on the exam, and concentrate on each question in turn.

144. A nurse states to a nurse co-worker, "The education coordinator and the charge nurse keep asking me for my new CPR and ACLS cards. I suppose that they will let me know when those certifications are about to expire." What is the appropriate response by the nurse co-worker regarding the nurse's responsibility for continuing education?

A. "They have a list of when your certifications expire and they continue to remind you until you recertify and bring them the new cards as proof of recertification."

B. "You will not be allowed to work if those certifications expire."

C. "Yes, they remind all of the nurses about certifications that are due to be renewed. You would think that they had more important things to accomplish."

D. "Renewal of certifications required for employment and your nursing license are your responsibility as a nurse. You are fortunate that they care and that they reminded you that your certifications were due for renewal."

Answer: D. Renewal of all nursing certifications required for employment and renewal of your nursing license is your responsibility as a professional nurse. It is not the responsibility of the charge nurse or the education coordinator to remind you, but they often do so as a courtesy.

TEST-TAKING STRATEGY: In questions that ask you to identify an "appropriate response," look first for obviously incorrect answer options that contain incorrect information or poor examples of communication to rule out the incorrect answer options.

145. Supervision of delegated client care responsibilities, tasks, and activities is essential to the delivery of quality, cost-effective, multidisciplinary client care. What is the correct definition of supervision?

A. Supervision is the process of transferring the responsibility for the performance of selected tasks or jobs from one person to another.

B. Supervision involves direct oversight of the work or work product of others.

C. Supervision is the coordination of care between members of the multidisciplinary health care team.

D. Supervision is an informal role based on professional knowledge and influence.

Answer: B. Supervision involves direct oversight of the work or work product of others. The process of transferring responsibility for the performance of selected tasks or jobs is incorrect, because this describes delegation. The coordination of care between members of the multidisciplinary health care team is a description of case management. An informal role based on professional knowledge and influence is a description of a leadership role.

TEST-TAKING STRATEGY: If you do not know the answer to a question, re-read the question carefully for cues to the correct answer. Use common sense and your best judgment to select the correct answer option.

146. A heath care facility uses the self-scheduling method for nursing schedules and individual unit staffing. Each nurse pencils in the preferred schedule by order of seniority, then all nurses are responsible to adjust scheduled days to cover that unit's target number of licensed nurses per schedule. The assistant nurse manager approves each finalized schedule and makes minor adjustments if necessary. What concepts of staff management does the assistant nurse manager employ to achieve completion of the nursing schedule?

   A. Delegation and supervision.

   B. Supervision and leadership.

   C. Management and leadership.

   D. Delegation and leadership.

   Answer: **A.** Delegation and supervision are the concepts of staff management used in completion of each nursing schedule. The responsibility for adjusting the preliminary schedule is *delegated* to each nurse. The assistant nurse manager *supervises* the process.

   TEST-TAKING STRATEGY: Focus on key words in the question stem to help select the correct answer.

147. Delegation and supervision are both used by nurses to manage time effectively and to deliver quality client care in a timely manner. Which statements are accurate regarding delegation and supervision? Select all that apply.

   A. Supervision of delegated client care is an essential part of appropriate delegation.

   B. Appropriate delegation of client care is part of a supervisor's responsibility.

   C. Delegation and supervision are the same thing.

   D. Accountability for delegated tasks and appropriate supervision of those tasks remains with the person who delegated the activity.

Answer: A, B, & D. Supervision of any delegated care or activity is an essential part of appropriate delegation. Appropriate delegation of client care is part of a supervisor's responsibility. Accountability for delegated tasks remains with the person who delegated the activity, as does the responsibility to adequately supervise the delegated activity.

TEST-TAKING STRATEGY: When answering "Select all that apply" questions, be sure and treat each answer as a true or false statement. There may be one correct answer or more.

148. Supervision is an important aspect of nursing staff development and staff skill level development. What are some of the components of appropriate staff supervision? Select all that apply.

   A. Delegation of client care to qualified staff with the appropriate skill levels.

   B. Direct evaluation of staff performance.

   C. Knowledge of each staff member's skill level and capabilities.

   D. Direct performance of all client-related care without delegation.

   Answer: A, B, & C. Supervision is an important aspect of nursing staff development and staff skill development. Appropriate staff supervision includes, but is not limited to, knowledge of each staff member's skill level and capabilities, delegation of client care to qualified staff members with the appropriate skill levels, and direct evaluation of staff work performance.

   TEST-TAKING STRATEGY: Read each question thoroughly, determine what you believe the answer will be before reading the answer options, select the answer that is closest to your own answer, then move on to the next question. Usually your first impression is the correct one. Do not change answers without conclusive proof that your original answer choice was incorrect.

149. An unstable, critically ill client in the intensive care unit has been assigned to a new nurse who has just completed the unit orientation and preceptorship programs. What is the role of the

unit charge nurse regarding supervision of the new nurse and the client's safety?

A. The unit charge nurse should observe the new nurse for care organization skills, prioritizing of care, nursing judgment, and critical thinking, but should not intervene. Client safety is the responsibility of the new nurse caring for the client.

B. The unit charge nurse should assume care of the client if the new nurse becomes overwhelmed. The client's safety is ultimately the responsibility of the charge nurse who delegated the client care assignments.

C. The unit charge nurse should carefully observe the new nurse for client care organization, prioritizing, nursing judgment, and critical thinking skills. The charge nurse should offer advice and assistance when necessary. The client's safety is ultimately the responsibility of the charge nurse who delegated the client care assignments.

D. The unit charge nurse should trust the judgment, critical thinking, and skill level of the new nurse and evaluate the nurse's client care at the end of the shift.

Answer: C. The unit charge nurse should carefully observe the new nurse for organization, prioritizing, nursing judgment, and critical thinking skills and should observe for any signs that the nurse is becoming overwhelmed. The client's safety is ultimately the responsibility of the supervising unit charge nurse who delegated the client care assignments. Offering advice and assistance when necessary will help to build the confidence and skill level of the new nurse.

TEST-TAKING STRATEGY: Often the longest answer option will be the correct answer, but not always. Read each answer option carefully and do not jump to the conclusion that the longest answer is correct.

150. Supervision is an essential component of the appropriate delegation of client care. Which example demonstrates inappropriate supervision?

A. The unit charge nurse evaluates each client's acuity level and then makes client care assignments based on the nurses' individual skill and competency levels.

B. A nurse has enrolled in a post-open heart surgery patient recovery course. The nurse is precepted by an experienced nurse on care and recovery of five post-open heart surgery clients for completion of the clinical portion of the course.

C. A registered nurse is newly assigned to a telemetry unit. The registered nurse is precepted for the first shift and oriented to the unit including policies, procedures, and safety equipment.

D. A student nurse in the final semester of nursing school is allowed to give intravenous medications unsupervised by either the nursing instructor or the nurse responsible for the client assignment.

Answer: D. The student nurse should be supervised during the delivery of all intravenous medications. This is an example of inappropriate supervision by both the nursing instructor and the nurse responsible for the client assignment.

TEST-TAKING STRATEGY: Read the instructions at the end of each question carefully to determine if the question is asking for a negative or a positive answer.

151. A nurse with less than 1 year of experience complains to an experienced nurse, "The charge nurses are always checking up on me and evaluating my client care. I feel as if the charge nurses do not trust me to give good care to my clients." Which response by the experienced nurse demonstrates an understanding of appropriate staff supervision?

A. "The charge nurses are accountable for supervising client care and client safety after delegating the client care assignments. The management staff may believe that they are being supportive by being available to you for help or advice."

B. "The charge nurses do that to everyone. It can be annoying sometimes, but I believe that they mean well."

C. "Why don't you speak to the charge nurses about your perception of not being trusted to care for your clients? This is probably not their intention."

D. "You are a new nurse, and the charge nurses know that you do not have the experience and knowledge base yet to handle some of your assignments."

Answer: A. The experienced nurse demonstrates an understanding of appropriate staff supervision by answering that the charge nurses are accountable for supervising client care and safety after they have made client care assignments and by clarifying that the charge nurses are probably attempting to be supportive of the new graduate nurse.

TEST-TAKING STRATEGY: Answers that would promote a hostile work environment or demonstrate poor communication skills will usually be incorrect.

152. Information technology and the computerization of health information bring additional confidentiality challenges to the multidisciplinary team. Which members of the health care multidisciplinary team are involved in ensuring the confidentiality of computerized health information data? Select all that apply.

A. Direct client care personnel accessing computerized client information on a need-to-know basis.

B. The client's physician accessing computerized client information stored in the health care facility's system from home for necessary client care.

C. The unit environmental services tech who finds a printed piece of client information on the floor.

D. The health care facility's information technology support team responsible for the integrity of the computer information system and client health information data entry when necessary.

Answer: A, B, & D. Information technology and computerized client health information bring new challenges for ensuring the confidentiality of health information. All health care organization personnel involved in both direct and indirect client care are responsible for the confidentiality of health information. The printed client health information, found by the environmental services tech, is not an example of computerized health information data.

TEST-TAKING STRATEGY: Read each answer selection carefully. Read each answer option twice if necessary to understand the meaning and content of each option.

153. Advances in information technology and computerized health information make ensuring the confidentiality of client information more of a challenge than ever. What actions can the nurse can take to ensure the confidentiality of computerized health information? Select all that apply.

A. Close out all monitor screens displaying client health information before leaving the computer work station.

B. Log off the health care facility's computerized client information system before leaving a computer work station.

C. Never share your password with anyone or allow anyone to log onto the health care facility's computer system with your password.

D. It is not important to log off the health care facility's computer system—the system will automatically log you off within a set time if left inactive.

Answer: A, B, & C.   It is important to close out all computer monitor screens displaying client health information and to log off the facility's computer system before leaving a computer work station. Never share your password with anyone as this should also be kept confidential. Never allow anyone to log onto the facility's computer system using your password.

TEST-TAKING STRATEGY: Read all of the answer options before you select one as the correct option. Do not make an answer selection before reading all answer options carefully.

154. A hospital co-worker states, "I can't remember my password for the computerized patient information system. May I please log on with your password to get some information that I need to care for one of my clients?" Which response to this request would be most appropriate and in compliance with confidentiality of computerized client health information?

   A. "You may log on using my password just this one time, but you need to call the information technology department and have them reset your password for you."

   B. "I am uncomfortable with someone using my password to access computerized client health information. I will log in for you and then you can access the information that you need. Look the other way while I log in."

   C. "I will log in and access the information for you. Which client are we talking about?"

   D. "I am uncomfortable with you using my password to access computerized client health information as this is a violation of client confidentiality. You will need to call the information technology department so that they can reset your computer access password for you."

Answer: D.   It is a violation of client confidentiality to allow another individual to use your personal computer access password to log into the health care facility's computer system. It is

also a violation of client confidentiality, as well as a federal HIPPA violation, to retrieve client information for another individual. Client health information is accessed on a need-to-know basis only.

TEST-TAKING STRATEGY: Information technology and the client privacy issues involved are relatively new issues in health care. Always select the answer that ensures the client's privacy and the confidentiality of health information. Use your common sense if you do not know the answer.

155. A physician has been looking up his client's morning laboratory test results. The nurse notices that the physician has walked away from the computer work station without logging out of the system, leaving a page of client medical information visible on the computer screen. Which action by the nurse is most appropriate to protect the confidentiality of the client's computerized health information?

   A. The nurse should immediately log the physician off the facility's health information system.

   B. The nurse should immediately shrink or hide the screen so that the client information is no longer visible, and then ask the physician if they will be returning to the computer work station. If not, suggest that the physician log off the health information system.

   C. The nurse should do nothing. The physician is a member of the health care team and is responsible for information accessed on the hospital's health information system and any consequences that come from a breach in health information confidentiality.

   D. The nurse should read the health information that the physician left visible on the computer screen to attempt to determine if the physician was finished accessing the system.

Answer: B. If you notice that another health care team member has walked away from a computer work station without logging out, or has left client health information visible on an unattended computer screen, it is appropriate and polite to initially minimize or shrink the screen so that the information is no longer visible and then inquire whether the user will be returning to the computer work station or not. Professionally remind them that they did not log out and left client health information visible to unauthorized persons. Simply logging the other person off the computer system could be a correct option if that person cannot be found, but it is professional and in the spirit of teamwork to attempt to discern if they will be returning to the computer shortly.

TEST-TAKING STRATEGY: You may find that the question does not offer a distinct clear answer, or that there are two possible correct answers. In this case, choose the most correct answer or the most complete correct answer.

156. A friend contacts a nurse at work and states, "Our friend, _____, has just been in a car accident and is in your emergency room. I am so worried. Can you check your hospital computer system and tell me the extent of the injuries?" What is the most appropriate response by the nurse to the concerned friend?

A. "I did not know about the accident, but I can't look that information up for you. Every client's health information is confidential and is protected by law. Unless I am caring for that person, I have no right to access their health information. I recommend that you contact the family for information."

B. "I will look the information up, but do not tell anyone that I did. Health information is confidential and is protected by law."

C. "OK, let me see here—the CAT scan looks terrible! You had better come to the emergency department as fast as you can!"

D. "I can't look that up for you. I will get into trouble. Call the emergency department and see if they will give you any information."

Answer: A. The nurse should inform the concerned friend that the client/friend's health information is confidential, protected by law, and cannot be accessed by the nurse without a treatment necessity or relayed to others without the client's consent. This appears harsh to concerned friends and family members calling to inquire about a loved one, but the HIPAA regulations for the confidentiality of health information were enacted to ensure the privacy of all health information. Medical personnel must be kind but firm while explaining and enforcing these regulations.

TEST-TAKING STRATEGY: Determine which response by the nurse will honor the confidential nature of client health information. This will guide you to the correct response.

157. A nurse has laboratory and radiology studies performed by the primary care physician's order at the health care facility where the nurse is employed. Curious about the test results, the nurse accesses the hospital's health information system and prints the lab and radiology studies. Are the actions taken by the nurse HIPAA violations? Select all that apply.

A. No. This does not violate HIPAA health information privacy regulations because the test result information belonged to the nurse personally.

B. No. This is not a HIPAA violation because the tests were performed on the nurse's own blood and the nurse's own body.

C. Yes. This is a HIPAA violation because the health information is the property of the health care facility until the nurse is either given the test results by the ordering physician or requests the test result information through the appropriate channels.

D. Yes. This is a HIPAA violation because the nurse is not accessing the information for client treatment or client necessity.

Answer: C & D. The nurse accessing the health care facility's client information system to discover the results of tests performed on their person is technically a HIPAA violation because the information is not being accessed on a need-to-know basis and is not being accessed for client necessity or treatment purposes. The study results are the confidential property of the health care facility until they are given to the nurse by the ordering physician, just as results would be given to any other client. The nurse can also have access to the test results by requesting them through the appropriate channels established by the facility.

TEST-TAKING STRATEGY: Do not become discouraged if you do not know the answer to a question. That is exactly why you are using sample exam questions as part of your study plan—to identify the areas that you need to clarify or learn before taking the exam. There is nothing wrong with not knowing an answer. Make a list of information that requires further study and correct your knowledge deficit.

158. Health care facilities store a large portion of their clients' health information on the facility's health information system. Each health care team member with a need to access health information is given a password or log-in code. How closely is access to a facility's health information system monitored?

A. Access is not monitored. After receiving a log in code and password, each employee accesses health information on the honor system.

B. Access is monitored intermittently.

C. Access of the health information system is monitored closely and constantly for inappropriate use of the system and health information stored on the system. There is a record of every log in, date, time, and the information accessed.

D. Access is monitored only during business office hours when the system usage is the highest.

Answer: C. Access to a health care facility's computerized health information system is monitored closely and constantly. Records of each health care team member's time and date of access, as well as the information that was accessed, are kept by the information technology services department. Access can be suspended, restricted, or revoked for unauthorized or inappropriate use of the health information system.

TEST-TAKING STRATEGY: Use information and cues from the question to identify obviously incorrect answer options. Read each question and answer thoroughly to ensure that you understood the context and what the question was asking.

159. How should computer monitors that display accessed client health information be positioned to ensure that no visitors to a health care facility or unauthorized persons will be able to view information stored on the facility's health information system?

A. Monitors should be positioned facing the client rooms so that health care personnel can access the information easily.

B. Monitors should face away from any visitor area or client care area where information displayed could possibly be viewed by unauthorized persons.

C. Monitors should be turned off unless in use.

D. Monitors should be positioned for quick access. Visitors and unauthorized personnel are responsible not to view information not intended for their knowledge.

Answer: B. Computer monitors that display accessed client health information should be positioned away from the view of any visitors or unauthorized persons. Even the best-guarded computer monitor with an authorized employee sitting in front of it could be a potential breach of confidentiality depending on the angle of the monitor screen and who was attempting to view the information on it. The responsibility for keeping health information safe is the responsibility of every member of the health care team.

TEST-TAKING STRATEGY: Use logic and common sense to select the correct answer in questions such as above if you do not know the answer.

160. The ability to navigate a computerized health information system is a daily necessity for nurses in the modern health care environment. Health care facilities are transitioning to a paperless, computerized documentation and health information system. What are the advantages of a computerized documentation and health information system? Select all that apply.

A. Enhanced security of health information by requiring each health care provider to use an individualized log-in code to access the system.

B. Increased access to client health information and medical records enabling authorized personnel to access portions of the same records from multiple computer terminals.

C. Increased client safety issues through decreasing or eliminating illegible penmanship on physician orders and all areas of documentation.

D. The ability to track and apprehend all unauthorized personnel who access health information without a direct need to know for client care purposes.

Answer: A, B, & C. Computerized health information systems offer advantages in the modern health care environment. A computerized health information and documentation system offers enhanced security through the use of individualized log-in codes for each member of the health care team. In theory, this system is more secure than a paper medical record left out on a desk for anyone to read. Computerized health information systems offer increased access to a client's health information by multiple members of the health care team. A paper medical record can only be accessed by one person at a time, but a computerized medical record may be accessed by multiple authorized personnel for multiple purposes at any time. A computerized medical record, health information, and documentation system reduces or eliminates the client safety issues that stem from illegible penmanship in physician orders and in documentation. Unauthorized users are typically not arrested by hospital security or the police. An investigation would occur and the employee would be given a chance to explain the access of the health information.

TEST-TAKING STRATEGY: Incorrect answer options often contain clues, such as absolutes like "always" or "never." "Select all that apply" indicates that there may be one or more than one correct answers.

161. The nurse is educating an older client who is status post-right total hip replacement on techniques to help prevent falls. The nurse knows that older adults can prevent falls by (select all that apply):

A. Exercising regularly.

B. Using sedatives to promote sleep.

C. Placing a grab bar in the tub.

D. Keeping the lights dim.

Answer: A & C. Exercising regularly will strengthen an older adult's bones, which can prevent falls. Sedatives should not be used because they can increase the risk of falls in older clients. Placing a grab bar in a slippery tub can assist the older adult in getting into and out of the tub. Keeping the lights bright ensures that the older adult can navigate safely, thus reducing the risk of falls.

TEST-TAKING STRATEGY: Use the process of elimination to rule out incorrect answer selections to help choose the correct answer.

162. The nurse working in a pediatrician's office teaches an adult client with three children that utilizing a booster seat in a vehicle is recommended for children of which age group?

A. 1 to 3 years of age.

B. 2 to 4 years of age.

C. 4 to 7 years of age.

D. 5 to 9 years of age.

Answer: C. According to the Center for Disease Control and Prevention (CDC), using a booster seat for children 4 to 7 years of age reduces injury risk by 59% compared to using safety belts alone.

TEST-TAKING STRATEGY: Use the process of elimination to rule out incorrect answer selections to help choose the correct answer.

163. The parent of a 5-year-old asks the nurse if the child is old enough to ride in the front passenger seat of the car. The nurse tells the parent that the recommended age for riding in the front seat of a vehicle is:

A. 10 years of age and younger.

B. 6 years of age and older.

C. 12 years of age and older.

D. 18 years of age.

Answer: C. All children ages 12 years and younger should ride in the back seat of a vehicle. This eliminates injury risk due to deployed front and passenger-side airbags and places children in the safest part of the vehicle in the event of a crash.

TEST-TAKING STRATEGY: Use the process of elimination to rule out incorrect answer selections to help choose the correct answer.

164. A nursing student is learning about suicide by poisoning in nursing school. The student knows that the group most likely to commit suicide by poisoning is:

A. Men.

B. Women.

C. Blacks.

D. Hispanics.

Answer: A. Among those who commit suicide by poisoning, men are 1.3 times more likely than women. Whites are more likely than blacks and Hispanics to commit suicide by poisoning.

TEST-TAKING STRATEGY: Terms like *most appropriately* and *most likely* mean that the undeniable correct answer is probably not present. Therefore, you must select the best answer choice from the selections provided.

165. The nurse working in a pediatrician's office is teaching an adult couple with small children about preventing poisoning in children. The nurse knows that strategies effective in preventing poisoning from occurring in children include (select all that apply):

A. Turning on the light when preparing medications for children.

B. Taking medicine in front of children, so that they may learn the correct way to swallow pills.

C. Calling medicine "candy," so the children will take the medicine without a fuss.

D. Taking the child with you to answer the ringing phone instead of leaving the child in the presence of an open bottle of cleaning solution.

Answer: A & D. Turning on the light when preparing medications for children will help eliminate medication administration errors. Never leaving a child in the presence of cleaning solutions or other chemicals may prevent a potentially fatal accident. Taking medicine in front of children is not recommended as children often try to imitate adult behavior. Calling medicine "candy" is inappropriate and misleading to the child.

TEST-TAKING STRATEGY: Look for similar answer choices and eliminate them.

166. An immigrant family regularly purchases imported candy for their children at the local market. A child can be exposed to lead by eating candy imported from which country?

A. Brazil.

B. Honduras.

C. Mexico.

D. Italy.

Answer: C. According to the CDC, the potential for exposure to lead from candy imported from Mexico prompted the FDA to issue warnings on the availability of lead-contaminated candy and to develop tighter guidelines for manufacturers, importers, and distributors of imported candy. Consuming even small amounts of lead can be harmful.

TEST-TAKING STRATEGY: Use the process of elimination to rule out incorrect answer selections to help choose the correct answer.

167. A home health nurse is caring for a client whose spouse smokes cigarettes. Knowing that smoking is the leading cause of fire-related deaths, the nurse includes which instructions when teaching the client and spouse how to prevent fires?

A. Smoking in bed is acceptable as long as the cigarette is extinguished prior to going to sleep.

B. Keep matches and lighters from children by storing them in a locked cabinet.

C. Test the smoke alarm every 6 months.

D. Place burning cigarettes into an ashtray while performing other duties.

Answer: B. Keeping matches and lighters from children by storing them in a locked cabinet can prevent fire-related deaths. Smoking in bed is never recommended. Smoke alarms should be tested every month and repaired or replaced immediately if malfunction occurs. Lit cigarettes should never be left unattended.

TEST-TAKING STRATEGY: The phrase "nurse includes which instructions when teaching" tells you to select the answer with accurate information.

168. The nurse working in a high school educates the students about car accident prevention. The nurse tells the students that teenagers at highest risk for a motor vehicle crash are:

A. Teenagers who recently turn 19 years of age.

B. Teenagers who recently acquired a driver's license.

C. Teenagers who carpool to the senior prom.

D. Teenagers who drive to weekly football games.

Answer B: According to the CDC, crash risk is particularly high during the first year that teenagers are eligible to drive. While teenagers who are 19 years old, carpool to the senior prom, and drive to weekly football games are also at risk for a motor vehicle crash, they are not the highest-risk teenage group.

TEST-TAKING STRATEGY: You may find that the question does not offer a distinct correct answer. In this case, choose the most correct answer.

169. A nurse enters a client's room to find the client in supine position on the floor thrashing about. The nurse should immediately:

A. Restrain the client.

B. Force a tongue blade in the client's mouth.

C. Assist the client back into the bed.

D. Place a towel or sheet under the client's head.

Answer: D. Placing a towel or sheet under the client's head prevents further injury to the client. Restraining the client may cause further injury to the client. Forcing an object into the client's mouth can result in choking the client or injuring the client's teeth and mouth. Lifting the client may cause injury to the nurse and client.

TEST-TAKING STRATEGY: Questions that ask you to prioritize your nursing actions use terms like *priority, first, best, initial, most important, immediate,* and *next.*

170. A client presents to the emergency department with complaints of fever, cough, malaise, and rash appearing as vesicles most prominently on the face, palms of the hands, and soles of the feet. The nurse's first reaction is to:

A. Send the client to the waiting room to wait for an available examination room.

B. Place the client into a negative pressure room implementing airborne precautions.

C. Notify the emergency department physician.

D. Place the client on contact precautions.

Answer: B. The client may have smallpox, which is very contagious. Smallpox can also be used in a biological incident. The first thing the nurse should do is place the client into a negative pressure room and implement airborne precautions, which require all persons to wear a fit tested N95 respirator. Wearing a surgical mask is not sufficient in this case. Doing this first will protect others from potential exposure to a very contagious disease. After the client is sequestered, the nurse should notify the emergency department physician for further treatment instructions.

TEST-TAKING STRATEGY: Questions that ask you to prioritize your nursing actions use terms like *priority, first, best, initial, most important, immediate,* and *next.*

171. During a mass casualty incident the hospital is faced with the arrival of multiple clients. Which use of gloves by the nurse during a mass casualty is appropriate? Select all that apply.

    A. Placing spare gloves in uniform pockets for immediate use.

    B. Donning three or four pairs of gloves at once.

    C. If gloves become scarce, using a 4 by 4 gauze to wipe the accumulated fluids off the gloves to decrease contamination between clients.

    D. Wearing gloves during a mass casualty event is only required if the casualty event is precipitated by a contagious illness.

    Answer: A, B, & C. Placing spare gloves in uniform pockets for immediate use, donning three or four pairs of gloves at once, using a shedding process to remove gloves as they become contaminated, and cleaning gloves—if they become scarce—between clients are all effective uses for gloves during a mass casualty. Gloves should be worn during all mass casualty events to prevent exposure to blood or body fluids.

    TEST-TAKING STRATEGY: When answering "Select all that apply" questions, be sure and treat each answer as a true or false statement. There may be one correct answer or more.

172. The nurse is selected to assist with emergency preparedness planning at the nurse's place of employment. The nurse knows that which action is most effective in this endeavor? Select all that apply.

    A. Developing a response plan.

    B. Developing different emergency response plans for each type of disaster.

    C. Educating all individuals to specifics of the response plan.

    D. Practicing the plan and evaluating the facility's level of preparedness.

    Answer: A, C, & D. Developing a response plan, educating individuals to the specifics of

the response plan, and practicing the plan and evaluating the facility's level of preparedness are effective means of implementing emergency preparedness. The basic principles of emergency preparedness are the same for all types of disasters. Only the response interventions vary to address the specific needs of the situation.

TEST-TAKING STRATEGY: When answering "Select all that apply" questions, be sure and treat each answer as a true or false statement. There may be one correct answer or more.

173. The nurse recently attended a facility seminar on pandemic flu planning. Hospitals preparing for the pandemic flu (select all that apply):

    A. Promote spatial separation in common areas.

    B. Mandate staff to wear a surgical mask when caring for infected clients.

    C. Implement contact and airborne precautions.

    D. Mandate staff to wear an N95 mask when in close contact with an infected client.

    Answer: A, C, & D. Using spatial separation, at least 3 feet apart, from potentially infectious clients helps decrease the spread of infection. Contact precautions—wearing gowns, gloves, mask, and protective eyewear—are used for contact with respiratory secretions. Airborne precautions are used, because flu is spread by airborne droplets. Wearing an N95 mask is suggested instead of wearing a surgical mask, because the pandemic flu involves a relatively new strain of virus.

TEST-TAKING STRATEGY: When answering "Select all that apply" questions, be sure and treat each answer as a true or false statement. There may be one correct answer or more.

174. A client is involved in a chemical exposure event. Decontamination efforts are performed. The majority of decontamination is accomplished by:

    A. Rinsing the client off with water.

    B. Removal of clothing.

    C. Washing the client off with soap and water.

    D. Flushing of the skin.

Answer B. Eighty percent of decontamination can be accomplished by removal of clothing. Complete decontamination involves clothing removal, complete flushing of the skin, and wrapping the client in a sheet or protective cover.

TEST-TAKING STRATEGY: Look for similar answer choices and eliminate them.

175. A chemical exposure event occurs during a football game. The hospital is notified and expects to receive clients. Which statement is most important regarding the decontamination of clients who are nonambulatory?

   A. The nurse should don appropriate personal protective equipment (PPE) prior to contact with the client.

   B. Clothes should not be removed and the client should be transported to an emergency department to receive life-saving interventions.

   C. Decontamination of the eyes is not required.

   D. Hot water should be used to decontaminate the client.

Answer: A. PPE should be donned prior to contact with the client to prevent contamination of the health care worker. All clothes, jewelry, and personal belongings should be removed and placed into appropriate containers. Decontamination of the eyes is performed using a saline solution via nasal cannula or Morgan lens. Hot water is unnecessary unless the client is hypothermic during decontamination procedures.

TEST-TAKING STRATEGY: Home in on the key words in the stem like "most important." Then eliminate the incorrect answers while focusing on the answer that provides information or an action that is the most important.

176. The nurse is preparing to administer medications to a client. To properly identify the client, the nurse must use two client identifiers. Which statement is an example of two client identifiers?

   A. The client's room number and the client's identification band.

   B. The client's date of birth and the client's identification band.

   C. The client's visitor and the client's identification band.

   D. Two identifiers are not required.

Answer: B. The client's date of birth and the client's identification band can be used as the two identifiers per Joint Commission standards. The client's room number or visitor are not considered a client identifier.

TEST-TAKING STRATEGY: Read the question twice to ensure that you understand what the question is asking, especially if the question is tricky or confusing. Focus on what the question is asking: two examples of client identifiers.

177. The nurse takes a telephone order from a physician. Which statement most appropriately applies to the implementation of the telephone order?

   A. The nurse records the order in the client's record at the end of the shift while performing all of other documentation.

   B. The nurse repeats the order back to the physician prior to transcribing the order.

   C. The nurse transcribes the order and repeats the order back to the physician.

   D. The nurse transcribes the order in the client's chart, and then phones the physician to repeat the order.

Answer C. Whenever a verbal or telephone order is given, the nurse is to transcribe the order, and then read it back to the ordering physician during the time the order is given. If the order is received and repeated back to the physician without transcribing the order first, an error may occur.

TEST-TAKING STRATEGY: Terms like *most appropriately* and *most accurately* mean that the undeniable correct answer is most likely not present. Therefore, you must select the best answer choice.

178. The nurse is about to receive a change-of-shift report. Which type report is acceptable?

  A. A taped report with all the client's information from the previous shift included.

  B. A taped report with the nurse from the previous shift available to answer questions.

  C. A taped report with the ability to call the nurse from the previous shift at home for questions.

  D. A taped report with one of the nurses on the previous shift available to answer questions.

Answer: B. A taped report is not acceptable unless it includes an opportunity to ask the nurse who left the report clarifying questions regarding the client's care. A process that relies on the option to call the nurse from a previous shift at home is not acceptable due to the possible unavailability of that nurse. Having only one nurse from the previous shift available to answer questions is not feasible because the nurse is not able to answer questions regarding clients the nurse did not care for during the previous shift.

TEST-TAKING STRATEGY: Look for similar answer choices and eliminate them.

179. An order is written to give MSO$_4$ 100 mg intramuscularly now. The nurse should:

  A. Check the order prior to sending it to the pharmacy.

  B. Notify the physician for clarification of the order.

  C. Notify the pharmacy that the order is needed immediately.

  D. Gather the supplies needed for an injection.

Answer: B. The nurse should notify the physician because MSO$_4$ is an abbreviation that is on the Joint Commission's "Do Not Use" list. MSO$_4$ can mean morphine sulfate or magnesium sulfate. Notifying the physician to clarify the order will prevent a medication error from occurring.

TEST-TAKING STRATEGY: Always pick the answer that is most life threatening or the nursing intervention that is most lifesaving.

180. The nurse cares for a client who undergoes a left total knee replacement. Before surgery begins, the "time-out" takes place. "Time-out" is a process:

  A. Where the nurses and technicians wait for the surgeon to perform a surgical scrub.

  B. Of active communication among the surgical team members to conduct a final verification of correct client, procedure, site, and implant.

  C. Performed to assure correct count of sponges and instrumentation.

  D. Performed to make sure the correct instrumentation has been opened for the procedure

Answer: B. Time out is a process that is performed immediately before the procedure to conduct a final verification of the correct client, procedure, site, and implant. Time out is active communication among all members of the surgical/procedural team, which is consistently initiated by a member of the team.

TEST-TAKING STRATEGY: Look for similar answer choices and eliminate them.

181. The nurse instructs the client having a left total knee replacement to mark the site where the surgery is to take place. In marking the site, the nurse should:

  A. Mark the right knee so that the mark will not hinder the operative incision.

  B. Have the client mark the site after the preoperative medication is administered.

  C. Mark the left knee with an "X."

  D. Assist the client in marking the left knee with "YES" while the client is awake and alert.

Answer: D. The nurse should assist the client in marking the left knee with an unambiguous mark such as "YES" while the client is awake and alert. The mark "X" may be considered ambiguous. The mark should be made at or near the incision site. Nonoperative sites should not be marked unless necessary for some other aspect of care.

TEST-TAKING STRATEGY: Look for similar answer choices and eliminate them.

182. The transporter is on the floor to take a client to the radiology department for a left lung tissue biopsy. The nurse is performing a final check before the client is transported to the radiology department. The nurse should ensure that:

A. The consent form is signed, any ordered pre-operative medication is given, and the operative site is marked.

B. The consent form is signed, any ordered pre-operative medication is given, and the operative site is prepped with a razor.

C. The consent form is signed, the lab work is in order, any ordered preoperative medication is given, and the operative site is marked.

D. The consent form is signed, the lab work is in order, and any ordered preoperative medication is given.

Answer: D. The nurse should ensure that the consent form is signed, the lab work is in order, and any ordered preoperative medication is given. The person who is performing the procedure should mark the site. The site should be prepped with clippers as opposed to a razor, which can cause injury to the client.

TEST-TAKING STRATEGY: Look for similar answer choices and eliminate them.

183. A newborn in a neonatal unit is to receive penicillin G benzathine intramuscularly. The dispensed dose is ten times the ordered dose. To minimize the number of injections the neonate receives, the nurse should:

A. Administer the drug intravenously.

B. Choose two injection sites and give the drug as ordered.

C. Question the order and consult with the pharmacy.

D. Read the available drug information to determine how to administer the medication.

Answer: C. Any time there is a discrepancy with the ordered drug, the order should be questioned. The nurse must consult with the pharmacy to receive further instructions. Because the drug is ordered intramuscularly, the route should not be changed to intravenous administration because this violates the order as written. The dose is

greater than the allowed volume to be given intramuscularly, which warrants clarification by the pharmacy. Although drug information may be available, there is a chance for misinterpretation by the nurse.

TEST-TAKING STRATEGY: Always pick the answer that is most life threatening or the nursing intervention that is most lifesaving.

184. A physician orders intravenous lipids to be administered to a critical-care client. The client has a triple-lumen subclavian central line, an epidural line, and an arterial line. Which line should the nurse choose to administer the intravenous lipids?

A. The line that is labeled at the connecting end.

B. The nurse should notify the physician regarding which line to choose.

C. None of the lines, because lipids should be given enterally.

D. The line that is not currently in use.

Answer: A. The nurse should choose the line that is labeled at the connecting end to administer the intravenous lipids to prevent administering the lipids into the epidural line. The nurse does not need to consult the physician regarding which line to use.

TEST-TAKING STRATEGY: Choose the answer selection that is the most life threatening or harmful to the client.

185. A 63-year-old male receives enalapril maleate-hydrochlorothiazide (Vaseretic) for 6 months for hypertension. Three days ago, the client began experiencing difficulty swallowing, mild difficulty breathing, and discomfort in the back of his throat. The client is seen in the emergency department where the physician diagnoses a drug reaction to the enalapril. The client's wife brings a bag of the client's medications to the hospital, and states the medication is administered to the client every day. The nurse should:

A. Notify the physician to give the client the medications.

B. Document the list of medications in the client's record for the physician to review.

C. Administer the medications to the client.

D. Instruct the wife to give the client the medications.

Answer: B. The nurse should document the list of medications in the client's record for the physician to review. If the nurse, spouse, or physician had given the medication, the client may have experienced an anaphylactic reaction and possible death.

TEST-TAKING STRATEGY: Determine which action will bring the most harm or help to the client. This helps determine the highest nursing priority.

186. A client receives a bed bath and bed linen change. The nurse knows that soiled linen should be:

   A. Held close to the body during a bed change to prevent contamination of the environment.

   B. Held close to the body only if the nurse is wearing gloves for protection.

   C. Placed into a leakproof container for transport.

   D. Placed on a cart in the unit's hallway.

Answer: C. Soiled linen should be placed in a leakproof container for transport off the unit to the laundry. Gloves should always be worn when handling soiled linen. Soiled linen should be carried away from the body to prevent contamination. Soiled linen should never be left in the unit's hallway.

TEST-TAKING STRATEGY: Look for similar answer choices and eliminate them.

187. The physician instructs the nurse to place body tissue obtained from a biopsy into a container with formalin prior to sending it to pathology. The nurse is not familiar with formalin and obtains the MSDS to read the precautions for handling formalin. MSDS stand for:

   A. Mechanisms for Safe Device Standard.

   B. Management of Safety Devices and Standard.

   C. Material Safety Data Sheet.

   D. Methods for Safe Distribution and Standard.

Answer: C. All hazardous materials come with an MSDS—Material Safety Data Sheet, which includes the identity of the chemical, the physical and chemical characteristics, the physical and health hazards, primary routes of entry, exposure limits, precautions for safe handling, controls to limit exposure, emergency and first-aid procedures, and the name of the manufacturer or distributor.

TEST-TAKING STRATEGY: Use the process of elimination to rule out incorrect answer selections to help choose the correct answer.

188. A nurse removes a small bandage from a client who received an injection. The nurse notices a speck of blood on the bandage. Where should the nurse dispose of the bandage?

   A. In a biohazard trash can lined with a biohazard trash liner.

   B. In a puncture-resistant biohazard container.

   C. In a biohazard trash can lined with a regular trash bag.

   D. In a regular trash can lined with a regular trash bag.

Answer: D. The small bandage should be disposed of in a regular trash can lined with a regular trash bag. The speck of blood on the bandage is not sufficient to cause an infection. If the bandage were soaked with blood, it would need to be discarded in a biohazard trash can lined with a biohazard trash bag. Puncture-resistant biohazard containers are used for sharp instrument disposal.

TEST-TAKING STRATEGY: Look for similar answer choices and eliminate them.

189. A nurse administers intravenous chemotherapeutic drugs to a client. When the infusion is complete, the nurse should:

   A. Remove the tubing from the IV bag.

   B. Wear shoe covers during disposal of the chemotherapeutic drugs.

   C. Place the disposable items directly into a chemotherapy waste container and close the lid.

   D. Remove outer PPE and bag it for disposal in the biohazardous waste.

Answer: C. The disposable items such as the IV bag and tubing should remain intact and disposed of into a securely sealed chemotherapy waste container. Tubing should never be disconnected from an IV bag containing a hazardous drug because the risk of splashing is increased. PPE (including double gloves, goggles, and protective gown) should be worn for all activities associated with chemotherapeutic drug administration. PPE used in chemotherapy drug administration should be disposed of in a chemotherapy—not biohazardous—waste receptacle.

TEST-TAKING STRATEGY: Read the question twice to ensure that you understand what the question is asking, especially if the question is tricky or confusing. Focus on what the question is asking: proper disposal of chemotherapy agents and equipment.

190. The nurse administers chemotherapeutic drugs to a client with breast cancer. Where should the nurse dispose of the medication vials?

   A. In a puncture-resistant biohazard container.

   B. In a chemotherapy sharps container.

   C. In a biohazard waste container.

   D. In a chemical container.

Answer: B. Empty vials and sharps such as needles and syringes used in delivering chemotherapy agents should be disposed of in a chemotherapy sharps container. These waste containers are designed to protect workers from injuries and are disposed of by incineration at regulated medical waste facilities. Hazardous, drug-contaminated sharps should not be placed in red biohazard sharps containers that are used for infectious wastes, since these are often autoclaved or microwaved.

TEST-TAKING STRATEGY: Look for similar answer choices and eliminate them.

191. A client recently diagnosed with diabetes is sent home with a prescription for subcutaneous insulin. The client and family are concerned about how they should discard the needles at home. The client and family demonstrate they understand the teaching when they state:

   A. "No special handling of the syringes is necessary."

   B. "A hospital-issued biohazard container must be used."

   C. "Any hard plastic container with a screw-on cap reinforced with heavy tape, may be used."

   D. "The needles must be brought to the nearest hospital for disposal."

Answer: C. At home, needles, syringes, and sharps may be disposed of in a hard plastic container placed into the regular trash. This protects the sanitation engineers from becoming injured by the sharps. The hospital need not be involved in sharps disposal in the home.

TEST-TAKING STRATEGY: The phrase "client understands the teaching" tells you to select the answer with accurate information.

192. A client preparing for discharge home is having difficulty urinating. The physician writes and an order for the client to receive instructions regarding intermittent urinary catheterization prior to being discharged home. The nurse knows that home intermittent catheterization is:

   A. Not recommended.

   B. A difficult procedure to teach.

   C. A clean procedure.

   D. A sterile procedure.

Answer: C. Home intermittent catheterization is a clean, not sterile technique when performed in the home environment. Home intermittent catheterization is preferred over continuous use of a Foley catheter, as a Foley catheter increases client risk of urinary tract infection. Home intermittent catheterization is best taught by return demonstration prior to the client being discharged home.

TEST-TAKING STRATEGY: You may find that the question does not offer a distinct correct answer. In this case, choose the most correct answer from the answer selections provided.

193. Home agents that are suitable for cleaning and disinfecting the home include (select all that apply):

A. Bleach.

B. Glutaraldehyde.

C. Hydrogen peroxide.

D. Boiling water.

Answer: A, C, & D. Bleach, hydrogen peroxide, and boiling water are suitable agents for cleaning and disinfecting the home. Glutaraldehyde is a disinfectant that is found only in health care facilities. Using this disinfectant in a home situation requires monitoring and can be a health hazard, so it is not the best choice for home cleaning.

TEST-TAKING STRATEGY: When answering "Select all that apply" questions, be sure and treat each answer as a true or false statement. There may be one correct answer or more.

194. A client is diagnosed with hepatitis B. When the client reveals this information to family members, the family becomes frightened to go home with the client. Teaching the family to decrease their risk of exposure to hepatitis B includes which information?

A. Do not share personal items with the client, such as razors or toothbrushes.

B. Wash dishes in separate water to decrease the risk of contamination.

C. Do not hug or kiss the client.

D. Use a separate bathroom from the client.

Answer: A. Hepatitis B is a blood-borne pathogen that can spread via sharing personal items, such as razors or toothbrushes. Hepatitis B is not spread via saliva or by sharing a bathroom. Hepatitis B is not spread by dirty dishwater.

TEST-TAKING STRATEGY: Look for similar answer choices and eliminate them.

195. Discharge instructions are written for a client admitted with cellulitis including a prescription for antibiotics. Which statement made by the nurse to the client is most accurate?

A. "Take most of the antibiotic until you feel better, but save some to take in case the infection returns."

B. "Follow the instructions on the label and finish the course of treatment."

C. "Double the prescription to get better sooner."

D. "If a dose is missed, double the dose of antibiotic at the time of the next dose."

Answer: B. Instruct the client to follow the instructions and finish the whole prescription. Not taking the whole prescription can lead to resistance of the organism and cause a relapse of the infection. Medication doses should never be doubled, even if one dose is missed.

TEST-TAKING STRATEGY: Terms like *most appropriately* and *most accurately* mean that the undeniable correct answer is probably not present. Therefore, you must select the best answer choice from the selections provided.

196. The home health nurse performs a culture of a client's urine. The results indicate vancomycin-resistant *Enterococcus* (VRE). The nurse prepares a fact sheet regarding VRE for the client and family. It is most important that the fact sheet include which instructions (select all that apply)?

A. Wash hands with hot water and soap when hands are soiled.

B. Frequently clean areas of the home that may become contaminated with VRE, such as the bathroom.

C. Gloves are not needed in the home, because contamination with VRE has already occurred.

D. Wash hands after using the bathroom and before preparing food.

Answer: B & D. The bathroom and kitchen should be cleaned with warm water and bleach to decrease contamination. The client and family should be instructed to wear gloves if they come into contact with VRE, such as in the stool. Hands should be washed with lukewarm water and soap after removing gloves. Instructing the client and family to wash with hot water can cause drying and cracking of the skin.

TEST-TAKING STRATEGY: When answering "Select all that apply" questions, be sure and treat each answer as a true or false statement. There may be one correct answer or more.

197. A community health nurse prepares a presentation about decreasing the risk of spreading influenza in the community. The presentation most likely includes which information?

   A. The flu is transmitted via the flu vaccine.

   B. Use a shirtsleeve when coughing or sneezing if tissue is not available.

   C. Tissues are not effective in decreasing the spread of the flu.

   D. Antibiotics are effective in treating the flu.

   Answer: B. A shirtsleeve should be used as a barrier when coughing or sneezing if tissue is not available. This prevents germs being spread via the hands. The flu vaccine contains a dead virus that is not capable of causing the flu. Clients may experience flu-like symptoms from the flu vaccine, but they won't contract the full-fledged virus. Tissues are effective in decreasing the spread of the flu if disposed of in the trash after use, while antibiotics are not effective in treating the flu. The flu is treated with antipyretics, fluids, and rest.

   TEST-TAKING STRATEGY: You may find that the question does not offer a distinct correct answer. In this case, choose the most correct answer.

198. In which ways may hollow-bore percutaneous injuries during injections or body fluid retrieval be prevented? Select all that apply.

   A. By using the two-handed recapping technique for syringes, only if no other alternative exists.

   B. By using a needleless system whenever possible.

   C. By using a blunt cannula to withdraw medication from a vial.

   D. By using an engineered sharp injury protective device whenever possible.

   Answer: B, C, & D. To prevent injury during injection administration or body fluid retrieval, use a one-handed recapping technique, needleless system, blunt cannula for medication withdrawal from a vial, and engineered sharp injury protective device whenever possible.

   TEST-TAKING STRATEGY: When answering "Select all that apply" questions, be sure and treat each answer as a true or false statement. There may be one correct answer or more.

199. In which way may a percutaneous injury occur in the operating room? Select all that apply.

   A. While the technician loads the needle into the needle holder using the suture packet to assist in mounting.

   B. When the technician passes the suture to the physician in the basin.

   C. When the surgeon ties the suture with the needle attached.

   D. When the technician retracts body tissue with the hands instead of an instrument.

   Answer: C & D. A percutaneous injury may occur in the operating room when the surgeon ties the suture with the needle attached. A percutaneous injury may also occur when a technician retracts body tissue with the hands instead of an instrument because the needle the physician uses can easily stick hands that are in the way. When using the hand to mount the needle, a stick may easily occur. The basin serves as a safety zone so that there is no hand-to-hand passing of a needle or sharp.

   TEST-TAKING STRATEGY: When answering "Select all that apply" questions, be sure and treat each answer as a true or false statement. There may be one correct answer or more.

200. During a staff inservice, the nurse describes the transmission process of hepatitis B and HIV. Which information by the nurse is most correct?

   A. HIV is transmitted via toilet seats whereas hepatitis B is not.

   B. HIV is transmitted by sexual contact whereas hepatitis B is not.

   C. Hepatitis B is more readily transmitted via needle sticks than HIV.

   D. Neither virus is transmitted via body fluids.

Answer: C. Studies show hepatitis B is more readily transmitted via needle sticks than HIV. Both hepatitis B and HIV are transmitted via body fluids through sexual contact. Neither virus is transmitted via toilet seats.

TEST-TAKING STRATEGY: Terms like *most appropriately, most accurately,* and *most correct* mean that the undeniable correct answer is most likely not present. Therefore, you must select the best answer choice from the selections provided.

201. A client experiences rapid and progressive dementia along with abnormal psychiatric behavior. The surgeon schedules the client for a brain biopsy to rule out Creutzfeldt–Jakob disease (CJD). Which action by the nurse is most important? Select all that apply.

    A. Notification of the operating room staff that the client may have CJD.

    B. Use of standard precautions while caring for the client.

    C. Use of contact precautions while caring for the client.

    D. Use of airborne and contact precautions while caring for the client.

Answer: A & B. The OR needs to know the client may have CJD so that either disposable instruments are used or the instruments are quarantined until a diagnosis is made. Regular sterilization techniques are not effective against the CJD organism. Standard precautions are used because CJD is not spread person to person, but rather through direct contact with the brain and spinal cord.

TEST-TAKING STRATEGY: Home in on the key words in the stem like "most important." Then eliminate the incorrect answers while focusing on the answer that provides information or an action that is the most important.

202. In order to prevent injury from a needle stick, the nurse should (select all that apply):

    A. Recap the needle after use to prevent injury.

    B. Clean used instrument trays carefully after every procedure.

    C. After drawing up saline to flush an IV, place the syringe in a pocket to prevent possible injury.

    D. Replace the puncture-resistant biohazard container when three-quarters full.

Answer: B & D. Instrument trays should be cleaned carefully after every procedure as sharp objects may be left behind, which can cause injury. Puncture- resistant biohazard containers should be replaced when three-quarters full to prevent hand injury when disposing of sharps. Needles should never be recapped due to the possibility of injury. Sharps should never be placed in a pocket.

TEST-TAKING STRATEGY: When answering "Select all that apply" questions, be sure and treat each answer as a true or false statement. There may be one correct answer or more.

203. A vase falls from a table located in the hallway of an assisted-living facility and shatters. Proper removal of the glass includes:

    A. Using a dustpan and broom to collect the glass and disposing of it into the garbage can.

    B. Using a dustpan and broom to collect the glass and disposing of it into a puncture-resistant sharps container.

    C. Donning gloves, picking up the glass, and disposing of it in a puncture-resistant sharps container.

    D. Using a wet mop to collect the glass and disposing of it into the garbage can.

Answer: B. Proper removal of glass includes using a dustpan and broom to collect the glass and disposing of it into a puncture-resistant sharps container. Placing glass into the garbage increases the housekeepers' potential for injury upon removal of the trash liner. Hands are never used to pick up glass even if they are gloved because of the increased risk of getting cut with the glass.

TEST-TAKING STRATEGY: Use the process of elimination to rule out incorrect answer selections to help choose the correct answer.

204. A nurse is at highest risk for blood-borne exposure during which situation?

A. When removing a needle from the syringe.

B. While placing a suture in the mechanical holder.

C. Prior to inserting the IV, the client moves, causing a needle stick to the nurse.

D. A clean needle sticks the nurse through blood-soiled gloves.

Answer: D. A clean needle that moves through blood-soiled gloves to stick the nurse is a blood-borne exposure. All other answers are considered a clean stick. Choose the answer selection that is the most life threatening or harmful to the client.

TEST-TAKING STRATEGY: Choose the answer selection that is the most life threatening or harmful to the client.

205. The nurse is working in the newborn nursery when the environmental services department states they would like to evaluate a new disinfectant on the unit. Which disinfectant should the nurse not recommend for the newborn nursery?

A. Bleach.

B. Phenolic.

C. Alcohol.

D. Iodophor.

Answer: B. Hyperbilirubinemia is a side effect of a phenolic, especially if used to clean a baby bassinet. Bleach, alcohol, and iodophor do not cause side effects in infants if utilized properly.

TEST-TAKING STRATEGY: Read the question twice to ensure that you understand what the question is asking, especially if the question is tricky or confusing. Focus on what the question is asking: the disinfectant that should not be used.

206. A nurse works in the operating room (OR) as a circulator with a focus on decreasing surgical site infections. Which action should the nurse perform to help prevent surgical site infections? Select all that apply.

A. Close the OR doors at all times during a surgical case.

B. Minimize traffic in the OR.

C. Ensure the room has laminar flow.

D. Monitor the sterile field at all times.

Answer: A, B, & D. Keeping the doors open impedes the air-exchange system in the OR. The air-exchange system is designed to decrease airborne contaminants in the OR. Limiting the traffic in the room decreases the amount of bacterial shedding, minimizes harmful air turbulence, and prevents accidental contamination of the sterile field. Laminar flow has not been proven to prevent surgical site infections.

TEST-TAKING STRATEGY: When answering "Select all that apply" questions, be sure and treat each answer as a true or false statement. There may be one correct answer or more.

207. Which personal protective equipment is required for nurses in the operating room? Select all that apply.

A. Mask.

B. Hair covering.

C. Surgical scrubs.

D. Shoe covers.

Answer: A, B, & C. A hair covering is donned first to prevent hair from falling on fresh surgical scrubs. A mask is worn to prevent dispelling droplets into the sterile field. Surgical scrubs are worn to prevent shedding. Scrub pants and tops are preferred over dresses to protect shedding from the perineum, which contaminates the sterile field. Shoe covers are worn as required by the Occupational Safety and Health Administration (OSHA). Therefore, when there are cases that may not involve blood, such as in the case of eye procedures, shoe covers are not required. Shoe covers are not used for the prevention of surgical site infections.

TEST-TAKING STRATEGY: When answering "Select all that apply" questions, be sure and treat each answer as a true or false statement. There may be one correct answer or more.

208. A nurse enters the operating room (OR) with artificial nails in place. Which statement best describes the use of artificial nails in the operating room? Select all that apply.

A. Pathogenic bacteria can be found on the fingertips of those who wear artificial fingernails.

B. Artificial nails are allowed to be worn in the OR.

C. Fungal growth can occur under the artificial nail, thus increasing the risk of surgical site infection to the client.

D. Nurses with artificial nails are more inclined to perform a more vigorous scrub than those who do not have artificial nails.

Answer: A & C. The variety and amount of pathogenic bacteria cultured from the fingertips of those wearing artificial nails is greater than from those with natural nails, both before and after hand-washing. Fungal growth occurs frequently under artificial nails because moisture gets trapped between the natural nail and artificial nail, providing a medium for growth. Artificial nails are not allowed in the OR. Nurses are less inclined to perform a vigorous scrub because of the potential for chipping, scratching, or breaking the artificial nails.

TEST-TAKING STRATEGY: When answering "Select all that apply" questions, be sure and treat each answer as a true or false statement. There may be one correct answer or more.

209. The nurse assists a physician in draining a client's large abscess at the bedside. The nurse holds the client to prevent the client from jerking during the procedure. The nurse should wear which personal protective equipment?

A. Sterile gloves and face shield.

B. Gloves and gown.

C. Gown, sterile gloves, and mask.

D. Gown, gloves, mask, and face shield.

Answer: D. During drainage of an abscess, there is the possibility of bodily fluids spraying the nurse. The nurse needs the protection of a gown, mask, and face shield. Gloves are worn to prevent touching contaminated material. Donning sterile items is not necessary, as the nurse is not assisting with the procedure, but holding the client instead.

210. The nurse preps a client's skin for a surgical procedure. The nurse notes the client has excessive body hair. Which is the preferred method of hair removal? Select all that apply.

A. Shaving the hair with a razor.

B. Removing the hair with clippers.

C. Lathering the skin with soap and water prior to shaving with a razor.

D. Using a depilatory cream.

Answer: B & D. Using a razor for hair removal is not recommended because it causes microabrasions of the skin. Bacteria multiply in the microabrasions increasing the risk of infection. Not removing the hair at all is preferred, but if this is not an option the use of clippers or a depilatory cream may be used.

TEST-TAKING STRATEGY: Determine which action brings the most help to the client.

211. The nurse prepares to insert a urinary catheter into a client. Which antiseptic is appropriate for the nurse to use for this procedure? Select all that apply.

A. Alcohol.

B. Ultradex.

C. Chlorhexadine.

D. Iodophor.

Answer: B & D. Ultradex and iodophor are used to safely prep the perineum prior to urinary catheter insertion. Alcohol and chlorhexadine are damaging to mucous membranes.

TEST-TAKING STRATEGY: Determine which action brings the least harm to the client.

212. The circulating nurse prepares the sterile field in the operating room (OR). Fifteen minutes later, the nurse is informed that the surgery is delayed for 20 minutes because the surgeon is working at another hospital. Which is the best action for the nurse to take?

A. Cover the sterile field with a sterile drape until the surgery is about to begin.

B. Close and tape the OR doors so that no one may enter.

C. Monitor the sterile field while awaiting the surgeon.

D. Tear down the sterile field until the surgeon arrives in the OR.

Answer: C. The nurse should monitor the sterile field while awaiting the surgeon. The nurse should not cover the sterile field because of the possibility of contamination during removal of the drape. A staff member should remain in the OR at all times to monitor the sterile field. It is unnecessary to tear down the sterile field as the delay is minimal.

TEST-TAKING STRATEGY: Questions that ask you to prioritize your nursing actions use terms like *priority, first, best, initial, most important, immediate,* and *next.*

213. During the middle of a surgical procedure, the technician informs the nurse that the biological indicator in the instrumentation pan does not indicate the instruments are sterilized. Which action should the nurse take first?

A. Tear down the entire sterile field and start over.

B. Nothing, because the instrument pan indicator may have been faulty.

C. Remove the instrument pan and involved instruments from the sterile field.

D. Complete an incident report.

Answer: C. The nurse should remove the instrument pan and involved instruments from the sterile field to prevent further contamination to the patient. Next, the nurse should complete an incident report. It is not necessary to tear down the entire sterile field. The instrument pan

indicator is placed to determine sterilization of the instruments inside of the pan. For this reason, it is important that the nurse who opens the sterile field look inside the trays to ensure the indicator has changed. If it has not changed, the instruments should not be placed on the sterile field because they are now considered contaminated. Indicators should be placed in the instrument pan so visualization can occur during opening of the instruments.

TEST-TAKING STRATEGY: Questions that ask you to prioritize your nursing actions use terms like *priority, first, best, initial, most important, immediate,* and *next.*

214. The nurse prepares to insert a peripheral intra-vascular catheter in a client requiring fluids. Which antiseptic is preferred for prepping the skin prior to insertion of the catheter?

A. Alcohol.

B. Iodophor.

C. Acetone.

D. Chlorhexadine.

Answer: D. Chlorhexadine is the desired antiseptic because it is broad spectrum. Chlorhexadine kills skin microorganisms immediately and continues to work (residual action) for several hours after application. It is not compromised when coming into contact with organic material, as is iodophor. Alcohol and acetone are drying to the skin.

TEST-TAKING STRATEGY: Use the process of elimination to rule out incorrect answer selections to help choose the correct answer.

215. The nurse knows that prevention of central line-associated bloodstream infection is crucial during insertion of venous central catheters. Which action by the nurse best prevents central line-associated bloodstream infection during central line insertion? Select all that apply.

A. Wearing a mask, cap, sterile gown, and sterile gloves.

B. Preparing the site prior to insertion with iodophor.

C. Using a sterile drape that covers the client's body.

D. Wearing a gown and gloves during insertion.

Answer: A & C. Wearing a mask, cap, sterile gown, and sterile gloves by the nurse prevents infection during central line insertion. A sterile drape should also be used to cover the client's body during insertion. Chlorhexadine antiseptic is used to prepare the skin prior to insertion.

TEST-TAKING STRATEGY: When answering "Select all that apply" questions, be sure and treat each answer as a true or false statement. There may be one correct answer or more.

216. The nurse prepares to flush a peripheral intravenous (IV) line with saline to prevent the IV from clotting. Prior to flushing, the nurse should (select all that apply):

    A. Swab the top of the sterile saline vial with alcohol before injecting the needle to aspirate the saline.

    B. Check the date of the sterile saline flush prior to use.

    C. Swab the port of the IV line with alcohol prior to flushing.

    D. Obtain a needle to flush the needleless port of the IV line.

    Answer: A, B, & C. The nurse should always swab the top of the saline vial and the port of the IV with alcohol to prevent the injection of microorganisms into the client's bloodstream. The date of the sterile saline flush should always be checked prior to use to prevent using a solution that is expired. A needle is not needed for a needleless port.

    TEST-TAKING STRATEGY: Use the process of elimination to rule out incorrect answer selections to help choose the correct answer.

217. A client is undergoing a total hip replacement when a screw that is going to be placed into the client is dropped on the floor. The nurse should:

    A. Prepare the instrument for flash sterilization for 3 minutes in a gravity-displacement steam sterilizer.

    B. Monitor the load with a biological indicator during sterilization and quarantine the device until results of the biological indicator are known.

    C. Soak the instrument in a disinfectant according to manufacturer recommendations.

    D. Check the availability of another sterilized screw to be used immediately.

    Answer: D. The nurse should check the availability of another sterilized screw so that the surgery is not delayed. Implantable devices like a screw should not be flash sterilized. Implants such as orthopedic devices require special handling before and during sterilization to prevent a contaminated device being placed into the client.

    TEST-TAKING STRATEGY: Use the process of elimination to rule out incorrect answer selections to help choose the correct answer.

218. The nurse knows negative pressure should be used in the operating room (OR):

    A. Always.

    B. Never.

    C. Sometimes.

    D. 50% of the time.

    Answer: A. The OR is designed to sustain positive pressure mode at all times. The air should flow out of the OR when the doors are opened to prevent air travel of organisms into the OR's sterile environment.

    TEST-TAKING STRATEGY: Look for similar answer choices and eliminate them ("sometimes" and "50% of the time").

219. Before using a bronchoscope from one client to the next, the bronchoscope must be cleaned. The nurse knows that minimal cleaning of the bronchoscope includes:

    A. Sterilization.

    B. High-level disinfection.

    C. Low-level disinfection.

    D. Washing with soap and water.

Answer: B. Disinfection and sterilization of client-care items or equipment are classified as critical, semi-critical, and noncritical. Bronchoscopes are an example of semi-critical items that come in contact with mucous membranes or nonintact skin. Semi-critical items should be free of all microorganisms, with the exception of high numbers of bacterial spores. Semi-critical items require high-level disinfection using wet pasteurization or chemical disinfectants.

TEST-TAKING STRATEGY: Use the process of elimination to rule out incorrect answer selections to help choose the correct answer.

220. The nurse prepares an intramuscular injection for a client who is HIV positive. After giving the client the injection, the client moves, causing the nurse to get stuck by the needle used for the injection. What should the nurse do first? Select all that apply.

   A. Immediately flush the exposed area with water and express blood from the puncture site.

   B. Notify employee health when the nurse's shift is over.

   C. Notify employee health immediately and complete an incident report.

   D. Notify the physician of the incident.

Answer: A & C. Flushing the area and expressing blood from the puncture site decreases the inoculum of the HIV. The employee health nurse should be notified immediately, because there are drugs available to prevent conversion to HIV-positive status. These drugs must be given within 2 hours of exposure to prevent conversion.

TEST-TAKING STRATEGY: When answering "Select all that apply" questions, be sure and treat each answer as a true or false statement. There may be one correct answer or more.

221. The nurse makes a client's bed when the nurse's index finger is caught between the bed coil and mattress. Two days later, the finger begins to swell, throb, and become red and warm. The nurse goes to the emergency department, where a fracture of the third right finger is diagnosed.

What action should the nurse have taken when the incident first occurred?

   A. Completed an incident report at the time of the incident.

   B. No action was required at the time of the incident.

   C. Completed an incident report while in the emergency department.

   D. Notified the physician that an incident occurred in the client's room.

Answer: A. The nurse should always notify the nurse manager and complete an incident report immediately after the incident. If no incident report is filed, there is no proof that the event occurred at the place of employment.

TEST-TAKING STRATEGY: Use the process of elimination to rule out incorrect answer selections to help choose the correct answer.

222. Prior to administering medication to a client, the nurse decides to check the dosage strength one more time. This check reveals a dosage error, and so the medication is not administered. What immediate action should the nurse take?

   A. Nothing, because an incident did not occur.

   B. Complete an incident report.

   C. Notify the physician of the potential error.

   D. Inform the client that the wrong dosage of medication was almost given.

Answer: B. Near misses are considered a potential serious consequence and should be reported. An incident report facilitates a process review of the incident. A process review can prevent the next health care provider from making an error.

TEST-TAKING STRATEGY: Questions that ask you to prioritize your nursing actions use terms like *priority, first, best, initial, most important, immediate,* and *next.*

223. When should the physician be notified by the nurse in the event of a medication incident? Select all that apply.

   A. 100% of the time.

   B. If the client is harmed or dies.

C. If the medication incident is a near miss.

D. If the nurse administers an incorrect dosage.

Answer: B & D. The physician should be notified if harm is brought to the client or death occurs as a result of the medication incident. The physician should be notified if the nurse administers an incorrect dosage to the client. An incident report needs to be completed in this situation. Near misses do not need to be reported to the physician.

TEST-TAKING STRATEGY: When answering "Select all that apply" questions, be sure and treat each answer as a true or false statement. There may be one correct answer or more.

224. The nurse completes an incident report after a client falls. Why must the nurse complete an incident report? Select all that apply.

A. For quality-assurance purposes.

B. To monitor client accident trends.

C. To monitor for potential serious consequences.

D. To inform the client that an injury has occurred.

Answer: A, B, & C. An incident report is completed for quality-assurance purposes and to monitor trends so that necessary steps can be taken to prevent further occurrences. Incident reports also serve to monitor for potential serious consequences, especially during a near-miss incident. The incident report is not used for informing the client of a potential injury.

TEST-TAKING STRATEGY: When answering "Select all that apply" questions, be sure and treat each answer as a true or false statement. There may be one correct answer or more.

225. The nurse completes an incident report after a client is given the incorrect dosage of a medication. Who should review the incident report? Select all that apply.

A. The client involved in the incident.

B. The unit manager or supervisor.

C. The risk management team.

D. The client's family.

Answer: B & C. The unit manager or supervisor should review the report before sending the report to the risk management team. The incident report is utilized to help the institution make the necessary improvements that are identified when an incident occurs.

TEST-TAKING STRATEGY: When answering "Select all that apply" questions, be sure and treat each answer as a true or false statement. There may be one correct answer or more.

226. A confused client falls out of the bed. When the nurse arrives, the side-rails are up, the client has urinated on the floor, and an abrasion is noted on the client's forehead. Which information should be included in the incident report? Select all that apply.

A. The abrasion on the client's forehead.

B. The nurse's opinion as to how the client fell.

C. The client's confused state.

D. The presence of urine on the floor

Answer: A, C, & D. The following should be included in an incident report detailing a client's fall: how the fall occurred (if observed); where the fall took place; how the nurse was notified of the fall; the environmental conditions (wet, dry, any obstructing conditions); presence of fall deterrents (side-rails, call light, nightlight); client vital signs; nurse's physical findings (confusion, abrasions); presence of family; and if toileting was an issue. Only facts, not opinions, should be stated.

TEST-TAKING STRATEGY: When answering "Select all that apply" questions, be sure and treat each answer as a true or false statement. There may be one correct answer or more.

227. An incorrect needle count is found during the closing of a surgical wound. Which action should the nurse take first?

A. Inform the Director of Surgery of an incorrect needle count.

B. Carry out steps to locate the missing needle.

C. Complete an incident report.

D. Inform the family of an incorrect needle count.

Answer: B. The nurse should carry out steps to locate the missing needle, such as notifying the surgeon and surgical team to begin manual inspection of the operative field and visual inspection of the area surrounding the surgical field. If the needle is not found, then an x-ray may be ordered by the surgeon and read before the client leaves the operating room. An incident report should also be completed.

TEST-TAKING STRATEGY: Questions that ask you to prioritize your nursing actions use terms like *priority, first, best, initial, most important, immediate,* and *next.*

228. Ultraviolet lights are placed in the waiting room of the emergency department. Care of the ultraviolet lights should include:

    A. Keeping the lights on while dusting.

    B. Ensuring that the lights are on at all times except during dusting and changing of the bulbs.

    C. Turning off the lights when the waiting room is empty.

    D. Changing the bulb only when it burns out.

    Answer: B. Ultraviolet lights should be turned off while dusting to prevent looking directly at the bulb. Looking directly at the bulb is the same as looking directly into the sunlight and could damage eyesight. The bulbs should be changed on a yearly basis and when the bulb burns out. The bulbs should remain on at all times. By turning the bulb on and off, the bulb could burn out sooner or have less power than needed to disinfect the air.

    TEST-TAKING STRATEGY: Use the process of elimination to rule out incorrect answer selections to help choose the correct answer.

229. A critical-are client is scheduled for computed tomography (CT) of the chest in the radiology department. The client currently receives 5 liters of oxygen via nasal cannula. The respiratory therapist is asked to bring an oxygen cylinder for client transport. The nurse knows the safe handling of oxygen cylinders includes:

    A. Allowing the cylinder to tip for proper transport.

    B. Placing the cylinder on the floor beside the client's bed to prevent it from falling.

    C. Dragging the cylinder to radiology.

    D. Using a cylinder cart or holder during transport.

    Answer: D. Gas cylinders must be secured at all times to prevent tipping and should never be rolled or dragged. Placing the cylinder on the floor beside the client's bed could be a fall hazard. Cylinders should be stored properly on a cylinder cart or in an approved cylinder holder. Oxygen cylinders should not be left unattended on the floor. Cylinders can explode if dropped or fractured.

    TEST-TAKING STRATEGY: Use the process of elimination to rule out incorrect answer selections to help choose the correct answer.

230. A nurse discovers that an IV pump is broken at the site where the IV tubing is placed. However, the nurse is still able to place the tubing into the pump without any complications. The nurse should:

    A. Continue to use the pump.

    B. Turn the pump off, disconnect the pump from the client, and tag the pump for repair.

    C. Turn the pump off, disconnect the pump from the client, and place the pump in the soiled utility room.

    D. Turn the pump off, repair the broken area, and continue using the pump.

    Answer: B. When there is a broken piece of equipment, the nurse should turn it off, disconnect it from the client, and tag it for repair so the equipment will not be used again until it has been repaired.

    TEST-TAKING STRATEGY: Use the process of elimination to rule out incorrect answer selections to help choose the correct answer.

231. The nurse who works in the newborn nursery notices that one of the babies is missing from the bassinet. Which action should the nurse take first?

A. Notify hospital security and the nurse manager, perform a head count of infants, and begin to look for the baby.

B. Notify the mother to inform her of the missing baby.

C. Notify the police that an infant abduction has occurred.

D. Notify the police, the mother, and the infant's family and provide comfort, answering questions as they arise.

Answer: A. The nurse should first notify hospital security and the nurse manager. Next, the nurse should perform a head count to ensure a baby is indeed missing and begin a search of the unit for the infant. During this time, a code word should be announced over the intercom alerting the staff to begin procedures to locate the baby. The nurse should then notify the mother.

TEST-TAKING STRATEGY: Questions that ask you to prioritize your nursing actions use terms like *priority, first, best, initial, most important, immediate,* and *next.*

232. A nurse who works on an oncology unit notices a respiratory technician (RT) carrying a baby down the hallway. The nurse should:

A. Do nothing.

B. Notify the nursery.

C. Notify the oncology nurse manger.

D. Ask the Director of RT to inform staff not to bring babies on the floor.

Answer: B. The nurse should become suspicious of possible abduction when sighting a staff member carrying a baby on the oncology floor. Although the staff member may be visiting a sick family member, the nurse needs to ensure that a baby has not been taken from the nursery. Babies have been abducted by people who dress in uniform to alleviate suspicion of wrongdoing.

TEST-TAKING STRATEGY: You may find that the question does not offer a distinct correct answer. In this case, choose the most correct answer.

233. Workplace violence is a growing concern for nurses. Major causes of violence in the hospital include:

A. Realistic client and staff expectations.

B. Increasing resources for mental health care.

C. The client's understanding of the plan of care.

D. Lack of communication between nurses and clients and visitors.

Answer: D. Clients and visitors often become enraged when ignored by busy nursing staff. Unrealistic client and staff expectations can escalate violence, as can a client's misunderstanding of the care received. Mental health care resource funding is decreasing.

TEST-TAKING STRATEGY: You may find that the question does not offer a distinct correct answer. In this case, choose the most correct answer.

234. During the hospital admission process, the client informs the nurse of $25.00 cash located in the client's wallet. The nurse should:

A. Instruct the client to place the money in the bedside table for safekeeping.

B. Document the amount of money on the client's record.

C. Instruct the client to send the money home with the family.

D. Lock the money in the safe.

Answer: C. The nurse should first instruct the client to send the money home with the family. If there is no family present or the client refuses, the nurse should follow the institution's protocol regarding client valuables.

TEST-TAKING STRATEGY: Use the process of elimination to rule out incorrect answer selections to help choose the correct answer.

235. At the end of the shift, the nurse is reviewing charting information on the computer when called to a client's room to assist with turning. The nurse should:

A. Ask another nurse to watch the computer screen as the first nurse leaves to assist with turning the client.

B. Do nothing because the computer will automatically turn off.

C. Set the computer screen to screen-saver mode.

D. Exit the chart and return to the computer password screen.

Answer: D. The nurse should exit the chart and return to the computer password screen to prevent others from viewing the client's chart. The nurse should not ask another nurse to view the client's record. Leaving the screen on screen-saver mode will allow someone to view the client's chart.

TEST-TAKING STRATEGY: Use the process of elimination to rule out incorrect answer selections to help choose the correct answer.

236. A 20-year-old college student who lives in a dormitory is admitted to the emergency department with complaints of headache, nausea, vomiting, stiff neck, and a rash. The nurse should perform which action based on the information given?

A. Wear a fit-tested N95 mask when caring for the client.

B. Implement droplet precautions when caring for the client.

C. Use airborne precautions and place the client into a negative-pressure room.

D. Implement standard precautions when caring for the client.

Answer: B. *Neisseria meningitidis* is usually found in college students, jails, or anywhere there is close contact among people. Headache, nausea, vomiting, stiff neck, and a rash are signs and symptoms of meningitis. The nurse should implement droplet precautions by wearing a surgical mask and eye protection during close contact with the client until a diagnosis is made. Placing the client in a negative-pressure room is

not necessary. Standard precautions do not protect the nurse against airborne transmission of meningitis.

TEST-TAKING STRATEGY: Use the process of elimination to rule out incorrect answer selections to help choose the correct answer.

237. While the nurse performs a hospital admission assessment, the client complains of night sweats, productive cough with blood-tinged sputum, fever, and weight loss. Chest x-ray shows an upper-lobe infiltrate. The nurse should implement which precautions?

A. Standard precautions only.

B. Standard precautions and airborne precautions.

C. Standard precautions and droplet precautions.

D. Standard precautions, airborne precautions, and use of a negative-pressure room.

Answer: D. When clients are admitted with signs and symptoms of tuberculosis, the nurse should implement standard precautions, airborne precautions, and the use of a negative-pressure room. In addition, the nurse should use good hand hygiene before and after caring for the client. Droplet precautions are not used because staff should wear a fit-tested NIOSH-approved mask and not a surgical mask when caring for clients with possible tuberculosis.

TEST-TAKING STRATEGY: Look for similar answer choices and eliminate them.

238. The nurse cares for a client who takes multiple antibiotics for treatment of an infection. The microbiology laboratory informs the nurse that the client's stool is positive for *Clostridium difficile*. Which action is most appropriate for the nurse to take? Select all that apply.

A. Use standard precautions.

B. Perform hand hygiene by using alcohol hand rub before and after caring for the client.

C. Implement contact precautions.

D. Perform hand hygiene by washing hands with soap and water before and after caring for the client.

Answer: A, C, & D. Because *Clostridium difficile* is a spore (killed only by sterilization), the friction performed during washing hands with soap and water rinses organisms off the hands. The nurse should also implement standard and contact precautions to protect the client and the nurse.

TEST-TAKING STRATEGY: When answering "Select all that apply" questions, be sure and treat each answer as a true or false statement. There may be one correct answer or more.

239. The nurse cares for a client who is diagnosed with methicillin-resistant *Staphylococcus aureus* (MRSA) infection. It is important for the nurse to:

A. Perform hand hygiene after care of the client.

B. Implement droplet precautions for the client.

C. Stock the client's room with dedicated equipment including a stethoscope, thermometer, and blood pressure cuff.

D. Eliminate dairy from the client's diet.

Answer: C. The client's room should be stocked with dedicated equipment just for that client to prevent the nurse from spreading MRSA to other clients through cross-contamination. The nurse should perform hand hygiene before and after client contact. Clients who are infected with MRSA should be placed on contact precautions. Eliminating dairy from the client's diet is not necessary.

TEST-TAKING STRATEGY: You may find that the question does not offer a distinct correct answer. In this case, choose the most correct answer.

240. The nurse cares for a client who recently delivered a baby. The client has a 10-mm reaction to a tuberculin (TB) skin test as measured on her left arm. The client does not have any symptoms, and chest x-ray is negative. The baby develops respiratory distress and is placed in the neonatal intensive care unit. The nurse should:

A. Place the mother on airborne precautions.

B. Place the baby on airborne precautions.

C. Leave the mother and baby in a regular, non-isolated hospital room.

D. Place a mask on the mother to prevent infecting the baby during visitation.

Answer: C. Since the mother had a negative chest x-ray, the mother probably is infected with TB. However, TB infection is not contagious. Only TB disease is infectious as evidenced by an abnormal chest x-ray showing upper lobe infiltrate, cavitation, or consolidation. Additionally, the mother does not have any signs or symptoms of active TB. The mother and baby do not need to be in isolation or on airborne precautions.

TEST-TAKING STRATEGY: Look for similar answer choices and eliminate them.

241. The nurse should implement which precautions for a client who has scabies?

A. Standard precautions only.

B. Contact precautions only.

C. Standard precautions and contact precautions.

D. No precautions are required.

Answer: C. Clients with scabies are highly contagious, requiring standard precautions and contact precautions. Gowns and gloves should be worn, and hand hygiene performed before and after client contact. Dedicated equipment must be placed in the client's room to prevent cross-contamination.

TEST-TAKING STRATEGY: Be wary of definitive terms like *only, always,* and *never.* These absolutes rarely if ever apply to nursing practice.

242. The nurse cares for a client diagnosed with HIV whose chest x-ray results are abnormal. The nurse suspects tuberculosis (TB). Which precautions should the nurse implement when caring for this client?

A. Standard precautions only.

B. Standard precautions and airborne precautions.

C. Standard precautions and droplet precautions.

D. Contact precautions only.

Answer: B. Clients who are HIV positive with an abnormal chest x-ray should be placed in isolation until tuberculosis (TB) has been ruled out. The nurse should implement standard precautions and airborne precautions to protect the client, family, and staff.

TEST-TAKING STRATEGY: Be wary of definitive terms like *only, always,* and *never.* These absolutes rarely if ever apply to nursing practice.

243. The pediatric nurse cares for a client diagnosed with cytomegalovirus (CMV). The nurse should take which precautions?

    A. Droplet precautions.

    B. Pediatric precautions.

    C. Standard precautions.

    D. Contact precautions.

    Answer: C. Using standard precautions with all clients is recommended to prevent transmission of any type of infection, including CMV.

    TEST-TAKING STRATEGY: You may find that the question does not offer a distinct correct answer. In this case, choose the most correct answer.

244. The home health nurse administers directly observed therapy (DOT) to a client who was diagnosed with pulmonary *Mycobacterium tuberculosis* (MTB) 9 days ago. At that time the client was started on TB chemotherapy regimen. Which personal protective equipment (PPE) should the nurse wear when making her first intake visit at the client's home?

    A. Eye shield and gloves.

    B. A surgical mask.

    C. No PPE is required.

    D. A fit-tested respirator.

    Answer: D. The client is considered contagious. Anyone coming in contact with the client must wear a fit-tested respirator until the client has three negative sputum smears, shows improvement in symptoms and chest x-ray, or has been on therapy for at least 2 weeks.

    TEST-TAKING STRATEGY: Use the process of elimination to rule out incorrect answer selections to help choose the correct answer.

245. Which statement describes the proper technique the nurse should implement for hand hygiene? Select all that apply.

    A. Wash hands with soap and water vigorously for at least 5 seconds, using friction covering all surfaces of the hand.

    B. Perform hand hygiene when hands are visibly soiled with an alcohol hand rub.

    C. Perform hand hygiene before and after direct contact with the client.

    D. Perform hand hygiene after touching a contaminated body area and before moving to a clean body area.

    Answer: C & D. The nurse should perform hand hygiene before and after direct contact with the client. Also, hand hygiene is performed after touching a contaminated body area and before moving to a clean body area. Hand-washing with soap and water should occur for at least 10 to 15 seconds and when hands are visibly soiled. An alcohol hand rub may be used when hands are contaminated but not visibly soiled.

    TEST-TAKING STRATEGY: When answering "Select all that apply" questions, be sure and treat each answer as a true or false statement. There may be one correct answer or more.

246. While performing a physical assessment, the nurse notices that the client has pustules on the arm from intravenous drug abuse. Cultures are taken of the pustules. The microbiology laboratory informs the nurse that the cultures are growing methicillin-resistant *Staphylococcus aureus* (MRSA). Which action should the nurse take? Select all that apply.

    A. Isolate the client immediately to prevent the spread of infection.

    B. Inform the client to remain in the room until the physician deems the infection cleared.

    C. Instruct the client on the importance of hand hygiene when leaving the room.

    D. Contain the pustules to prevent drainage from contaminating the environment.

    Answer: C & D. In a behavioral health situation such as drug abuse, client activities are important for recovery. Usually these clients are ambulatory and isolation is not necessary. It is important that the nurse instruct the client on proper hand hygiene when leaving the room to prevent the spread of infection. Covering the pustules prevents wound drainage from contaminating the environment. If the client refuses to follow instructions, then isolation precautions are warranted.

TEST-TAKING STRATEGY: When answering "Select all that apply" questions, be sure and treat each answer as a true or false statement. There may be one correct answer or more.

247. A client has a past history of vancomycin-resistant *Enterococcus* (VRE). The nurse knows that for isolation precautions to be discontinued for this client, which must occur?

A. The client must no longer complain of headache.

B. Results from rectal swab testing must be negative for 3 weeks.

C. Chest x-ray must be negative for infiltrates.

D. Nothing, because the client will have VRE indefinitely.

Answer: B. Clients diagnosed with VRE should be placed on isolation precautions. Before discontinuing isolation precautions, rectal swabs should be obtained once weekly for 3 weeks. Results for each swab should be negative prior to discontinuing isolation precautions. Headache and chest x-ray results do not impact discontinuation of isolation precautions in this scenario.

TEST-TAKING STRATEGY: Use the process of elimination to rule out incorrect answer selections to help choose the correct answer.

248. A client is diagnosed with *Mycobacterium tuberculosis* (MTB) and is placed in a negative-pressure room. Which compromises the negative pressure in the client's room? Select all that apply.

A. An open door.

B. An open window.

C. A shower.

D. An open vent.

Answer: A & B. In order for negative pressure to be established, the door and window must be kept closed and the vents inside the room must be opened. Negative pressure is used to prevent the air inside the room from flowing out into the hallway.

TEST-TAKING STRATEGY: When answering "Select all that apply" questions, be sure and treat each answer as a true or false statement. There may be one correct answer or more.

249. A client is placed on contact precautions. A dietary worker brings the client's lunch using regular dishes. The nurse's first reaction should be:

A. Send the tray back to the dietary department and request the dishes be replaced with disposables

B. Allow the client to eat the lunch.

C. Notify the nurse manager immediately.

D. Prevent the dietary tray from being taken into the client's room.

Answer: B. Clients placed on contact precautions can eat from regular dishes. Disposable dishes are not required, because during the cleaning of the dishes, the water temperature is high enough to kill dangerous organisms.

TEST-TAKING STRATEGY: Questions that ask you to prioritize your nursing actions use terms like *priority, first, best, initial, most important, immediate,* and *next.*

250. A client who has been on contact precautions during hospitalization is discharged. Environmental services performs cleaning of the room prior to admission of another client. Which action applies in cleaning an isolation room? Select all that apply.

A. The floor should be stripped of wax and a new coat placed on the floor.

B. All rooms should be cleaned in the same manner.

C. Surfaces that come in close contact with the client should be thoroughly cleaned.

D. Environmental cultures should be taken after the room is cleaned to ensure cleaning of the room.

Answer: B & C. All rooms should be cleaned in the same manner, because clients can be infected with organisms without staff knowledge. Surfaces that come in close contact with the client, such as bed-rails, telephones, bedside tables, and faucet handles, should be thoroughly cleaned. Environmental cultures are not necessary unless there is epidemiological evidence that transmission occurs due to the environment.

TEST-TAKING STRATEGY: When answering "Select all that apply" questions, be sure and treat each answer as a true or false statement. There may be one correct answer or more.

251. The critical-care nurse performs active surveillance cultures on all client admissions. Which is an example of an active surveillance culture?

    A. Culture of the client's room for vancomycin-resistant *enterococcus* (VRE).

    B. Culture of the client's room for methicillin-resistant *Staphylococcus aureus* (MRSA).

    C. Culture of the client for VRE and MRSA.

    D. Culture of the client's equipment for VRE and MRSA.

Answer: C. Active surveillance cultures are used to identify clients who may be infected or colonized with organisms. These clients are placed into isolation immediately to prevent the transmission of multidrug-resistant organisms such as MRSA and VRE.

TEST-TAKING STRATEGY: Look for similar answer choices and eliminate them.

252. The nurse cares for a client who is diagnosed with methicillin-resistant *Staphylococcus aureus* (MRSA) and is placed in isolation. The nurse needs to perform an assessment of the client's wound and administer prescribed medications to the client. The nurse should wear which personal protective equipment (PPE)?

    A. Gown and gloves.

    B. Gloves only.

    C. Gown, gloves, and mask.

    D. Gown only.

Answer: C. The nurse should wear a gown to prevent contamination of clothing, gloves to prevent contamination of hands, and a mask to prevent touching and colonizing the nose with MRSA.

TEST-TAKING STRATEGY: Be wary of definitive terms like *only, always,* and *never.* These absolutes rarely if ever apply to nursing practice.

253. The nurse cares for a client who has undergone a bone marrow transplant. While the nurse assesses the client's IV site, the client's sister complains of a low-grade fever. The nurse should:

    A. Encourage the sister to wash hands frequently while visiting.

    B. Encourage the sister to seek medical attention.

    C. Encourage the sister to go home.

    D. Encourage the sister to wear a mask while visiting.

Answer: C. The nurse should inform the sister to go home because clients who undergo bone marrow transplant are severely immuno-compromised. The sister's low-grade fever is an indication of illness that could easily be transmitted to the client. The sister may resume visiting when the fever has subsided.

TEST-TAKING STRATEGY: Use the process of elimination to rule out incorrect answer selections to help choose the correct answer.

254. A client is admitted to the hospital with influenza. Which action should the nurse take when caring for this client?

    A. Put the client on droplet precautions.

    B. Put the client on airborne precautions in a negative-pressure room.

    C. No special precautions are needed for this client.

    D. Wear an N95 fit-tested mask.

Answer: A. The nurse should place the client on droplet precautions because influenza is spread via droplets. Airborne precautions, an N95 fit-tested mask, and a negative-pressure room are not necessary in caring for a client with influenza. The nurse should wear a surgical mask and wash hands before and after contact with the client and the client's environment.

TEST-TAKING STRATEGY: Use the process of elimination to rule out incorrect answer selections to help choose the correct answer.

255. In which order should the nurse remove personal protective equipment (PPE)?

A. Mask, gloves, goggles, gown.

B. Goggles, mask, gloves, gown.

C. Gloves, goggles, gown, mask.

D. Gown, mask, gloves, goggles.

Answer: C. The sequence for removing PPE is intended to limit opportunities for self-contamination. The gloves are considered the most contaminated pieces of PPE and are removed first. Goggles or face shields are next, because they are the most cumbersome and interfere with the removal of other PPE. The gown is next, followed by the mask or respirator. PPE should be removed inside of the client's room, with the exception of the respirator, which needs to be removed outside of the client's room to prevent breathing in airborne contaminants.

TEST-TAKING STRATEGY: Use the process of elimination to rule out incorrect answer selections to help choose the correct answer.

256. The nurse cares for a client with a history of falls and who continues to attempt to get out of bed. The family is not able to sit with the client, and medications are ineffective in calming the client. After all efforts are exhausted, it is determined restraints are needed. Which action should the nurse take first?

A. Notify physician to obtain an order for restraints.

B. Place the restraints on the client as soon as possible.

C. Assess limb strength for restraint use.

D. Notify the nursing supervisor of the client's need for restraints.

Answer: A. The nurse should notify the physician first to obtain an order for restraints. Next, the nurse should don the restraints and notify staff of the presence of restraints. Assessing limb strength is not a requirement for restraints.

TEST-TAKING STRATEGY: Questions that ask you to prioritize your nursing actions use terms like *priority, first, best, initial, most important, immediate,* and *next.*

257. An elderly client with severe dementia is not able to communicate the most basic needs. How may the nurse improve the client's comfort? Select all that apply.

A. Assess the client for pain on a regular basis.

B. Establish a toileting schedule for the client.

C. Increase observation of the client.

D. All four side-rails engaged.

Answer: A, B, & C. Establishing a toileting schedule, administering pain medication as scheduled or as needed, and increasing observation of the client, can enhance healing and promote comfort. Having all four side-rails engaged is considered a restraint and requires a physician order.

TEST-TAKING STRATEGY: When answering "Select all that apply" questions, be sure and treat each answer as a true or false statement. There may be one correct answer or more.

258. When implementing restraints, nurses should:

A. Choose the least restrictive device.

B. Assess the client's response every 2 hours.

C. Remove the restraint every hour.

D. Renew the physician order for the restraints every 48 hours after evaluation.

Answer: A. The nurse should choose the least restrictive device when restraining a client. Side-rails are less restrictive than arm or leg restraints. The client's response to restraints should be assessed every hour; the restraints should be removed every 2 hours; and the physician order for restraints should be renewed every 24 hours after evaluation.

TEST-TAKING STRATEGY: Use the process of elimination to rule out incorrect answer selections to help choose the correct answer.

259. Which statement most accurately describes the use of restraints?

   A. The potential to discontinue or reduce restraint use should be considered every 8 hours.

   B. Clients should be monitored for the development of complications from restraint use at every shift.

   C. New orders should be written after 36 hours if restraint use is to be continued.

   D. Restraints should be used prior to medicating the client.

Answer: A. The potential to discontinue or reduce restraint use should be considered every 8 hours. The client should not be left in restraints any longer than absolutely necessary. The client should be monitored for the development of complications from restraint use every 4 hours. New orders should be written every 24 hours if restraint use is to be continued. Physical restraint is the last option for maintaining client safety. Medications may be tried prior to physically restraining a client.

TEST-TAKING STRATEGY: Terms like *most appropriately* and *most accurately* mean that the undeniable correct answer is most likely not present. Therefore, you must select the best answer choice from the selections provided.

260. A client becomes violent and is in need of restraint. After all efforts to prevent the use of restraints are exhausted, the physician orders a vest restraint. While applying the vest restraint, the nurse should:

   A. Assess the client for proper fit of the vest.

   B. Place the client in prone position while administering the vest.

   C. Secure the straps tightly to ensure the client's safety.

   D. Tie the strap to the top of the bed to ensure the client is unable to wiggle out of the restraint.

Answer: A. The client should be assessed for proper fit of the vest. If the vest does not fit properly, a different size should be obtained. A client is never to be placed face down in a restraint. The straps should be secured loosely and placed in a manner that can be released quickly and easily in an emergency. The straps should never be tied to the top of the bed because this could cause hanging of the client.

TEST-TAKING STRATEGY: Look for similar answer choices and eliminate them.

261. An order is written to restrain a client that is thrashing in the bed. Which type of restraint should the nurse choose for this client?

   A. Leather restraint.

   B. Metal handcuffs.

   C. Kerlix bandage.

   D. Plastic handcuffs.

Answer: C. Thick roller bandages (Kling or Kerlix) work well in restraining a client and do not cause harm to the client. Metal or plastic handcuffs and leather restraints may cause injury to the client.

TEST-TAKING STRATEGY: Always pick the nursing intervention that is most helpful to or safe for the client.

262. During a visit to the emergency department, a client requires physical restraint to prevent harm to the staff. Which method effectively disables the client's ability to use the abdominal muscles?

   A. Restrain both arms together.

   B. Restrain one arm up and one arm down.

   C. Restrain the right arm to the right side-rail and the left arm to the left side-rail of the stretcher.

   D. Restrain the right arm to the right side-rail and the left arm to the left side-rail of the stretcher.

Answer: B. Position the client to limit strength and range of motion. Restraint with one arm up and one arm down disables the client's ability to use the abdominal muscles to resist restraint procedures.

TEST-TAKING STRATEGY: Look for similar answer choices and eliminate them.

263. The nurse admits a client to the hospital who was involved in an automobile accident. Upon assessment, the nurse notes the client is wearing soft restraints. The client continues to be combative and is compromising the airway. Which type of restraint is most appropriate for this client?

    A. Chemical restraint.

    B. Physical restraint.

    C. Leather restraint.

    D. Mechanical restraint.

    Answer: A. Chemical restraint should be used for restraining a violent and combative client who presents a danger to themselves or others. Chemical restraint prevents clients from further injury caused by physical restraints.

    TEST-TAKING STRATEGY: Terms like *most appropriate* and *most accurate* mean that the undeniable correct answer is most likely not present. Therefore, you must select the best answer choice.

264. A client is given haloperidol (Haldol) as a form of chemical restraint. During physical assessment, the client has a blood pressure of 80/50 mm Hg, heart rate of 120 beats/minute, and experiences an acute dystonic reaction. Which statement is most accurate?

    A. The client is experiencing a side effect of haloperidol (Haldol).

    B. The nurse should administer furosemide (Lenadryl) to treat the dystonic reaction.

    C. The nurse should monitor the client for increased excitability.

    D. The nurse should turn the client to the left side to increase blood flow.

    Answer: A. Side effects of Haldol include hypotension, tachycardia, and acute dystonic reaction (distorted twisting of the body). Dystonic reaction is treated with Benadryl 25 to 50 mg IM or IV. The client should be monitored for increased sedation. Turning the client to the left side does not resolve side effects of Haldol.

    TEST-TAKING STRATEGY: Terms like *most appropriate* and *most accurate* mean that the undeniable correct answer is most likely not present. Therefore, you must select the best answer choice.

265. The nurse cares for a 15-year-old who is placed in restraints due to combative behavior. Based on this information, which statement is correct?

    A. Evaluation of restraint reorders should be conducted every 12 hours since the client is a youth.

    B. Evaluation of the youth in restraints should be conducted every 4 hours.

    C. It is against the law to chemically or physically restrain a youth.

    D. A family member must be present while the youth is placed in physical restraints.

    Answer: B. Evaluation of the youth in restraints is the same as an adult in restraints: every 4 hours. Evaluation of restraint reorders should be conducted every 24 hours for youths and adults alike. It is not against the law to restrain youths, nor must a family member be present while physical restraints are placed on the youth.

    TEST-TAKING STRATEGY: Use the process of elimination to rule out incorrect answer selections to help choose the correct answer.

266. When applying soft arm and leg restraints to a client, the nurse should (select all that apply):

    A. Apply the limb restraint above the IV site.

    B. Secure all four restraints to the same side of the bed.

    C. Tie the restraint to immovable parts of the bed.

    D. Maintain the client in supine position.

    Answer: C & D. The restraint must be tied to an immovable part of the bed to prevent injury to the client. Tying a restraint above an IV site could cause the IV to occlude or infiltrate. Restraints should not be secured to one side of the bed for safety reasons. The client must remain in supine, not prone, position.

TEST-TAKING STRATEGY: When answering "Select all that apply" questions, be sure and treat each answer as a true or false statement. There may be one correct answer or more.

267. The physician orders a urinary catheter for the client stat. After gathering supplies, which action should the nurse take first?

    A. Lower the bed to prevent injury to the client.

    B. Adjust the bed to a workable position.

    C. Place both side-rails up to prevent the client from falling out of bed.

    D. Place the items to be used for the procedure on the bed.

    Answer: B. The height of the bed should be at a workable position to prevent back injury to the nurse. Stretching over raised side-rails to perform the procedure can cause injury to the nurse. The items can be placed on the bed but only after the bed and client are positioned. This prevents the equipment from being knocked to the floor.

    TEST-TAKING STRATEGY: Questions that ask you to prioritize your nursing actions use terms like *priority, first, best, initial, most important, immediate,* and *next.*

268. The nurse cares for an obese paraplegic client. The client needs to be repositioned in the bed. In order to position the client, the nurse should (select all that apply):

    A. Obtain assistance from a co-worker.

    B. Place the bed in the lowest position.

    C. Adjust the bed to a workable position and move close to the client.

    D. Use a draw sheet with the assistance of a co-worker and pivot the hips while pulling the draw sheet upward.

    Answer: A, C, & D. The nurse should solicit a co-worker for help; adjust the bed to a workable position; move close to the client; use a draw sheet with the assistance of a co-worker, and pivot the hips while pulling the draw sheet upward. These steps will prevent injury to the nurse and client.

    TEST-TAKING STRATEGY: When answering "Select all that apply" questions, be sure and treat each answer as a true or false statement. There may be one correct answer or more.

269. While preparing to move a client higher up on the stretcher, the nurse should first:

    A. Move the bed into a workable position.

    B. Place a draw sheet under the client.

    C. Lock the stretcher.

    D. Reposition the client.

    Answer: C. The stretcher should be locked prior to taking other steps to reposition the client. Locking the stretcher ensures the safety of both the client and the nurse.

    TEST-TAKING STRATEGY: Questions that ask you to prioritize your nursing actions use terms like *priority, first, best, initial, most important, immediate,* and *next.*

270. The nurse prepares to assist the client from a wheelchair to the bed. Which action should the nurse take when assisting the client? Select all that apply.

    A. Use the back muscles to aid lifting.

    B. Bend the back to prevent injury.

    C. Bend the arms to keep the client close to the nurse.

    D. Lock the wheelchair.

    Answer: C & D. Constant abuse of the spine from moving and lifting clients is the leading cause of injury to nurses. The nurse should lift using the legs instead of the back and should bend the legs, not the back when lifting. The leg muscles are stronger than the back muscles. The client should be kept close to the nurse's body as the nurse bends the arms. This puts less strain on the back when moving a client.

    TEST-TAKING STRATEGY: When answering "Select all that apply" questions, be sure and treat each answer as a true or false statement. There may be one correct answer or more.

271. Elderly clients who take several medications are at risk for adverse drug reactions and interactions. The most important nursing action to prevent such risk is:

A. Implementing a thorough client assessment.

B. Instructing the client about adverse drug reactions.

C. Explaining to the client that approximately 12% of hospital admissions of older adults are due to a drug reaction.

D. Teaching the client that the chances of adverse drug reactions are directly proportional to the number of medications taken.

Answer: A. To prevent complications of medication administration, such as adverse drug reactions and interactions, careful planning is a priority. A thorough assessment of the client is vital when planning care. Instructing the client about adverse drug reactions, explaining the prevalence of drug reactions in the elderly, and teaching the client that risk increases with the number of medications taken are true statements that support client education.

TEST-TAKING STRATEGY: Home in on the key words in the stem like "most important." Then eliminate the incorrect answers while focusing on the answer that provides information or an action that is the most important.

272. An adult client presents with a new onset of a chronic disease. The nurse can benefit the client most by:

A. Teaching the client that the disease will never resolve.

B. Instructing the client that lifestyle changes must be made.

C. Treating the client as a competent manager of the disease.

D. Encouraging the client to prepare for custodial care.

Answer: C. Viewing the client as a manager of care demonstrates respect for the client, dispels stereotyping, and establishes trust between client and caregiver. A chronic disease will not resolve, but may be managed. Often, lifestyle changes are necessary when disease develops, but there are instances when this is not applicable. Many chronic diseases can be managed without the need for custodial care, especially at the onset.

TEST-TAKING STRATEGY: Home in on the key words in the stem like "most." Then eliminate the incorrect answers while focusing on the answer that provides information or an action that is the most beneficial.

273. The older client who lives in a rural setting is most likely to (select all that apply):

A. Exhibit healthy behaviors.

B. Experience longevity.

C. Be underserved by health care workers.

D. Fail to engage in health-promoting activities.

Answer: C & D. The average client living in a rural setting experiences geographic isolation and a higher level of poverty than those living in metropolitan or suburban areas. Health care access is diminished by the lower number of health care workers in a rural setting and the decreased availability of public transportation. This limits health screening, frequent client–physician counseling, and early detection of disease. The client living in a rural area is more likely to engage in activities that do not promote health, such as smoking and driving without a seatbelt.

TEST-TAKING STRATEGY: In "select all that apply" questions, there may be more than one correct answers. Terms like *most likely* mean that the undeniably correct answer is probably not present. Therefore, you must select the best answer from the choices presented.

274. Ageism is a negative attitude toward older adults. To prevent ageism when working with older adult clients, the nurse should:

A. Have knowledge about normal aging while maintaining contact with healthy, independent, older clients.

B. Speak slowly with increased volume while providing educational pamphlets and brochures.

C. Limit the client's activities to prevent injury and promote rest.

D. Involve the family in decision-making and financial concerns.

Answer: A. By understanding the normal aging process and being familiar with older clients, the nurse avoids ageism. Myths and stereotypes are often supported by media reports of needy, problematic, older clients. Such misconceptions may lead to errors in assessment and unnecessary limitation to interventions. Speaking slowly with increased volume, limiting client activity, and involving the family in decision-making and financial concerns are inappropriate.

TEST-TAKING STRATEGY: Read the question twice to ensure that you understand what the question is asking, especially if the question is tricky or confusing. Focus on what the question is asking: preventing ageism.

275. Cellular damage related to oxidative stress (free radicals) is associated with degenerative diseases that affect older clients, such as atherosclerosis and cancer. Antioxidants may slow the oxidative process. The client obtains benefit from antioxidants by:

    A. Avoiding harmful substances such as tobacco smoke and radiation.

    B. Taking a multivitamin daily and eating a balanced diet.

    C. Engaging in regular exercise and physical activity.

    D. Maintaining a normal body weight.

Answer: B. Several vitamins—such as A, C, E, β-carotene, selenium, and lycopene—are just some of the antioxidants found in a multivitamin and a balanced diet rich in colorful fruits and vegetables. Antioxidants capture the free radial, an electron emitted as part of the cellular process of oxidation, thus limiting cellular damage. Although avoiding harmful substances, exercising regularly, and maintaining a normal body weight are all beneficial lifestyle goals, they do not answer the question directly.

TEST-TAKING STRATEGY: Read the question twice to ensure that you understand what the question is asking, especially if the question is tricky or confusing. Focus on what the question is asking: the benefits of antioxidants, not the benefits of lifestyle changes.

276. A client with gestational diabetes delivers a macrosomic infant. The nurse understands that the most vital component of the infant's assessment is:

    A. Evaluation of the infant for tethered spinal cord.

    B. Determining if the infant sustained a clavicle fracture.

    C. Observing for arm movement to evaluate for Erb's palsy.

    D. Frequent blood glucose monitoring to ensure stable values.

Answer: D. Infants of diabetic mothers are at risk for hypoglycemia following birth. Hypoglycemia can trigger seizures, hearing impairment, and cognitive deficits. Assessing for clavicle fracture, Erb's palsy, and tethered cord are important in macrosomic infants, but not as vital as ensuring stable glucose levels.

TEST-TAKING STRATEGY: Questions that ask you to prioritize your nursing actions use terms like *priority, first, best, initial, most important, most vital,* and *next.* Terms like *most vital* mean that the undeniably correct answer is probably not present. Therefore, you must select the best answer choice available.

277. A pregnant client is admitted to the hospital. On initial assessment the client is determined to be febrile. The nurse should:

    A. Administer aspirin, an antipyretic agent.

    B. Ascertain simultaneous and separate fetal and maternal heart rates.

    C. Hydrate the mother by infusing intravenous fluids.

    D. Institute isolation procedures until the etiology of the fever is determined.

Answer: B. Fetal and maternal heart rate determination is part of the admission process and initial assessment. The mother may be tachycardic as a result of the fever, and her elevated heart rate may be misinterpreted as the fetal heart rate. Simultaneous and separate fetal and maternal heart rate determinations ensure accuracy. Medications and intravenous fluids require a physician's order. Isolation may be considered for a client with a fever of unknown origin.

TEST-TAKING STRATEGY: Questions that ask you to prioritize your nursing actions use terms like *priority, first, best, initial, most important,* and *next.*

278. A client is determined to be newly pregnant and is prescribed prenatal vitamins by the physician. The nurse knows further teaching is necessary when the client states:

A. "My husband is not the father of this baby."

B. "My first baby was perfectly normal."

C. "I eat a balanced diet. I don't need vitamins."

D. "I only eat organic foods. Are vitamins organic?"

Answer: C. Although eating a balanced diet is commendable, it is not generally achieved 100% of the time. In addition, the growing fetus imposes further nutritional requirements on the mother. Prenatal vitamins help to meet the nutritional requirements of the mother and fetus, thus preventing deficiencies and some anomalies such as neural tube defects. The fact that the client's husband is not the father of the baby is not applicable to the test question. The statements regarding the first baby's health and the organic diet do not require further teaching by the nurse.

TEST-TAKING STRATEGY: Determine which action will bring the most harm or help to the client. This helps determine the highest nursing priority. The phrase "further teaching is necessary" tells you to select an answer with inaccurate information.

279. A pregnant client in labor receives an epidural and anesthetic for pain control. The most important, initial nursing action is to:

A. Perform a thorough skin prep of the insertion site.

B. Obtain the client's consent for the procedure.

C. Assure the client that residual effects of the procedure won't be felt.

D. Monitor maternal blood pressure.

Answer: D. Epidural anesthesia may result in distal vasodilation and a precipitous drop in maternal blood pressure, which will adversely affect placental blood flow. Obtaining consent and preparing the insertion site are responsibilities of the physician. Residual effects of epidural anesthesia include infection and headache.

TEST-TAKING STRATEGY: Determine which action will bring the most harm or help to the client. This helps determine the highest nursing priority. Choose the answer selection that is the most life threatening or harmful to the client.

280. A pregnant client in labor is placed on an external fetal monitor. Later, the fetal strip shows late fetal heart decelerations. The nurse should (select all that apply):

A. Turn the client to the left side and administer oxygen.

B. Start an intravenous line.

C. Prep the mother for caesarian section.

D. Notify the physician.

Answer: A & D. Late fetal heart rate decelerations are associated with fetal hypoxia and acidosis. Positioning the mother on her left side prevents compression of the vena cava. Oxygen administration increases maternal, then fetal blood levels, thus treating current and preventing further development of hypoxia and acidosis. Failure to recognize fetal monitoring strip abnormalities and failure to report abnormalities to the physician are deviations from the standard of care.

TEST-TAKING STRATEGY: In "select all that apply" questions, there may be more than one correct answer. Determine which action will bring the most harm or help to the client. This helps determine the highest nursing priority.

281. In the office for a yearly physical examination, a 30-year-old client reports that she and her husband used to be very happy before the children were born. Now the client is struggling with the current situation. The nurse understands that:

A. The client is probably having an extramarital affair.

B. The developmental task at this stage is adjusting to the needs of more than two family members.

C. A relative or close friend should be consulted for help so the client can pursue activities outside the home.

D. The client should be referred to a psychotherapist for evaluation and care.

Answer: B. When children are born or adopted into a family, the established couple must adjust to supporting the physical and emotional needs of the additional family member. Additionally, the couple is engaged in developing an attachment with the child(ren) and coping with energy depletion and lack of privacy. These requirements may lead to a sense of unhappiness and frustration on the part of one or both parents. The answer choice that the client is having an extramarital affair is inappropriate. Although receiving assistance from family and friends is a good option, it is not the best answer choice. The client's feelings are normal and do not require the client to be referred to a psychotherapist.

TEST-TAKING STRATEGY: Use Maslow's hierarchy of needs to determine the correct answer.

282. An elderly client is approaching death and expresses intense despair and anxiety. Based on Erikson's theory of ego integrity versus despair, this client's despair and anxiety may be based on:

A. An inappropriate desire for youthfulness and staying young.

B. The decision to never marry.

C. Lack of a sense of wholeness, purpose, and a life well-lived.

D. The fear of experiencing a painful death.

Answer: C. Older adults who view their lives as purposeful and full have an increased ability to view death as a meaningful part of life. Conversely, older adults who view their lives as meaningless and full of lost opportunities view their approaching death with despair and conflict.

TEST-TAKING STRATEGY: Use Maslow's hierarchy of needs to determine the correct answer. Use the process of elimination to rule out incorrect answer selections to help choose the correct answer.

283. As individuals move through life, predictable changes occur. When the nurse assists the client in understanding these predictable changes, the client:

A. Accepts biologic aging.

B. Experiences a reduced risk of chronic illness.

C. Looks forward to retirement and "letting go" of work-related responsibility.

D. Redirects growth and goals.

Answer: D. Life structure is dynamic; individuals transition as they go through the various stages of life. These transitions present an opportunity to refocus growth toward objectives. Understanding transitions may assist the client to accept biologic aging—the progressive loss of function and acclimation to retirement. Understanding transitions may not reduce chronic illness, but may assist the client to accept and deal with it.

TEST-TAKING STRATEGY: Use Maslow's hierarchy of needs to determine the correct answer. Use the process of elimination to rule out incorrect answer selections to help choose the correct answer.

284. A 2-year-old client is seen in the clinic for a well-child visit. Which denotes an abnormal finding for an average client of this age?

A. The client pulls a toy across the room.

B. The client uses one- to two-word sentences.

C. The client shows defiant behavior.

D. The client imitates the behavior of others.

Answer: B. A 2-year-old client should demonstrate language skills using 2- to 4-word sentences. Pulling a toy, exhibiting defiant behavior, and imitating behavior are normal in the average 2-year-old.

TEST-TAKING STRATEGY: Focus on key words like *abnormal finding* in the question stem. Use the process of elimination to rule out incorrect answer selections to help choose the correct answer.

285. In young adulthood, the expected developmental tasks include:

    A. Satisfying and supporting the next generation.

    B. Formulating a sense of oneself and feeling fulfilled.

    C. Developing peer relationships.

    D. Giving and sharing with an individual without asking what will be given or shared in return.

Answer: D. In young adulthood, the developmental tasks involve intimacy versus isolation. Intimacy relates more to sharing and not sex. Intimacy produces feelings of safety, closeness, and trust. Parenting is a task of middle adulthood. During the mature stage (age 65 and above), a sense of self and fulfillment are found. Developing peer relationships occurs during adolescence.

TEST-TAKING STRATEGY: Use the process of elimination to rule out incorrect answer selections to help choose the correct answer.

286. Parents are reluctant to immunize their child. They feel that because the majority of children with whom their child will interact have been vaccinated, there is no need for their child to be immunized. The nurse:

    A. Files a report with social services.

    B. Understands that the organisms that cause disease are still prevalent in the environment and may cause illness in this child.

    C. Counsels the parents that refusal to vaccinate their child may result in legal charges.

    D. Notifies the school system that the child is not in compliance with immunization regulations.

Answer: B. With few exceptions (smallpox, polio), bacteria and viruses that cause disease have not been eradicated in the United States. An unvaccinated child is at risk for developing a vaccine preventable disease if exposed to the causative organism. Unless state law requires notification of social services when a parent refuses to have a child vaccinated, no report is made. Unless social services file neglect charges against the parents, no legal charges are warranted. The school system is responsible for verifying required immunizations.

TEST-TAKING STRATEGY: Use the process of elimination to rule out incorrect answer selections to help choose the correct answer.

287. A middle-aged client has a strong positive family history of type 2 diabetes mellitus. The best method to prevent or delay the development of this disease in this client is to:

    A. Test serum glucose values monthly.

    B. Avoid starches and sugars in the diet.

    C. Obtain a normal body weight and exercise regularly.

    D. Maintain a normal serum lipid panel.

Answer: C. Genetics and body weight are the most important factors in the development of type 2 diabetes mellitus. The client cannot alter his genetics. Therefore, a normal body weight is imperative. Regular exercise reduces insulin resistance and permits increased glucose uptake by cells. This serves to lower insulin levels and reduce hepatic production of glucose. Monthly glucose monitoring is not sufficient. Starch and sugar intake should be decreased, not avoided. Maintaining a normal serum lipid panel may not be achievable in some clients, but it is always the goal.

TEST-TAKING STRATEGY: Determine which action will bring the most help to the client.

288. At a health fair, a nurse encourages an older adult male to be screened for prostate cancer. The client is apprehensive and asks the nurse about the methods used to detect prostate cancer. The nurse explains that the detection process involves:

A. An abdominal x-ray to detect lesions and masses.

B. A serum calcium test to detect elevated levels, which may indicate bone metastasis.

C. A digital rectal exam (DRE) and prostate-specific antigen (PSA) test to evaluate the prostate.

D. A magnetic resonance image (MRI) study to detect tumors and other abnormal growths.

Answer: C. Prostate cancer is the second most common type of cancer and the second leading cause of cancer death in men. Early detection improves outcome. DRE and PSA should be offered annually beginning at age 50 to men who have a life expectancy of at least 10 years and at age 45 in high-risk groups. The DRE estimates the size, symmetry, and consistency of the prostate gland, while the PSA measures for elevated levels consistent with prostatic pathology, although not necessarily cancer. Declining PSA levels are useful in determining efficacy of treatment for prostate cancer. Radiologic studies are not screening tools for this disease. Hypercalcemia may indicate cancerous bone involvement, but is not a screening tool. MRI is a diagnostic tool, not a screening tool.

TEST-TAKING STRATEGY: Use the process of elimination to rule out incorrect answer selections to help choose the correct answer. Home in on the key words in the stem like "screening." Then eliminate the incorrect answers while focusing on the answer that provides information or an action that is the most relevant.

289. As a nurse working in a chronic obstructive pulmonary disease (COPD) clinic, you advise clients daily about health care matters. The most important factor in prevention and treatment of COPD is:

A. Controlling asthma.

B. Receiving an influenza shot annually.

C. Taking a daily multivitamin containing antioxidants.

D. Ceasing cigarette smoking.

Answer: D. Cigarette smoking is the major risk factor for developing COPD. Clinically significant airway obstruction (inflammation, edema, increased mucus production, and diminished ciliary activity) is followed by a long period of debilitation, then death. The disease process is reversible if smoking cessation occurs early. The disease process is halted if smoking cessation occurs later. Controlling asthma, receiving flu vaccination, and taking a daily multivitamin are all positive measures in preventing and treating COPD, but they are not the most important factor.

TEST-TAKING STRATEGY: Home in on the key words in the stem like "most important." Then eliminate the incorrect answers while focusing on the answer that provides information or an action that is the most important. Choose the answer selection that is the most life threatening or harmful to the client.

290. The most effective method to decrease morbidity and mortality of stroke is prevention. What is the most effective method of stroke prevention?

A. Administering platelet inhibitors to prevent clot formation.

B. Undergoing transluminal angioplasty to open a stenosed artery and improve blood flow.

C. Maintaining normal weight, exercising, and controlling co-morbid conditions.

D. Administering tissue plasminogen activator (tPA).

Answer: C. Although administering platelet inhibitors and tPA and undergoing transluminal angioplasty may improve cerebral blood flow, the best stroke prevention includes controlling obesity and its co-morbidities, such as hypertension and type 2 diabetes mellitus. Exercise improves cardiac function and helps lower serum lipids and glucose levels.

TEST-TAKING STRATEGY: Home in on the key words in the stem like "most important." Then eliminate the incorrect answers while focusing on the answer that provides information or an action that is the most important.

291. New parents ask the nurse how to predict the adult height of their new baby. The nurse knows that the major factors that determine adult height are:

A. Intrauterine growth and maternal health.

B. Chromosome abnormalities in the parents.

C. Genetics and chronic illness.

D. Parental genetics and nutrition.

Answer: **D.** Genetics that influence parental growth and development are inherited by the infant. Nutrition is a major factor in growth after birth. Before birth, the size of the baby is related to maternal influences such as age, health, and diet. By age 2 years, the genetic effects of both parents becomes evident. A simple formula to calculate predicted adult height is: Add the height of both parents (in centimeters) and divide by 2. Add 7 centimeters for a boy. Subtract 7 centimeters for a girl. Malnutrition, chronic illness, and chromosome abnormalities lead to poor somatic growth.

TEST-TAKING STRATEGY: Home in on the key words in the stem like "major factors." Then eliminate the incorrect answers while focusing on the answer that provides information or an action that are major factors.

292. A 10-year-old female client is seen in the clinic. The client's mother asks the nurse when puberty will begin and what corresponding signs will be evident. The nurse replies:

A. "It is difficult to predict since each child develops at her own rate."

B. "Your daughter should already have breast buds and sparse genital hair."

C. "Between ages 10 and 14 years, expect papilla elevation and short 'peach fuzz' genital hair."

D. "The average age for puberty is approximately 11 years old. Breast buds, enlarged aerolae, and a small amount of pigmented labial hair are typically seen."

Answer: **D.** Females enter stage 2 of Tanner development on average at 10.9 years of age. Evidence of this maturation includes palpable breast buds, enlargement of aerolae, and sparse, coarse, pigmented hair predominately on the labia. Elevation of papilla and "peach fuzz" genital hair are normal characteristics of stage 1 Tanner development (prepubertial).

TEST-TAKING STRATEGY: Use the process of elimination to rule out incorrect answer selections to help choose the correct answer.

293. A 40-year-old client is curious about visible appearance changes related to menopause. In general, menopausal clients experience:

A. Bone loss and fractures.

B. Loss of muscle mass and increased fat tissue.

C. Improved skin tugor and elasticity.

D. A reduction in waist size.

Answer: **B.** Visible changes associated with menopause include loss of muscle mass, increased fat tissue leading to a thicker waist, dryness of the skin and vagina, hot flashes, sleep abnormalities, and mood changes. Bone loss is dependent on bone mass, weight-bearing exercise, and nutrition. Some bone loss may occur, but may not lead to fractures.

TEST-TAKING STRATEGY: Use the process of elimination to rule out incorrect answer selections to help choose the correct answer.

294. A client reports a diminished ability to visually focus on close objects and has also noticed a need for a well-lit environment to enhance vision. The nurse is aware that:

A. These are normal changes associated with aging.

B. A cataract is the likely etiology for these symptoms.

C. This client may be experiencing symptoms of a brain tumor.

D. These changes are precipitated by diabetic retinopathy.

Answer: A. Aging results in stiffening of the lens, thus lessening the ability to focus. The retina is less sensitive to light, making accurate vision in low-light situations more difficult. Pupillary response diminishes affecting the ability to adjust to changing light levels. Cataracts present with blurred vision and a glare from lights. Brain tumors increase intracranial pressure, resulting in blurring of vision. Diabetic retinopathy is caused by changes in retinal blood vessels and results in blurred vision and outright impairment in some fields.

TEST-TAKING STRATEGY: Use the process of elimination to rule out incorrect answer selections to help choose the correct answer.

295. A pregnant client comes to the clinic with complaint of hemorrhoids and constipation. The nurse explains (select all that apply):

A. Increased rectal pressure from the gravid uterus may result in hemorrhoids.

B. Hormones decrease maternal GI motility resulting in constipation.

C. The client needs more fluid and fiber in the diet.

D. A mild laxative is recommended to alleviate constipation.

Answer: A, B, & C. As pregnancy progresses, the enlarging uterus increases abdominal and rectal pressure. GI motility slows due to hormonal influences. Pregnant clients may benefit significantly from dietary changes including adequate hydration and increased fiber intake. Medications, including laxatives, should not be taken by pregnant women unless prescribed by the physician. If needed, the physician may prescribe a stool softener, but rarely a laxative because of possible fluid and electrolyte shifts.

TEST-TAKING STRATEGY: In "select all that apply" questions, there may be one or more than one correct answer. Determine which action will bring the most help to the client. This helps determine the highest nursing priority.

296. A female client comes to the family planning clinic. The client is a smoker and doubts her ability to stop smoking. The nurse recommends which form of birth control based on the client's history?

A. Female sterilization.

B. Depo-Provera injection.

C. Oral contraceptive pills.

D. The Ortho Evra patch.

Answer: B. Depo-Provera is a synthetic progesterone injection taken every 3 months. It prevents pregnancy by stopping ovulation and increasing the thickness of cervical mucous to block sperm entry into the uterus. This agent can be used in clients who smoke while other hormones are not recommended for smokers.

TEST-TAKING STRATEGY: Use the process of elimination to rule out incorrect answer selections to help choose the correct answer.

297. A female client comes to the student health clinic with concerns about unprotected sex experienced last night. The nurse:

A. Reassures the client that the chances of pregnancy are exceedingly small and that the client should not worry.

B. Asks the client to return to clinic if she experiences a missed menstrual period.

C. Obtains a pregnancy test on the client.

D. Knows that emergency contraception is an option to prevent pregnancy.

Answer: D. Emergency contraception (EC) consists of taking high-dose oral progestin pills as soon after unprotected sex as possible. EC is most effective within 12 hours, but may be administered up to 72 hours after unprotected intercourse. EC interferes with egg development, prevents ovulation, and inhibits fertilization. It does not terminate an already established pregnancy. EC is marketed under the trade name Plan B in the United States. Reassurance and delay in treatment may be harmful, not helpful, to the client. A pregnancy test is not warranted.

TEST-TAKING STRATEGY: Never delay treatment. Choose an answer that addresses the client's problem immediately.

298. A male client and his partner have decided not to have more children. The client requests information about permanent, male birth control options. The nurse explains:

A. Vasectomy is a highly effective and safe surgical procedure.

B. Abstinence should be considered rather than vasectomy.

C. Permanent solutions, such as vasectomy, cannot be reversed.

D. Vasectomy is a surgical procedure covered by insurance.

Answer: A. Vasectomy is a simple, quick, and safe surgical procedure that blocks the entry of sperm into ejaculated seminal fluid. In general, it is considered permanent, but surgical reversal is available. Some insurance companies consider it to be a form of elective surgery and require the client to pay out of pocket. Abstinence is not a viable option in this case as the client is interested in preventing pregnancy but not becoming sexually inactive.

TEST-TAKING STRATEGY: Read the question twice to ensure that you understand what the question is asking, especially if the question is tricky or confusing. Focus on what the question is asking: birth control, not abstinence.

299. A female client considers using spermicidal agents because she wants both birth control and protection from sexually transmitted infections (STIs). The nurse educates the client that spermicidal agents:

A. Are also effective in reducing vaginal fungal infections, such as *Candida albicans.*

B. Eliminate bacterial and viral STIs.

C. Are more effective when used in conjunction with barrier methods, such as the diaphragm or condom.

D. Are used on an "as needed" basis and exhibit few side effects.

Answer: C. Spermicidal agents alone have an approximately 25% failure rate in preventing pregnancy. These agents (nonoxynol 9 and octoxynol) kill sperm by destroying the protective surface of sperm and preventing metabolic activities necessary for survival. They have some cidal effect on viruses in vitro but need to be studied in vivo. They do not kill fungi such as *Candida albicans,* even in high concentrations. Spermicidal agents are used only when sexual intercourse is expected, but side effects include vaginal and penile irritation, lesions, and ulcerations due to the detergent effect. Disruption of normal protective vaginal flora results in an increased risk of opportunistic vaginal infections and urinary tract infections.

TEST-TAKING STRATEGY: Use the process of elimination to rule out incorrect answer selections to help choose the correct answer.

300. A female client has used Depo-Provera injections for birth control for several years. For the past 6 months, attempts to become pregnant have been unsuccessful. The nurse advises the client:

A. To be seen in the fertility clinic.

B. To have a sperm count performed on the client's partner.

C. Ovulation may not occur for many months after using Depo-Provera.

D. To ensure proper nutrition and rest.

Answer: C. Ovulation ceases with Depo-Provera use. It may take 6 to 18 months to reestablish normal ovulation and menstruation. A fertility workup for the client and her partner may be warranted after adequate time to reestablish ovulation has passed. Good nutrition and rest are important for all individuals.

TEST-TAKING STRATEGY: Read the questions twice to ensure that you understand what the question is asking, especially if the question is tricky or confusing. Focus on what the question is asking: immediate advice to the client, not long-term options.

301. A home health nurse visits a recently discharged client with right-sided paresis due to a stroke. The nurse discovers the spouse has been feeding the client. The nurse:

A. Instructs the spouse to require the client to feed independently.

B. Suggests the spouse hire an aide to feed and bathe the client.

C. Advises the spouse to consider an extended-care facility for the client.

D. Determines why the spouse is not encouraging self-care by the client.

Answer: D. Because family members are important in promoting client self-care and preventing further illness, it is important to include family members in the teaching plan for the client. In a family support model, the goal is client self-care activities through formal and informal support systems. Simply instructing the spouse to require the client to perform self-care activities may result in an affirmative verbal response from the spouse without actual follow-through after the home health nurse leaves. Hiring others to perform care activities that the client can do independently does not contribute to the self-care model.

TEST-TAKING STRATEGY: Determine which action will bring the most harm or help to the client. This helps determine the highest nursing priority.

302. A family member is involuntarily admitted to the psychiatric mental health unit. As a psychiatric mental health nurse you know that clients are involuntarily admitted when behavior is driven by mental illness and:

A. An imminent threat of self-harm.

B. Refusal to bathe.

C. Anger toward government officials.

D. Refusal to take prescribed psychiatric medications.

Answer: A. In the presence of mental illness, threats of suicide and physical harm to others warrant involuntary commitment and evaluation. Anger at others, including government officials, is not sufficient to lead to hospitalization. Refusing to bathe or take prescribed psychiatric medications is the client's right unless it leads to imminent threats of harm. The Mental Health and Developmental Disabilities Code protects the basic liberties and freedoms of all citizens.

TEST-TAKING STRATEGY: Choose the answer selection that is the most life threatening or harmful to the client.

303. As a disaster relief nurse, you counsel parents of young clients (select all that apply):

A. To act as if things are normal.

B. That young children may exhibit separation fears and clinging.

C. To sedate the client until the crisis is resolved.

D. That nightmares and sleep disturbances may occur in young children.

Answer: B & D. Following a disaster, children exhibit a range of emotional and physiological reactions including separation fear and sleep issues. They may also appear confused, passive, fearful, and have somatic symptoms. They have difficulty talking about the event or identifying feelings. Acting as if nothing happened is a nontherapeutic parental response. Sedation may be an emergent need, but more therapeutic responses are quickly warranted.

TEST-TAKING STRATEGY: When answering "Select all that apply" questions, be sure and treat each answer as a true or false statement. There may be one correct answer or more.

304. The spouse of an elderly client dies. The nurse understands that this client faces the task of:

A. Balancing freedom and responsibility.

B. Adjusting to living alone.

C. Promoting joint decision-making.

D. Considering the economic ramifications.

Answer: B. The client must adjust to living alone due to the loss of the spouse. Balancing freedom and responsibility, joint decision-making, and economic costs are tasks associated with earlier stages in family life.

TEST-TAKING STRATEGY: Use the process of elimination to rule out incorrect answer selections to help choose the correct answer.

305. The definition of "family" has evolved as society has changed. The most comprehensive definition of the term includes:

A. A unit of people related by birth or adoption or by marriage.

B. Two or more emotionally involved people.

C. Related people who live in close proximity to each other.

D. A changing group of people.

Answer: B. Significant others who may be related or bonded to the client by friendship are considered "family." In our society, even pets can be considered family members, because of the emotional bond between client and animal. Related people living in close proximity was a previous definition of family, which has since evolved to be more inclusive. A changing group of people is not a specific classification, and is therefore an incorrect answer choice.

TEST-TAKING STRATEGY: Read the question twice to ensure that you understand what the question is asking, especially if the question is tricky or confusing. Focus on what the question is asking: evolved definition, not previous definition.

306. A client delivers healthy twin infants. In educating the client on how to care for twins, the nurse:

A. Teaches the client to feed one infant while propping the bottle for the other infant to minimize feeding time, thus allowing the client more time to rest.

B. Instructs the client to add cereal to the night-time bottle so the infants will sleep longer.

C. Educates the client to feed each infant individually rather than simultaneously.

D. Informs the client that warming bottles in the microwave is rapid and provides more time to bond with the infant.

Answer: C. Each infant should receive individual attention to enhance parent–child bonding, ensure adequate intake, and prevent complications associated with bottle propping. Cereal in the bottle is not recommended by the American Academy of Pediatrics. Formula can easily be overheated in the microwave, leading to injury of the infant.

TEST-TAKING STRATEGY: Determine which action will bring the most harm or help to the client. This helps determine the highest nursing priority.

307. To enhance adaptive language skills in a young client, the nurse educates parents to foster appropriate language in social situations. An example is:

A. Effective persuasion, such as polite versus impolite language.

B. Direct versus indirect language when demanding action.

C. Correction of pronunciation or grammar errors.

D. Introduction of new topics.

Answer: A. Using polite terms is more persuasive that using impolite terms. This helps the child understand more effective ways to present a message. Demanding language is improper in social adaptive language situations. Respond to the child's intended message rather than correct him. Comment on the current topic before moving to a new topic.

TEST-TAKING STRATEGY: Read the question twice to ensure that you understand what the question is asking, especially if the question is tricky or confusing. Focus on what the question is asking: language in social situations.

308. Growth and development includes not only the physical changes that occur from birth onward but also (select all that apply):

A. Language skills.

B. Changes in personality and emotions.

C. Athletic strength and agility.

D. Height acceleration associated with puberty.

Answer: A & B. Language and personality and emotional changes are evident as a child develops understanding and interacts with the world. Athletic ability and height increases are physical attributes.

TEST-TAKING STRATEGY: Read the question twice to ensure that you understand what the question is asking, especially if the question is tricky or confusing. Focus on what the question is asking: growth and development, which is not a physical concept.

309. The most accurate information to give parents regarding when to engage a child in an organized athletic activity is:

A. Participation depends on the ability to run without falling.

B. A child with impaired vision should not play sports.

C. The parents should wait until the child asks to play sports.

D. The average child is ready to participate in sports at 6 to 7 years of age.

Answer: D. At about 6 to 7 years of age most children have developed the physical skills necessary to play sports—the ability to run and throw at the same time. In addition, a child of this age will have the attention span needed to listen to directions and grasp the rules of the sport. Sports activities prior to this age should be just for fun without a competitive edge. Engaging too early can lead to frustration and reluctance on the part of the child to further participate.

TEST-TAKING STRATEGY: Use the process of elimination to rule out incorrect answer selections to help choose the correct answer.

310. A 3-year-old child refuses to take a prescribed medication. The nurse is aware that parental education is necessary when the mother makes the following statement(s). Select all that apply.

A. "He is trying to make me angry."

B. "I feel like such a bad mother when he acts this way."

C. "I promised him a reward for taking his medication."

D. "I am unfazed by his actions."

Answer: A & B. If the mother feels the child is trying to "make her angry," she may respond with inappropriate discipline. The nurse can help the mother understand that developing independence is one of the developmental tasks of a child this age and that the movement toward independence reflects good, not bad parenting.

TEST-TAKING STRATEGY: In "select all that apply" questions, there may be more than one correct answers. The phrase "further teaching is necessary" or something similar ("parental education is necessary") tells you to select an answer with inaccurate information.

311. A nurse moves to a rural area and becomes aware that medical services are limited. An initial method to improve the health of rural clients includes:

A. Apply for a grant from the Department of Health and Human Services, which will allow for the hiring of additional health care providers.

B. Use innovative models of care including videotapes, health fairs, radio, and church social events to promote healthful practices.

C. Organize a van pool to transport clients to urban medical facilities for care.

D. Conduct door-to-door visits to assess the needs of clients in the community.

Answer: B. The use of videotapes, health fairs, radio, and church events can be instituted quickly and reach numerous constituents. Obtaining federal funds is time consuming and not guaranteed. A van pool is costly and serves a limited number of clients. Door-to-door assessments are time consuming and reach a limited segment of the population.

TEST-TAKING STRATEGY: Questions that ask you to prioritize your nursing actions use terms like priority, first, best, initial, most important, and next.

312. A client delivered a healthy newborn. As part of discharge teaching, the nurse informs the client about the need for well child check-ups. The client asks for an explanation. A well child check-up is:

A. A clinic visit of a sick child in an attempt to return him to health.

B. A rapid in-and-out visit where only the child's weight and height are determined and plotted on a growth chart.

C. The administration of routine childhood vaccinations.

D. Regularly scheduled clinic visits encompassing various aspects of health promotion.

Answer: D. In addition to physician visits when the child is sick or needs an examination to participate in a particular activity, routine well child check-ups (WCCs) are recommended. WCCs include physical examination, immunizations, tracking growth and development, detecting problems early, and education for both parent and child. Measurements of height and weight and the administration of vaccines are only part of a WCC.

TEST-TAKING STRATEGY: Use the process of elimination to rule out incorrect answer selections to help choose the correct answer.

313. Infants who are breastfed until a year of age show an interesting pattern of health and wellness. From an epidemiologic standpoint these clients (select all that apply):

A. Have negligible episodes of illness during the first year of life.

B. Are less prone to hypertension and diabetes as adults.

C. Are rarely diagnosed with autism spectrum disorder.

D. Have a lower body mass index than formula-fed infants at 12 months.

Answer: B & D. Infants breastfed for 12 months have a lower BMI at 12 months. This effect continues into childhood and adulthood. The incidence of hypertension and diabetes is also lower in this group. As adults, these subjects demonstrate fewer incidences of cholesterol abnormalities and allergies and a higher IQ. Breast milk contains maternal antibodies and IgA and reduces the infection rate in infants. However, illness is not nearly or entirely reduced. The etiology of autism is unknown and there are no studies to suggest that breastfeeding prevents autism.

TEST-TAKING STRATEGY: Use the process of elimination to rule out incorrect answer selections to help choose the correct answer.

314. A pregnant client with a positive history for untreated gonorrheal infection delivers a full-term infant. Initially, the most important nursing action is to:

A. Notify the health department of this reportable sexually transmitted infection (STI).

B. Determine all sexual contacts of the infected client.

C. Instill erythromycin (0.5%) ophthalmic ointment or silver nitrate (0.1%) aqueous solution into the infant's eyes.

D. Administer prescribed antibiotics to the mother.

Answer: C. An infant may acquire gonorrheal ophthalmitis by descending through an infected birth canal. Untreated gonorrheal eye infection in the newborn leads to permanent blindness. The administration of prophylactic ophthalmic antibiotics prevents blindness caused by the gonococcus.

TEST-TAKING STRATEGY: Determine which action will bring the most harm or help to the client. This helps determine the highest nursing priority. Choose the answer selection that is the most life threatening or harmful to the client.

315. At the beginning of the 20th century the average lifespan was 45 years. One hundred years later, the average lifespan increased to 78 years. The most accurate reason for this is:

A. Decreasing infant and childhood mortality.

B. Improved sanitation.

C. Better nutrition.

D. The ability to access health care more easily.

Answer: A. Advances in health care during the 20th century focused on preventing early death. This was especially true for infants and young children. The perinatal death rate for infants decreased from 15 percent to 1 percent. The development of vaccines decreased the death rate of children. Overcoming the risks of dying youth has resulted in lengthening the lifespan. Improved sanitation, nutrition, and access to health care are important but are not the most accurate reasons for increased lifespan.

TEST-TAKING STRATEGY: Terms like *most appropriately* and *most accurately* mean that the undeniably correct answer is most likely not present. Therefore, you must select the best answer choice from the selection provided.

316. A healthy client with no physical or mental problems asks the nurse why the physician recommends a yearly physical examination for the client. The nurse understands that the value of the physical examination includes (select all that apply):

A. A routine assessment using the 5 senses and minimal invasiveness, such as the ophthalmoscope, otoscope, and stethoscope.

B. An efficient and effective means of diagnosing illness.

C. Provision of a physical connection between physician and client leading to establishment of trust.

D. Billing requirements of Medicaid and Medicare that mandate a physical examination.

Answer: B & C. The physician–client relationship is extremely valuable. The history, observation, and physical examination of the client have essentially led to medicine being viewed as an art. In addition to diagnosing a problem and promoting health, strong connections form between physician and client. The client permits the physician to touch his body, and the physician demonstrates fidelity to the relationship by taking time to see, hear, and feel what the client's body reveals. Trust is fostered and is beneficial to both parties. A routine assessment is the definition of a physical examination. Medicaid and Medicare do require a certain portion of a physical examination for physician reimbursement for services.

TEST-TAKING STRATEGY: Read the question twice to ensure that you understand what the question is asking, especially if the question is tricky or confusing. Focus on what the question is asking: what is valuable about the physical examination, not what is the definition of a physical examination.

317. Female clients are encouraged to receive regularly scheduled health care screenings and examinations throughout each pregnancy. The primary value of prenatal care is to:

A. Detect clients who are at risk for preterm delivery.

B. Assess the client and baby for genetic defects.

C. Monitor the health of the mother and baby.

D. Determine if a vaginal birth is expected.

Answer: C. Monitoring the health status of both client and baby provides support and education, detects problems, and allows timely intervention and planning. Prenatal care includes a comprehensive assessment to detect high-risk issues for both client and baby.

TEST-TAKING STRATEGY: Terms like *primary value* mean that the undeniably correct answer is most likely not present. Therefore, you must select the best answer choice.

318. A client asks the nurse, "Will my immune system be weaker by relying on a vaccine for protection?" The nurse informs the client that:

A. The immune system works in healthy people but not in those with illness.

B. A vaccine offers some degree of immunity for a limited time.

C. Exposure to the natural disease strengthens the immune system better than a vaccine.

D. The immune system makes antibodies against a germ whether the germ is encountered naturally or by receiving a vaccine.

Answer: D. The immune system mounts a response to an antigen. The immune system does not differentiate between antigens occurring in the environment and those administered in a vaccine. People with an illness will have varying degrees of immune system activity depending on what type of illness they have. Some vaccines require booster doses while others impart lifetime immunity.

TEST-TAKING STRATEGY: Read the question twice to ensure that you understand what the question is asking, especially if the question is tricky or confusing. Focus on what the question is asking: will a vaccine weaken the immune system.

319. A client who will be flying nonstop from New York to Tokyo is seen in the travel clinic today. The nurse knows the client understands the teaching regarding deep vein thrombosis (DVT) prevention when he replies:

A. "I will take an aspirin prior to departure."

B. "I need to stretch and move about the plane every 1 to 2 hours."

C. "I should drink 8 ounces of water midway through the flight."

D. "I should drink an alcoholic beverage to relax me."

Answer: B. To prevent venous stasis and DVT formation, the client should flex and extend the foot, move each foot in a circular pattern, and contract the lower extremity muscles frequently throughout the flight. In addition, walking the aisle enhances venous and lymphatic return. Aspirin prevents platelet aggregation but is not recommended therapy to prevent DVT.

Maintaining adequate hydration is healthy. Eight ounces of water is not an adequate intake for such a flight. Alcoholic beverages do not precipitate DVT but may make the client sleepy, resulting in failure to exercise the lower extremities.

TEST-TAKING STRATEGY: The phrase "client understands the teaching" tells you to select an answer with accurate information. Determine which action will bring the most help to the client.

320. The nurse understands that the best predictor of health behavior and long-lasting successful behavior change is the:

A. Culture in which a client lives.

B. Age of the client.

C. Reading level and education of the client.

D. Diagnosis of a chronic illness.

Answer: A. Most health-promotion strategies assist the individual to change risky behaviors, but the long-term failure rate is high. The most successful strategies change the community culture to one of health promotion by involving the client, family, media, employers, educators, faith communities, organizations, health care, and government. Factors in the community culture that continue to place individuals at risk are changed. Age is not a deterrent to positive change. Literacy is important, but illiterate individuals can adapt to positive change by learning methods other than reading. Chronic illness may motivate a client initially, but the reversion rate to old habits is high. Health promotion is focused basically on healthy people to prevent illness, disability, and death.

TEST-TAKING STRATEGY: Terms like *best predictor* mean that the undeniably correct answer is most likely not present. Therefore, you must select the best answer choice from the selections provided.

321. As the nurse in a primary care clinic, you teach self-breast exams to all women. What do you advise them about breast cancer screening? Select all that apply.

A. Women at increased risk for breast cancer include those with a positive family history, genetic tendency, or past breast cancer.

B. Obtain a mammogram yearly starting at age 40.

C. Women at increased risk may require additional tests such as ultrasound or MRI.

D. Mammograms expose the client to considerable doses of radiation and should only be done when abnormalities in the self-breast exam are noted.

Answer: A, B, & C. The American Cancer Society recommends a yearly mammogram for all women beginning at age 40. The organization defines women at increased risk of breast cancer and recommends earlier mammograms and additional testing if warranted.

TEST-TAKING STRATEGY: When answering "Select all that apply" questions, be sure and treat each answer as a true or false statement. There may be one correct answer or more.

322. All 50 states perform some type of newborn screening on each newborn client. The main purpose of this blood test procedure is:

A. Assessment of the visual acuity of the newborn client.

B. Screening the newborn client for hearing loss.

C. Evaluation of each newborn client for autism.

D. Detection of disorders not readily apparent at birth.

Answer: D. Newborn screening programs identify newborn clients with rare disorders, which may cause developmental delay, mental retardation, serious medical problems, or death. Some disorders currently have no treatment. However, for those disorders for which treatment is available, serious morbidity and mortality can be avoided. The test requires a few drops of blood from a heel stick. This test does not assess vision, hearing, or autistic tendencies.

TEST-TAKING STRATEGY: Terms like *main purpose* mean that the undeniably correct answer is most likely not present. Therefore, you must select the best answer choice from the selections provided.

323. The incidence of melanoma rises rapidly in Caucasians after age 20. Clients at high risk require screening. The greatest risk for melanoma development is in clients with:

A. Fair skin who experience sun exposure.

B. Pigmented lesions such a dysplastic or atypical nevi.

C. Several large nondysplastic nevi.

D. Many small nevi or moderate freckling.

Answer: A. The best defense against any skin cancer, especially melanoma, is protection from the sun and ultraviolet light. Melanoma accounts for 75% of skin cancer deaths. The number of pigmented lesions also shows a relationship with the incidence of melanoma.

TEST-TAKING STRATEGY: Terms like *greatest risk* mean that the undeniably correct answer is most likely not present. Therefore, you must select the bet answer choice from the selections provided.

324. The most prevalent screening procedure for colorectal cancer includes:

A. Exploratory laparotomy.

B. Sigmoidoscopy.

C. DNA stool test for genetic changes.

D. Laparoscopic examination.

Answer: B. A thin, tube-like instrument with a light and lens for viewing is inserted into the rectum and sigmoid colon to ascertain the presence of polyps, abnormal areas, or cancer. The tool is equipped to remove polyps or tissue samples. A laparotomy and laparoscopic examination are not screening procedures. The DNA stool test for genetic changes in cells is being evaluated as a possible tool in colorectal cancer detection.

TEST-TAKING STRATEGY: Terms like *most prevalent* mean that the undeniably correct answer is most likely not present. Therefore, you must select the best answer choice from the selections provided.

325. A monthly testicular self-exam is recommended for males to permit early detection and treatment of testicular cancer. Testicular cancer is more prevalent:

A. As male clients age, with the highest incidence in the elderly.

B. In male clients who have a second type of cancer.

C. Among young, adult male clients between 20 and 35 years of age.

D. In male clients with mental retardation.

Answer: C. Testicular cancer is rare, but in young adult males the incidence is the most common type of cancer. Risk factors include positive family history, gonadal dysgenesis or Klinefelter's syndrome, cancer in one testicle, and white race. Although some testicular cancers are discovered by routine physical examination, the majority are detected by the patient. Therefore, routine self-examinations are recommended. Older clients are at less risk for testicular cancer. Clients with testicular cancer are at a higher risk for a second type of cancer, but another type of cancer does not predispose the client to testicular cancer. Male clients with mental deficits not attributable to chromosome abnormalities are not at an increased risk for testicular cancer.

TEST-TAKING STRATEGY: Terms like *more prevalent* mean that the undeniably correct answer is most likely not present. Therefore, you must select the best answer choice from the selections provided.

326. A client reports to the nurse in a college student health clinic for minor injuries associated with a fall. Upon further questioning, the client states he is a freshman and that he also misses class usually on Monday mornings. The nurse should screen this client for:

A. Binge drinking.

B. Sleep disorder.

C. Unsafe sex practices.

D. Suicidal tendency.

Answer: A. Young adults away from home for the first time may engage in high-risk behaviors. Over 40% of college students report binge drinking, and half of them report frequent binge drinking. Injuries such as falls and inability to attend class are signs of binge drinking.

TEST-TAKING STRATEGY: Use the process of elimination to rule out incorrect answer selections to help choose the correct answer.

327. The nurse overhears the spouse of an alcoholic client telling the client to "be quiet and don't tell the physician anything about your drinking problem." The nurse recognizes:

A. The spouse is exhibiting co-dependent behavior.

B. The spouse is the person of authority in this marriage.

C. The client has no choice but to follow the spouse's instructions.

D. The nurse must pretend not to have overheard this private conversation.

Answer: A. The spouse is exhibiting co-dependent behavior by refusing to change her own attitudes and by focusing on controlling the alcoholic client. The nurse can benefit the couple by helping the spouse to disregard the alcoholic client's promises, developing less dependence on the opinions of others, learning to set boundaries, expressing feelings, living in the present moment, and moving toward serenity, self-esteem, and independence.

TEST-TAKING STRATEGY: Look for similar answer choices and eliminate them. Determine which action will bring the most harm or help to the client. This helps determine the highest nursing priority.

328. The adventure-seeking teenager who gets bored easily and requires action, movement, and quick changes is at risk for drug and sexual experimentation. The nurse counsels the client and family to avert these high-risk behaviors by:

A. Getting an after-school job.

B. Working with a mental health specialist.

C. Engaging in physical activities that allow the client to push the limits.

D. Volunteering at a homeless shelter.

Answer: C. High-risk teenagers push the limits in everything they do. The novelty-seeking teenager benefits from activities like rock climbing, mountain biking, kayaking, and team sports. These activities provide healthy stimulation while teaching delayed gratification, consequences for actions, and how to get along with others in society. Although an after-school job and volunteer work may be positive behaviors, they don't provide the sense of independence and accomplishment needed by adventure-seeking teenagers. Counseling may help a high-risk teenager to understand his urges and consequences but again, does not provide the excitement the high-risk teenager seeks.

TEST-TAKING STRATEGY: Determine which action will bring the most harm or help to the client. This helps determine the highest priority.

329. When screening a client for high-risk behaviors the nurse should (select all that apply):

A. Use medical jargon to educate the client about proper terminology.

B. Appear nonjudgmental and comfortable.

C. Initially use questions that are direct and target specific behaviors.

D. Open with a statement such as "I discuss behaviors with all clients as part of their medical care."

Answer: B & D. Introductory statements that are nonthreatening prevent the client from feeling targeted. Open-ended questions produce detailed client responses and should begin with less threatening questions and then move to

more direct questions. A nonjudgmental, comfortable demeanor establishes trust.

TEST-TAKING STRATEGY: When answering "Select all that apply" questions, be sure and treat each answer as a true or false statement. There may be one correct answer or more.

330. A female, teenage client is seen in clinic today for a routine physical examination. During the screening for high-risk behaviors the client tells the nurse that while she does not drink alcoholic beverages, her boyfriend does prior to driving an automobile. The nurse counsels the client to:

A. Quit dating the boyfriend.

B. Refuse to ride with anyone who has been drinking alcoholic beverages.

C. Drive herself home even though the client does not have a valid driver's license yet.

D. Threaten to call the police.

Answer: B. A client should never ride with a driver who has been drinking. Alcohol impairs judgment and places all riders at risk for injury or death. Alternate methods to arriving home include calling a sober, responsible person. Not dating the boyfriend is an option if the boyfriend refuses to change his behavior. Driving without a valid license is illegal. Threatening the boyfriend is not therapeutic.

TEST-TAKING STRATEGY: Determine which action will bring the most harm or help to the client. This helps determine the highest nursing priority.

331. A client is perimenopausal. She asks the nurse about the need for birth control. The nurse knows:

A. Birth control should continue until menstrual periods have been absent for at least 1 year.

B. The client requires evaluation of follicle stimulating and leutinizing hormone levels.

C. Estrogen replacement therapy is warranted.

D. Sexual activity should be avoided during this time.

Answer: A. Irregular menstrual periods associated with perimenopause leave the client vulnerable to an unplanned pregnancy if the client is sexually active. Hormone levels are useful to determine if the client is perimenopausal. Hormone measurement and hormone replacement therapy are not forms of birth control. Being perimenopausal does not preclude sexual activity.

TEST-TAKING STRATEGY: Determine which action will bring the most harm or help to the client. This helps determine the highest nursing priority.

332. The nurse counsels a post-menopausal client:

A. It would be advisable to continue to use birth control.

B. The risk of sexually transmitted infections decreases as age increases.

C. Abstinence from sexual intercourse is advised.

D. After menopause, sexually transmitted infections can still occur.

Answer: D. Sexually transmitted infections (STIs) do not discriminate based on age or sexual orientation. Post-menopausal clients who are sexually active should use precautions, such as condoms, to prevent STIs. Statistics show the rate of HIV infection in people over 50 years old is increasing. Birth control is no longer needed in the post-menopausal client. Abstinence will prevent STIs, but abstinence is not an option in a client who remains sexually active.

TEST-TAKING STRATEGY: Choose the answer selection that is the most life threatening or harmful to the client.

333. A male client asks the nurse about the use of withdrawal (coitus interruptus) as a method for birth control. The nurse advises the client:

A. To use this method as a reliable form of birth control.

B. The effectiveness of this method is poor.

C. The sexual experience will not be altered.

D. Coitus interruptus prevents sexually transmitted infections.

Answer: B. In coitus interruptus, the couple engages in penile-vaginal intercourse. The penis is withdrawn from the vagina and female genital area when ejaculation is about to occur. It involves no cost, devices, or chemicals. However, the chance of pregnancy is higher (80% to 90%) than with any other method. Some men cannot gage ejaculation and may not withdraw in sufficient time. Interruption of the sexual response may decrease pleasure. There is no protection from sexually transmitted infections.

TEST-TAKING STRATEGY: Use the process of elimination to rule out incorrect answer selections to help choose the correct answer.

334. Teenagers who make virginity pledges begin engaging in vaginal intercourse later than those who have not made such pledges. The nurse is aware that (select all that apply):

A. Teenagers who take virginity pledges are more likely to engage in oral or anal sex than nonpledging, virgin teenagers.

B. Both groups have an equal number of sexual partners.

C. Pledgers have similar rates of sexually transmitted infections (STIs) as nonpledging teenagers.

D. Teenagers who make virginity pledges are more likely to use condoms when they become sexually active.

Answer: A & C. Teenagers who take virginity pledges initiate sexual activity 18 months later than nonpledgers and have fewer sexual partners. However, they are less likely to use condoms once they become sexually active, undergo STI testing, and know their STI status. They view oral and anal sex as not "real sex," placing them at risk of contracting STIs. They exhibit rates of STIs similar to nonpledgers.

TEST-TAKING STRATEGY: When answering "Select all that apply" questions, be sure and treat each answer as a true or false statement. There may be one correct answer or more.

335. Human sexuality education for clients with special needs:

A. Is not appropriate, especially for clients with intellectual disabilities.

B. Is time consuming and often frustrating for client and educator.

C. Should focus on genital sex rather than the expanded attributes of body image and social relationships.

D. Improves social skills, reduces the risk of sexual abuse and sexually transmitted disease, and prepares clients for adulthood.

Answer: D. Like all children, clients with developmental disabilities grow into adolescence with physically maturing bodies and emerging social and sexual feelings and needs. It is important that parents, educators, and health care personnel overcome cultural barriers to healthy sexuality in clients with special needs and prepare them for adulthood by providing information in a positive and constructive way that is both clear and educationally appropriate.

TEST-TAKING STRATEGY: Use the process of elimination to rule out incorrect answer selections to help choose the correct answer.

336. A client is exposed to an organism that causes disease. The physician prescribes an immunoglobulin to prevent illness. This is an example of:

A. Passive immunity.

B. Active immunity.

C. Acquired immunity.

D. Herd immunity.

Answer: A. Passive immunity is provided by the administration of antibodies (immunoglobulins) produced by other people or animals. With active and acquired immunity, the client is exposed to the antigen and produces his own antibodies. With herd immunity, the individual is not immunized but the people around him are. This greatly decreases the chances the individual will develop the disease.

TEST-TAKING STRATEGY: Use the process of elimination to rule out incorrect answer selections to help choose the correct answer.

337. A client asks the nurse how she can be protected against a particular disease. The nurse explains acquired/active immunity to the client in the following manner (select all that apply):

A. The client develops the disease.

B. A live, attenuated vaccine is administered.

C. A vaccine manufactured from killed organisms is administered.

D. An immunoglobulin is administered.

Answer: A, B, & C. Acquired/active immunity occurs when the client is exposed to a bacterial or viral antigen. This exposure can be the result of naturally acquired disease or the administration of a vaccine. Vaccines are manufactured from live, attenuated (weakened) or killed organisms. An immunoglobulin is an example of passively acquired immunity. Passive immunity occurs with the administration of antibodies produced by other persons or animals.

TEST-TAKING STRATEGY: When answering "Select all that apply" questions, be sure and treat each answer as a true or false statement. There may be one correct answer or more.

338. The nurse explains to a client that a vaccine is a:

A. Medication that prevents an immune response.

B. Serum protein noted with immunologic deficiencies.

C. Suspension of bacteria or viruses that are nonpathogenic.

D. Substance that destroys invading organisms.

Answer: C. A vaccine is nonpathogenic. It induces, not prevents, an immune response. The total serum protein measures albumin and globulins. Decreased levels are present with malnutrition, liver disease, and immunologic deficiencies. A substance that destroys invading organisms is an immunoglobulin.

TEST-TAKING STRATEGY: Use the process of elimination to rule out incorrect answer selections to help choose the correct answer.

339. The most common side effects of vaccine administration are:

A. Unconsolable crying for several hours and refusal to eat.

B. Anaphylaxis and shock.

C. Soreness at the injection site and fever.

D. Sleepiness and mild rash.

Answer: C. The most common side effects of immunizations are minor and include injection site redness and discomfort, elevated temperature, and mild rash. Unconsolable crying, anaphylaxis, and shock are adverse events, not side effects. They are uncommon events with vaccine administration.

TEST-TAKING STRATEGY: Terms like "most common" mean that the undeniably correct answer is most likely not present. Therefore, you must select the best answer choice from the selections provided.

340. A student nurse asks the clinical instructor where there is an accurate place to obtain information regarding immunizations. The instructor recommends:

A. Looking up each vaccine in a current drug handbook.

B. The Centers for Disease Control and Prevention website.

C. Seeking information from the pharmaceutical manufacturer of each vaccine.

D. Asking a physician colleague.

Answer: B. The Centers for Disease Control and Prevention (CDC) website contains a wealth of information on each vaccine and updates information throughout the year as it becomes available. The site also publishes vaccine recommendations for children, adults, individuals who need to "catch-up" vaccinations, travelers to foreign countries, state-by-state school requirements, and special considerations such as recommendations for immunocompromised clients and clients with allergies to ingredients in a particular vaccine. A drug handbook and manufacturer information contain data about a specific vaccine. It does not contain the remainder of information available from the CDC website. A physician may be an incomplete source of information.

TEST-TAKING STRATEGY: Read the questions twice to ensure that you understand what the question is asking, especially if the question is tricky or confusing. Focus on what the question is asking: accurate information source for immunizations.

341. The component of a person's lifestyle that primarily affects health status is:

A. Patterns of eating.

B. Having earned at least a high-school diploma.

C. Owning a pet.

D. Possessing computer skills.

Answer: A. The diet is influential in promoting health by providing necessary nutrients for growth and repair. Unhealthy patterns of eating lead to obesity, hypertension, diabetes, and cancer. Studies have shown a correlation between education and caring for a pet and health of the individual. Computer skills may permit an individual to obtain information about health and disease.

TEST-TAKING STRATEGY: Read the question twice to ensure that you understand what the question is asking, especially if the question is tricky or confusing. Focus on what the question is asking: component that primarily affects health status.

342. A client tells the nurse, "There's no point in quitting cigarette smoking at my age. I have smoked for 40 years." The nurse:

A. Understands that this is accurate, because the client already has pulmonary disease.

B. Tells the client that the progression of pulmonary disease may be halted with smoking cessation.

C. Encourages the client to switch to smokeless tobacco use.

D. Discusses the combination of pulmonary diseases that are the result of cigarette smoking.

Answer: B. Cessation of smoking interrupts the progression of processes such as chronic obstructive pulmonary disease. It cannot stop cancer that is present but contributes to cancer therapy by eliminating vasoconstriction, thus permitting chemotherapeutic agent penetration. Cessation of smoking prevents further injury. Tobacco usage in any form is detrimental to health. Discussing pulmonary complications of smoking is informative to the client.

TEST-TAKING STRATEGY: Read the question twice to ensure that you understand what the question is asking, especially if the question is tricky or confusing. Focus on what the question is asking: the client is asking what the point of smoking cessation is now. Determine which action will bring the most help to the client. This helps determine the highest nursing priority.

343. During a yearly physical examination, a client tells the nurse that the client "is stressed to the max" by work and family obligations. First, the nurse:

    A. Encourages the client to speak with the physician.

    B. Suggests the client obtain a prescription for sleep aid medication.

    C. Discusses positive options for stress reduction.

    D. Counsels the client to consider a career change.

Answer: C. Positive options for stress reduction include healthy diet, normal weight, regular exercise, and sufficient rest and sleep. It is important to educate the client that overeating, sedentary lifestyle, and chemical agents such as alcohol, nicotine, and caffeine are detrimental to health and have negative effects on stress reduction. While discussing the client's stress with the physician is beneficial, it is not the nurse's first action. Sleep aids and career changes do not address the complete problem.

TEST-TAKING STRATEGY: Questions that ask you to prioritize your nursing actions use terms like *priority, first, best, initial, most important,* and *next.*

344. Altered responses to lifestyle choices include (select all that apply):

    A. Hypertension in an obese client.

    B. Balding in a male client.

    C. Black lung (pneumoconiosis) in a coal miner.

    D. Skin cancer in a farmer.

Answer: A, C, & D. The association between obesity and hypertension, inhaling coal dust and black lung, and sun exposure and skin cancer are well known. These disease processes are a direct result of the client's lifestyle choices.

TEST-TAKING STRATEGY: When answering "Select all that apply" questions, be sure and treat each answer as a true or false statement. There may be one correct answer or more.

345. A young, adult client has a family history of chronic lung disease. He wants to avoid these processes and asks the nurse for information. The nurse replies:

    A. "There is nothing that can alter your genetic makeup."

    B. "Chronic lung disease affects the elderly."

    C. "You will not have lung disease if you do not smoke cigarettes."

    D. "Occupational exposure to inhaled toxic agents leads to lung disease."

Answer: D. The environment has a major influence on health. Inhaled toxic agents such as asbestos and coal dust lead to debilitating pulmonary disease and death. Genetics cannot be altered, but this response does not provide the information that the client seeks. Many forms of lung disease begin with chronic exposure to agents as a teenager or young adult and manifest well before becoming elderly. Cigarette smoking is a leading cause of lung disease, but individuals who have never smoked also develop pulmonary disease.

TEST-TAKING STRATEGY: Determine which action will bring the most harm or help to the client. This helps determine the highest nursing priority.

346. A nurse works in a clinic where the nurse is responsible for client education. Which principle is a factor in client education?

A. Every client is a learner throughout life.

B. Learning is difficult for the very young and very old client.

C. Middle-aged clients are busy with work and family and cannot focus on learning.

D. Clients learn best when they are faced with a serious illness.

Answer: A. Each client learns throughout his or her lifetime within social and cultural contexts and interactions with others. All clients including the young, middle aged, and elderly can and do learn. A serious illness poses severe stress on a client and actually may interfere with learning.

TEST-TAKING STRATEGY: Use the process of elimination to rule out incorrect answer selections to help choose the correct answer.

347. The nurse understands that one of the most vital aspects of teaching includes:

A. Relaying accurate information to the client.

B. Asking the client what the client feels and needs to know.

C. Identifying the way a client learns best.

D. Having the client take a short pre- and post test on the material.

Answer: C. The nurse can target client education when the way a client learns is utilized. Visual learners need pictures or diagrams while others learn best by listening to information. Accurate information is imperative, but if not provided in a way the client learns best, vital information may never be learned. The nurse should teach the information that the client needs to know. Taking tests is time consuming and not warranted. Assessment of the client's knowledge base before teaching begins can be accomplished by asking direct and indirect questions. At the conclusion of the education session, the nurse can ask the client to summarize what he has learned.

TEST-TAKING STRATEGY: Home in on the key words in the stem like "most vital." Then eliminate the incorrect answers while focusing on the answer that provides information or an action that is the most important.

348. The nurse is most likely to be an effective educator of clients when:

A. The nurse has complete content expertise.

B. The nurse displays listening skills and receives feedback.

C. The relationship between nurse and client is formal and impersonal.

D. The nurse understands that good educators are born, not made.

Answer: B. In establishing a relationship with the client learner, the nurse develops interaction and understands communication is from nurse to client and client to nurse. Two-way communication is invaluable. The nurse educator has considerable knowledge regarding a topic. However, if content expertise is lacking the effective educator will refer the client to someone with the necessary information. The nurse facilitates and has expertise but does not need to know everything. The relationship between the nurse and client can be professional without being impersonal. Educators improve their skills when they learn and apply principles of learning and communication.

TEST-TAKING STRATEGY: Terms like *most likely* mean that the undeniably correct answer is probably not present. Therefore, you must select the best answer choice from the selections provided.

349. For a client to learn information, which must be present? Select all that apply.

A. The learning experience must have a clear purpose.

B. The learner can regain his health.

C. The learning experience is inclusive of all necessary information.

D. The learner must be actively engaged.

Answer: A & D. The client must see the activity as purposeful with focused objectives and outcomes. Relevant information is better received and assimilated. Active, hands-on, concrete experiences that employ a variety of media allow the client to learn by doing and by analogy. These activities are engaging to the client and are highly effective in promoting education. Education benefits the client, but may not restore health. Educational sessions that are too long may tire and overwhelm the client. Depending on the amount of material needing to be covered and the client's condition, it may be more beneficial to break the content into shorter sessions with a direct focus.

TEST-TAKING STRATEGY: When answering "Select all that apply" questions, be sure and treat each answer as a true or false statement. There may be one correct answer or more.

350. The nurse educator knows that a client will understand and recall material better if the learning environment includes problem-based as well as knowledge-based activities. Which is an example of a problem-based activity?

   A. The client recalls the symptoms of the client's disease.

   B. The client comprehends the client's medication regimen.

   C. The client can analyze the client's glucometer value and determine what action is needed.

   D. The client performs a self-care activity accurately.

Answer: C. Problem-based learning involves higher-order thinking skills such as analysis, synthesis, and evaluation. Knowledge-based learning involves recall, comprehension, and application.

TEST-TAKING STRATEGY: Read the question twice to ensure that you understand what the question is asking, especially if the question is tricky or confusing. Focus on what the question is asking: recognizing and solving a problem, not recalling information.

351. A client has asthma. The nurse is aware that:

   A. A written asthma plan and peak expiratory flow measurements foster self-care.

   B. Asthma education (information) improves health outcomes in adults.

   C. Regular, ongoing reviews of client education are not necessary or beneficial.

   D. Clients with asthma have the same incidence of hospital admissions, unscheduled physician visits, and missed days of work as clients without asthma.

Answer: A. Education regarding the disease, self-management, and regular review by health care providers improves health outcomes for adults with asthma. Self-monitoring by peak expiratory flow or symptoms together with a written action plan produces positive results. Information alone does not improve outcomes. Clients with asthma are more likely to require unplanned care.

TEST-TAKING STRATEGY: Determine which action will bring the most help to the client. This helps determine the highest nursing priority.

352. As winter approaches, the nurse counsels an elderly client:

   A. To remain indoors as much as possible.

   B. That he needs thermal protection when outdoors.

   C. To consider spending the winter in a milder climate.

   D. That he will likely become ill if he does not remain in an environment with a constant temperature.

Answer: B. Clients, especially the older adult, require attention to environmental temperature variations. Winter temperatures can quickly lead to hypothermia in an elderly client due to reduced subcutaneous fat, skin thinning, and reduced sensation, especially in the extremities. Hyperthermia is an opposite concern in the summer.

TEST-TAKING STRATEGY: Use the process of elimination to rule out incorrect answer selections to help choose the correct answer.

353. Self-monitoring of blood glucose is an important part of diabetes management because:

  A. An elevated blood glucose level prompts the client to exercise and thus lower the value.

  B. An abnormal blood glucose value indicates the client is ingesting too many carbohydrates.

  C. It enables the client to make self-management decisions.

  D. Monitoring alerts the client that his insulin is not effective, and he should open a new vial.

Answer: C. By being aware of the blood glucose value, the client can adjust diet, exercise, and medications. This process also informs the client of episodes of hyperglycemia and hypoglycemia, which is important in fostering tight control of blood glucose values and preventing complications of the disease process. Elevated levels may indicate a worsening condition but may also represent stress and infection.

TEST-TAKING STRATEGY: Use the process of elimination to rule out incorrect answer selections to help choose the correct answer.

354. Self-care behaviors are vital to health promotion because (select all that apply):

  A. They are a complement to professional health care.

  B. Self-care makes the client completely responsible for her behaviors and outcomes.

  C. The client is empowered to actively participate in fostering her own health.

  D. Employers do not raise health care premiums for healthy employees.

Answer: A & C. Self-care decisions improve health or assist with a health problem. Such decisions include diet, exercise, rest and stress reduction, substance reduction or elimination, and education. It also includes the client's learning from past experience. These activities are empowering. Coupled with regular professional care the health, well-being, and quality of life of the client is promoted.

TEST-TAKING STRATEGY: When answering "Select all that apply" questions, be sure and treat each answer as a true or false statement. There may be one correct answer or more.

355. As clients age, the nurse should remember that self-care practices by the client:

  A. Result in a failure of the client to utilize medical services.

  B. Have little or no effect on mortality, but do reduce the overall rate of illness.

  C. Are limited in the ability to influence health and well-being.

  D. Promote health of the client now and in the future.

Answer: D. Self-care is the enhancement of health and independent functioning through self-initiated behaviors. The health of elderly clients is significantly determined by patterns of living in young adulthood through middle age. Health behaviors now influence present and future morbidity and mortality. Self-care is intertwined with professional health care in meeting the needs of the individual.

TEST-TAKING STRATEGY: Look for similar answer choices and eliminate them.

356. A 75-year-old client exhibits diminished but equal peripheral pulses and cool hands and feet. The nurse's most appropriate action is to:

  A. Immediately notify the physician.

  B. Place the client on a cardiorespiratory monitor and assess the client for possible atrioventricular block.

  C. Understand these are normal gerontological changes caused by diminished inotrophy and arterial rigidity.

  D. Initiate oxygen therapy and call the code team.

Answer: C. Gerontologic differences in cardiovascular assessment include decreased contractility (decreased myocardium, ventricular wall thickening, slow ventricular relaxation) and increasing arterial rigidity (reduction in elastin and smooth muscle). Notification of the physician is not urgent. A cardiorespiratory monitor, oxygen therapy, and resuscitation are not indicated.

TEST-TAKING STRATEGY: Terms like *most appropriate* and *most accurate* mean that the undeniably correct answer is probably not present. Therefore, you must select the best answer choice from the selections provided.

357. When performing a physical examination on a 2-year-old client, the nurse:

   A. Performs a head-to-toe examination in the same manner as a physical examination performed on an adult client.

   B. Sedates the client to achieve cooperation.

   C. Performs the minimally invasive maneuvers such as the examination of the ears and eyes at the beginning of the exam.

   D. Listens to the heart, lungs, and bowel sounds first.

Answer: D. A pediatric client requires a complete physical examination just like the adult client. However, initially when the client is generally quieter, listening to various sounds using the stethoscope is recommended. Sedation is not warranted. Invasive procedures that may scare the client and result in loss of cooperation and initiation of resistant behaviors or crying should be performed last.

TEST-TAKING STRATEGY: Determine which action will bring the most harm or help to the client. This helps determine the highest nursing priority.

358. A student nurse is having difficulty determining the liver span of a client. The experienced nurse educates the student:

   A. Because the liver span varies considerably between individuals, its measurement is of little value.

   B. To percuss in the midclavicular line from the nipple line downward and the iliac crest upward.

   C. To palpate the position of the liver first, and then attempt to percuss its position.

   D. That having the client flex his knees will relax the abdominal musculature.

Answer: B. In normal clients the liver is located in the midclavicular line on the right. The average liver span is 2.5 to 5 inches (6 to 12 cm). By percussing from the nipple line downward and the iliac crest upward, the examiner can accurately assess liver span. This value is useful in determining normalcy versus a disease state and is part of the physical examination. The correct order of abdominal examination is inspection, auscultation, percussion, and palpation. Knee flexion relaxes abdominal muscles but may hinder liver span measurement.

TEST-TAKING STRATEGY: Read the question twice to ensure that you understand what the question is asking, especially if the question is tricky or confusing. Focus on what the question is asking: how to determine liver span.

359. When assessing the cardiovascular system the nurse inspects and palpates blood vessels. A rigid (hard) blood vessel will vibrate. The correct term for a palpable vibration of a blood vessel is:

   A. Bruit.

   B. Murmur.

   C. Thrill.

   D. Heave.

Answer: C. The pulse in a normal vessel feels like a tap. In a narrow or bulging vessel, the pulse feels like a vibration and is called a thrill. A bruit and a murmur are sounds due to turbulent blood flow. A heave is a bounding pulse that moves the examiner's finger, hand, or stethoscope upward and outward away from the body.

TEST-TAKING STRATEGY: Use the process of elimination to rule out incorrect answer selections to help choose the correct answer.

360. When performing a physical examination on an elderly client, the nurse:

   A. Assesses the musculoskeletal system by asking the client to hop on one foot and perform deep knee bends.

   B. Limits distractions because of the client's sensory deficits in vision and hearing.

C. Evaluates the pulmonary status with deep breaths, breath-holding, and forced expirations.

D. Focuses on different walking maneuvers (heel-to-toe, tandem, heel walking) to evaluate neuromuscular function.

Answer: B. Many elderly clients have sensory deficits, and distractions can be confusing and limit the ability to thoroughly assess the client. Hopping, deep knee bends, and walking maneuvers can be difficult due to limited range of motion, decreased reflexes, and diminished sense of balance. Pulmonary changes in the elderly include decreased force of expiration, weakened cough reflex, and shortness of breath. Deep breaths, breath-holding, and forced expiration may compound respiratory difficulty.

TEST-TAKING STRATEGY: Determine which action will bring the most harm or help to the client. This helps determine the highest nursing priority.

361. The Neuman's Systems Model maintains that each person (or group of persons) constitutes a system of five variables: physiological, psychological, sociocultural, developmental, and spiritual. These variables exist along a developmental continuum. The spiritual continuum can range from lack of awareness or denial of spirituality to a highly developed spiritual consciousness. A nurse who allows Neuman's Systems Model to guide practice should address the client's level of spiritual awareness or development and address any identifiable spiritual needs occurring in reaction to the:

A. Attitude clients choose in response to suffering.

B. Availability and efficacy of resources for coping with the stressor.

C. Meaning of this experience for the client.

D. Stress of surgery.

Answer: D. The Neuman's Systems Model addresses any identifiable spiritual needs occurring in reaction to the stress of surgery. Travelbee's theory of nursing makes an effort to ascertain the meaning of this experience for the client. Frankl's theory suggests that people are able to find meaningfulness and can do so by what they take from the world, what they give to the world, and the attitude they choose for themselves in response to suffering.

TEST-TAKING STRATEGY: Use the process of elimination to rule out incorrect answer selections to help choose the correct answer.

362. The theoretical support for spiritual caregiving is recognized by professional organizations that influence nursing practice and education. Some professional organizations have issues mandating that nurses offer spiritual care to clients and teach spiritual care to nursing students. Which organization meets these criteria?

A. American Nurses Association's (ANA) *Code for Nurses*.

B. Department of Health Services (DHS).

C. Joint Commission on Accreditation for Healthcare Organizations (JCAHO).

D. State Nurses Association's *Policy & Procedure*.

Answer: C. JCAHO specifies that all clients be assessed for spiritual beliefs and practices and have access to spiritual support. The ANA's *Code for Nurses* states that nurses will respect the dignity and uniqueness of each client regardless of personal attributes. There is no state nurses association's *Policy & Procedure*. DHS does not issue mandates for spiritual care.

TEST-TAKING STRATEGY: Use the process of elimination to rule out incorrect answer selections to help choose the correct answer.

363. Nurses sometimes perceive barriers to providing spiritual care. These barriers include (select all that apply):

A. Ability.

B. A perceived lack of time.

C. Confusion about what spiritual care is.

D. Lack of knowledge and preparation for spiritual caregiving.

Answer: A, B, C, & D. All of the answer choices are correct. Nurses sometimes perceive barriers to providing spiritual care. These barriers include a perceived lack of time, ability, lack of knowledge and preparation for spiritual caregiving, orientation to nursing care that emphasizes the biologic, and confusion about what spiritual care is.

TEST-TAKING STRATEGY: When answering "Select all that apply" questions, be sure and treat each answer as a true or false statement. There may be one correct answer or more.

364. Ethical principles to guide spiritual care include: Select all that apply.

   A. Autonomy.

   B. Beneficence.

   C. Justice.

   D. Nonmaleficence.

Answer: A, B, C, & D. Several ethical principles to guide spiritual care include:
   • Beneficence (doing good for clients).
   • Nonmaleficence (doing no harm to clients).
   • Autonomy (respecting and supporting others' rights to self-determination).
   • Justice (or fairness).
   • Fidelity (or faithfulness to previous agreements).
   • Veracity (or truth-telling).

TEST-TAKING STRATEGY: When answering "Select all that apply" questions, be sure and treat each answer as a true or false statement. There may be one correct answer or more.

365. Which quality is essential for a nurse to be an effective spiritual care provider?

   A. Love.

   B. Motivation.

   C. Patience.

   D. Self-awareness.

Answer: D. Self-awareness is essential for nurses if they are to be effective spiritual care providers. Developing spiritual self-awareness is an essential part of learning how to provide spiritual care to nursing clients. The nurse's awareness of his sense of the spiritual has a profound influence on the ability to provide effective spiritual care.

TEST-TAKING STRATEGY: Use the process of elimination to rule out incorrect answer selections to help choose the correct answer.

366. Effective communication requires the nurse to recognize and respond to the client's nonverbal as well as verbal messages. Nonverbal communication generally provides more accurate information about emotions than verbal communication. Nonverbal communication includes (select all that apply):

   A. Body movements.

   B. Facial expressions.

   C. Gestures.

   D. Touch.

Answer: A, B, C, & D. Nonverbal communication includes touch, body movements, facial expressions, gestures, posture and gait, and even the way people dress or otherwise decorate themselves.

TEST-TAKING STRATEGY: When answering "Select all that apply" questions, be sure and treat each answer as a true or false statement. There may be one correct answer or more.

367. Listening is an essential element of nursing activities that promote spiritual health. Key aspects of listening empathetically are:

   A. Helping clients listen to the nurse.

   B. Translating what the nurse said.

   C. Recognizing the client's inner response.

   D. Striving to hear all aspects of the client's message.

Answer: D. Key aspects of listening empathically are striving to hear all aspects of the client's message, recognizing the nurse's inner response, and helping clients to listen to themselves and make sense of the information they have received.

TEST-TAKING STRATEGY: Use the process of elimination to rule out incorrect answer selections to help choose the correct answer.

368. Techniques for empathic listening include:

A. Assuming an attitude of superiority or savior.

B. Attending to nonverbal messages as well as verbal messages.

C. Changing the topic of conversation to avoid emotional discomfort.

D. Offering responses that preach or attempt to fix the client's emotional pain.

Answer: B. Techniques for empathic listening include maintaining an attitude of caring, placing full attention in the present moment and on the client to be present to their deepest moods, refraining from personal issues and stories, attending to clients' feelings as well as thoughts, attending to nonverbal messages as well as verbal messages, being aware of inner responses to a client, allowing silence, accepting tears, and integrating verbal and nonverbal client messages when forming responses. Assuming an attitude of superiority, changing the topic of conversation, and offering responses that preach are not conducive to empathic listening.

TEST-TAKING STRATEGY: You may find that the question does not offer a distinct correct answer. In this case, choose the most correct answer from the answer selections provided.

369. In the Buddhist religion, the use of drugs and alcohol is:

A. Believed to be necessary.

B. Discouraged.

C. Encouraged.

D. Not addressed.

Answer: B. In the Buddhist religion, the use of drugs and alcohol is strongly discouraged.

TEST-TAKING STRATEGY: Look for similar answer choices and eliminate them.

370. Which religion believes that physical disease results from good or bad karma (result of acts previously committed)?

A. Buddhism.

B. Catholicism.

C. Hinduism.

D. Judaism.

Answer: A. Buddhists believe that physical disease results from good or bad karma (result of acts previously committed). Hinduism believes that health results when body elements are balanced by consuming food and drink in the right way and time. Jews believe that sickness and suffering is explained by sin, physical and psychological causes, or even demons.

TEST-TAKING STRATEGY: Read the question twice to ensure that you understand what the question is asking, especially if the question is tricky or confusing. Focus on what the question is asking: the religion that believes disease results from acts previously committed.

371. Which religion believes in final judgment that determines heaven or hell?

A. Buddhism.

B. Christianity.

C. Hinduism.

D. Judaism.

Answer: B. Christianity believes in final judgment that determines heaven or hell. Buddhism believes in reincarnation until Nirvana is attained. Hinduism believes in reincarnation. Judaism has no official stance on existence of an afterlife.

TEST-TAKING STRATEGY: Use the process of elimination to rule out incorrect answer selections to help choose the correct answer.

372. Which religion worships Allah, performs ritual prayers five times per day with ablutions prior, and attends mosque or gathers with groups at noon on Fridays?

A. Hinduism.

B. Islam.

C. Judaism.

D. Mormons.

Answer: B. Muslims worship Allah, address their lay religious leaders as Imam, perform ritual prayers five times per day with ablutions prior, attend mosque or gather with a group at noon on Fridays, and do not eat pork. Hinduism, Judaism, and the Mormons do not share these restrictions.

TEST-TAKING STRATEGY: Use the process of elimination to rule out incorrect answer selections to help choose the correct answer.

373. Which religious group may decline unnecessary health care procedures on Shabbat?

A. Christians.

B. Christian scientists.

C. Jews.

D. Mormons.

Answer: C. Jews may decline unnecessary health care procedures on Shabbat. Christian scientists refuse many medical interventions and prefer to see their own practitioners. Christians and Mormons do not share this restriction.

TEST-TAKING STRATEGY: Use the process of elimination to rule out incorrect answer selections to help choose the correct answer.

374. Unique and salient religious beliefs and practices found across many different faith traditions include (select all that apply):

A. After life in some form.

B. Use of religious objects and worship practices to commune with higher spiritual beings or a deity.

C. Vegetarianism and abstention from pork or certain other meats.

D. Weekly holy days or sabbaths when persons attend religious services.

Answer: A, B, C, & D. All should be considered in addition to solemn and festive annual holy days that commemorate an important historical event significant to the religious tradition. Prohibition of actions that are considered disrespectful of the sanctity of life are also beliefs found across many different faith traditions.

TEST-TAKING STRATEGY: When answering "Select all that apply" questions, be sure and treat each answer as a true or false statement. There may be one correct answer or more.

375. Which form of communication most likely informs a client about how sincere, interested, and receptive a nurse is toward the client?

A. Body language.

B. Presencing.

C. Silence.

D. Touching.

Answer: A. Body language reveals much about a client's emotional state. Conversely, body language informs clients about how sincere, interested, and receptive a nurse is toward them.

TEST-TAKING STRATEGY: Terms like *most appropriately* and *most likely* mean that the undeniably correct answer is most likely not present. Therefore, you must select the best answer choice from the selections provided.

376. The nurse knows that family coping is influenced by the family's (select all that apply):

A. Function.

B. Genders.

C. Process.

D. Structure.

Answer: A, C, & D. Family coping is influence by the family's structure, function, and process. The family's resources such as time, energy, money, knowledge, skills, and past experiences also influence the ways members solve problems and cope with stress and crisis. Gender is not listed as an influence on family coping.

TEST-TAKING STRATEGY: Use the process of elimination to rule out incorrect answer selections to help choose the correct answer.

377. The nurse teaches the client who has recently lost a spouse that a number of factors influence grief and mourning. These factors include (select all that apply):

A. Characteristics of death.

B. Characteristics of the mourner.

C. Nature and meaning of the loss.

D. Social factors.

Answer: A, B, C, & D. A number of factors influence grief and mourning. These include the nature and meaning of the loss, characteristics of the mourner, characteristics of the death, social factors, and psychological factors.

TEST-TAKING STRATEGY: When answering "Select all that apply" questions, be sure and treat each answer as a true or false statement. There may be one correct answer or more.

378. In every household, members have to decide the ways in which work and responsibilities will be divided and shared. Different roles include:

A. Bidder.

B. Gender.

C. Provider.

D. Student.

Answer: C. Different household roles include provider role, housekeeping and child care roles, socialization role, sexual and therapeutic roles, recreation role, and kinship role. Bidder, gender, and student do not describe ways in which responsibilities will be divided and shared.

TEST-TAKING STRATEGY: Read the question twice to ensure that you understand what the question is asking, especially if the question is tricky or confusing. Focus on what the question is asking: the roles involved in the division of household responsibilities.

379. Interactional sources of role strain are related to difficulties in the delineation and enactment of familial roles. Five sources of difficulties in the interaction process include (select all that apply):

A. Inability to define the situation.

B. Lack of role consensus.

C. Lack of role knowledge.

D. Role conflict.

Answer: A, B, C, & D. Five sources of difficulties in the interaction process include inability to define the situation, lack of role knowledge, lack of role consensus, role conflict, and role overload.

TEST-TAKING STRATEGY: When answering "Select all that apply" questions, be sure and treat each answer as a true or false statement. There may be one correct answer or more.

380. The nurse is giving a facility inservice on the topic of domestic abuse. Health effects of domestic violence include (select all that apply):

A. Chronic health problems.

B. Higher rates of psychological disorders.

C. Higher rates of sexually transmitted infections.

D. Injuries from assault.

Answer: A, B, C, & D. Health effects of domestic violence include injuries from assaults; chronic health problems such as irritable bowel syndrome, backache, and headaches; increased unintended pregnancies, pregnancy terminations, and low-birthweight babies; higher rates of sexually transmitted infections, including HIV; and higher rates of depression, anxiety, post-traumatic stress disorder, self-harm, and suicide.

TEST-TAKING STRATEGY: When answering "Select all that apply" questions, be sure and treat each answer as a true or false statement. There may be one correct answer or more.

381. A nurse working in a Planned Parenthood clinic routinely asks clients about experiencing possible domestic violence. The advantage of this line of questioning is that it:

A. Alienates victims of abuse, thus increasing cooperation with members of the health care team.

B. Assists the local police in maintaining local inmate populations.

C. Assures that the truth is revealed.

D. Maintains the safety of women experiencing domestic violence.

Answer: D. The advantages of routinely inquiring about domestic violence include uncovering hidden cases of domestic violence; changing perceived acceptability of violence in relationships; increasing ease of women to access support services earlier; changing health professionals' knowledge and attitudes toward domestic violence and reducing social stigma; and maintaining the safety of women experiencing domestic violence.

TEST-TAKING STRATEGY: Determine which action will bring the most harm or help to the client. This helps determine the highest nursing priority.

382. The nurse working in a long-term care facility knows that elder abuse most often consists of:

    A. Financial exploitation.

    B. Neglect.

    C. Physical abuse.

    D. Sexual abuse.

    Answer: B. Elder abuse mostly consists of neglect, followed by physical abuse, financial or material exploitation, psychological or emotional abuse, and sexual abuse.

    TEST-TAKING STRATEGY: You may find that the question does not offer a distinct correct answer. In this case, choose the most correct answer from the selections provided.

383. An example of internal family coping strategies include:

    A. Maintaining active links with community groups and organizations.

    B. Role flexibility.

    C. Seeking and using spiritual supports.

    D. Seeking information and professional help.

    Answer: B. Internal family coping strategies include family group reliance including delegation; the use of humor and stress management tactics; increased sharing together—maintaining cohesiveness; controlling the meaning of the stressor/demand—cognitive refraining and passive appraisal; joint family problem-solving; role flexibility; normalizing; limiting leisure time and recreational activities; and accepting stressful events as a fact of life. Maintaining community relationships, seeking spiritual supports, and seeking professional help are examples of external family coping strategies.

TEST-TAKING STRATEGY: Read the questions twice to ensure that you understand what the question is asking, especially if the question is tricky or confusing. Focus on what the question is asking: example of internal family coping strategies.

384. An example of external family coping strategies includes:

    A. Joint family problem-solving.

    B. Limiting leisure time and recreational activities.

    C. Sharing concerns and experiences with relatives, friends, and neighbors.

    D. The use of humor and stress management tactics.

    Answer: C. External family coping strategies include seeking information and professional help; maintaining active links with community groups and organizations; seeking and using social supports (informal and formal social support systems and self-help groups); seeking and using spiritual supports; and sharing concerns and experiences with relatives, friends, and neighbors. Joint family problem-solving, limiting leisure time and recreational activities, and the use of humor and stress-management tactics are examples of internal family coping strategies.

    TEST-TAKING STRATEGY: Read the questions twice to ensure that you understand what the question is asking, especially if the question is tricky or confusing. Focus on what the question is asking: example of external family coping strategies.

385. The nurse knows that traits of healthy families include (select all that apply):

    A. Developing a sense of trust.

    B. Balancing the interaction between members.

    C. Sharing leisure time.

    D. Valuing service to others.

Answer: A, B, C, & D. Traits of healthy families include communication and listening; fostering time table and conversation; affirming and supporting each member; teaching respect for others; developing a sense of trust, play, and humor; balancing the interaction among members; sharing leisure time; and exhibiting a sense of shared responsibility and service to others.

TEST-TAKING STRATEGY: When answering "Select all that apply" questions, be sure and treat each answer as a true or false statement. There may be one correct answer or more.

386. At different stages of life, families must master certain developmental tasks in order to maintain psychological health. Families with young adults who are launching into society have family developmental tasks to master including:

    A. Coping with energy depletion.

    B. Maintaining kinship ties.

    C. Maintaining a supportive home base.

    D. Thinking about the future, education, and work.

    Answer: A. Families with young adults launching into society have developmental tasks including maintaining a supportive home base, maintaining parental couple intimacy and relationship, and after a member moves out, reallocating roles, space, power, and communication. Families with adolescents have developmental tasks including thinking about the future, education, job, and work. Families with middle-aged parents have developmental tasks including maintaining kinship ties. Families with preschool children have developmental tasks include coping with energy depletion.

    TEST-TAKING STRATEGY: Use the process of elimination to rule out incorrect answer selections to help choose the correct answer.

387. Family structure is the ordered set of relationships among family parts and between the family and other social systems. In determining the family structure, the nurse needs to identify the:

    A. Age of the individual family members.

    B. Gender of the individual family members.

    C. Individuals that compose the family.

    D. Living arrangements of family members.

    Answer: C. In determining the family structure, the nurse needs to identify the individuals that compose the family and the relationships between them; the interactions between the family members; and the interactions with other social systems. Age, gender, and living arrangements of the members of the family are not factors that need to be identified.

    TEST-TAKING STRATEGY: Use the process of elimination to rule out incorrect answer selections to help choose the correct answer.

388. The technology-driven, critical care environment is fast paced and directed toward monitoring and treating life-threatening changes in client conditions. To the families of critical care clients, four behaviors indicate caring. These include:

    A. Closed communication.

    B. Open visiting hours.

    C. Touch.

    D. Withholding information.

    Answer: C. The major types of behavior that indicate caring to family members of critical care clients are touch; providing information; open, honest communication; and an intuitive ability to detect changes in both physiologic and psychosocial status.

    TEST-TAKING STRATEGY: Use Maslow's hierarchy of needs to determine the correct answer.

389. Complementary and alternative therapies are proven effective in helping clients. Which are examples of complementary and alternative therapies? Select all that apply.

    A. Animal-assisted therapy.

    B. Guided imagery.

    C. Massage.

    D. Prescription medications.

Answer A, B, & C. Alternative therapy denotes that a specific therapy is an option or alternative to what is considered conventional treatment of a condition or state. The term complementary reflects that the therapy can be used as complementary or supportive to the conventional therapy. Animal-assisted therapy, guided imagery, and massage are examples or complementary and alternative therapies. Prescription medications are a conventional treatment.

TEST-TAKING STRATEGY: When answering "Select all that apply" questions, be sure and treat each answer as a true or false statement. There may be one correct answer or more.

390. Guided imagery is a form of alternative therapy. Guided imagery can frequently be used by the nurse to decrease stress, pain, and anxiety. Additional benefits of guided imagery include:

A. Decreased client satisfaction.

B. Decreased side effects.

C. Increased length of stay.

D. Increased hospital costs.

Answer: B. Additional benefits of guided imagery are shown to decrease side effects, decrease length of stay, reduce hospital costs, enhance sleep, and increase client satisfaction. Guided imagery is a low-cost intervention that is relatively simple to implement. The client's involvement in the process offers a sense of empowerment and accomplishment and motivates self-care.

TEST-TAKING STRATEGY: Read the questions twice to ensure that you understand what the question is asking, especially if the question is tricky or confusing. Focus on what the question is asking: benefits of guided imagery.

391. Acutely ill clients often experience high levels of physiologic and psychologic stress. Sources of physiologic stress in the acutely ill client are:

A. Learning new concepts.

B. Level of nursing staff.

C. Pain.

D. Payment of bills.

Answer: C. Sources of physiologic stress in the acutely ill client include medications, pain, hypoxia, decreased cerebral and peripheral perfusion, hypotension, fluid and electrolyte imbalances, infection, sensory alterations, fever, and neurologic deficits. Experiencing one or more of these stressors can completely consume all the client's available energy and thoughts, thus affecting his or her ability to interact, comprehend, and respond to teaching.

TEST-TAKING STRATEGY: Use Maslow's hierarchy of needs to determine the correct answer.

392. When confronted with life-altering situations, both clients and families can experience emotional stress. Which are sources of emotional stress? Select all that apply.

A. Fear of cure.

B. Role change.

C. Self-image change.

D. Uncertain prognosis.

Answer: B, C, & D. Sources of emotional stress are fear of illness, role change, self-image change, and uncertain prognosis. Other sources of emotional stress are isolation from other family members, disruption in daily routines, financial concerns, and unfamiliar critical care environments.

TEST-TAKING STRATEGY: When answering "Select all that apply" questions, be sure and treat each answer as a true or false statement. There may be one correct answer or more.

393. During the initial phases of a critical illness, feelings of disbelief and denial are common. Fear of death, loss, powerlessness, and helplessness may be experienced. Which educational techniques are most effective when teaching the client who experiences these emotions?

A. Develop the client's awareness.

B. Explain all procedures and activities.

C. Orient teaching to the present.

D. Teach during other nursing activities.

Answer: A, B, C, & D. Education during this phase should be aimed at reduction of immediate stress, anxiety, and fear rather than future lifestyle alterations or rehabilitation needs. Clients and families may need to be refocused on the present and encouraged to not dwell on what might happen in the future.

TEST-TAKING STRATEGY: When answering "Select all that apply" questions, be sure and treat each answer as a true or false statement. There may be one correct answer or more.

394. During which stage of illness should the nurse orient teaching to meet the client's family's needs?

A. Developing awareness.

B. Disbelief.

C. Identifying change.

D. Reorganization and resolution.

Answer: D. As families begin to understand and become more aware of the client's current situation, feelings of hopelessness, anger, frustration, resentment, and guilt can occur. Eventually signs of hope and acceptance will emerge, signaling entrance into the reorganization and resolution phase. During this phase, the client's family is more receptive to teaching and learning new information.

TEST-TAKING STRATEGY: Read the questions twice to ensure that you understand what the question is asking, especially if the question is tricky or confusing. Focus on what the question is asking: the client's stage of illness that is most conducive to client education.

395. When admitting a new client to the unit, the nurse should (select all that apply):

A. Explain reasons for equipment, monitors, and associated alarms.

B. Orientate to the unit environment: for example, call light and bed controls.

C. Orient to unit routines and plan of care.

D. Orient to the various care providers and services they deliver.

Answer: A, B, C, & D. All of the above should be performed by the nurse including explaining all procedures and their expected sensations or discomforts both in the unit and off the unit. The client should also be oriented to medications given including name, purpose of administration, and side effects to report to the nurse or health care team.

TEST-TAKING STRATEGY: When answering "Select all that apply" questions, be sure and treat each answer as a true or false statement. There may be one correct answer or more.

396. Which action should be a part of the teaching by the nurse during a client's discharge planning? Select all that apply.

A. Diet.

B. Medications.

C. Financial assistance.

D. Activity allowances and restrictions.

Answer: A, B, & D. Discharge planning should include teaching of: medications, diet, activity, pathophysiology of disease, symptom management, special procedures and associated equipment, when to call the health care provider, and available community resources.

TEST-TAKING STRATEGY: When answering "Select all that apply" questions, be sure and treat each answer as a true or false statement. There may be one correct answer or more.

397. Several skin conditions that are of most importance in African-American clients include:

A. Cardiomyopathy.

B. Diverticulosis.

C. Keloids.

D. Sarcoidosis.

Answer: C. Several skin conditions that are of most importance in African-American clients include:

- Keloids—scars that form at the site of a wound and grow beyond the normal boundaries of the wound. They are sharply elevated and irregular and continue to enlarge.
- Pigmentary disorders—areas of either post-inflammatory hypopigmentation or hyperpigmentation, appear as dark or light spots.
- Pseudofolliculitis—"razor bumps" and "ingrown hairs" are caused by shaving too closely with an electric razor or straight razor. The sharp point of the hair, if shaved too close, enters the skin and induces an immune response as to a foreign body. The symptoms include papules, pustules, and sometimes keloids.
- Melasma—the "mask of pregnancy" is a patchy tan to dark brown discoloration of the face more prevalent in dark pregnant women.

TEST-TAKING STRATEGY: Use the process of elimination to rule out incorrect answer selections to help choose the correct answer.

398. Which factor is most accurately linked to stress?

   A. Breakdown disorder.

   B. Decreased life satisfaction.

   C. Improvement of mental disorders.

   D. Increased immunologic functioning.

Answer: B. Decreased life satisfaction, the development of mental disorders, the occurrence of stress-related illnesses—such as cardiovascular disease, gastrointestinal disorders, low back pain, and headaches—and decreased immunologic functioning, which has been implicated in a diagnosis of cancer, are linked to stress.

TEST-TAKING STRATEGY: Terms like *most appropriately* and *most accurately* mean that the undeniably correct answer is most likely not present. Therefore, you must select the best answer choice from the selections provided.

399. Environmental and social stressors that place children and adolescents at high risk for poor adjustment include (select all that apply):

   A. Community violence.

   B. Increased availability of drugs.

   C. Personal safety concerns.

   D. Prolonged affluence.

Answer A, B, & C. Environmental and social stressors that place children and adolescents at high risk for poor adjustment are personal safety concerns, community violence, prolonged poverty, increased availability of drugs, homelessness, and AIDS.

TEST-TAKING STRATEGY: When answering "Select all that apply" questions, be sure and treat each answer as a true or false statement. There may be one correct answer or more.

400. The primary mode of intervention for stress management consist of:

   A. Avoiding all stress.

   B. Conditioning to avoid physiologic arousal resulting from stress.

   C. Decreasing resistance to stress.

   D. Minimizing the frequency of stress-inducing situations.

Answer: D. The primary mode of intervention for stress management consist of minimizing the frequency of stress-inducing situations; increasing resistance to stress; and counterconditioning to avoid physiologic arousal resulting from stress. Changing the environment to decrease the incidence of stressors should be the "first line of defense." When that is not possible, individual and family coping resources need to come into play to reinterpret stress as a challenge, increase resilience against stress, or decrease the health-threatening effects of stressors.

TEST-TAKING STRATEGY: Questions that ask you to prioritize your nursing actions use terms like *priority, first, best, initial, most important, primary, immediate,* and *next.*

401. The nurse teaches a client who complains of stress that the most proactive approach to minimizing the frequency of stress-inducing situations is to (select all that apply):

A. Embrace excessive change.

B. Change the stressful environment.

C. Control others.

D. Manage time effectively.

Answer: B & D. Changing the environment, when it is possible, is the most proactive approach to minimizing the frequency of stress-inducing situations. Other approaches include avoiding excessive change and managing time effectively. Stress is increased by exposure to excessive change and by attempting to control the behaviors and actions of others.

TEST-TAKING STRATEGY: When answering "Select all that apply" questions, be sure and treat each answer as a true or false statement. There may be one correct answer or more.

402. Psychologic conditioning to increase resistance to stress focuses on:

A. Building physical resources.

B. Decreasing assertiveness.

C. Enhancing self-esteem.

D. Exercise.

Answer: C. Resistance to stress is achieved through either physical or psychological conditioning. Physical conditioning for stress resistance focuses on exercise. Psychological conditioning to increase resistance resources focuses on enhancing self-esteem, enhancing self-efficacy, increasing assertiveness, setting realistic goals, and building coping resources.

TEST-TAKING STRATEGY: Use the process of elimination to rule out incorrect answer selections to help choose the correct answer.

403. General coping strategies identified to enhance stress resistance include: Select all that apply.

A. Resistance.

B. Self-doubt.

C. Problem solving.

D. Stress monitoring.

Answer: C & D. General coping resources identified to enhance stress resistance are self-disclosure, self-directedness, confidence, acceptance, social support, financial freedom, physical health, physical fitness, stress monitoring, tension control, structuring, and problem-solving.

TEST-TAKING STRATEGY: When answering "Select all that apply" questions, be sure and treat each answer as a true or false statement. There may be one correct answer or more.

404. Social networks that provide support to a client can be categorized by (select all that apply):

A. Composition.

B. Density.

C. Intensity.

D. Size.

Answer: A, B, C, & D. Social networks can be defined with *size* (actual number of individuals), *composition* (types of persons in the network, such as spouse or friends), *geographic dispersion* (distances separating network members), *intensity* (frequency and extent of contact with network members), *density* (extent to which members know and interact with each other), and *homogeneity* (similarity of network members on various characteristics).

TEST-TAKING STRATEGY: When answering "Select all that apply" questions, be sure and treat each answer as a true or false statement. There may be one correct answer or more.

405. Which are sources of client support? Select all that apply.

A. Church.

B. Family.

C. Peers.

D. Self-help groups.

Answer: A, B, C, & D. Social support is defined as a network of interpersonal relationships that provide companionship, assistance, and emotional nourishment. Several social support systems relevant to health have been identified: natural support systems (families), peer support systems, organized religious support systems, organized professional support systems, and organized self-help support groups not directed by health professionals.

TEST-TAKING STRATEGY: When answering "Select all that apply" questions, be sure and treat each answer as a true or false statement. There may be one correct answer or more.

406. Nurses work with dying clients and their families every day. The needs of the families of dying clients are:

   A. To allow the nurse to provide all of the care to the dying person.

   B. To chastise the physician and health care staff.

   C. To shun the dying person.

   D. To ventilate emotions.

   Answer: D. Needs of families of dying clients are to be with the dying person and to provide help to the dying person; to be informed of the dying person's changing condition and to understand what is being done to the client and why; to be assured of the client's comfort and to be comforted; to ventilate emotions and to be assured that their decisions regarding care are sound; to find meaning in the dying of their loved one; and to be fed, hydrated, and rested.

   TEST-TAKING STRATEGY: Read the question twice to ensure that you understand what the question is asking, especially if the question is tricky or confusing. Focus on what the question is asking: the needs of the client's family during the dying process.

407. Many facilities allow the client's family to be present during resuscitative efforts. What is the advantage to having family present during resuscitation of a client?

   A. The client's obstruction of the grieving process.

   B. The client's denial of death.

   C. The family's feelings of helplessness.

   D. The family's recognition that the client is dying.

   Answer: D. Advantages to having family present to watch nurses and physicians carry out resuscitative efforts of the client include recognizing that the client is dying; feeling helpful and supportive to the client and the staff; knowing that everything possible is being done to resuscitate the client; being able to touch the client while he or she is warm; saying whatever they need to say while there is still a chance that the client can hear; recognizing the futility of further resuscitation efforts; facilitating the grieving process; and accepting the reality of death.

   TEST-TAKING STRATEGY: Use the process of elimination to rule out incorrect answer selections to help choose the correct answer.

408. The nurse should communicate the news about the death of a client to the family:

   A. By voice-mail.

   B. By messenger.

   C. By telephone.

   D. In person.

   Answer: D. Communicating news about the death of a client to the family should be done in person whenever possible. The ideal setting is in a private room that has seating available for everyone.

   TEST-TAKING STRATEGY: Look for similar answer choices and eliminate them.

409. The nurse should demonstrate compassion and empathy when communicating news about the death of a client to the family. Which is an example of appropriate communication skills by the nurse during this situation?

   A. "He was on the vent for a short time."

   B. "I am very sorry for your loss."

   C. "It's okay. He is at peace now."

   D. "We coded him. He just didn't make it."

   Answer: B. Avoiding clichés and unfamiliar jargon such as "code" and "vent" are important communication skills for the nurse. Stating a simple condolence and offering to answer any questions is appropriate.

   TEST-TAKING STRATEGY: Use the process of elimination to rule out incorrect answer selections to help choose the correct answer.

410. The nurse discusses organ donation with a family whose loved one has suddenly passed. Common courtesy and sensitivity to the family's grief are important. Which action facilitates the family's option of organ donation?

A. Assuring the family that the decision is not theirs to make.

B. Asking the family about organ donation immediately following the client's death.

C. Using a private area to discuss organ donation with the family.

D. Communicating about the loved one's death after organ donation forms are signed.

Answer: C. Using a private area to discuss organ donation with the family facilitates the option of organ donation. The family should be assured that organ donation is their decision to make. The family should be allowed time to absorb the news regarding their loved one's death before addressing donation or signing donation forms. Informing the family of the possible benefits of donation, providing information that will assuage the family's fears about donation, and providing time for families to be with their loved ones and deciding about their options also facilitate offering of the option of organ donation.

TEST-TAKING STRATEGY: Use the process of elimination to rule out incorrect answer selections to help choose the correct answer.

411. Some health care providers believe there are disadvantages to having families observe cardiopulmonary resuscitation (CPR). These disadvantages are: Select all that apply.

A. CPR is traumatic and frightening to watch.

B. Families may interfere with protocols and procedures.

C. Staff may become too stressed and distracted when family is present.

D. There is not enough space at the client's bedside for the CPR team as well as the family.

Answer: A, B, C, & D. All of the above are correct. Some health care providers also believe that there is an increased risk of liability, and staff is not available to provide family information and support during the resuscitation.

TEST-TAKING STRATEGY: When answering "Select all that apply" questions, be sure and treat each answer as a true or false statement. There may be one correct answer or more.

412. Which are the four factors that are helpful in readying families for hospital discharge? Select all that apply.

A. Availability of social support.

B. Ignorance of what to expect.

C. Misuse of coping strategies.

D. Accessibility to public resources.

Answer: A & D. Four factors that are helpful in readying families for hospital discharge are availability of social support, use of coping strategies, accessibility to personal resources, and knowledge of what to expect after discharge.

TEST-TAKING STRATEGY: When answering "Select all that apply" questions, be sure and treat each answer as a true or false statement. There may be one correct answer or more.

413. The nurse knows that families require coping skills to manage illness recovery at home. Which is an appropriate coping skill of the family?

A. Inability to acquire needed information.

B. Inability to manage worry and anxiety.

C. Inability to seek help if needed.

D. Problem-solving ability.

Answer: D. Coping skills of the family during a client's illness recovery at home are problem-solving ability, ability to seek help if needed, ability to manage worry and anxiety, and ability to acquire needed information. Nurses need to assess family coping strategies to devise interventions that will fit the individual family's needs.

TEST-TAKING STRATEGY: Look for similar answer choices and eliminate them.

414. Four categories of personal resources can help family members feel ready to take a client home from the hospital. Which should the nurse address with the client and family during discharge teaching? Select all that apply.

A. Health and energy.

B. Positive health beliefs.

C. Self-confidence.

D. Time.

Answer: A, B, C, & D. Health and energy, positive health beliefs, self-confidence, and time are categories that need to be addressed by the nurse during discharge teaching.

TEST-TAKING STRATEGY: When answering "Select all that apply" questions, be sure and treat each answer as a true or false statement. There may be one correct answer or more.

415. Which have influenced clients' treatment needs and the system of care delivery in psychiatric and mental health treatment? Select all that apply.

A. Decreased outpatient care.

B. Increased hospital stays.

C. Increased outpatient care.

D. Shortened hospital stays.

Answer: C & D. Increased outpatient care and shortened hospital stays along with more manageable medication protocols have influenced clients' treatment needs and the system of care delivery in psychiatric and mental health treatment.

TEST-TAKING STRATEGY: When answering "Select all that apply" questions, be sure and treat each answer as a true or false statement. There may be one correct answer or more.

416. Which percentage of those with mental illness receive treatment in the health care system?

A. 25%.

B. 33%.

C. 40%.

D. 50%.

Answer: A. Only 25% of those with mental illness receive treatment in the health care system

despite the prevalence of mental illness, its many consequences, and the existence of effective treatment.

TEST-TAKING STRATEGY: Use the process of elimination to rule out incorrect answer selections to help choose the correct answer.

417. One theory commonly used in family mental health nursing is Bowen's family systems theory. The central assumption in this theory is that chronic anxiety is the underlying basis for dysfunction. The theory consists of eight interlocking concepts that address anxiety and emotional processes. These include:

A. Differentiation of self.

B. Quadriceps.

C. The family process system.

D. The nuclear family spiritual system.

Answer: A. Bowen's family systems theory concepts include: differentiation of self, triangles, the family projection process, the nuclear family emotional system, multigenerational transmission process, sibling position, emotional cutoff, and societal regression.

TEST-TAKING STRATEGY: Use the process of elimination to rule out incorrect answer selections to help choose the correct answer.

418. Major depression most prominently affects:

A. The employed.

B. The educated.

C. More women than men.

D. Affluent women.

Answer: C. Major depression affects approximately twice as many women as men. Women who are poor, less educated, unemployed, or on welfare are at highest risk for experiencing a major depression.

TEST-TAKING STRATEGY: Look for similar answer choices and eliminate them.

419. The nurse is caring for a client who experiences battered women's syndrome. The nurse knows that the four forms of abuse are (select all that apply):

A. Emotional.

B. Neglect.

C. Physical.

D. Sexual.

Answer: A, B, C, & D. The four forms of abuse are emotional, neglect, physical, and sexual.

TEST-TAKING STRATEGY: When answering "Select all that apply" questions, be sure and treat each answer as a true or false statement. There may be one correct answer or more.

420. Three sets of factors place families at risk for child abuse and neglect. Parental risk factors that place families at risk for child abuse and neglect include:

   A. The behavior issues of the child.

   B. The parent's belief in emotional punishment.

   C. The parent's strong friendships in the community.

   D. The abuse or neglect the parent suffered as a child.

Answer: D. Research indicates that there are three sets of factors that place families at risk for child abuse and neglect: parental characteristics, child characteristics, and family ecosystem characteristics. Parental factors include the parent's abuse or neglect suffered as a child; the parent's belief in physical punishment; the parent's unrealistic expectations of the child; the parent's level of stress; the parent's loner behavior with few friends; the parent's vision that the child is willful and purposely "bad"; and the parent's substance abuse.

TEST-TAKING STRATEGY: Read the question twice to ensure that you understand what the question is asking, especially if the question is tricky or confusing. Focus on what the question is asking: parental risk factors for engaging in child abuse.

421. Which factor most accurately reflects characteristics of the child that place families at risk for child abuse and neglect?

   A. The child is healthy.

   B. The child has a difficult personality.

C. The family is socially isolated.

D. The parent believes in physical punishment.

Answer: B. Research indicates there are three sets of factors that place families at risk for child abuse and neglect: parental characteristics, child characteristics, and family ecosystem characteristics. Characteristics of the child that place the family at risk for child abuse and neglect are the child being different as a result of illness, prematurity, or disability; and the child being difficult (e.g., fussy, hyperactive, demanding).

TEST-TAKING STRATEGY: Read the question twice to ensure that you understand what the question is asking, especially if the question is tricky or confusing. Focus on what the question is asking: characteristics of a child that places the family at risk for engaging in child abuse.

422. Which is a familial factor that most accurately places a family at risk for child abuse and neglect?

   A. The child has a difficult personality.

   B. The family has no history of abuse.

   C. The family is socially isolated.

   D. The parent experiences tremendous stress.

Answer: C. Research indicates that there are three sets of factors that place families at risk for child abuse and neglect: parental characteristics, child characteristics, and family ecosystem characteristics. Familial factors include the family's level of stress, social isolation of the family, a patriarchal (male-dominated) household, and history of abuse in the nuclear or extended family.

TEST-TAKING STRATEGY: Terms like *most appropriately* and *most accurately* mean that the undeniable correct answer is most likely not present. Therefore, you must select the best answer choice from the selections provided.

423. Primary prevention of domestic abuse involves:

  A. Conduct community classes to teach parents about normal developmental challenges.

  B. Early intervention to prevent or stop the violence.

  C. Identification of families at risk for violence.

  D. Strengthening individuals and families to enable them to better cope with life stressors.

Answer: D. Primary prevention of abuse involves strengthening individuals and families to enable them to better cope with multiple life stressors. For example, nurses can conduct community classes to teach parents about normal developmental challenges, such as toilet training; ways to discipline without physical punishment; and methods of conflict resolution. Secondary prevention involves identification of families at risk for violence and those who are beginning to use violence, followed by early intervention to prevent or stop the violence.

TEST-TAKING STRATEGY: Use the process of elimination to rule out incorrect answer selections to help choose the correct answer.

424. When the family is faced with impending loss of a member, unresolved conflicts and relational patterns may become intensified. In assisting the family, the family mental health nurse may intervene by (select all that apply):

  A. Eliciting the family's multigenerational history of loss to better understand the meaning of the impending loss to the family.

  B. Guiding the family in constructively addressing unresolved conflicts and issues between family members and the dying individual.

  C. Helping the family to convey its feelings to the dying person and to say good-bye.

  D. Supporting family members through the bereavement process, while remaining alert to symptoms that suggest complicated bereavement and the need for additional intervention.

Answer: A, B, C, & D. All of these are interventions that can be made by the mental health nurse when assisting the family that experiences impending loss of a member.

TEST-TAKING STRATEGY: When answering "Select all that apply" questions, be sure and treat each answer as a true or false statement. There may be one correct answer or more.

425. Sensitive and skilled end-of-life care for clients and family members is critical for gerontological family nurses. Which is a common concern for clients and families experiencing the end of life?

  A. Communication about relationships.

  B. Making preparations for the living.

  C. Maintaining public identity.

  D. Management of symptoms.

Answer: D. Six common concerns for clients and families experiencing the end of life are management of symptoms, communication about treatment, making preparations for death, completing and contributing, maintaining personal identity, and perpetuating a trusting relationship with the nurse and physician.

TEST-TAKING STRATEGY: Use the process of elimination to rule out incorrect answer selections to help choose the correct answer.

426. Which questionnaire should the nurse use to screen a male client for alcohol abuse?

  A. CAGE.

  B. COPE.

  C. FACT.

  D. TACE.

Answer: A. The CAGE questionnaire is used to screen a client for alcohol abuse. There is no such thing as the COPE questionnaire. There is no such thing as the FACT questionnaire. TACE is a four-item questionnaire based on CAGE but for use with pregnant women.

TEST-TAKING STRATEGY: Use the process of elimination to rule out incorrect answer selections to help choose the correct answer.

427. Which is a self-help group for families of alcoholics?

  A. Al-Anon.

  B. Al-Avert.

C. Alcoholics Anonymous.

D. Narc-Anon.

Answer: A. Al-Anon is for families who are at risk for alcohol problems, or who have a problem drinker or alcohol-dependent individual in the family. Al-Avert is not a self-help group. Alcoholics Anonymous is a self-help group for clients who are alcohol-dependent. Narc-Anon is for clients who are narcotic dependent.

TEST-TAKING STRATEGY: Use the process of elimination to rule out incorrect answer selections to help choose the correct answer.

428. Clients who are alcohol dependent usually require a two-phase treatment regimen. Which is an example of an effective two-phase treatment regimen?

A. Detoxification and rehabilitation.

B. Detoxification and purging.

C. Rehabilitation and depression.

D. Rehabilitation and reformation.

Answer: A. Detoxification ameliorates the symptoms of withdrawal. Rehabilitation helps the client avoid future problems with alcohol.

TEST-TAKING STRATEGY: Look for similar answer choices and eliminate them.

429. In a client with anorexia nervosa, the nurse expects to see:

A. Amenorrhea.

B. Insistence on maintaining weight.

C. Intense fear of weight loss.

D. Recurrent episodes of binge eating.

Answer: A. Diagnostic criteria for anorexia nervosa are the refusal to maintain weight at or above a minimally normal weight for age and height; intense fear of weight gain even though the client is underweight; amenorrhea; and a severe body-image disturbance in which weight has undue influence on feelings of self-worth. Recurrent episodes of binge eating occurs with bulimia nervosa.

TEST-TAKING STRATEGY: Use the process of elimination to rule out incorrect answer selections to help choose the correct answer.

430. In a client with bulimia nervosa, the nurse expects to see (select all that apply):

A. Amenorrhea.

B. Feelings of self-worth unduly influenced by weight.

C. Recurrent episodes of binge eating.

D. Recurrent inappropriate compensatory behavior to prevent weight gain.

Answer: B, C, & D. Diagnostic criteria for bulimia nervosa are recurrent episodes of binge eating; recurrent inappropriate compensatory behavior to prevent weight gain such as laxative, diuretic, or enema use, induced vomiting, fasting, and excessive exercise; and feelings of self-worth unduly influenced by weight. Amenorrhea is found in anorexia nervosa.

TEST-TAKING STRATEGY: When answering "Select all that apply" questions, be sure and treat each answer as a true or false statement. There may be one correct answer or more.

431. Which is a behavioral intervention that the nurse can use to assist the client who wishes to quit smoking?

A. Assist with proper performance of spirometry.

B. Perform complete examination of lungs.

C. Provide assistance with application of transdermal nicotine replacement patches.

D. Provide practical counseling.

Answer: D. A behavioral intervention the nurse can employ to assist the client who wishes to quit smoking is providing practical counseling. Assisting with proper performance of spirometry, performing a complete examination of the lungs, and providing assistance with application of transdermal nicotine replacement patches are not behavioral interventions.

TEST-TAKING STRATEGY: Use the process of elimination to rule out incorrect answer selections to help choose the correct answer.

432. Clients with primary anxiety disorders are most responsive to pharmacotherapy or a combination of pharmacotherapy and psychotherapy in the form of cognitive-behavioral therapy. Which is a therapeutic technique that can be utilized by the nurse for clients with primary anxiety disorders? Select all that apply.

A. Activity assignments.

B. Careful monitoring.

C. Goal setting.

D. Relaxation techniques.

Answer: A, B, C, & D. Therapeutic techniques that can be utilized by the nurse for clients with primary anxiety disorders include activity assignments, careful monitoring, goal setting, and relaxation techniques. Other therapeutic techniques include assisting clients to use "self-talk" to help deal with anxiety-provoking stressors.

TEST-TAKING STRATEGY: When answering "Select all that apply" questions, be sure and treat each answer as a true or false statement. There may be one correct answer or more.

433. A 24-year-old client undergoes a traumatic below-the-knee amputation. The nurse assesses the client for risk of suicide. Which is a risk factor for suicide?

A. Age.

B. Female.

C. Hopelessness.

D. Living with family.

Answer: C. Risk factors for suicide are hopelessness, Caucasian race, male gender, age greater than 65 years, living alone, personal and family history of suicide attempts, and personal and family history of alcohol or substance abuse.

TEST-TAKING STRATEGY: Use the process of elimination to rule out incorrect answer selections to help choose the correct answer.

434. A client's family experiences acute grief. Which action by the nurse offers the most comfort to the family?

A. The nurse speaks about the philosophy of death.

B. The nurse tells the family, "I care."

C. The nurse offers advice about which action the family should take next.

D. The nurse relates a personal anecdote detailing the nurse's coping strategies during a similar situation.

Answer: B. The nurse's presence and empathy is the most important comfort to the family. Speaking about a philosophy of death or relating personal anecdotes is not helpful to the family.

TEST-TAKING STRATEGY: Questions that ask you to prioritize your nursing actions use terms like *priority, first, best, initial, most important, immediate,* and *next.*

435. A 74-year-old client is seen by the physician for treatment of cataracts. The nurse teaches the client about the signs and symptoms of cataracts. Which statement by the client indicates that the client understands the teaching?

A. "I may experience altered color perception and image distortion."

B. "My vision should improve with the cataracts."

C. "Where do I buy a seeing eye dog?"

D. "My nighttime driving should improve with the cataracts."

Answer: A. Cataracts can cause decreased vision, glare, distortion, and altered color perception. Nighttime vision decreases with cataracts making driving a challenge. Cataract surgery can improve a client's vision, thus making the purchase of a seeing eye dog unnecessary.

TEST-TAKING STRATEGY: The phrase "client understands the teaching" tells you to select the answer with accurate information.

436. The nurse knows that risk factors for glaucoma include:

A. Asian-American race.

B. Decreased intraocular pressure.

C. Diabetes.

D. Younger age.

Answer: A & C. Risk factors for glaucoma include high intraocular pressure (IOP); older age; African-American race; family history of glaucoma, myopia, diabetes, and hypertension.

TEST-TAKING STRATEGY: Use the process of elimination to rule out incorrect answer selections to help choose the correct answer.

437. Bilateral progressive hearing loss in a 27-year-old female was first noticed 2 years ago when she was pregnant with her second child. Which illness is most likely the cause of the client's progressive hearing loss?

    A. Acoustic neuroma.

    B. Cholesteatoma.

    C. Otosclerosis.

    D. Serous otitis media.

    Answer: C. Otosclerosis is associated with slow, progressive hearing loss (usually bilateral) beginning in the second or third decade of life. In women, hearing loss is often first noticed during pregnancy. Acoustic neuroma presents with tinnitus, unilateral, unexplained hearing loss, and disequilibrium. Cholesteatoma is a benign, slowly growing lesion in the middle ear or mastoid that destroys bone and normal ear tissue. Serous otitis media is the most frequent cause of hearing loss in children and an important factor of hearing loss in adults.

    TEST-TAKING STRATEGY: Terms like *most appropriately* and *most likely* mean that the undeniably correct answer is probably not present. Therefore, you must select the best answer choice from the selections provided.

438. A client experiences a transient ischemic attack (TIA). The nurse informs the client upon discharge that which factor is associated with an increased risk of stroke after a TIA?

    A. Clear speech.

    B. Diabetes mellitus.

    C. Symptoms lasting less than 10 minutes.

    D. Younger age.

Answer: B. Factors associated with an increased risk of stroke after a TIA include advanced age, diabetes mellitus, symptoms lasting more than 10 minutes, weakness, and impaired speech.

TEST-TAKING STRATEGY: Use the process of elimination to rule out incorrect answer selections to help choose the correct answer.

439. The nurse who works in a rehabilitation facility knows that client risk factors for alcohol and other drug abuse are (select all that apply):

    A. Affiliating with alcohol- and drug-using peers.

    B. Depression.

    C. Family trauma.

    D. Poor interpersonal relationships.

    Answer: A, B, C, & D. Affiliating with alcohol- and drug-using peers, depression, family trauma, and poor interpersonal relationships are risk factors for alcohol and other drug abuse.

    TEST-TAKING STRATEGY: When answering "Select all that apply" questions, be sure and treat each answer as a true or false statement. There may be one correct answer or more.

440. Clients who have substance use disorders fall into one of five stages. These stages occur along a continuum that provides a useful framework for monitoring progress. A client admits to the nurse that substance use is causing difficulties in the client's life. Which stage is the client experiencing?

    A. Action.

    B. Contemplation.

    C. Maintenance.

    D. Precontemplation.

    Answer: B. Contemplation occurs when the client reflects on the consequences substance use is causing. Action occurs when the client acts. Maintenance occurs when the client has internalized change and is maintaining the change. Precontemplation occurs prior to contemplation when the client is assessing the effects of substance use.

TEST-TAKING STRATEGY: Use the process of elimination to rule out incorrect answer selections to help choose the correct answer.

441. The nurse who works in a rehabilitation facility knows that psychosocial interventions for substance abuse include:

    A. Behavioral therapy.

    B. Group therapy.

    C. Pharmacotherapies.

    D. Self-help groups.

    Answer: **B.** A psychosocial intervention for substance abuse includes group therapy. Behavioral therapy, pharmacotherapies, and self-help groups are not forms of psychosocial intervention.

    TEST-TAKING STRATEGY: Use the process of elimination to rule out incorrect answer selections to help choose the correct answer.

442. The nurse teaches an alcoholic client the signs and symptoms of alcohol withdrawal. Which statement by the client indicates that he understands the teaching?

    A. "My heart rate may slow down during withdrawal."

    B. "I will become very sleepy during withdrawal."

    C. "My hands may begin to shake once I quit drinking."

    D. "My blood pressure will drop once I quit drinking."

    Answer: **C.** The most common signs and symptoms of alcohol withdrawal are hand tremor, tachycardia, nervousness, and hypertension.

    TEST-TAKING STRATEGY: The phrase "client understands the teaching" tells you to select the answer with accurate information.

443. The nurse teaches a narcotic addict the signs and symptoms of opioid withdrawal. Which statement by the client indicates further teaching by the nurse is necessary? Select all that apply.

    A. "My heart rate will slow down when I quit using."

    B. "My breathing rate will speed up when I quit using."

    C. "My blood pressure will drop when my body craves more drugs."

    D. "My pupils can dilate for a long time when I quit using."

    Answer: **A & C.** Signs and symptoms of opioid withdrawal include tachycardia, tachypnea, hypertension, and mydriasis (prolonged dilation of the pupils).

    TEST-TAKING STRATEGY: The phrase "further teaching is necessary" tells you to select an answer with inaccurate information.

444. If disulfiram (Antabuse) is prescribed and the client drinks alcohol, which of the following symptoms will likely occur? Select all that apply.

    A. Chest pain.

    B. Nausea.

    C. Sweating.

    D. Throbbing headache.

    Answer: **A, B, C, & D.** If a client is taking disulfiram (Antabuse) and drinks alcohol, the client will likely experience chest pain, nausea, sweating, and a throbbing headache.

    TEST-TAKING STRATEGY: When answering "Select all that apply" questions, be sure and treat each answer as a true or false statement. There may be one correct answer or more.

445. Clients unlikely to abstain from alcohol are not appropriate candidates for treatment with disulfiram (Antabuse), nor are clients with:

    A. A sedentary occupation.

    B. Chronic hepatitis.

    C. Latex allergy.

    D. Significant cardiac disease.

    Answer: **D.** Clients unlikely to abstain from alcohol are not appropriate candidates for treatment with disulfiram (Antabuse), nor are clients with significant cardiac disease. Disulfiram can worsen cardiac disease. A sedentary occupation, chronic hepatitis, and latex allergy have no effect on the use of disulfiram.

TEST-TAKING STRATEGY: Use the process of elimination to rule out incorrect answer selections to help choose the correct answer.

446. A client is diagnosed with obsessive-compulsive disorder. Which behavior would the nurse expect to observe in this client? Select all that apply.

A. Compulsions.

B. Excessive symptoms.

C. Recurrent obsessions.

D. Unreasonable symptoms.

Answer: A, B, C, & D. Obsessive-compulsive disorder is characterized by recurrent obsessions (intrusive and inappropriate thoughts, impulses, and images) and/or compulsions (behaviors or mental health acts performed in response to obsessions or rigid application of rules) that consume less than 1 hour a day or cause marked impairment or distress. These symptoms are perceived as excessive and unreasonable.

TEST-TAKING STRATEGY: When answering "Select all that apply" questions, be sure and treat each answer as a true or false statement. There may be one correct answer or more.

447. Which disease process is characterized by anxiety about and avoidance of places or situations in which the ability to escape is limited or embarrassing?

A. Agoraphobia.

B. Arachnophobia.

C. Sociophobia.

D. Trypanophobia.

Answer: A. Agoraphobia is the fear of public places. Arachnophobia is fear of spiders. Trypanophobia is fear of injections. Sociophobia is fear of social evaluation.

TEST-TAKING STRATEGY: Read the question twice to ensure that you understand what the question is asking, especially if the question is tricky or confusing. Focus on what the question

is asking: the disease characterized by fear of inability to escape a place or situation.

448. Every crisis model is based on the behavioral problem-solving model. Which are steps of the behavioral problem-solving model? Select all that apply.

A. Brainstorming alternatives.

B. Defining the problem.

C. Following up.

D. Reviewing past actions to correct the problem.

Answer: A, B, C, & D. There are actually five steps of the behavioral problem-solving mode: defining the problem, reviewing past actions to correct the problem, deciding the desired outcome of the solved problem, brainstorming alternatives, selecting alternatives and committing to following through with them, and following up.

TEST-TAKING STRATEGY: When answering "Select all that apply" questions, be sure and treat each answer as a true or false statement. There may be one correct answer or more.

449. The ABC model of crisis intervention is a convenient way to organize a crisis interviewing session. The focus of the ABC model is to identify the client's (select all that apply):

A. Thoughts about the precipitating event.

B. Failed coping mechanisms.

C. Ideas regarding precipitating events.

D. Subjective distress.

Answer: A, B, C, & D. The ABC model identifies the client's thoughts regarding the precipitating event, failed coping mechanisms, ideas regarding precipitating events, and subjective distress. Another focus is the client's impaired function. These are the aspects of a crisis. The goal is to help the client integrate the precipitating event into daily functioning and return to pre-crisis levels emotionally, occupationally, and interpersonally. Key concepts include developing and maintaining contact, identifying the problem, and coping.

TEST-TAKING STRATEGY: When answering "Select all that apply" questions, be sure and treat each answer as a true or false statement. There may be one correct answer or more.

450. The foundation of crisis intervention is the development of a state of understanding and comfort between client and nurse. This is known as:

    A. Attending behavior.

    B. Paraphrasing.

    C. Rapport.

    D. Reflection.

    Answer: C. Before delving into the client's personal world, the nurse must achieve personal contact and establish rapport. Attending behavior includes eye contact, warmth, body posture, and vocal style. Paraphrasing includes restating in your own words to clarify the client's message. Reflection includes talking about painful feelings, positive feelings, and ambivalent feelings.

    TEST-TAKING STRATEGY: Use the process of elimination to rule out incorrect answer selections to help choose the correct answer.

451. A client arrives in the physician's office complaining of insomnia, decreased appetite, and weight loss due to a recent job loss. The physician diagnoses the client with generalized anxiety disorder and prescribes two common anti-anxiety medications. The client expresses concern to the nurse about taking medication for the symptoms and asks about alternatives for treating the anxiety. The nurse's best action is to:

    A. Instruct the client to begin yoga and provide the times and locations of local classes in the area.

    B. Instruct the client in basic rhythmic breathing techniques as well as a simple modified autogenic relaxation exercise.

    C. Educate the client in various relaxation techniques while determining which seems most appealing to the client.

    D. Refer the client to a local financial advisor.

Answer: C. Educating the client in various relaxation techniques, while determining which seems most appealing to the client, helps to alleviate the client's anxiety while allowing the client to maintain control by making choices.

TEST-TAKING STRATEGY: This question asks for the best nursing action. Focus on the diagnosis and determine what nursing action is the most appropriate for this client.

452. Which are considered complementary and/or alternative therapies? Select all that apply.

    A. Digoxin (Lanoxin)

    B. Zone diet

    C. Tai Chi

    D. Reiki

    Answer: B, C, & D. The Zone diet, Tai Chi, and Reiki are all considered complementary and/or alternative therapies. Digoxin, although originally derived from the foxglove plant and used for centuries, has become a staple of Western medicine for the treatment of cardiac disorders and is not considered a complementary or alternative therapy.

    TEST-TAKING STRATEGY: When answering "Select all that apply" questions, be sure and treat each answer as a true or false statement. There may be one correct answer or more.

453. A client is admitted to the hospital with a blood pressure of 85/53 mm Hg and is complaining of light-headedness and near syncope. The client's current medications include carvedilol (Coreg), amiodarone (Cordarone), warfarin (Coumadin), lanoxin (Digoxin), furosemide (Lasix), potassium (K-Dur), and a daily vitamin. The client also reports using both St. John's wort and cat's claw. Based upon this information, what is the nurse's best action?

    A. Notify the physician immediately reporting the client is critically ill and needs transfer to the ICU.

    B. Notify the physician that the client's use of cat's claw may interact with some of the other heart medications that the client is taking, resulting in hypotension.

C. Notify the physician that the client's use of St. John's wort may interact with the diuretic the client is taking, resulting in light-headedness.

D. Notify the physician that the client's use of cat's claw may interact with the anticoagulant the client is taking, resulting in near syncope.

Answer: B. Notify the physician that the client's use of cat's claw may interact with some of the other heart medications the client is taking, resulting in hypotension.

TEST-TAKING STRATEGY: Use the process of elimination to determine the most inappropriate actions. Then focus on the client's presenting complaints to determine which herb may be causing a potential interaction.

454. A client is having a CAT scan and is worried about being in an enclosed space for the test. The client also states that anti-anxiety medications cause confusion. The client asks if there are other ways of helping control the fear while the scan is being done. The client reports attending yoga classes and finds guided imagery very relaxing. What is the nurse's best action to take with this client?

A. Discuss the use of the breath work that the client does during yoga and inform the client that music headphones are available in the radiology department.

B. Discuss the use of Reiki therapy and therapeutic touch during the CAT scan. Provide instruction in the use of these two methods during the CAT scan.

C. Discuss use of the "zone diet" and meditation during the CAT scan as alternatives to yoga and guided imagery.

D. Discuss the use of hypnotherapy as an alternative to the guided imagery that the client does during yoga.

Answer: A. Music therapy and breath work are appropriate for use during a CAT scan and provide alternatives that are similar to the methods of relaxation that are familiar to the client. Reiki therapy, hypnotherapy, and therapeutic touch are inappropriate during a CAT scan because

they require the physical presence of a person who is providing the therapy.

TEST-TAKING STRATEGY: Carefully consider the procedure for a CAT scan. Use critical thinking to determine which therapies allow the client to remain motionless and do not require additional practitioners.

455. What is the main goal of herbal therapy?

A. To treat a specific disease or symptom by taking prescription medications.

B. To restore balance within the body by supporting the client's self-healing ability.

C. To avoid the use of toxic chemicals within the body.

D. To incorporate Eastern healing practices into Western medicine.

Answer: B. The main goal of herbal therapy is to restore balance within the body by supporting the client's self-healing ability. Drug therapy's main goal is the treatment of a specific disease or symptom.

TEST-TAKING STRATEGY: Carefully consider the *main goal* of herbal therapy when answering the question.

456. Which type of therapy uses substances found in nature?

A. Energy therapies.

B. Mind-body interventions.

C. Body-based methods.

D. Biologically based therapies.

Answer: D. Biologically based therapies use substances found in nature such as herbs, foods, and vitamins. Energy therapies use energy fields. Mind-body interventions use the mind to help affect the function of the body. Body-based methods use movement of the body.

TEST-TAKING STRATEGY: Carefully consider which of the complementary and alternative medicine therapies fit the short description provided, and then use the process of elimination to determine the correct answer.

457. Which client would benefit most from therapeutic touch therapy?

 A. A pregnant client suffering from backache and anxiety.

 B. A client with cancer and a history of physical abuse.

 C. A client hospitalized with cardiovascular disease and anxiety.

 D. A client with septic shock and anemia in the ICU.

Answer: C. Therapeutic touch has been shown to be effective in the treatment of anxiety in hospitalized patients with cardiovascular disease. The remaining clients are not good candidates for therapeutic touch therapy.

TEST-TAKING STRATEGY: Use the process of elimination to reduce the number of choices. Then focus on the client who would *most* benefit from therapeutic touch.

458. Which client would most benefit from an integrative medicine health care strategy?

 A. A client with chronic fatigue syndrome who has had no relief of fatigue.

 B. A client with diabetes whose blood sugars are out of control and refuses to take the prescribed oral and injection medications.

 C. A client with cholecystitis who wants surgery to definitively treat the symptoms.

 D. A client with a history of a cough for 4 days with green sputum production, fever of 104.2°F, and chest pain with inspiration.

Answer: A. Chronic fatigue syndrome is a chronic health problem that is difficult to treat using only traditional allopathic medicine and responds well to the use of an integrative medicine health care strategy, using a combination of traditional and holistic therapies. Clients with acute illness symptoms are more appropriately treated with traditional medicine strategies.

TEST-TAKING STRATEGY: Use critical thinking to determine how each client would benefit from an integrative medicine health care strategy and then determine which client would *most* benefit from this health care strategy.

459. A client arrives at the physician's office with a history of heart failure, coronary artery disease, fibromyalgia, and hypertension. The client complains of weight gain of 5 pounds in the past week with ankle swelling. The client also reports unresolved pain in the neck, back, shoulders, hips, and knees despite the alternated use of ibuprofen and acetaminophen for pain. The pain has led to feelings of constant fatigue and anxiety. Vital signs are: 130/85-75-24-36.0°C. The physician prescribes additional furosemide (Lasix) and potassium (K-Dur) and adds carvedilol (Coreg) to the client's medication regimen. What suggestion should the nurse make to the physician that would be most helpful in resolving the symptoms listed above which were not addressed by the physician?

 A. Consultation with a cardiologist.

 B. Consultation with a local physician specializing in complementary and alternative medicine (CAM) therapy.

 C. Referral to a local chronic fatigue syndrome support group.

 D. Referral to a pain specialist.

Answer: B. Consultation with a local physician specializing in CAM therapy is the most helpful for the client. Fibromyalgia is difficult to treat with traditional allopathic medicine. CAM therapy, in addition to traditional medical treatments, can provide better treatment for this chronic condition.

TEST-TAKING STRATEGY: Carefully consider the symptoms treated and the other unaddressed symptoms. Choose the option that would be *most helpful* based upon your knowledge of fibromyalgia and its treatment.

460. According to traditional Chinese medicine, what is defined as the vital energy of the human body?

 A. Meridians.

 B. Yin and yang.

 C. Acupoints.

 D. Qi.

Answer: D. Qi is defined as the vital energy of the human body. Meridians are channels of energy that run through the body. Yin and yang represent the inner and outer parts of the body, and the balance between the two, which maintains health in the body. Acupoints are holes along the energy channels where Qi can be influenced.

TEST-TAKING STRATEGY: Use the process of elimination to exclude those terms that do not fit the definition.

461. A client with a recent ACL reconstruction has just received education on crutch use and safety. Which statement best indicates that the client has a complete understanding of the education?

   A. During return demonstration of crutch use, the client's axillas are free of pressure.

   B. The client states principles of crutch safety and use and then demonstrates these principles while using the crutches in the hallway.

   C. The client correctly uses the crutches in the hallway.

   D. The client verbally repeats instructions given regarding the safe use and maintenance of crutches.

   Answer: B. The client both verbally states the principles of crutch safety and use and then demonstrates these principles in practice.

   TEST-TAKING STRATEGY: Look for the most complete answer.

462. A client needs crutches. How does the nurse choose the correct size?

   A. Turn the crutches upside down and measure from the heel to the shoulder.

   B. Obtain a set of crutches and then adjust the height until the client can stand comfortably while resting the axilla on the crutch pad.

   C. Measure the client while standing upright from the axilla to the heel. Then adjust the crutches so that the elbow flexion is a 30-degree angle when the client's hands are placed on the handgrips.

   D. Measure the client from three finger-widths below the axilla to 6 inches lateral to the client's heel.

   Answer: D. Measuring the client from three finger-widths below the axilla to 6 inches lateral to the client's heel is correct to measure for crutches.

   TEST-TAKING STRATEGY: Look for the most complete answer and focus on what the question is asking.

463. The nurse is instructing a client in the use of a cane. Which is the best description of correct cane technique?

   A. Place the cane on the weaker side of the body to help support the weaker leg. Using the cane for support, step forward with the good leg, and then move the weaker leg and the cane forward to the good leg.

   B. Place the cane on the stronger side of the body. The cane is placed forward 6 to 10 inches while the client stands with the body weight divided between the two legs. Then the weaker leg is advanced to the cane, with the body weight divided between the good leg and the cane. Finally, the stronger leg is advanced past the cane and the weaker leg, with the body weight divided between the cane and the weaker leg.

   C. Place the cane on the weaker side of the body. The cane is placed forward 6 to 10 inches while the client stands with the body weight divided between the two legs. The weaker leg is then advanced to the cane, with the body weight divided between the good leg and the cane. Finally, the stronger leg is advanced past the cane and the weaker leg, with the body weight divided between the cane and the weaker leg.

   D. Place the can on the stronger side of the body to help support the weaker leg. Using the cane for support, step forward with the good leg, and then move the weaker leg and the cane forward to the good leg.

Answer: B. Place the cane on the stronger side of the body. The cane is placed forward 6 to 10 inches while the client stands with the body weight divided between the two legs. The weaker leg is then advanced to the cane, with the body weight divided between the good leg and the cane. Finally, the stronger leg is advanced past the cane and the weaker leg, with the body weight divided between the cane and the weaker leg. The cane should be on the stronger side of the body to create a wider base for balance as the client advances the good leg and must use the weaker leg for support with the cane. If the cane is placed on the weaker side of the body, this would create a narrower base for support and balance and increase the risk of falling.

TEST-TAKING STRATEGY: Look for the most complete answer. Consider the body mechanics of the cane on each side of the body. Safety first!

464. Which patient would benefit most from a quad cane?

   A. A recent stroke victim with partial left leg paralysis.

   B. A client with recent right total knee replacement.

   C. A client with an unsteady gait requiring two people to assist with walking.

   D. A recent stroke victim with complete right hemiplegia.

Answer: A. A recent stroke victim with partial left leg paralysis would most benefit from a quad cane. The quad cane provides the best support when there is partial leg paralysis. The other clients would most likely require other types of assistive devices for walking, such as a walker or wheelchair.

TEST-TAKING STRATEGY: Consider the type of support a quad cane provides. Determine the type of assistive device each client may require and use the process of elimination to determine which client would *most* benefit from the quad cane.

465. A client has just been admitted to the medical unit and the nurse is performing an initial physical assessment. The nurse finds that the client has difficulty hearing questions. The nurse also notices an empty glasses case that was sent up with the client from the emergency department. Based on this information, which action should first be taken by the nurse?

   A. Determine out of which ear the client hears best and if there is a hearing deficit in both ears. Then ask the client about the empty glasses case.

   B. Ask the client about use of any "assistive devices" and document the client's response.

   C. Look through the client's belongings to determine if there is a pair of glasses and a hearing aid.

   D. Notify the physician of the client's difficulty hearing and the empty glasses case.

Answer: A. Determine out of which ear the client hears best and if there is a hearing deficit in both ears. If there is a hearing deficit in both ears, use a low-pitched voice that is slightly elevated in volume directed into the better ear and ask the client if the client uses a hearing aid, and if so, if it works. Ask if the client uses glasses and how often the glasses are used at home. Finally, ask if the client brought any of these assistive devices to the hospital. Determining out of which ear the client hear out of best will facilitate verbal communication. The use of the low-pitched voice will assist the client in hearing out of the good ear. Asking about the glasses will determine if the client actually has glasses and when they are used. Finally, asking if these devices were brought to the hospital determines if they should be with the client and might be potentially lost.

TEST-TAKING STRATEGY: Determine the most complete answer. Use your common sense to determine which action should be taken first.

466. A client has a broken lower leg with a non–weight-bearing cast. Which crutch gait would be most appropriate for the nurse to teach?

   A. Swing-through.

   B. Two-point.

   C. Three-point.

   D. Four-point alternating.

Answer: C. Three-point gait. All of the weight-bearing is done by the unaffected leg and the crutches. The injured leg does not touch the ground during the performance of this gait. This is most appropriate for this client with a lower leg cast. The swing-through, two-point, and four-point alternating gaits would require some form of weight-bearing on the broken leg and would therefore not be acceptable forms of crutch-walking for this client.

TEST-TAKING STRATEGY: Visualize how each crutch gait would be performed and then determine which would be appropriate for this client based upon the client's inability to bear weight on the broken leg.

467. A client comes to the physician's office for a follow-up appointment. The nurse notes that the client is using correct cane walking technique. However, the nurse also notes that the client appears to loose balance each time the quad cane is lifted off of the floor and, upon examination, finds bruises on the client's arms and legs. The nurse asks the client about use of the cane at home. The client reports a history of recent falls. The client asks the nurse not to tell the physician because the client does not want to end up in "a home." What is the best action for the nurse to take?

   A. Reassure the client that there are other assistive devices that are options for use at home, such as a walker, and that the nurse and physician will work to find one that will allow the client to remain at home. Inform the physician of the observations made regarding the quad cane.

   B. Inform the client that there are only a few assistive devices available to help with ambulation.

   C. Reassure the client that "homes" are not so bad.

   D. Do not notify the physician of the observations due to patient confidentiality and hope the physician picks up on the client's unstable gait with the quad cane.

Answer: A. Reassure the client that there are other assistive devices that are options for use at home, such as a walker, and that the nurse and physician will work to find one that will allow the client to remain at home. Inform the physician of the observations made regarding the quad cane. This client would most likely benefit from a walker. Discussing the observations with the physician would not be a breach of patient confidentiality and the failure to do so may prove detrimental to the client's safety.

TEST-TAKING STRATEGY: Find the most detailed answer that accurately addresses both the client's concerns of wanting to remain at home and the nurse's concern regarding the client's unsteady gait.

468. A client is being instructed in ascending and descending stairs using crutches. The client cannot bear any weight on the injured leg. Which are appropriate techniques for ascending the stairs? Select all that apply.

   A. All body weight is placed on the crutches.

   B. The body weight is transferred from the crutches to the uninjured leg on the stair.

   C. Body weight is on the affected leg as crutches move to the next stair.

   D. Body weight is transferred to the crutches on the next stair down.

Answer: A & B. All body weight is placed on the crutches and then the body weight is transferred from the crutches to the uninjured leg on the stair. Transferring body weight to the crutches on the next step down is an appropriate technique for *descending* the stairs.

TEST-TAKING STRATEGY: Note that the question refers to appropriate techniques for *ascending* the stairs. Use the process of elimination to rule out inappropriate answers. "Select all that apply" indicates that there may be more than one correct answer.

469. A client is being discharged from the hospital. The client has an unsteady gait and has weakness in the right leg. What assistive device would be most appropriate for the client?

A. Quad cane.

B. Single straight-legged cane.

C. Walker.

D. Lofstrand crutches.

Answer: **C.** A walker—with four wide, sturdy legs—would provide the most stable assistive device for a client with an unsteady gait. The quad cane, single straight-legged cane, or crutches would not provide enough support for this client.

TEST-TAKING STRATEGY: Consider each device and how it would be used by a client with an unsteady gait. Determine which device would best allow the client to ambulate safely.

470. A client has just had knee surgery and is being instructed in how to descend stairs using crutches. The client cannot bear weight on the injured leg. Which instructions should be given to the client? Select all that apply.

A. The body weight is transferred from the crutches to the uninjured leg on the stairs.

B. The uninjured leg is aligned with the crutches on the stair.

C. The body weight is transferred to the crutches on the next stair.

D. All of the body weight starts on the uninjured leg.

Answer: **B, C, & D.** The uninjured leg is aligned with the crutches on the stairs. Transferring the body weight from the crutches to the uninjured leg on the stairs is an instruction for *ascending* the stairs using crutches.

TEST-TAKING STRATEGY: "Select all that apply" indicates that there may be more than one correct answer option. Remember that the steps in a process may not be presented in the correct order.

471. Which part of the kidney forms the urine?

A. Glomerulus.

B. Proximal convoluted tubule.

C. Loop of Henle.

D. Nephron.

Answer: **D.** The nephron is the functional unit of the kidney that forms the urine. The glomerulus, proximal convoluted tubule, and loop of Henle are all parts of the nephron that contribute to the formation of urine.

TEST-TAKING STRATEGY: Make sure you are clear on what the question is asking.

472. The nurse is assisting a client to the bedside commode to urinate. Which brain structures influence the client's bladder function? Select all that apply.

A. Cerebral cortex.

B. Thalamus.

C. Hypothalamus.

D. Brainstem.

Answer: **A, B, C, & D.** The cerebral cortex, thalamus, hypothalamus, and the brainstem all coordinate the muscles that control urination.

TEST-TAKING STRATEGY: When answering "Select all that apply" questions, be sure and treat each answer as a true or false statement. There may be one correct answer or more.

473. A client was admitted to the medical unit after having abdominal surgery. The nurse questioned the client during the morning assessment about the passage of flatus. The client stated that flatus had been passed early in the morning. In anticipation of defecation, what is the most important instruction for the nurse to give the client?

A. Please call the nurse if you need to go to the bathroom.

B. If you feel the urge to have a bowel movement, please call for assistance before getting up to the toilet. When having a bowel movement, be sure to breathe out to prevent straining. Do not hold your breath.

C. To prevent the Valsalva maneuver, contract the stomach muscles while holding your breath and push. This will assist in the passage of the stool and will decrease the amount of time required to have a bowel movement.

D. Your bowels will be moving soon. Please report any abdominal pain.

Answer: B. If you feel the urge to have a bowel movement, please call for assistance before getting up to the toilet. When having a bowel movement, be sure to breathe out to prevent straining. Do not hold your breath.

TEST-TAKING STRATEGY: Focus on what is most important for a client, with an abdominal surgical wound, to know regarding defecation. Consider the client's safety by instructing the client to request assistance when getting out of bed.

474. A client has come to the physician's office complaining of recent constipation. The nurse takes a health history. Which statement made by the client suggests a likely cause of the constipation?

A. "I walk with a group of friends every day at the mall for an hour."

B. "My spouse died 20 years ago, but my family is very loving and supportive. They live just around the corner and come over a few times a week to visit."

C. "The fast food place near my home has really good food. I eat there most of the time."

D. "What is a laxative?"

Answer: C. The fast food place near my home has really good food. I eat there most of the time. A low-fiber diet that is high in animal fats and refined sugar, as is common in fast food, can cause constipation. Walking is a good way to prevent constipation. Stress can cause constipation, but the history does not suggest that the client is having stress at this time. The client's lack of knowledge of laxatives suggests the client does not take one and therefore is not abusing laxatives.

TEST-TAKING STRATEGY: Use your knowledge and common sense to determine the correct response.

475. A client presents to the emergency department (ED) via ambulance with SOB for the past 3 days. After spending 4 hours in the ED, the client is admitted to the intensive care unit (ICU) with pulmonary edema requiring intubation and ventilation. The ED nurse reports to the ICU nurse that a Foley catheter was placed and that the client has had a total of 25 mL of urine output. The labs from the ED reveal BG of 300, BUN of 100, and creatinine of 5.0. The client has a medical history of CAD, CHF, diabetes, COPD, and asthma. What is the most likely cause of the client's low urine output?

A. Acute and chronic renal failure due to diabetes and a decreased blood flow to the kidneys due to heart failure.

B. Renal failure due to decreased coronary output secondary to heart failure.

C. Decreased blood flow to the kidneys due to congestive heart failure (CHF) secondary to noncompliance with home fluid restriction.

D. Severe dehydration.

Answer: A. Acute and chronic renal failure due to diabetes and a decreased blood flow to the kidneys due to heart failure. Renal failure can be caused by both decreased blood flow to the kidneys, as is common in heart failure and damage to the glomeruli, as is common in uncontrolled diabetes. The blood glucose taken in the ED suggests that the client's diabetes is not well-controlled. The BUN and creatinine are elevated showing renal failure. The patient is in pulmonary edema, suggesting a fluid overload, not a deficit.

TEST-TAKING STRATEGY: Concentrate on the mechanisms that cause decreased urine output.

476. A client presents to the clinic with complaints of nausea and occasional vomiting. As the nurse reviews the client's medical records, the nurse notes that the client has a 4-year history of renal insufficiency. The client has been on fluid restrictions and a renal diet. A review of the client's labs shows a steady increase in the BUN, creatinine, and potassium. The client's spouse accompanies the client to the appointment and pulls the nurse aside stating that the client has episodes of confusion each day. The spouse is very concerned and wants to know if the client is having small strokes. Based upon the information provided, what is the nurse's best response to this question?

A. "Confusion is a common sign of transient ischemic attacks. Thank you for informing me of this. The client will need a CAT scan of the head."

B. "The client's kidneys are not working very well. However, confusion is not a common symptom. I will inform the physician of the confusion and have him assess the situation further with the client."

C. "The elevated potassium is causing the confusion. The client will need some medication to decrease the potassium level."

D. "The client is experiencing worsening uremic syndrome. This is associated with kidney failure and is a sign that the client's kidney function is becoming worse. I will notify the physician about the confusion. There are a couple of treatment options to consider. The physician will discuss the treatment options with the client and you."

Answer: D. "The client is experiencing worsening uremic syndrome. This is associated with kidney failure and is a sign that the client's kidney function is becoming worse. I will notify the physician about the confusion. There are a couple of treatment options to consider. The physician will discuss the treatment options with the client and you." The clinical picture is of uremic syndrome and the client is in need of dialysis. Confusion is a common symptom of uremic syndrome.

TEST-TAKING STRATEGY: The most complete answer is usually the correct answer. Use the process of elimination to remove those answers that are obviously incorrect.

477. An elderly client is complaining if increasing trips to the bathroom to urinate. The client's estimated coffee intake is 3 cups per day. What is the best explanation the nurse can provide to the client?

A. The increased urine production is most likely due to a urinary tract infection.

B. Coffee is causing the increased urination due to your increased fluid intake. This is completely normal and nothing to be concerned about.

C. Coffee is causing the increased urination. Coffee contains caffeine, which causes diuresis, or increased urine formation. Simply decreasing the number of cups of coffee you drink each day, and limiting the consumption of caffeinated beverages to the morning hours, should help decrease your trips to the bathroom.

D. Drinking coffee increases the circulating plasma in the body and this increases the urine formation. Simply decreasing the number of cups of coffee you are drinking should help.

Answer: C. Coffee is causing the increased urination. Coffee contains caffeine that causes diuresis or increased urine formation. Simply decreasing the number of cups of coffee you drink each day and limiting the consumption of caffeinated beverages to the morning hours, should help decrease your trips to the bathroom. The increase in urination is due to the diuretic effect of the caffeine. There is nothing in the question to suggest that the client has a UTI.

TEST-TAKING STRATEGY: Look for the answer that contains the best information to give the client. Make sure to focus on the client's concerns.

478. The nurse is receiving shift report on a client. The client has a urinary catheter with a closed urinary drainage system. Which sites have the greatest potential for introducing infection in the closed urinary drainage system?

A. Catheter insertion site and the spigot.

B. Catheter insertion site, the drainage bag, and the junction of the drainage tube and the bag.

C. Catheter, catheter insertion site, drainage bag, the spigot, tube junction, and the junction of the tube and the bag.

D. Catheter insertion site, drainage bag, the spigot, tube junction, and the junction of the tube and the bag.

Answer: D. The catheter insertion site, drainage bag, the spigot, tub junction, and the junction of the tube and the bag are all sites for introducing potential infection in a closed urinary drainage system. The catheter itself poses a risk for infection at the time the catheter is placed. Thereafter, the insertion site is where bacteria most likely will be introduced.

TEST-TAKING STRATEGY: Read the question carefully. Make sure to choose the most complete answer.

479. The nurse at the beginning of the shift is assessing a client. The nurse notes the client has a Foley catheter connected to a collection bag. What are the best routine catheter care actions for the nurse to take while caring for this client?

A. Encourage increased oral fluid intake and observe for any opacity in the urine suggesting bacterial infection.

B. Carefully wash the perineal area with soap and water after each bowel movement.

C. Avoid touching the tip of the spigot to any surfaces when emptying the collection bag.

D. Encourage the client to drink at least 2000 mL each day and carefully wash the perineal area, with soap and water, at least twice daily and with each bowel movement.

Answer: D. Encourage the client to drink at least 2000 mL each day and carefully wash the perineal area, with soap and water, at least twice daily and with each bowel movement. Observing for opacity in the urine is not part of routine

catheter care. Careful management of the drainage bag spigot, when emptying the urine, is a good infection control practice but is not part of routine catheter care.

TEST-TAKING STRATEGY: Focus on the root of the question. Eliminate answers that do not directly pertain to the question.

480. The client has just arrived at the physician's office for follow-up regarding a new colostomy. The client states that the home health nurse changed the pouch 4 days ago. The physician requests that the pouch and skin barrier be removed for a better assessment of the stoma. Which nurse's note contains all of the major elements of assessment for the client's colostomy?

A. The client has active bowel sounds in all four quadrants. The colostomy bag is removed and noted to contain semi-formed brown stool. The skin barrier is removed per physician request.

B. There are active bowel sounds in all four quadrants. The colostomy bag is removed. The stoma is moist and dark pink. The skin barrier is removed revealing reddened skin with areas of excoriation.

C. The abdomen is soft and round with active bowel sounds in all four quadrants. The colostomy is noted in the lower left quadrant. No leakage of feces is noted with intact skin barrier. Semi-formed, brown stool is noted in the pouch. The stoma is budlike, moist, dark pink, oval-shaped, and measures 29 by 26 mm. There is a healed midline incision scar noted just below the stoma. The skin under the skin barrier is reddened with areas of excoriation. The client has an adult child who has been helping with colostomy care at home.

D. The colostomy is noted in the lower left quadrant without leakage of feces. The skin barrier appears to be intact. There is semi-formed, brown stool noted in the pouch. The stoma is budlike, moist, dark pink, oval shaped, and measures 29 by 26 mm.

Answer: C. The abdomen is soft and round with active bowel sounds in all four quadrants. The colostomy is noted in the lower left quadrant. No leakage of feces is noted with intact skin barrier. Semi-formed, brown stool is noted in the pouch. The stoma is budlike, moist, dark pink, oval-shaped, and measures 29 by 26 mm. There is a healed midline incision scar noted just below the stoma. The skin under the skin barrier is reddened with areas of excoriation. The client has an adult child who has been helping with colostomy care at home. This is the only answer option that contains all of the major elements of assessment for this client's colostomy.

TEST-TAKING STRATEGY: Look for the longest and most complete answer.

481. Which statement best describes Instrumental activities of daily living (IADL)?

   A. Activities that are usually performed in the course of a normal day. These activities include ambulating, eating, dressing, bathing, brushing the teeth, and grooming.

   B. Activities that assist the client in recognizing and managing stress. These activities include facilitating interpersonal relationships, allowing adequate time for rest, and providing regular, nutritious meals.

   C. Activities that allow the client to be independent in society. These activities include shopping, preparing meals, paying bills, and taking medications appropriately.

   D. Activities that support the effectiveness of direct care interventions. These activities include checking equipment, directing the maintenance of the client's room, and managing the supply of materials needed for client care.

Answer: C. Instrumental activities of daily living (IADL) allow a client to be independent in society beyond the home environment. These activities include shopping, preparing meals, paying bills, and taking medications appropriately. Activities of daily living (ADL) are those basic activities that are usually performed in the course of a normal day. These activities include ambulating, eating, dressing, bathing, brushing the teeth, and grooming.

TEST-TAKING STRATEGY: Read the question carefully. Be sure to differentiate between IADL and ADL.

482. A client has arrived in the preoperative area for knee surgery. The nurse asks the client to put an elastic stocking on the nonoperative leg. The client asks the nurse the purpose of the stockings. The nurse's best response is:

   A. "The stockings promote return of venous blood to the heart and assist in preventing the blood from clotting in the legs."

   B. "The operating room is very cold. The stockings assist in maintaining a healthy core body temperature during the operation."

   C. "The stockings promote joint mobility."

   D. "The stockings promote the return of arterial blood to the heart and prevent blood from clotting in the legs."

Answer: A. "The stockings promote return of venous blood to the heart and assist in preventing the blood from clotting in the legs."

TEST-TAKING STRATEGY: Use the process of elimination to determine the correct answer. Use your knowledge and critical thinking skills to correlate circulation to the promotion of blood return to the heart.

483. What are the complications of immobility? Select all that apply.

   A. Primary osteoporosis.

   B. Foot drop.

   C. Urinary stasis.

   D. Pressure ulcer.

Answer: B, C, & D. Foot drop, urinary stasis, and pressure ulcers are all direct complications of immobility. Foot drop occurs due to disuse, atrophy, and shortening of the muscle fibers causing a decrease in the ROM of the joint. Primary osteoporosis is not a result of immobility. Disuse osteoporosis, a process of bone reabsorption, is directly related to immobility but is not a complication of immobility.

TEST-TAKING STRATEGY: Read each answer carefully. "Select all that apply" indicates that there may be more than one correct answer.

484. A client has been on strict bed rest for 6 days and now has orders from the physician to begin getting up to the chair. As the client stands up for the first time at the bedside preparing to pivot to the chair, the client complains of dizziness and "almost passing out." The nurse assists the client back to a supine position and takes a blood pressure. The blood pressure is 122/75. The client feels much better after lying down. The nurse once again assists the client to a standing position. The nurse once again takes a blood pressure which is now 89/60. How should the nurse describe the events when informing the physician?

A. "I stood the client up at the bedside. The client had orthostatic hypotension."

B. "I assisted the client to stand at the side of the bed. The client was hypotensive."

C. "I assisted the client to a standing position at the side of the bed. The client complained of dizziness and "almost passing out." I took the client's blood pressure which was 89/60. The client appears to be hypotensive."

D. "I assisted the client to a standing position at the side of the bed. The client complained of dizziness and "almost passing out." I assisted the client back to a supine position and obtained a set of orthostatic blood pressures. The blood pressures were: 122/75 supine and 89/60 standing. The client appears to have orthostatic hypotension."

Answer: D. "I assisted the client to a standing position at the side of the bed. The client complained of dizziness and "almost passing out." I assisted the client back to a supine position and obtained a set of orthostatic blood pressures. The blood pressures were 122/75 supine and 89/60 standing. The client appears to have orthostatic hypotension." The client has orthostatic hypotension. The nurse reports the action being taken, assisting the client to stand, the client's complaints, the nurse's action, assisting the client back to bed, taking a set of orthostatic blood pressures both supine and standing, and the nurse's analysis of the situation.

TEST-TAKING STRATEGY: Look for the answer with the most detail.

485. A client has just been admitted to the intensive care unit (ICU) and is chemically sedated and paralyzed. What is the best description of the precautions that need to be taken to prevent skin breakdown in this client?

A. No precautions are needed. This client is too critically ill to be moved. Keep the client supine to promote circulation to all areas of the body.

B. The client needs to be turned at least every 2 hours and should be placed in a 30-degree lateral position if the client becomes too unstable to be turned for more than two hours.

C. No precautions are needed. The client is in the ICU and is not at risk for skin breakdown.

D. The client needs to be turned at least every 2 hours.

Answer: B. The client needs to be turned at least every 2 hours and should be placed in a 30-degree lateral position if the client becomes too unstable to be turned for more than two hours.

TEST-TAKING STRATEGY: Look for the most detailed answer. Carefully consider the critical needs of the client in the ICU when selecting the best answer.

486. The nurse's client is ready to get up to the chair for the first time. Before assisting the client to the chair, which should be included in the nurse's assessment? Select all that apply.

A. Muscle strength.

B. Joint mobility.

C. Cognition.

D. Vision.

Answer: A, B, C, & D. Muscle strength, joint mobility, cognition, and vision should be assessed before assisting the client up to the chair for the first time. Muscle strength assists the nurse in determining how much of the physical transfer the client can perform. Joint mobility assessment assists the nurse in knowing if there are joints that will be nonfunctional or partially functional during the transfer. The client's cognitive status affects how well the client can follow directions for the transfer. The client's visual status determines the need for transfer techniques adapted to assist with visual deficits.

TEST-TAKING STRATEGY: Make sure to choose all of the answers that apply. Use critical thinking to correlate each of the potential answers to the needs of the client described.

487. A client has just been admitted to the medical surgical floor after having a total knee replacement. The nurse is reviewing the admission orders from the surgeon and notes the following order: "Please set up trapeze bar on hospital bed." What is the best definition of a trapeze bar?

   A. A bar that hangs from a frame fastened to the bed that is used by the nurse and assistive personnel to help the client turn in bed.

   B. A bar that helps prevent external rotation of the hips when the client is lying supine in bed and can be positioned at various points to promote positioning or promote bone alignment.

   C. A bar that hangs from a frame fastened to the bed that is used by the client for pulling with the arms to raise the trunk off of the mattress to assist with repositioning, upper body exercises, and with transfers to a bedside chair.

   D. A bar that is triangular in shape and is used to maintain the legs in abduction after surgery.

Answer: C. A bar that hangs from a frame fastened to the bed that is used by the client for pulling with the arms to raise the trunk off of the mattress to assist with repositioning, upper body exercises, and with transfers to a bedside chair. The trapeze bar is not used by the nurse or assistive personnel to assist with turning. A trochanter roll prevents external rotation of the

hips. A wedge pillow is a triangular-shaped pillow and is used to maintain the legs in abduction after hip surgery.

TEST-TAKING STRATEGY: Use a process of elimination to eliminate incorrect answers.

488. A client had cardiothoracic surgery. After a long stay in the cardiovascular recovery unit (CVRU), the client has not yet been out of bed. The client's medical history reveals that the client lives in a one-story home alone and drives a car. The nurse notes that the client has been lethargic, unwilling to participate in basic ADLs, and needs one-on-one encouragement to eat. What is the most logical rationale for the client's unwillingness to participate in self-care and what is the best plan of care for the nurse to follow to promote independence?

   A. The client has been immobile in the CVRU for an extended period of time and is most likely experiencing grief, withdrawal, and fear of not being able to return to an independent lifestyle upon discharge. The nurse should encourage discussion with the client regarding the client's feelings about the hospitalization and the client's fears. The nurse should compassionately dispel any irrational fears, encouraging and praising all attempts by the client to regain independence.

   B. The client has been immobile in the CVRU for an extended period of time and is most likely experiencing grief, withdrawal, and fear of not being able to return to an independent lifestyle upon discharge. The nurse should allow the client plenty of quiet time, isolated and alone, to reflect and to grieve. The nurse should promote proper hygiene by performing all ADL activities for the client.

   C. The client is experiencing "ICU syndrome." The nurse should notify the physician of the nurse's observations and request anti-anxiety medication. The nurse should then monitor the client closely.

   D. The client is experiencing "ICU syndrome." The nurse should notify the physician of the nurse's observations and request anti-anxiety medication. The nurse should then encourage discussion with the client regarding the client's feelings about the hospitalization and the client's fears. The nurse should compassionately dispel any irrational fears; encouraging and praising all attempts by the client to regain independence.

Answer: A. The client has been immobile in the CVRU for an extended period of time and is most likely experiencing grief, withdrawal, and fear of not being able to return to an independent lifestyle upon discharge. The nurse should encourage discussion with the client regarding the client's feelings about the hospitalization and the client's fears. The nurse should compassionately dispel any irrational fears, encouraging and praising all attempts by the client to regain independence. Extended immobility may lead to grief, withdrawal, and fear. The client should not be isolated for reflection. The client should be encouraged to perform ADLs as independently as possible. The client is not experiencing "ICU syndrome."

TEST-TAKING STRATEGY: Look for answers with similar choices and consider the questions for possible elimination to assist in narrowing down the possible correct answers.

489. Which complication of immobility is most potentially life-threatening?

A. Orthostatic hypotension.

B. Urinary tract infection.

C. Pressure ulcer.

D. Deep vein thrombosis.

Answer: D. A venous thrombus has the potential to dislodge and travel to the lungs and heart, impairing circulation and oxygenation. A venous thrombus can be life threatening.

TEST-TAKING STRATEGY: Chose the answer that is most life threatening to the client. Remember the ABCs.

490. A physician has ordered bed rest for a client who has just had a massive heart attack. The client complains of chest pain with most activities and complains of feeling tired all of the time. The client's family asks about why the client is unable to get up from the bed. What are appropriate rationales for bed rest for this client? Select all that apply.

A. Reducing the oxygen needs of the body.

B. Allowing an exhausted client the opportunity for uninterrupted rest.

C. Allowing an ill or debilitated client to rest.

D. Reducing pain and the need for large doses of analgesics.

Answer: A, B, C, & D. Reducing the oxygen needs of the body, allowing an exhausted client the opportunity for uninterrupted rest, allowing an ill or debilitated client to rest, and reducing pain and the need for large doses of analgesics are appropriate rationales for bed rest for this client.

TEST-TAKING STRATEGY: Make sure to choose all of the answers that apply.

491. The nurse is administering medication to an elderly client who has no visitors. The nurse enters the room, quickly giving the client a cup of medications and pouring some water. The client takes the pills and, as the client hands the medication cup back to the nurse, grabs onto the nurse's hand tightly. What is the most logical rationale for the client's action?

A. The client is confused and wants help.

B. The client is scared and lonely and grabs the nurse's hand for comfort.

C. The client would like to talk with the nurse and initiates this communication by grabbing the nurse's hand.

D. The client is would like to reminisce with the nurse.

Answer: B. This elderly client with no visitors is most likely scared and lonely. The touch of the nurse's hand is comforting for the client.

TEST-TAKING STRATEGY: Use your common sense to determine the correct answer.

492. A client has just returned from surgery. In anticipation of the client having pain, what nursing action would be most effective in helping to prevent or control the client's pain?

   A. The nurse discusses with the client and the available family how the client generally controls pain at home, carefully inquiring about pharmacological and nonpharmacological pain control methods. The client states that soft music, a heating pad, and lying on the right side help reduce pain. The nurse documents the findings and arranges for a headset with soft music to be brought in from home and a heating pad from the hospital.

   B. The nurse discusses with the client and the available family how the client generally controls pain at home. The client states that ibuprofen (Advil) generally helps the most. The nurse documents the findings and checks the physician's orders to make sure that ibuprofen is one of the medications ordered for pain control.

   C. The nurse discusses with the client and the available family how the client generally controls pain at home, carefully inquiring about pharmacological and nonpharmacological pain control methods. The client states that soft music, a heating pad, and lying on the right side help reduce pain. The nurse documents the findings.

   D. The nurse carefully inquires about pharmacological and nonpharmacological pain control methods. The client states that soft music, a heating pad, and lying on the right side help reduce pain. The nurse arranges for ice packs, and a headset with the nurse's favorite music.

Answer: A. The nurse discusses with the client and the available family how the client generally controls pain at home, carefully inquiring about pharmacological and nonpharmacological pain control methods. The client states that soft music, a heating pad, and lying on the right side help reduce pain. The nurse documents the findings and arranges for a headset with soft music to be brought in from home and a heating pad from the hospital. The nurse should open a discussion with the client and available family regarding all types of successful pain control methods used at home and should document the findings and arrange for those comfort methods that can be used in the hospital. In addition to medication, the nurse should arrange for nonpharmacological pain control methods that are helpful to the client; not ones that the nurse likes or randomly decides upon.

TEST-TAKING STRATEGY: Focus on the most detailed answer, making sure it is the best answer.

493. A client has just returned home and the hospice nurse is visiting for the first time. The client complains of a lot of pain. In addition to the physician and the nurse, what member of the care team will assist in providing comfort therapies for this client?

   A. The physical therapist.

   B. The nutritionist.

   C. The massage therapist.

   D. The occupational therapist.

Answer: C. The massage therapist provides alternative therapies that complement the medical pain control therapies being provided by the physician and the nurse.

TEST-TAKING STRATEGY: Focus on the root of the question and consider which care team member would be most effective in providing these services.

494. A client has arrived for abdominal surgery. The nurse takes a medical history and finds that the client has never had surgery before and denies any major illnesses, hospitalizations, or injuries. The client received education in the physician's office only regarding the operative procedure. Based upon this information, what is the nurse's best action in preparing the client for postoperative pain control?

   A. The nurse provides the client with a pamphlet on pain control to read while waiting for the operating room to be ready.

   B. The nurse asks the client about what the client expects after surgery. The nurse educates the client on the pain scale, when to request pain medication, and explains that pain, a normal part of the postoperative course, will be controlled.

C. The nurse educates the client on the pain scale and when to request pain medication.

D. The nurse reports the findings from the medical history to the operating room nurse, who takes the client back to surgery, and requests that the operating room nurse pass along the information to the nurse who will be caring for the client after surgery.

Answer: B. The nurse asks the client about what the client expects after surgery in regard to pain. The nurse educates the client on the pain scale, when to request pain medication, and explains that pain, a normal part of the postoperative course, will be controlled. The client's lack of previous experience with major illness or surgery could result in an impaired ability to cope with pain after surgery.

TEST-TAKING STRATEGY: Look for the most complete answer that provides the best nursing action for this client.

495. The nurse reassesses the client's pain level after administering an oral analgesic. The client states that the pain is better, but continues to complain of a backache. Which actions may help the client's backache? Select all that apply.

A. Educating the client regarding pain and pain control.

B. Assisting the client into a side lying position.

C. Providing a back massage.

D. Providing a heating pad.

Answer: B, C, & D. Assisting the client to a side lying position, providing a back massage, and providing heat therapy could help the client's backache. Education regarding pain control does not directly help the client's complaint of pain.

TEST-TAKING STRATEGY: Carefully choose all of the options that apply.

496. A client is complaining of pain rated an 8 out of 10 on the numeric pain scale. The nurse administers an oral pain medication to the client and starts a CD of the client's favorite relaxing music. Fifteen minutes later, the client rates the pain as 2 out of 10 on the numeric pain scale. What type of nonpharmacologic pain relief intervention has the nurse used?

A. Distraction.

B. Biofeedback.

C. Progressive relaxation.

D. Cutaneous stimulation.

Answer: A. The nurse uses distraction, in the form of music, while the oral analgesic takes effect. Biofeedback is a behavioral therapy that trains individuals to take control of the physiological responses to stressors. Progressive relaxation uses a combination of breathing exercises and muscle group contractions and relaxation. Cutaneous stimulation uses stimulation of the skin through heat, cold or even electrical nerve stimulation to decrease or eliminate pain.

TEST-TAKING STRATEGY: Carefully think through which nonpharmacologic pain relief method uses music.

497. Which outcome is a goal of cognitive behavioral pain intervention?

A. To provide pain relief.

B. To correct physical dysfunction.

C. To reduce fear of pain-related immobility.

D. To change the client's perceptions of pain.

Answer: D. One of the goals of cognitive behavioral pain interventions is to change the client's perceptions of pain. Pain relief, correcting physical dysfunction, and reduction of fear of pain-related immobility are all goals of physical pain relief agents.

TEST-TAKING STRATEGY: Re-read the question to be sure that you have a clear understanding of what this question is asking.

498. A client has recently been transferred to the medical surgical floor from the ICU after sustaining multiple system traumas. The client has been to the operating room three times in the past 5 days and will require more operations in the coming weeks to repair further injuries. The client is very anxious, rates the current pain as a 6/10 on the numeric pain scale, and states the pain medication is not very effective. The client is receiving large doses of both intravenous and oral narcotic and nonsteroidal-type analgesics. The nurse discusses the pain further with the client. The client states a willingness to try anything that might help the pain. What pain control intervention would be most appropriate for this client based upon the information provided?

A. Progressive relaxation.

B. Increased analgesic dosages.

C. Distraction.

D. Herbals.

Answer: A. Progressive relaxation is the most appropriate pain intervention to try with this client. The client is anxious and is already receiving large doses of analgesics. Distraction may help this client, but due to the client's anxiety, would not be the best choice. Herbals are not FDA approved and are not typically utilized in the hospital setting.

TEST-TAKING STRATEGY: Select the most appropriate pain intervention. Focus on which method would be most effective in helping a client with anxiety.

499. The nurse is instructing a client on relaxation and begins with the proper body positioning. Which positioning instructions would be given to the client? Select all that apply.

A. Keep legs separated with toes pointed slightly outward.

B. Place feet flat on the floor.

C. Allow arms to hang loosely at the sides or rest comfortably on supports.

D. Use a small pillow, or other small support, under the head.

Answer: A & D. The client should keep the legs separated with toes pointed slightly outward and use a small pillow, or other small support, under the head. Placing the feet flat on the floor and allowing the arms to hang loosely at the sides or rest comfortably on supports are instructions for proper relaxation positioning while sitting.

TEST-TAKING STRATEGY: Choose all of the answers that apply; focusing on relaxation in the *supine* position.

500. Which is the best example of a nurse preventing painful stimuli?

A. Encouraging the client to hit the PCA button before ambulating in the hall.

B. Instructing the client in deep breathing exercises while the nurse performs a painful dressing change.

C. Arranging for an elevated toilet seat in the bathroom of a client with knee arthritis.

D. Placing an ice pack on the hip of a client who recently had a hip replacement.

Answer: C. Arranged for an elevated toilet seat in the bathroom of a client with knee arthritis. The nurse is preventing pain by arranging for an elevated toilet seat so that the client does not need to bend the knees deeply, causing pain. The PCA provides an intravenous analgesic that pretreats the client for pain during walking, but does not prevent the pain. The deep-breathing exercises help the client tolerate pain during the dressing change, but are not intended to prevent pain. The ice packs on the hip of a client with a hip replacement use cutaneous stimulation to relieve but not prevent pain.

TEST-TAKING STRATEGY: Focus on what the question is asking. Concentrate on the difference between treating pain and preventing pain.

501. Which client would be an appropriate candidate for oral hydration?

A. A pregnant client with uncontrolled nausea and vomiting.

B. A client with aspiration pneumonia.

C. A client who has had a stroke, has right-sided facial droop, and coughs when trying to swallow oral secretions.

D. A client who has had knee surgery.

Answer: D. The client who has had knee surgery has no contraindications to oral hydration. A client with nausea and vomiting is unable to maintain adequate hydration and needs intravenous therapy. The client with aspiration pneumonia has already aspirated and oral hydration would be contraindicated. The client who has had a stroke, has right-sided facial droop, and coughs when trying to swallow oral secretions is at high risk for aspiration.

TEST-TAKING STRATEGY: Use the process of elimination to narrow down the potential correct answers.

502. An elderly client is admitted with dehydration and has a pitcher of water at the bedside. The nurse assesses the client's thirst with every visit to the room and the client denies thirst each time. While calculating the end-of-shift intake and output, the nurse notes the client has had very little to drink. What is the best explanation for this finding?

    A. The client has had enough to drink.

    B. The thirst mechanisms of elderly clients are depressed.

    C. The client does not like the choices of fluids offered.

    D. The client's family is bringing in fluids for the client to drink that are not included in the intake and output totals.

    Answer: B. The thirst mechanisms of elderly clients are depressed.

    TEST-TAKING STRATEGY: More than one answer may be correct. Choose the best answer. Focus on the client's age.

503. A client has just delivered a baby and is successfully breast feeding. How many extra kilocalories per day does the client need to consume to compensate for the increased energy requirements of lactation?

    A. 1000.

    B. 300.

    C. 500.

    D. 800.

    Answer: C. The client needs an extra 500 kcal/day above the usual allowance.

    TEST-TAKING STRATEGY: Use the process of elimination to determine the correct answer.

504. What is the main source of energy in the diet?

    A. Fats.

    B. Water.

    C. Carbohydrates.

    D. Minerals.

    Answer: C. Carbohydrates are the main source of energy in the diet. Fats are the most energy dense nutrients in the diet. Water provides no energy for the body. Minerals do not provide energy.

    TEST-TAKING STRATEGY: Use a process of elimination to determine the correct answer. Consider which source of energy composes the greatest proportion of a healthy diet.

505. A client is admitted with an open sore on the coccyx. Which nutrient is most important for healing this sore?

    A. Protein.

    B. Water.

    C. Fats.

    D. Vitamins.

    Answer: A. Proteins are essential to body repair. Water is critical for cell function. Fats are not the most important nutrient for body repair. Vitamins are used in biochemical reactions in the body.

    TEST-TAKING STRATEGY: Remember to focus on the nutrient that is most important for healing.

506. How much of the total body weight is composed of water?

A. 80–90%.

B. 70–80%.

C. 60–70%.

D. 50–60%.

Answer: C. The total body weight is composed of 60 to 70% water.

TEST-TAKING STRATEGY: Use your knowledge and a process of elimination to determine the correct answer.

507. A client has just had a nasogastric tube placed. What is the best method for verifying correct placement of the tube in the stomach?

A. X-ray.

B. Gastric aspiration and pH testing.

C. Auscultation.

D. Visualization of the tube markings.

Answer: A. X-ray verification of tube placement is the most reliable method for verifying correct placement of the nasogastric tube in the stomach. Visualization of the tube markings does not provide a reliable verification of placement of the tube in the stomach. Coiling of the tube can occur preventing the tip from reaching the stomach.

TEST-TAKING STRATEGY: Choose the best answer. More than one answer may be correct.

508. A client has just returned from an EGD, where the client was diagnosed with peptic ulcers. The client does not have a history of taking NSAIDs. During the procedure, biopsies and cultures were taken. What lab results can the nurse anticipate?

A. Negative biopsies.

B. Cultures positive for *Helicobacter pylori*.

C. Cultures showing normal gastric flora.

D. Cultures positive for *Staphylococcus*.

Answer: B. The nurse can anticipate cultures positive for *Helicobacter pylori,* the bacteria that causes peptic ulcers.

TEST-TAKING STRATEGY: Immediately eliminate the "normal" results. Then focus on the bacteria that cause peptic ulcers.

509. Which of the following patients would most benefit from parenteral nutrition?

A. A client with neck cancer.

B. A client with a CVA.

C. A client with severe pancreatitis.

D. An intubated client.

Answer: C. The client with severe pancreatitis needs parenteral nutrition to provide nutrients until malabsoption in the gastrointestinal tract can be corrected. The client with neck cancer, a CVA, or an intubated client can all be safely started on enteral nutrition, which is the preferred method of meeting nutritional needs for a client.

TEST-TAKING STRATEGY: Eliminate problems that do not effect the functioning of the gastrointestinal tract.

510. The physician has written discharge orders for the client that includes a no-salt-added diet. What is the best education the nurse can provide the client at discharge regarding this type of diet?

A. When preparing foods, do not add any salt or salt-containing spice preparations to the food. Look for spice preparations that do not contain sodium. Do not add salt to foods after preparation.

B. Do not use canned or processed foods while cooking. Use salt substitutes to put on food at the table.

C. Eat a healthy, well-balanced diet at home that is rich in fruits, vegetables, and whole grains.

D. Eat a healthy, well-balanced diet at home that is rich in fruits, vegetables, and whole grains. When preparing foods, do not add any salt or salt-containing spice preparations to the food. Look for spice preparations that do not contain sodium. Do not add salt to foods after preparation.

Answer: D. Eat a healthy, well-balanced diet at home that is rich in fruits, vegetables, and whole grains. When preparing foods, do not add salt or salt-containing spice preparations to the food. Look for spice preparations that do not contain sodium. Do not add salt to foods after preparation. This education provides the most comprehensive information for the client.

TEST-TAKING STRATEGY: Choose the answer that best educates the client on the low sodium diet. Look for the answer with the most detail.

511. What are goals of palliative care? Select all that apply.

   A. Preventing disease symptoms.

   B. Relieving disease symptoms.

   C. Curing a disease.

   D. Treating a disease.

   Answer: A & B. Both preventing and relieving disease symptoms are goals of palliative care. Curing a disease and treating a disease are goals of disease management.

   TEST-TAKING STRATEGY: Choose all of the answers that apply and remember that the focus of palliative care is symptom control.

512. A client is currently under the care of the palliative care service of home health and has been experiencing nausea. What nursing actions will most likely promote comfort in this client?

   A. Educate the patient and family in the use of prescribed anti-emetics; providing oral care every 2 to 4 hours; consuming a diet of clear liquids and ice chips; and avoiding liquids such as coffee, milk, and citrus juices.

   B. Administer additional pain medication.

   C. Provide education to the patient and family regarding oral care and anti-emetic medication.

   D. Take a detailed medical history to determine the cause of the nausea.

   Answer: A. Educate the patient and family in the use of prescribed anti-emetics; providing oral care every 2 to 4 hours; consuming a diet of clear liquids and ice chips; and avoiding liquids

such as coffee, milk, and citrus juices. Providing oral care every 2 to 4 hours assists in keeping oral mucous membranes moist and prevents bad tastes in the mouth that could increase nausea. Consuming a diet of clear liquids and ice chips helps keep the mucous membranes moist and prevents gastric stimulation. Coffee, milk, and citrus juices increase stomach acidity. Administering additional pain medication may exacerbate the nausea further and there is no indication that the client is in pain. A detailed medical history may not provide a specific cause of the nausea and does not directly help promote comfort.

TEST-TAKING STRATEGY: Look for the most detailed answer that describes the nursing action most likely to promote comfort.

513. Which list contains common symptoms of terminally ill clients?

   A. Hunger, thirst, fatigue, and diarrhea.

   B. Dehydration, nausea, effective breathing, and adequate nutrition.

   C. Discomfort, nausea, ineffective breathing, and fatigue.

   D. Urinary continence, thirst, dehydration, and diarrhea.

   Answer: C. Discomfort, nausea, ineffective breathing, and fatigue are all common symptoms of terminally ill clients. Urinary continence and thirst are more common in healthy clients, while dehydration and diarrhea are common seen in the terminally ill.

   TEST-TAKING STRATEGY: Use the process of elimination to determine the correct answer.

514. What is the best definition of palliative care?

   A. Care for terminally ill clients.

   B. Symptom management for a client when a disease no longer responds to cure-focused treatment.

   C. Aggressive cure-focused disease treatment and management.

   D. Comfort care.

Answer: B. Symptom management for a client when a disease no longer responds to cure-focused treatment is the best definition of palliative care. Care for terminally ill clients is a definition of hospice care. Aggressive cure-focused disease treatment and management describes active medical disease management. Comfort care, a synonym for palliative care, does not define this care philosophy.

TEST-TAKING STRATEGY: The longest and most detailed answer is usually the correct answer.

515. A terminally ill client is being cared for at home by family members. Based upon the client's physical assessment, the nurse is aware that the client's death is imminent. What is the nurse's most important role in the care of the family at this time?

    A. Providing temporary relief of care giving duties to allow the family to rest.

    B. Providing education regarding the symptoms the client will likely experience.

    C. Coordinating a visiting schedule for the family.

    D. Communicating news of the client's impending death to the family while they are together.

Answer: D. Communicating news of the client's impending death to the family while they are together. The nurse's most important role in the care of the family is compassionate communication. The family needs to be informed about the situation so that they are prepared for the client's death and can provide support to one another.

TEST-TAKING STRATEGY: In determining the nurse's most important role, consider the needs of the family within the context of the situation.

516. Which is the most accurate statement regarding pain?

    A. Pain has been extensively studied and is well understood.

    B. Pain is one of the most common symptoms in medicine.

    C. Pain perception is very objective; every client feels pain the exact same way.

    D. Pain is only a result of physical bodily damage.

Answer: B. Pain is one of the most common symptoms in medicine. Pain, although extensively studied, is not well understood. Pain perception is very subjective; not every client will experience pain in the same way. Psychological pain can manifest itself as physical pain.

TEST-TAKING STRATEGY: Avoid answer options that use words such as *every, always,* or *never*. These answers are usually incorrect.

517. Which are types of pain? Select all that apply.

    A. Pain tolerance.

    B. Chronic pain.

    C. Idiopathic pain.

    D. Pseudoaddiction.

Answer: B & C. Chronic pain and idiopathic pain are types of pain. Chronic pain lasts longer than expected, and may not have a clear cause. Idiopathic pain is a type of chronic pain that does not have a clinically identifiable cause. Pain tolerance refers to the amount of pain a client is able to endure. Pseudoaddiction refers to clients in pain who go from doctor to doctor seeking pain relief. These clients may be labeled as being drug-seeking.

TEST-TAKING STRATEGY: "Select all that apply" indicates that there may be more than one correct answer. Similar phrasing may provide hints to the correct answer options.

518. Which is a common misconception about pain?

    A. The severity of a client's illness indicates the amount of pain the client should be experiencing.

    B. Psychogenic pain is real.

    C. Clients are the best authorities on the nature and level of their pain.

    D. Drug abusers and alcoholics can provide accurate information regarding their pain experience.

Answer: A. That the severity of a client's illness indicates the amount of pain the client should be experiencing is a common misconception about pain. Every client experiences pain differently. The other answer options are accurate statements regarding pain.

TEST-TAKING STRATEGY: Read the question carefully. Determine which answer option describes a common *misconception* regarding pain.

519. The nurse is assessing pain in a 3-year-old client after surgery. Which pain scale should the nurse use to assess this client's pain level?

    A. Numerical scale.

    B. Verbal descriptive scale.

    C. Visual analog scale.

    D. FACES scale.

    Answer: D. The nurse should use the FACES scale as a tool to assess this client's pain level. Children as young as 3 years of age can use the FACES scale to communicate their pain level to the medical team.

    TEST-TAKING STRATEGY: Focus on the age of the client. Select the pain scale that is most appropriate for the client.

520. A client fell at home and sustained a back injury. The client reports back pain and the inability to play golf or go to the store. The client remains at home most of the time due to the pain. Which nurse's note includes all of the elements of a complete pain assessment?

    A. The client's back pain began 6 months ago and has been constant since the fall. The pain is located in the mid lower back area, is rated a 6 out of 10 on the numeric pain scale, and is described as a constant, dull ache. The pain is made worse by ambulating or standing for more than 5 minutes. The client uses a hot-water bottle over the back for some relief at night. The client denies other symptoms related to the back pain. The client reports being unable to play golf since the fall or go to the store, and remains at the home most of the time due to the pain.

    B. The pain is rated a 6 out of 10, and is a constant, dull ache. The client uses a hot-water bottle over the back for some relief at night. The client reports being unable to play golf since the fall or go to the store, and remains at the home most of the time due to the pain.

    C. The client's back pain began 6 months ago after a minor fall in the kitchen. The pain has been constant since the fall. The pain is located in the mid lower back area and is rated a 6 out of 10 on the numeric pain scale.

    D. Client reports pain began after a fall and the pain has limited his physical activity and does not seen to be improving.

    Answer: A. A complete pain assessment should include onset and duration, location, intensity, quality, pain pattern, relief measures, contributing symptoms, and effects of the pain on the client. The remaining answers do not include all of these elements.

    TEST-TAKING STRATEGY: Choose the most complete answer. The longest answer is often the correct answer.

521. The nurse is bathing a comatose client. Which nurse's note best describes additional nursing activities that can be done during the bed bath?

    A. Client bathed; tolerated well; range-of-motion exercises done; client turned to left side.

    B. Client bathed; tolerated well; no skin lesions noted. IV flushes well; site is clear. Dressing is clean, dry, and intact. Leg, arm, and neck range-of-motion exercises done; no contractures or joint swelling noted.

    C. Client bathed; tolerated well; no skin lesions noted.

    D. Client bathed; tolerated well; no skin lesions noted. IV flushes well; site is clear. Dressing is clean, dry, and intact. Leg, arm, and neck range-of-motion exercises done; no contractures or joint swelling noted. Physician in to see client. Assisted physician with placement of chest tube.

Answer: B. Client bathed; tolerated well; no skin lesions noted. IV flushes well; site is clear. Dressing is clean, dry, and intact. Leg, arm, and neck range-of-motion exercises done; no contractures or joint swelling noted. The nurse can include assessments, ROM exercises, dressing changes, and IV site inspection and care during bathing. Chest tube placement would not be done during a bed bath.

TEST-TAKING STRATEGY: Read the question carefully. Note that the question refers to activities that can be done *during the bed bath*.

522. Which client is at the greatest risk for ineffective oral hygiene?

A. A client who has just had knee surgery after a skiing accident.

B. A right-handed client who has had a stoke causing mild weakness on the left side of the body.

C. A client with breast cancer who is experiencing severe nausea and vomiting after chemotherapy.

D. An independent, elderly client having elective surgery.

Answer: C. A client with severe nausea and vomiting after chemotherapy is at an increased risk for ineffective oral hygiene problems due to vomiting, decreased oral intake, and the effects of the chemotherapy on the normal bacterial flora of the mouth.

TEST-TAKING STRATEGY: Look for answers that describe direct issues related to hygiene care.

523. Which client is at the highest risk for periodontal disease?

A. An 18-year-old client who reports regularly brushing teeth and has a medical history that includes acne, and asthma.

B. A 45-year-old client who brushes regularly, does not like flossing, and has a medical history that includes hypertension and an appendectomy.

C. A 55-year-old client who brushes regularly and has a medical history that includes multiple surgeries for broken bones and one case of pneumonia at age 8.

D. A 75-year-old client who brushes regularly, has a partial plate, and has a medical history that includes hypertension, diabetes, coronary artery disease, and a CABG 3 years ago.

Answer: D. The 75-year-old client who brushes regularly, has a partial plate, and has a medical history that includes hypertension, diabetes, coronary artery disease, and a CABG 3 years ago has the greatest risk for periodontal disease. Diabetes and cardiovascular disease increase the risk of periodontal disease in the older adult. The combination of the client's age and medical history make this client the highest risk for periodontal disease.

TEST-TAKING STRATEGY: Consider the client's age and medical history when assessing for risk of periodontal disease.

524. Which client has the greatest need for perineal care?

A. An elderly client who needs assistance with ADLs and has a catheter.

B. A male client who is very independent, well groomed, and is uncircumcised.

C. A female client who is 2 days postpartum and ready for discharge to home.

D. A paraplegic female client who is currently menstruating.

Answer: A. An elderly client who needs assistance with ADLs and has a catheter has the greatest risk for infection and therefore has the greatest need for perineal care.

TEST-TAKING STRATEGY: Identify the client who is at the greatest risk of infection if perineal care is not performed.

525. The nurse is preparing to perform foot care on a client. Which client would most likely require a physician's order to trim the toenails?

A. A client with coronary artery disease.

B. A client with diabetes mellitus.

C. A client with hypertension.

D. A client with hemiplegia.

Answer: B. A client with diabetes mellitus, due to the increased risk of foot complications, will most likely require a physician's order to trim the toenails. Some institutions may require a podiatry consult for toenail trimming.

TEST-TAKING STRATEGY: Focus on the condition that holds the greatest risk for foot complications.

526. Which conditions are signs of vascular insufficiency? Select all that apply.

A. Decreased pedal pulses.

B. Thickened toenails.

C. Chronic foot wounds.

D. Hairy legs.

Answer: A, B, & C. Decreased pedal pulses, thickened toenails, and chronic foot wounds are all signs of vascular insufficiency. Decreased blood flow to the legs creates a thickened appearance to the toenails. Decreased blood flow to the legs impairs the strength of the pulses, causes a thickening of the toenails, and impairs wound healing. Hairy legs are not a sign of vascular insufficiency. A client with decreased blood flow would not have enough oxygen or nutrients flowing to the area to support a large number of hair follicles.

TEST-TAKING STRATEGY: When answering "Select all that apply" questions, be sure and treat each answer as a true or false statement. There may be one correct answer or more.

527. What is the best way for the nurse to assess a client with a dark skin tone?

A. The family may perceive that the nurse is culturally insensitive if asked about the client's baseline skin tone.

B. There is never a need to assess for changes in dark skin tone.

C. The use of a bright, florescent light assists in better visualization of the skin.

D. The areas of the skin with the least melanin provide the best locations for baseline skin color identification.

Answer: D. The areas of the skin with the least melanin provide the best locations for baseline skin color identification. Asking family to assist in identifying patches of skin that are of normal color for the client is not culturally insensitive and is an important assessment tool for the nurse while caring for the client. Clients with dark skin tones should be assessed frequently due to the increased difficulty in observing subtle changes that can be early signs of disease processes. Natural light should be used, if at all possible, to assess the skin. Florescent lights cast a bluish hue on skin with a dark skin tone.

TEST-TAKING STRATEGY: Use your knowledge and common sense to eliminate incorrect answer options.

528. Which initiative is a Healthy People 2010 initiative to improve dental health?

A. Decrease tooth loss caused by tooth decay or periodontal disease for the economically disadvantaged.

B. Reduce the number of older adults who have lost their natural teeth.

C. Increase the use of proper flossing techniques.

D. Reduce the rate of periodontal disease in the economically disadvantaged.

Answer: B. Reducing the number of older adults who have lost their natural teeth is one of four Healthy People 2010 initiatives to improve dental health in the United States.

TEST-TAKING STRATEGY: Note that two of the incorrect answer options both use the term *economically disadvantaged*. This can help eliminate these two answer options and help narrow down potentially correct answers.

529. The nurse is providing oral care to an unconscious client. What is the most important step in the care of this client?

A. Performing hand hygiene.

B. Pulling the curtain around the bed.

C. Positioning the client in a side-lying position.

D. Cleaning the teeth using a soft brush.

Answer: C. Positioning the client in a side-lying position allows secretions to drain from the mouth and prevents aspiration. The most important aspect of care is the protection of the airway of this unconscious client. This is accomplished through proper positioning of the client in a side-lying position.

TEST-TAKING STRATEGY: Remember the ABCs: airway, breathing, and circulation.

530. The nurse wants to promote comfort and relaxation after giving the client a bed bath. Which action best meets this goal?

A. Providing the client with a back rub.

B. Dimming the lights in the room.

C. Providing warm milk and cookies.

D. Playing soft music.

Answer: A. Providing the client with a back rub promotes comfort, relieves muscle tension, and promotes relaxation. The conclusion of a bed bath is the best time to perform this action. Dimming the lights or playing soft music can help promote a more relaxed atmosphere, but can be done at any time during the day or night.

TEST-TAKING STRATEGY: Focus on the timing of activity. Critically analyze each answer to determine which action best promotes comfort and relaxation at this specific time.

531. Which brain structures regulate sleep and wakefulness?

A. Thalamus and hypothalamus.

B. Reticular activating system and bulbar synchronizing region.

C. Cerebral cortex and reticular activating system.

D. Hypothalamus and bulbar synchronizing region.

Answer: B. The reticular activating system and bulbar synchronizing region regulate sleep. The reticular activating system contains neurons that release catecholamines, which stimulate wakefulness. The bulbar synchronizing region then takes over, decreasing the action of the reticular activating system, causing sleep.

TEST-TAKING STRATEGY: Read the question carefully. While the brain structures mentioned in the answer options contribute to sleep and wakefulness, the question asks which pair *regulates* sleep and wakefulness.

532. A male client is seen in the physician's office with complaints of ongoing sleepiness during the day requiring napping. The client reports that he has "nodded off" at the wheel of his car during the day and snores loudly at night. The client is 6'0" tall and weighs 300 pounds. What is the most likely diagnosis for this client?

A. Obstructive sleep apnea.

B. Narcolepsy.

C. Insomnia.

D. Delayed sleep phase syndrome.

Answer: A. The client most likely has obstructive sleep apnea, which is caused by the muscles of the oral cavity or throat relaxing during sleep, creating a partial or complete upper airway blockage. The client struggles to breathe around the airway blockage, which creates loud snoring noises and may cause brief periods of apnea. Men are more likely than women to experience obstructive sleep apnea, especially in combination with obesity.

TEST-TAKING STRATEGY: Focus the details provided to match the disorder to the symptoms described.

533. Which factors can most negatively affect the quantity and quality of a client's sleep? Select all that apply.

A. Diuretics.

B. Stressful work environment.

C. One cup of coffee in the morning.

D. Weight gain.

Answer: A & B. Diuretics can cause a client to need to get up to the bathroom multiple times during the night, interrupting quality sleep. A stressful work environment can disrupt a client's ability to relax and fall to sleep and may decrease the quality and quantity of sleep.

TEST-TAKING STRATEGY: "Select all that apply" indicates that there may be more than one correct answer option. Carefully consider how each factor affects sleep.

534. An elderly client comes to the physician's office with complaints of sleep deprivation. What is the best action the nurse can take to help the client promote sleep?

A. Provide the client with a free gym membership trial.

B. Recommend the client take a mid-afternoon nap.

C. Instruct the client to decrease oral fluids 2 to 4 hours before bedtime.

D. Encourage the client to sleep later in the morning.

Answer: C. The elderly client has a higher likelihood of nocturia due to decreased bladder tone. Decreasing oral fluids 2 to 4 hours before bedtime will help decrease the amount of urine produced by the kidneys during the night and the amount of urine in the bladder.

TEST-TAKING STRATEGY: Choose the best nursing action. Consider factors that promote sleep as well as the age of the client.

535. Which question best assesses a client for symptoms of insomnia?

A. Where do you sleep?

B. How often do you have trouble sleeping?

C. Do you currently have specific stressors in your life?

D. What time do you go to bed?

Answer: B. The question "how often do you have trouble sleeping?" gives the nurse a history of sleep problems that can help assess the client for insomnia.

TEST-TAKING STRATEGY: Read the question carefully. Focus on what the question is asking.

536. A client has a history of drinking 4 cups of coffee a day, does not exercise, and works a stressful job for 16 hours a day. Which nursing intervention will be most helpful to a middle-aged client experiencing insomnia?

A. Instruct the client to initiate an exercise routine during the day.

B. Educate the client on ways to adjust the sleep environment.

C. Educate the client on progressive relaxation techniques to be used just before bedtime.

D. Instruct the client to decrease caffeine intake.

Answer: C. Instruct the client on progressive relaxation techniques to be used just before bedtime. The client works a stressful job for 16 hours a day. The use of progressive relaxation techniques would help the client relax just before bedtime and promote sleep. Instructing the client to decrease caffeine intake would help the client, but the current caffeine consumption is confined to the morning hours.

TEST-TAKING STRATEGY: Make sure to choose the most helpful intervention for sleep promotion in this client.

537. In the intensive care unit, which intervention will best promote sleep for a critically ill client?

A. Administer a sleeping medication.

B. Allow the family to remain at the bedside to talk with client.

C. Keep the television on to block the noise of other alarms.

D. Cluster care and avoid awakening client for nonessential tasks.

Answer: D. Cluster care and avoid awakening client for nonessential tasks. This intervention provides the client with greater periods of uninterrupted sleep. Sleep medications do not promote quality sleep.

TEST-TAKING STRATEGY: Recognize the barriers to sleep that are present in the ICU. Consider how each intervention promotes sleep in this unique environment.

538. What is the best nursing intervention for preventing sudden infant death syndrome (SIDS) in a newborn client?

A. Place the infant in a supine position for sleep.

B. Keep the infant in a bassinet during the day.

C. Use baby oil on the scalp just before bathing.

D. Keep a knit cap on the infant's head.

Answer: A. Placing the infant in the supine position for sleep has been shown to decrease the incidence of SIDS.

TEST-TAKING STRATEGY: Use a process of elimination to eliminate the answer options that do not apply.

539. Which conditions describe a state of rest? Select all that apply.

A. Mental relaxation.

B. Lack of anxiety.

C. Inactivity.

D. Calmness.

Answer: A, B, & D. Mental relaxation, lack of anxiety, and calmness are all descriptions of a state of rest. A state of inactivity does not necessarily relate to rest.

TEST-TAKING STRATEGY: Note that the correct answer options describe mental states as opposed to physical states.

540. Which activity describes a good sleep hygiene habit?

A. Exercising after work until 7:30 PM and then going to bed at 9 PM.

B. Getting up and doing a quiet activity if unable to fall asleep after 30 minutes.

C. Sleeping in on Saturday and Sunday.

D. Reviewing projects needing to be completed the following day just before bed.

Answer: B. When unable to fall to sleep within 30 minutes of lying down, getting up and doing a quiet activity, such as reading, until feeling tired enough to return to bed keeps the bed a restful place without the stress of being unable to fall to sleep.

TEST-TAKING STRATEGY: The longest answer option is often correct.

541. A client provides a list of medications for the nurse. The medications include atorvastatin (Lipitor), clopidogrel bisulfate (Plavix), and phenelzine sulfate (Nardil). Which statement indicates that the client requires further education regarding medications?

A. "I'm looking forward to my birthday celebration tonight. I'm even going to have wine with my meal!"

B. "I've finally begun using an electric razor to shave. That was hard to change over."

C. "My doctor took me off my other blood thinner when he started me on that cholesterol medication."

D. "I wish I could have chocolate again. I miss having a candy bar every once in a while."

Answer: A. Phenelzine (Nardil) is an MAO inhibitor which cannot be taken with tyramine-containing foods. Wine, especially red wine, contains tyramine and must be avoided. A hypertensive crisis can occur with this type of reaction. Other foods that must be avoided in patients taking this medication are cheese, bananas, raisins, yeast, yogurt, broad beans, meat tenderizers, and bean curd. Chocolate can also be implicated in the hypertensive reaction. Warfarin (Coumadin) should not be used with atorvastatin (Lipitor) because an interaction can occur, causing muscle pain and inflammation. Clopidogrel bisulfate (Plavix) can increase the potential for bleeding; therefore using an electric razor would be a good choice for this client.

TEST-TAKING STRATEGY: When the stem asks for information regarding potential further education related to a statement the patient makes, you must look for an incorrect statement.

542. A client who takes tranylcypromine (Parnate) is changed to fluoxetine (Prozac). Which manifestation indicates a serious interaction between these two medications?

    A. Decreased salivary secretions.

    B. Complete heart block.

    C. Hyperthermia.

    D. Hypoactive reflexes.

    Answer: C. When an MAO inhibitor (such as tranylcypromine [Parnate]) and a selective-serotonin reuptake inhibitor (such as fluoxetine [Prozac]) are interchanged, a period of time must pass before stopping one drug and starting the other. Both of these medications increase the amount of serotonin in the body. Manifestations of serotonin syndrome include increased salivation, tachycardia, hyperreflexia, and hyperthermia as well as mental status changes, seizures, hypertension, tremors, rigidity, and nystagmus.

    TEST-TAKING STRATEGY: Once you read the stem, stop and determine what you think the answer should be. Then read the options and choose the right one. Knowing what you are looking for will help you to choose the right one.

543. A client complains of an urticarial rash, itching, and dyspnea after receiving an intramuscular injection of penicillin G benzathine (Bicillin L-A). Which medication is the most appropriate primary intervention in this circumstance?

    A. Epinephrine (adrenaline) 1:1000 to 0.3 mL IV.

    B. Diphenhydramine (Benadryl) 50 mg IV.

    C. Methylprednisolone sodium succinate (Solu-Medrol) 125 mg IV.

    D. Atropine sulfate (atropine) 0.5 mg IV.

    Answer: B. Administration of diphenhydramine (Benadryl) is the first priority. It works by competing with the histamine on receptor sites. Epinephrine (adrenaline) would

be the first priority, except that the dilution is incorrect for the route—1:1000 is given subcutaneously, not intravenously. Methylprednisolone sodium succinate (Solu-Medrol) is an appropriate medication, but is not the first priority because it takes longer to take effect. Atropine sulfate (atropine) is not appropriate for an allergic reaction.

TEST-TAKING STRATEGY: Be sure to read the entire options, especially questions that ask about medications and dosages. Just because the medication is correct does not mean that the dosage/dilution is appropriate.

544. Which adverse reaction can be attributed to a medication in the classification of tricyclic antidepressants?

    A. Increased temperature.

    B. Miosis.

    C. Hypersecretions.

    D. Pallor.

    Answer: A. Hyperthermia is one of the anticholinergic effects that can take place as either an adverse reaction or an overdose situation. Anticholinergic effects include mydriasis, flushed skin, dry mucous membranes, anxiety, psychoses, tachycardia, hyperthermia, and urinary retention. A mnemonic that is helpful in remembering the anticholinergic effects of tricyclic reaction or overdose is: "Blind as a Bat, Red as a Beet, Dry as a Bone, Mad as a Hatter, and Hotter than Hades." Miosis, hypersecretions, and pallor are not manifestations of tricyclic antidepressants.

    TEST-TAKING STRATEGY: Know what terminology, such as "miosis," means. Not understanding terminology can cause you to choose the wrong response.

545. A client receives a dose of furosemide (Lasix) 120 mg intravenously for treatment of congestive heart failure. Which symptom indicates that an adverse reaction is most likely occurring?

A. Bradycardia.

B. Weight gain.

C. Hypotension.

D. Crackles.

Answer: C. Excessive diuresis can occur with large doses of furosemide (Lasix). The client should be monitored for manifestations of hypovolemia, which include hypotension and tachycardia. Weight gain and crackles or rales are indicative of retaining too much fluid and are not manifestations of an adverse reaction to the medication.

TEST-TAKING STRATEGY: Questions will not always be straightforward regurgitations of facts. You must be able to apply your knowledge to assess and manage problems that can occur.

546. A client receives an injection of promethazine hydrochloride (Phenergan). Which manifestation can occur if the patient has an adverse reaction to this medication?

A. Torticollis.

B. Nystagmus.

C. Excessive salivation.

D. Hyperthermia.

Answer: A. Phenothiazines can cause extrapyramidal symptoms such as torticollis, oculogyric crises, and dystonic type of movements. Nystagmus, excessive salivation, and hyperthermia are not manifestations of adverse reactions associated with phenothiazines.

TEST-TAKING STRATEGY: Be sure to know your terminology. Questions can not be answered correctly if you don't understand the answer choices provided.

547. Which statement by the client indicates proper knowledge of the use of the medication phenazopyridine hydrochloride (Pyridium)?

A. "Once I have taken this medication for 24 hours, my infection should be gone."

B. "I know I must abstain from sexual intercourse while I am on this medication."

C. "I know that I am not allergic to this particular antibiotic."

D. "This medication will turn my urine orange and will stain fabrics."

Answer: D. Phenazopyridine hydrochloride (Pyridium) is used as a urinary tract analgesic. One of the side effects is the discoloration of urine to an orange or reddish hue, which will also stain anything in which it comes into contact. It is not an antibiotic, and the medication itself has nothing to do with the practice of sexual intercourse.

TEST-TAKING STRATEGY: When two responses are similar and different from the other two options, you should be able to rule them out.

548. In which client is the use of the drug tetracycline hydrochloride (tetracycline) appropriate?

A. A 22-year-old female who is breast feeding.

B. A 32-year-old female who is pregnant.

C. A 58-year-old female who has 6 children.

D. A 7-year-old female who is premenarche.

Answer: C. Tetracycline hydrochloride (tetracycline) is contraindicated in children under the age of 8 because it can discolor permanent teeth. It is also contraindicated in pregnant women and those who are breast feeding for the same reason.

TEST-TAKING STRATEGY: Look for similarities in options when you must determine a trait or outcome that is "appropriate" for a certain population of client.

549. The nurse administers promethazine hydrochloride (Phenergan) intravenously to a client. Which action by the nurse is appropriate when the client complains of pain in the arm being used for the intravenous site?

A. Administer at a faster rate to finish the injection sooner.

B. Stop administration of the medication immediately.

C. Continue administration at a slower rate of speed.

D. This is normal, and no change in administration is needed.

Answer: B.   Promethazine hydrochloride (Phenergan) is irritating to the intima (inner layer) of the vein. Administration should be stopped when the patient describes pain associated with the injection in a peripheral intravenous line. Poor outcomes have occurred with the administration of this medication. This is not a normal reaction and the administration should not be sped up or slowed down.

TEST-TAKING STRATEGY: Use the process of elimination to rule out incorrect answer selections to help choose the correct answer.

550. Sublingual nitroglycerin is given to a client who experiences chest pain. Which symptom can occur with this medication?

A. Tachycardia.

B. Tinnitus.

C. Diarrhea.

D. Diplopia.

Answer: A.   One of the side effects of nitroglycerin is reflex tachycardia. Other common side effects include hypotension and headache. Tinnitus, diarrhea, and diplopia are not side effects of nitroglycerin.

TEST-TAKING STRATEGY: The process of elimination to rule out incorrect answer selections to help choose the correct answer.

551. A client with chronic low back pain receives injections of meperidine hydrochloride (Demerol) every other day for 4 weeks. Which symptom exhibited by this patient could be an adverse reaction caused by this medication?

A. Increased salivation.

B. Polyuria.

C. Seizure activity.

D. Mydriasis.

Answer: C.   Meperidine   hydrochloride (Demerol) should not be used for long-term pain relief. The accumulation of the toxic metabololite, normeperidine, can cause seizures. Other adverse reactions for this medication include urinary retention (not polyuria), hypotension, bradycardia, and respiratory depression. Increased salivation and mydriasis are not adverse reactions to meperidine hydrochloride (Demerol).

TEST-TAKING STRATEGY: Have in mind the correct response once the stem of the question is read. Do not read the answer choices until you have the correct answer in your mind.

552. Standard orders on the nurse's unit include an intravenous infusion of 1000 mL of normal saline with 20 mEq potassium chloride to run at 100 mL per hour. In which client should this order be questioned?

A. 42-year-old female diagnosed with Addison's disease.

B. 56-year-old male diagnosed with hypertension.

C. 32-year-old male diagnosed with abdominal cramping.

D. 52-year-old female diagnosed with Graves' disease.

Answer: A.   Clients with Addison's disease can have hyperkalemia if they experience an addisonian crisis due to lack of aldosterone. When aldosterone is not secreted, sodium and water are released and potassium levels elevate in response to the hyponatremia. Patients with hypertension, abdominal pain, and Graves' disease do not have contraindications to this therapy.

TEST-TAKING STRATEGY: Having a basic understanding of the pathophysiology associated with disease processes can help to choose the correct response.

553. A client admitted to the hospital takes isoniazid (INH), metoprolol succinate (toprol-XL), and paroxetine hydrochloride (Paxil). Which lab test indicates a contraindication to the continuation of isoniazid (INH)?

A. SGOT elevated.

B. Sodium decreased.

C. TSH normal.

D. Creatinine elevated.

Answer: A. Isoniazid (INH), a medication used to treat tuberculosis, can cause hepatic disease. It is important to have baseline and follow-up liver panel studies in clients taking this medication. Sodium, TSH, and creatinine levels do not change with adverse reactions to isoniazid (INH).

TEST-TAKING STRATEGY: Be cautious with lab values that are out of range that do not have anything to do with the question. Focus on what the stem is asking.

554. The physician's order states: Ceftriaxone sodium (Rocephin) 50 mg/kg IM now. The client, a child, weighs 22.5 pounds. According to the manufacturer's instructions, after adding the appropriate diluent the concentration is 100 mg/mL. Which dose in milliliters should the nurse administer?

A. 2.25 mL.

B. 3.0 mL.

C. 5.1 mL.

D. 11.25 mL.

Answer: C. A weight of 22.5 pounds is equal to 10.22 kilograms. At 50 mg/kg, this child would need 511 milligrams of medication. At 100 mg/ml, the proper dose in milliliters is 5.1 milliliters.

TEST-TAKING STRATEGY: With dosage calculations, be sure to change pounds into kilogram and then calculate the problem.

555. The toxic dose of acetaminophen is 140 mg/kg. How many tablets (strength equals 325 milligrams per tablet) should a client weighing 275 pounds need to take to attain a toxic level?

A. 28 tablets.

B. 35 tablets.

C. 54 tablets.

D. 118 tablets.

Answer: C. The equation of 275 pounds divided by 2.2 pounds equals 125 kilograms. At 140 mg/kg, the client would need to take the equivalent of 17,500 milligrams to reach the toxic dose. With tablets equaling 325 milligrams, the client would need to take 54 tablets to attain toxicity.

TEST-TAKING STRATEGY: Be sure to perform all the mathematical steps necessary to obtain the correct response when answering questions regarding dosage calculations.

556. A 46-year-old client is prescribed 1.5 grams of levodopa (Larodopa) daily. Available forms of this drug include tablets of 250 milligrams. How many tablets (250 mg) should this client be given to receive the proper amount of medication?

A. 2 tablets.

B. 4 tablets.

C. 6 tablets.

D. 8 tablets.

Answer: C. Changing 1.5 grams to milligrams equals 1500 milligrams as a daily dosage. Dividing 1500 milligrams by 250 milligrams equals 6.

TEST-TAKING STRATEGY: Always change different measurements to the same unit of measure. Grams must be changed to milligrams or vice versa to begin calculations in order to find the correct response.

557. Physician orders for a client instruct the nurse to give lanoxin (Digoxin) 0.125 milligrams intravenously as a one-time dose. The available medication is in a concentration of 0.5 milligrams in 2 milliliters. How many milliliters should the nurse give?

A. 0.25 mL.

B. 0.5 mL.

C. 0.75 mL.

D. 1.0 mL.

Answer: B. To give 0.125 milligrams of a concentration of 0.5 milligrams in 2 milliliters, multiply 0.125 times 2 and then divide by "X" which would be 0.5X. This equals 0.5 mL.

TEST-TAKING STRATEGY: Be wary of decimal points! Keep them in the proper place in order to obtain the correct response.

558. A client is admitted to the hospital with carbon monoxide poisoning at a level of 32. If the client is not given oxygen, how many hours will it take for the carbon monoxide to dissipate down to a level of 1 at a half-life rate of 4 hours?

A. 4 hours.

B. 5 hours.

C. 16 hours.

D. 20 hours.

Answer: D. The carbon monoxide will be half the level in 4 hours, then half the level again in another 4 hours, etc. At this rate it will take 5 cycles to reduce the client's level to 1. Four hours times 5 cycles (of 4-hour increments) equals 20 hours.

TEST-TAKING STRATEGY: With math problems, be sure to think your way through to the final answer. Don't stop prematurely.

559. A client is admitted to the hospital with a lanoxin (digoxin) level of 5.6 mg/mL. Digoxin immune fab (Digibind) is ordered. Because the digoxin level is known, the formula to determine the number of vials needed is digoxin level times client weight in kilograms divided by 100 (digoxin level × kg /100). If the client weighs 185 pounds, how many vials should the nurse give? Round to the nearest whole number.

A. 2 vials.

B. 4 vials.

C. 5 vials.

D. 10 vials.

Answer: C. A client weighing 185 pounds equals 84 kilograms. Multiplying 84 kilograms

by the digoxin level of 5.6 equals 470.4. Divide this by 100, which equals 4.7. Then round up to the nearest whole number, which is 5.

TEST-TAKING STRATEGY: Always be sure to change pounds into kilograms. Medications are given according to kilogram weight.

560. A client is admitted to the hospital after being bitten by a bat. Rabies immune globulin, human (BayRab) is ordered as an injection. The drug leaflet instructs to administer 20 IU/kg. This medication comes in vials of 150 IU/mL. The client weighs 220 pounds. How many milliliters should the nurse administer?

A. 4.6 mL.

B. 9.2 mL.

C. 13.3 mL.

D. 29.3 mL.

Answer: C. A client weighing 220 pounds equals 100 kilograms. Multiply 100 kilograms by 20 IU to equal 2000 IU. If the vial dosage is 150 IU/mL, the proper dose is 13.3 milliliters (2000 divided by 150).

TEST-TAKING STRATEGY: Always make sure the proper mathematical component (multiplication, division, etc.) is used at the right time. Set the formulas up correctly and follow through with the correct math application.

561. An intravenous infusion of normal saline is ordered at 150 milliliters per hour. Using tubing that has a drip rate factor of 15, how many drops per minute should the nurse deliver?

A. 15 drops.

B. 20 drops.

C. 24 drops.

D. 38 drops.

Answer: D. The formula to use for drip rates is the total amount of milliliters divided by the total number of minutes multiplied by the drip factor. Divide 150 by 60 minutes to equal 2.5. Multiplying 2.5 by the drip factor of 15 equals 37.5. Because partial drops cannot be counted, always round to the nearest whole number, which is 38.

TEST-TAKING STRATEGY: Have basic drug calculation formulas memorized. The NCLEX® will not always provide the formula.

562. An intravenous infusion of 0.45 normal saline is ordered at a rate of 1000 milliliters in 24 hours. The tubing has a drip factor of 15. How many drops per minute are delivered?

   A. 11 drops.

   B. 35 drops.

   C. 120 drops.

   D. 240 drops.

   Answer: A. The formula used to calculate drip rates is the total amount of milliliters divided by the total number of minutes multiplied by the drip factor. In this circumstance, the minutes portion must be figured first—that is, 24 hours equals 1440 minutes. Then, dividing 1000 by 1440 equals 0.69, rounded to 0.70. This is multiplied by the drip factor, which is 15. Multiplying 15 by 0.70 equals 10.5, which rounds to 11. The nurse could also divide 1000 by 24, which gives the amount of infusion per hour. This equals 42 milliliters per hour. Using the formula, 42 divided by 60 minutes equals 0.7, and this multiplied by the drip factor of 15 equals 10.5. Round this to 11.

   TEST-TAKING STRATEGY: When tackling numbers and formulas, always be sure that the right number is in the correct place in the formula. First, steps may need to be taken to change a number into its proper format.

563. The following physician order states: Give bolus of 250 mL normal saline in 45 minutes. What would the drip rate be with tubing that has a drip factor of 10?

   A. 10 drops.

   B. 45 drops.

   C. 60 drops.

   D. 80 drops.

   Answer: C. The formula to use for drip rates is the total number of milliters divided by the total number of minutes multiplied by the drip factor. In this case, the number of minutes is less than 60. Dividing 250 milliliters by 45 equals 5.55, which is rounded to 6. The drip factor is 10. Multiplying 10 by 6 equals 60.

   TEST-TAKING STRATEGY: Understand how numbers are plugged into formulas.

564. The physician writes the following order: Give 20 mL per kg bolus of normal saline over 60 minutes. The client, a child, weighs 32 pounds. What number of drops should be delivered per minute? The tubing has a drip factor of 10.

   A. 30 drops.

   B. 50 drops.

   C. 110 drops.

   D. 150 drops.

   Answer: B. This question requires several steps to determine the correct answer. First, determine the proper amount of normal saline to be given. Change the child's weight to kilograms. Dividing 32 by 2.2 equals 14.54 kilograms, which is rounded to 15 kilograms. Multiplying 15 kilograms by 20 (20 milliliters per kilogram) equals 300 milliliters to be given as the bolus. Divide 300 milliliters by 60 minutes to equal 5. Multiplying 5 times the drip factor of 10 equals 50 drops per minute.

   TEST-TAKING STRATEGY: When calculating mathematical problems, perform all of the necessary steps.

565. A 500-milliliter bag of 5% dextrose in water contains 2 grams of lidocaine. What is the concentration of this medication?

   A. 0.25 mg/mL.

   B. 2 mg /mL.

   C. 4 mg /mL.

   D. 8 mg/mL.

   Answer: C. The formula to use to determine the concentration of a medication in mg/mL is milligrams (mg) of medication divided by the amount of fluid in milliliters (mL). With this formula, the 2 grams is changed to milligrams. If there are 1000 milligrams in 1 gram, then there are 2000 milligrams in 2 grams. Dividing

2000 milligrams by 500 milliliters equals a concentration of 4 mg/mL.

TEST-TAKING STRATEGY: When tackling mathematical questions, be sure to change numbers into their proper format for inclusion in the formula.

566. The client, a child, is prescribed erythromycin base (ERYC). The client is to take 75 milligrams four times a day. The medication has a concentration of 125 mg/5 mL. How many milliliters will provide enough medication for 1 week?

   A. 21 mL.

   B. 60 mL.

   C. 75 mL.

   D. 84 mL.

Answer: D. In this question, first determine how many milliliters the child needs each day. Set up the equation as: $\frac{75\ mg}{X\ mL} = \frac{125\ mg}{5\ mL}$ and then cross-multiply so that 75 times 5 equals 375. This is then divided by X, so 375 divided by 125 equals 3 milliliters. Each dose the child receives is 3 milliliters. The child receives this dose four times a day, so 3 milliliters multiplied by 4 times a day equals 12 milliliters. The child requires 12 milliliters. Multiply the 12 milliliters per day by 7 days to equal 84 milliliters for the entire week.

TEST-TAKING STRATEGY: Always be sure that you are aware of what the question is asking. In this case, how much medication is needed for 1 week.

567. A 24-year-old male enters the emergency department with a chief complaint of seizure activity that lasted approximately 45 seconds. The client's vital signs are blood pressure 118/64 mm Hg, pulse 84 beats/minute, respiratory rate 16 breaths/minute, and a pulse oximetry reading of 100% on room air. The client has a past medical history of tonic-clonic seizures. Due to loss of employment for the past 2 weeks, the client has not taken antiseizure medication. Which medication should the nurse administer to this client?

   A. Furosemide (Lasix).

   B. Fosinopril sodium (Monopril).

   C. Fosphenytoin sodium (Cerebyx).

   D. Famotidine (Pepcid).

Answer: C. Fosphenytoin sodium (Cerebyx) is used to treat seizures, status epilepticus, and is a short-term replacement for oral phenytoin (Dilantin). Furosemide (Lasix) is a loop diuretic. Fosinopril sodium (Monopril) is an ACE inhibitor used to treat hypertension, and famotodine (Pepcid) is an H$_2$-receptor antagonist used for ulcers (both prevention and treatment), GERD, heartburn, and allergic reactions.

TEST-TAKING STRATEGY: Read the answer selections carefully when they are similar in spelling and sound, especially medications.

568. An 82-year-old female client who recently relocated to the United States from a small Caribbean island is treated for a laceration to the right forearm. The physician orders both tetanus immune globulin human (Baytet) (TIG), and diptheria-tetanus (DT). Which is a true statement regarding this client's medication care?

   A. Tetanus immune globulin, human, provides active immunity for the patient.

   B. Diptheria-tetanus (DT) provides passive immunity for this patient.

   C. The TIG and the diptheria-tetanus should be given in opposite arms.

   D. Other vaccinations can be given once a week after receiving these medications.

Answer: C. Tetanus immune globulin (TIG) provides passive immunity and diptheria-tetanus (DT) provides active immunity (which produces antibodies). Both must be given if the patient has never been immunized before. These should be given in opposite arms so that they do not interfere with the actions of one another. Other live virus vaccinations should not be given for 3 months after the administration of these medications.

TEST-TAKING STRATEGY: Make sure you read the entire stem of the question to gather all the information prior to making an answer selection.

569. A 24-year-old female client is admitted for an elective cholecystectomy. The client is complaining of a severe, pounding headache and vomiting. Vital signs are blood pressure 136/88 mm Hg, pulse 86 beats/minute, respiratory rate 20 breaths/minute, temperature 99.6°F, and pulse oximetry 96% on room air. The client has a history of migraine headaches, hypertension, and fibromyalgia. The nurse expects the physician will order which medication for this client?

A. Nifedipine (Procardia) 60 mg PO.

B. Sumatriptan succinate (Imitrex) 6 mg subcutaneous.

C. Ribavirin (Rebetol) 1000 mg PO.

D. Propylthiouracil (PTU) 100 mg PO.

Answer: B. Sumaptriptan succinate (Imitrex) is used for migraine headaches. Migraines are usually a throbbing type of pain associated with nausea, vomiting, and photophobia. Nifedipine (Procardia) is a calcium-channel blocker used for variant angina and hypertension. Ribvavirin is an antiviral usually used in children with respiratory syncytial virus (RSV) and adults with hepatitis C. Propylthiouracil (PTU) is a thyroid hormone antagonist used for hyperthyroidism.

TEST-TAKING STRATEGY: Read the question carefully to derive important information needed to answer the question.

570. The physician writes an order that states: methimozole (Tapazole) 15 mg daily PO. Which disease process is most likely being treated with this medication?

A. Addison's disease.

B. Hyperthyroidism.

C. Rheumatoid arthritis.

D. Parkinison's disease.

Answer: B. Methimozole (Tapazole) is an antithyroid medication used to treat forms of hyperthyroidism. Addison's disease, rheumatoid arthritis, and Parkinson's disease are not treated with methimozole (Tapazole).

TEST-TAKING STRATEGY: Use the process of elimination to rule out incorrect answer selections to help choose the correct answer.

571. A client awaiting surgery is accidentally given a double dose of morning medication, which includes metformin hydrochloride (Glucophage) 1000 mg and aspirin 81 mg. Which step should the nurse take to ensure that no ill effects occur as a result of this incident?

A. Observe for Kussmaul respirations.

B. Monitor closely for hypertension.

C. Test for blood glucose levels.

D. Document temperature readings.

Answer: C. Metformin hydrochloride (Glucophage) is an antidiabetic medication that lowers glucose levels. Kussmaul respirations are seen in diabetic ketoacidosis, which accompanies hyperglycemic reactions. Hypertension and temperature are not significant side effects of Glucophage or the daily dose of aspirin.

TEST-TAKING STRATEGY: Use your critical thinking skills to determine the correct answer.

572. A client takes the following medications: labetolol hydrochloride (Normodyne) 100 milligrams twice a day, ketorolac tromethamine (Toradol) 10 milligrams as needed, and mirtazapine (Remeron) 15 milligrams at bedtime. Which nursing diagnosis is most appropriate for this client?

A. Risk for trauma related to drug-induced hypotension.

B. Risk for fluid volume deficit related to adverse reactions.

C. Risk for trauma related to lowered seizure threshold.

D. Risk for impaired skin integrity related to dermatologic reactions.

Answer: A. The expected outcome of the medication labetolol hydrocholoride (Normodyne) is lowered blood pressure. Mirtazapine (Remeron) can cause orthostatic hypotension. Fluid volume deficit, seizures, and dermatologic reactions are not effects (or side effects) of these medications.

TEST-TAKING STRATEGY: Use the process of elimination to rule out incorrect answer selections to help choose the correct answer.

573. Which statement by the nurse indicates a positive outcome for a client who takes sodium polystyrene sulfonate (Kayexalate)?

A. "The client's urine output is good."

B. "The client's nausea is gone."

C. "The client's affect has improved."

D. "The client's potassium level has decreased."

Answer: D. Sodium polystyrene sulfonate (Kayexalate) is used to treat hyperkalemia. It can be given orally, via nasogastric tube, or rectally. Urine output, nausea, and affect are not related to this medication.

TEST-TAKING STRATEGY: Use the process of elimination to rule out incorrect answers when searching for the correct answer.

574. Timolol maleate (Timoptic) is ordered for a client with a diagnosis of open-angle glaucoma. The nurse knows this medication reduces intraocular pressure through which expected action?

A. Timolol maleate (Timoptic) helps to decrease inflammation.

B. Timolol maleate (Timoptic) works to reduce aqueous humor production.

C. Timolol maleate (Timoptic) acts as an antifibrinolytic.

D. Timolol maleate (Timoptic) is an optic analgesic.

Answer: B. Timolol maleate (Timoptic) reduces intraocular pressure by reducing aqueous humor production. It does not decrease inflammation, as an anti-fibrinolytic or as an analgesic.

TEST-TAKING STRATEGY: Relate possible answers to the pathophysiology of the disease process stated in the stem. Choose the answer that best relates to the pathophysiology.

575. Hydrochlorthiazide (Microzide) is ordered for a client as an antihypertensive. Which should the nurse expect to be included in the client's list of current medications?

A. Sodium thiosulfate.

B. Potassium chloride (K-Dur).

C. Magnesium citrate (Citrate of Magnesia).

D. Calcium gluconate.

Answer: B. Hydrochlorthiazide (Microzide) is a diuretic and an antihypertensive. As a result of its action, hypokalemia is a concern. Clients should take oral potassium replacement during therapy with hydrochlorothiazide (Microzide). Sodium thiosulfate is used for cyanide toxicity. Magnesium citrate (Citrate of Magnesia) is a laxative. Calcium gluconate is a calcium adjunct that is not needed with hydrochlorthiazide.

TEST-TAKING STRATEGY: Use the process of elimination to rule out incorrect answer selections to help choose the correct answer.

576. A 52-year-old client is seen in the local clinic after positive seroconversion of a tuberculin (TB) test. The nurse expects the client to be placed on which medication?

A. Doxycycline hydrochloride (Vibramycin).

B. Fluconazole (Diflucan).

C. Isoniazid (INH).

D. Oseltamivir phosphate (Tamiflu).

Answer: C. Isoniazid (INH) is used for treatment and prevention of tuberculosis (TB). Doxycycline hydrochloride (Vibramycin) is an antibiotic used to treat gram-positive and gram-negative organisms and anthrax. Fluconazole (Diflucan) is an antifungal used to treat candidiasis. Oseltamivir phosphate (Tamiflu) is an antiviral utilized in the treatment of influenza.

TEST-TAKING STRATEGY: Do not read into the question. Answer the question based on the information presented.

577. A client is admitted for minor injuries sustained in a motorcycle accident. The physician order reads: desmopressin acetate (DDAVP) 0.3 mcg/kg IV × 1 dose. The nurse knows this medication is ordered to manage the client's:

A. Christmas disease.

B. Disseminated intravascular coagulation (DIC).

C. Sickle-cell anemia.

D. Von Willebrand's disease.

Answer: D. Desmpression acetate (DDAVP) is a hemostatic medication used to treat hemophilia A and Von Willebrand's disease. It works by causing the release of factor VIII. Christmas disease is a deficiency of factor IX. Disseminated intravascular coagulation is a disorder of both bleeding and clotting with a variety of treatments not including desmopressin acetate (DDAVP). Sickle-cell anemia is a genetic disorder not treated with desmopressin acetate (DDAVP).

TEST-TAKING STRATEGY: Use the process of elimination to rule out incorrect selections to help choose the correct answer.

578. Which evaluation statement by the nurse is most accurate for a client who has been taking colchicine (Colgout)?

    A. "The client is free of pain."

    B. "The client's platelet level is increased."

    C. "The client's cardiac output is improved."

    D. "The client is free from infection."

    Answer: A. Colchicine (Colgout) is an anti-gout medication that relieves gout-related symptoms such as pain. Platelet level, cardiac output, and infectious processes are not impacted.

    TEST-TAKING STRATEGY: Once you read the stem, think of the correct answer prior to reading the answer selections. Then read the answer selections to determine the correct answer.

579. The medication indomethacin (Indocin) is used in the management of which symptom? Select all that apply.

    A. To reduce pain.

    B. To relieve inflammation.

    C. To treat fever.

    D. To suppress cough.

    Answer: A, B, & C. Indomethacin (Indocin) is used to treat pain, inflammation, and fever. It does not have any cough-suppressant actions.

    TEST-TAKING STRATEGY: When answering "Select all that apply" questions, be sure and treat each answer as a true or false statement. There may be one correct answer or more.

580. A client is prescribed the following medications: cefprazil (Cefzil) 500 mg PO twice a day, digoxin (Lanoxin) 0.125 mg PO daily, magaldrate (Riopan) 10 mL PO at meals, and zolpidem tartrate (Ambien) 10 mg HS. Which medications should not be given together?

    A. Digoxin (Lanoxin) and zolpidem tartrate (Ambien).

    B. Digoxin (Lanoxin) and magaldrate (Riopan).

    C. Magaldrate (Riopan) and zolpidem tartrate (Ambien).

    D. Cefprazil (Cefzil) and zolpidem tartrate (Ambien).

    Answer: B. Antacids such as magaldrate (Riopan) taken at the same time as digoxin (Lanoxin) can decrease the absorption of the digoxin (Lanoxin). Cefprazil (Cefzil) and zolpidem tartrate (Ambien) taken together do not have interactions. Digoxin (Lanoxin) and zolpidem tartrate (Ambien) do not interact. Magaldrate (Riopan) and zopidem tartrate (Ambien) also do not interact.

    TEST-TAKING STRATEGY: When multiple medications are present in a question, be sure to read both the stem and the potential answers very carefully.

581. A 32-year-old female client who is 5 months pregnant is diagnosed with pelvic inflammatory disease and given a prescription for metronidazole (Flagyl). Which substance should be avoided in this client in order to prevent an interaction with Flagyl?

    A. Furosemide (Lasix).

    B. Alcohol.

    C. Doxycycline (Vibramycin).

    D. St. John's Wort.

    Answer: B. Metronidazole (Flagyl) and alcohol can interact with each other causing severe nausea and vomiting as well as cramping and flushed appearance. Fuorsemide (Lasix), doxycycline (Vibramycin), and St. John's wort do not interact with metronidazole (Flagyl).

TEST-TAKING STRATEGY: Look for similar answer choices and eliminate them.

582. For which client would the use of acetaminophen (Tylenol) pose the highest risk?

    A. A 42-year-old female who abuses cocaine.

    B. A 54-year-old male who abuses alcohol.

    C. A 23-year-old female who has asthma.

    D. A 34-year-old male with sickle-cell anemia.

    Answer: B. The use of acetaminophen (Tylenol) poses the highest risk for the client who abuses alcohol due to interaction with the liver. Clients should be educated to be cautious if using acetaminophen (Tylenol) due to the hepatotoxicity that can occur with liver dysfunction and failure. Clients who use cocaine or who have a history of asthma or sickle-cell anemia do not have a higher risk.

    TEST-TAKING STRATEGY: Utilize your core content knowledge to help you assess the answer options.

583. A client admitted to the unit for treatment of an upper respiratory infection receives erythromycin lactobionate (erythromycin). The client has a history of renal transplant and is taking cyclosporine (Neoral). These two medications can interact at which pharmacological phase?

    A. Absorption.

    B. Distribution.

    C. Metabolism.

    D. Excretion.

    Answer: C. Erythromycin   lactobionate (eythromycin) and cyclosporine (Neoral) interact during the metabolism phase through competition for the same hepatic enzyme. The absorption, distribution, and excretion phases are not affected.

    TEST-TAKING STRATEGY: Use the process of elimination to rule out incorrect answer selections to help choose the correct answer.

584. Which is a true statement regarding medication interactions and the phases of pharmacologic actions? Select all that apply.

    A. Antacids combined with certain medications can cause harmful interactions in the absorption phase due to a decreased pH.

    B. When two medications compete for the same hepatic enzyme, the effects can be deleterious due to possible toxic levels.

    C. Distribution of medications is affected by protein-binding sites and can result in toxic levels of certain medications.

    D. When two medications interact at the excretion level causing decreased elimination, this can produce a beneficial result.

    Answer: B, C, & D. Two medications, when competing for the same hepatic enzyme for metabolism purposes, can cause increased levels of the medications and therefore toxic levels can occur. Medications that cannot bind with proteins are then "free" and can increase the actions of that medication. Beneficial results can occur from medication interactions if the desired effect is to achieve increased levels in the body. If elimination of the medication is discouraged, the medication level remains elevated. Antacids increase the level of pH in the gastric secretions.

    TEST-TAKING STRATEGY: When answering "Select all that apply" questions, be sure and treat each answer as a true or false statement. There may be one correct answer or more.

585. An immigrant from the Kurdish Jewish population is admitted for fever of unknown origin, generalized body aches, and dyspnea. The following medication regimen is ordered: albuterol sulfate (Proventil) inhaler 2 puffs four times a day as needed for dyspnea; acetylsalicylic acid (aspirin) 650 mg PO every 4 hours as needed for pain or fever; celecoxib (Celebrex) 200 mg PO daily; and fosinopril sodium (Monopril) 10 mg PO daily. Which order should the nurse question?

    A. Albuterol sulfate (Proventil) inhaler 2 puffs four times a day as needed for dyspnea.

    B. Acetylsalicylic acid (aspirin) 650 mg PO every 4 hours as needed for pain or fever.

    C. Celecoxib (Celebrex) 200 mg PO daily.

    D. Fosinopril sodium (Monopril) 10 mg PO daily.

Answer: B. Clients of the Kurdish Jewish population have a 50% occurrence of glucose-6-phosphate dehydrogenase (G6PD) deficiency. When acetylsalicylic acid (aspirin) is taken in the presence of this genetic deficiency, hemolysis of red blood cells can occur, which can be fatal. Albuterol sulfate (Proventil), celecoxib (Celebrex), and fosinopril sodium (Monopril) do not pose a problem to Kurdish Jews.

TEST-TAKING STRATEGY: Use the process of elimination to rule out incorrect answer selections to help choose the correct answer.

586. An elderly client receives instructions regarding the use of warfarin sodium (Coumadin). Which statement indicates the client understands the possible food interactions which may occur with this medication?

   A. "I'm going to miss having my evening glass of wine now."

   B. "I told my daughter to buy bananas for me. I'll have to eat more of those now."

   C. "I will have to watch my intake of salads, something that I really love."

   D. "I am going to begin eating more fish and pork and leave beef alone now."

Answer: C. Clients taking warfarin sodium (Coumadin) must watch their intake of vitamin K, which is present in leafy green vegetables, tomatoes, fish, and bananas. Wine does not affect the use of warfarin sodium (Coumadin).

TEST-TAKING STRATEGY: Use the process of elimination to rule out incorrect answer selections to help choose the correct answer.

587. Which electrolyte imbalances should be of concern for the client taking digoxin (Lanoxin)?

   A. Hypokalemia.

   B. Hyponatremia.

   C. Hypomagnesemia.

   D. Hypocalcemia.

Answer: A. Hypokalemia can interact with digoxin (Lanoxin) by predisposing the client to digitalis toxicity. Hyponatremia, hypomagnesemia, and hypocalcemia do not interfere with

digoxin (Lanoxin). Hypercalcemia does predispose the client to digoxin (Lanoxin) toxicity.

TEST-TAKING STRATEGY: Think of the correct answer after reading the stem and before looking at the answer selections.

588. A client complains of increasing fatigue and pain due to rheumatoid arthritis currently being treated with sulfasalizine (Azulfidine). The client's history includes diabetes mellitus type 2 and chronic obstructive pulmonary disease (COPD). The client's medications include glipizide (Glucotrol) and estradiol (Estrace). Which symptom should the nurse expect to find as a result of medication interactions?

   A. Pathological fractures.

   B. Hot flashes.

   C. Increased dyspnea.

   D. Hypoglycemia.

Answer: D. Sulfonamides such as sulfasalizine (Azulfidine) can interact with sulfonylureas, such as glipizide (Glucotrol), thus producing hypoglycemic reactions. Pathological fractures, hot flashes, and increasing dyspnea are not potential interactions associated with this client.

TEST-TAKING STRATEGY: Use the process of elimination to rule out incorrect answer selections to help choose the correct answer.

589. An elderly client is prescribed spironolactone (Aldactone) with the addition of potassium chloride (Kaochlor). Which is a true statement regarding the use of these two medications together?

   A. Spironolactone (Aldactone) should not have potassium chloride (Kaochlor) added to the regimen because it is a potassium-sparing diuretic.

   B. Potassium is necessary when clients are placed on spironolactone (Aldactone) because it is a loop diuretic.

   C. Spironolactone (Aldactone) and potassium chloride (Kaochlor) have no additive or antagonistic effects with each other.

D. Potassium chloride (Kaochlor) added to spironolactone (Aldactone) causes renal failure.

Answer: **A.** Spironolactone (Aldactone) is a potassium-sparing diuretic and should not have potassium supplements added to it. This can cause hyperkalemia. Spironolactone (Aldactone) is not a loop diuretic. Spironolactone (Aldactone) and potassium chloride (Kaochlor) do not cause renal failure.

TEST-TAKING STRATEGY: Use the process of elimination to rule out incorrect answer selections to help choose the correct answer.

590. A 62-year-old male client has nitroglycerin (Nitrostat) added to his medication regimen. Which statement made by this client indicates that further education is needed?

A. "I will take this medication if I have an episode of chest pain."

B. "I will wait at least 1 hour after I take my sildanefil (Viagra) before using Nitrostat."

C. "I can take up to 3 tablets every 5 minutes if my angina occurs."

D. "I know that I must put this tablet under my tongue for it to work."

Answer: **B.** Nitrates should not be used with sildanefil (Viagra), as extreme hypotension may occur. Nitroglycerin (Nitrostat) should be used for chest pain. Up to 3 tablets every 5 minutes given sublingually is the recommended dose.

TEST-TAKING STRATEGY: The phrase "further teaching is necessary" tells you to select an answer with inaccurate information.

591. Which dietary change must a client make when starting treatment with the medication spironolactone (Aldactone)?

A. Eat extra helpings of bananas.

B. Increase intake of water.

C. Avoid salt substitutes .

D. Increase intake of green leafy vegetables.

Answer: **C.** Spironolactone (Aldactone) is a potassium-sparing diuretic and should not be

used with increased potassium intake. Salt substitutes have potassium instead of sodium and should be avoided. Bananas have potassium and thus should be avoided. Water intake does not affect the use of Aldactone. Green, leafy vegetables contain vitamin K and are not contraindicated.

TEST-TAKING STRATEGY: Use the process of elimination to rule out incorrect answer selections to help choose the correct answer.

592. A client is given a prescription for amiodarone (Cordarone) in addition to digoxin (Lanoxin). Which action should the nurse take?

A. No action is necessary.

B. Contact the physician.

C. Encourage the patient to take the medications at the same time.

D. Instruct the client to only take a half dose of digoxin (Lanoxin).

Answer: **B.** Amiodarone (Cordarone) and digoxin (Lanoxin) taken together can cause increased digoxin levels by as much as two times. Digoxin levels must be reduced when given together with amiodarone (Cordarone) due to a decreased clearance of the digoxin.

TEST-TAKING STRATEGY: Determine which action brings the most help to the client. This determines the highest nursing priority.

593. A client tells the nurse that her religious preference is Jehovah's Witness. Which is a true statement regarding the use of blood products for this client? Select all that apply.

A. Packed red cells are allowed in emergency and critical situations.

B. Blood may be used with heart-lung equipment as long as it does not leave the circulation of the body.

C. The client may be given doses of erythropoietin (Epogen) to assist in the creation of new blood cells.

D. Blood may be accepted if it is taken from a blood relative and used immediately.

Answer: B & C. Jehovah's Witnesses may receive blood if it is the client's own blood, and if the blood is used in either a heart-lung machine or dialysis. The blood should not at any time remain outside of the patient's circulation. Erythropoietin (Epogen) is used synthetically to stimulate growth of red blood cells. Jehovah's Witnesses do not allow blood in any form, whether packed red cells or whole blood from a relative.

TEST-TAKING STRATEGY: When answering "Select all that apply" questions, be sure and treat each answer as a true or false statement. There may be one correct answer or more.

594. Hypocalcemia can occur when large amounts of blood are used in critical patient situations. Which statement is true regarding the cause of hypocalcemia?

A. The citrate contained in the blood bags combines with calcium ions, making them unusable.

B. The pH of banked blood is alkalinic, creating an environment that is not stable for the calcium ions.

C. A shift to the right on the oxyhemoglobin dissociation curve occurs, causing calcium to be excreted more quickly from the renal system.

D. Increased amounts of 2.3 DPG are found in banked blood, which antagonizes calcium.

Answer: A. Citrate is a preservative used in banked blood. It attaches to the free calcium ions in the body. When these ions are bound, they are not usable for cellular functions. The pH of banked blood is acidic and has nothing to do with the calcium ions. Shifts on the oxyhemoglobin dissociation curve, which might occur due to blood transfusions, are usually to the left and do not interfere with the calcium ions. The substance 2.3 DPG is found on the hemoglobin molecule. When present in adequate amounts, it allows the oxygen to drop off of the hemoglobin molecule faster. Banked blood has decreasing amounts of 2.3 DPG.

TEST-TAKING STRATEGY: When you are asked to identify "true" statements, you are looking for the answer selection that offers accurate information.

595. A client has no antibodies in the blood when tested for cross-match. Which blood type is this client?

A. Type A.

B. Type B.

C. Type AB.

D. Type O.

Answer: C. No antibodies in the blood means that the client is Type AB. Type A blood has anti-B antibodies, type B has anti-A antibodies, and type O has both anti-A and anti-B antibodies.

TEST-TAKING STRATEGY: Look for similar answer choices and eliminate them.

Blood Group	Antigen	Antibody
A	A	Anti-B
B	B	Anti-A
AB	A & B	None
O	None	Anti-A and Anti-B

596. A client has a history positive for HIV with onset of acquired immunodeficiency syndrome (AIDS). The client receives 2 units of whole blood. Which transfusion reaction is this client most likely to have?

A. Acute hemolytic reaction.

B. Graft-versus-host disease.

C. Allergic reaction.

D. Febrile transfusion reaction.

Answer: B. Graft-versus-host disease occurs frequently in those clients who are immunocompromised or immunosuppressed. This occurs because of an attack on the host tissues from donor lymphocytes. Acute hemolytic reaction, allergic reaction, and febrile transfusion reaction can occur, but immunosuppressed clients are not especially prone to them.

TEST-TAKING STRATEGY: When the words "most likely" are used, you must select the most correct answer choice. All of the responses could be true, but one will outweigh the others.

597. The nurse receives a unit of blood at 0800 for transfusion. This unit of blood must be infused by what time?

   A. 1000.

   B. 1200.

   C. 1400.

   D. 1600.

Answer: B. A unit of blood must be given within 4 hours of receipt by the hospital unit.

TEST-TAKING STRATEGY: Perform the calculation in your mind prior to selecting an answer option.

598. A client with a diagnosis of neutropenia would most likely be transfused with which substance?

   A. Cyroprecipitate.

   B. Fresh-frozen plasma.

   C. Granulocytes.

   D. Platelets.

Answer: C. Granulocyte infusion may be used for clients who are neutropenic. Cryoprecipitate is used in clients with hemophilia. Fresh-frozen plasma is used in patients with increased pro-times and partial thromboplastin times. Platelets are given to patients who are thrombocytopenic.

TEST-TAKING STRATEGY: Understanding terminology is important in test-taking. Be sure to have a good command of general medical terms.

599. A client is in need of a transfusion of platelets. Which statement is true regarding this blood product infusion? Select all that apply.

   A. Platelets do not have to be typed to each particular client.

   B. Platelets should be given slowly over a 2- to 4-hour period of time.

   C. Special transfusion sets should be used with platelet infusions.

   D. Filters are used when clients receive multiple units of platelets.

Answer: A, C, & D. Platelets are obtained from multiple donors. Typing is not necessary for this blood product. Special transfusion sets

are used, which have smaller filters and shorter lengths, to prevent platelets from catching on the bigger filter and adhering to the longer tubing. When clients receive multiple units of platelets, it is best to utilize a special filter, which will trap white blood cells and decrease the chances of reactions. Platelets should be given over a very short time period: 15 to 60 minutes because of the fragility of the platelet cells.

TEST-TAKING STRATEGY: When answering "Select all that apply" questions, be sure and treat each answer as a true or false statement. There may be one correct answer or more.

600. A client who receives a blood transfusion complains of chest and low back pain. Vital signs are blood pressure 94/62 mm Hg, pulse 140 beats/minute, respiratory rate 32 breaths/minute. Which nursing action takes priority?

   A. Contact the physician immediately.

   B. Turn off the blood.

   C. Place the client in Trendelenburg position.

   D. Open the saline on the blood tubing.

Answer: B. This client exhibits signs and symptoms of a hemolytic blood transfusion reaction. The blood product must be turned off immediately so that no more blood is infused into the client. The physician should be contacted, but it is not the priority in this circumstance. Trendelenburg position is not recommended at this time because it can intensify hypotension. Placing the client in modified Trendelenburg position is acceptable, but is not the priority action. Opening the saline on the blood tubing continues to infuse blood into the client until the tubing is cleared. The tubing should be changed at the hub and saline can be infused with the new tubing.

TEST-TAKING STRATEGY: Never delay treatment, especially when the situation is life threatening. Choose the answer that addresses the client's problem immediately.

601. Which is an advantage of using packed red cells for a client in need of a blood transfusion?

A. It provides added clotting factors.

B. It decreases the chance of overload.

C. It has a longer shelf life.

D. It reduces the chance of allergic reactions.

Answer: B. The advantage of using packed red cells is the reduced potential for cardiac overload. Packed red cells do not include the plasma and other cells, thus decreasing the volume infused into the client. Clotting factors are found in fresh-frozen plasma. Packed red cells have a shorter shelf life and can cause allergic reactions.

TEST-TAKING STRATEGY: Use the process of elimination to rule out incorrect answer selections to help choose the correct answer.

602. A client receives a unit of packed red blood cells. Which is appropriate nursing care for this client?

A. Give a bolus of 50 mL of blood to start the process.

B. Take vital signs prior to the start of administering blood and again in 15 minutes.

C. Measure the client's blood pressure, pulse, and pulse oximetry only.

D. A nurse and nurse's aide can check the blood prior to administration.

Answer: B. Always take full vital signs prior to administering blood and then again in 15 minutes. Blood should be started slowly and gradually increased. Vital signs include temperature and respiratory rate as well as blood pressure, pulse, and pulse oximetry. Two nurses should check the unit of blood prior to its administration.

TEST-TAKING STRATEGY: Eliminate answers that have incomplete information, such as answer C (blood pressure, pulse, and pulse oximetry), which leaves out respiratory rate.

603. A 22-year-old female client receives $Rh_o(D)$ immune globulin, human (Rhogam) after a sudden miscarriage. Which statement is true regarding this blood product?

A. Rhogam should be given to females who are Rh positive after miscarriage or delivery.

B. Rhogam provides active immunity to women exposed to Rh-positive blood from the fetus.

C. Epinephrine should be available, because Rhogam can cause anaphylaxis.

D. Rhogam increases antibody response to Rh-negative exposure.

Answer: C. $Rh_o(D)$ immune globulin, human (Rhogam) can cause anaphylaxis, and epinephrine should be available for use should anaphylaxis occur. Rhogam is given to women who are Rh negative and who have a pregnancy associated with an Rh-positive fetus. Rhogam produces passive immunity to women who are exposed to Rh-positive blood. The antibody response is decreased in women who have Rh-positive exposure.

TEST-TAKING STRATEGY: When the words "positive" and "negative" are used, be careful not to confuse the two.

604. A client involved in a major vehicle accident has type O blood. Which blood types can this client receive?

A. Type A.

B. Type B.

C. Type AB.

D. Type O.

Answer: D. Type O is the universal donor, meaning a client with type O blood can only receive type O blood. Type A clients can receive type A and type O blood. Type B clients can receive type B and type O blood. Type AB clients can receive type A, type B, type AB, and type O blood.

TEST-TAKING STRATEGY: When several letters are used to identify potential answers, think these through very carefully.

605. A client with type A-positive blood receives type A-negative blood. Which action should the nurse take when this discrepancy is noted?

A. The blood bank and the physician should be notified, but there is no danger in Rh-positive individuals receiving Rh-negative blood.

B. Blood should be drawn immediately from the client, and the blood bag sent to the blood bank.

C. Oxygen should be given by partial rebreather mask at 10 liters per minute so the adverse effects from this incident can be reversed.

D. The client needs to be closely monitored for the next 24 hours with attention to vital signs and level of consciousness.

Answer: A. A client who is Rh positive can receive Rh-negative blood. However, those who are Rh negative can never receive Rh-positive blood. There is no need to draw blood, provide oxygen, or closely monitor this client.

TEST-TAKING STRATEGY: If you don't know the answer, think through the pathophysiology of the question to select the appropriate answer.

606. A client receives an implanted port. After insertion, an x-ray is performed to determine proper positioning. The tip of the catheter should be located in which vascular structure?

A. Inferior vena cava.

B. Superior vena cava.

C. Left atrium.

D. Aortic arch.

Answer: B. The tip of an implanted port should be located in the superior vena cava, which feeds into the right atrium. The tip will not be in the inferior vena cava, the left atrium, or the aortic arch, which is an arterial vascular component.

TEST-TAKING STRATEGY: Picture normal anatomy and physiology in your mind prior to answering the question.

607. A client has a Groshong central venous access device. The nurse prepares to flush the device. Which information is correct regarding the flushing?

A. Administer 10 mL of heparin 100 units/mL on a weekly basis.

B. Administer normal saline 2 mL on a weekly basis.

C. Administer 1 to 2 mL of heparin solution 1000 units/mL daily.

D. Administer normal saline 5 to 10 mL weekly.

Answer: D. The Groshong catheter should be flushed with 5 to 10 mL of normal saline on a weekly basis. Heparin solution, which has a concentration of 100 units/mL, is used to flush PICC lines, tunneled devices other than the Groshong, and implanted ports. Normal saline is used for peripheral nontunneled devices. Heparin solution at a concentration of 1000 units/mL is used for pheresis and hemodialysis catheters.

TEST-TAKING STRATEGY: The presence of many numbers in the list of potential answers means you must be careful not to get the numbers confused.

608. The nurse gathers supplies needed to access an implanted port in a client. Which equipment is appropriate for use in this client?

A. 19-gauge butterfly needle.

B. Straight 20-gauge needle.

C. 20-gauge noncoring needle.

D. 20-gauge over-the-needle catheter.

Answer: C. A noncoring needle must be used to access implanted ports. A butterfly needle is used to access a peripheral site for blood draws. A straight needle is used to deliver an intramuscular injection. An over-the-needle catheter is used to insert a peripheral intravenous line.

TEST-TAKING STRATEGY: Use the process of elimination to rule out incorrect answers to help choose the correct answer.

609. A peripherally inserted central catheter (PICC) line is ordered for a client. Which statement made by the nurse indicates an understanding of the proper insertion information for this intravenous access device?

   A. "This intravenous line should be used only for antibiotics. No one should give anything else through this line."

   B. "I watched one of these being placed last week. I think I can do it without disturbing anyone."

   C. "Once I get this line in, it will need to be checked with an x-ray. The line should be in the superior vena cava.

   D. This is useful for about 2 weeks. After that, another line will need to be inserted to maintain patency."

Answer: C. PICC line placement should be verified with an x-ray for proper placement (in the superior vena cava). Once placed, the line can be used for any intravenous therapy including antibiotics. Nurses must be specially trained to insert this device and must have a minimum of 8 hours of education and observation prior to performing the procedure independently. PICC lines can be left in place for prolonged periods of time. Some last up to 12 months.

TEST-TAKING STRATEGY: The phrase "indicates an understanding" tells you to select the answer with accurate information.

610. When accessing a Groshong tunneled venous access device, the nurse notes there is no clamp on the end. Which action should the nurse take?

   A. Utilize a bulldog clamp, and notify the physician who inserted the device.

   B. Realize that no clamp is needed on this device due to the three-way valve.

   C. Have another nurse provide pressure on the tubing while the physician is notified.

   D. Bend the tubing and place a rubber band to hold it closed.

Answer: B. A Groshong catheter does not have a clamp. A three-way valve on the end of the catheter allows for both aspiration of blood and infusion of fluids and medications. The valve

prevents bleeding or infiltration of outside air if it is pulled apart. No clamp is necessary, so utilizing a metal clamp, putting pressure on the tubing, or using a rubber band is incorrect.

TEST-TAKING STRATEGY: Look for similar answer choices and eliminate them.

611. A client receives a blood transfusion through a peripherally inserted central catheter (PICC) line. The blood runs very slowly. Which action by the nurse helps the blood run faster through the line? Select all that apply.

   A. Utilize an infusion or pressure pump.

   B. Add 50 mL of normal saline to the blood.

   C. Run normal saline with the blood.

   D. Push the blood manually with a 60-mL syringe.

Answer: A, B, & C. When blood does not run well through a PICC line, a pressure pump or infusion pump may be necessary. Also, adding normal saline to the blood or running normal saline through the same tubing as the blood can help to decrease the viscosity. Pushing blood with a syringe is not appropriate.

TEST-TAKING STRATEGY: When answering "Select all that apply" questions, be sure and treat each answer as a true or false statement. There may be one correct answer or more.

612. The nurse finds the client with a disconnected central venous access device. The client complains of chest pain and dyspnea. The client's blood pressure is 84/52 mm Hg and pulse is 150 beats/minute. Which nursing action takes priority?

   A. Contact the physician immediately.

   B. Turn the client to the left side.

   C. Place the client in reverse Trendelenburg position.

   D. Monitor the pulse oximetry reading.

Answer: B. The nurse should immediately turn the client to the left side. The physician should be contacted next. The client should be placed in Trendelenburg position, not reverse Trendelenburg position. The pulse oximetry readings should be monitored, but not as a first priority.

TEST-TAKING STRATEGY: Questions that ask you to prioritize your nursing actions use terms like *priority, first, best, initial, most important, immediate,* and *next.*

613. The nurse who is accessing a client's central line notices the infusion rate is difficult to maintain. The nurse notes the rate is affected when the client raises an arm or moves a shoulder. The nurse should be concerned with which possible complication?

A. Extravasation.

B. Pinch-off syndrome.

C. Central vein thrombosis.

D. Phlebitis.

Answer: B. Pinch-off syndrome occurs when the catheter becomes pinched between two structures—the first rib and the clavicle. When the arm or shoulder is moved, the pinch is either made worse or relieved. Intermittent aspiration of blood or intermittent infusion of fluids indicates pinch-off syndrome. Symptoms of extravasation are pain and swelling of the area and a decrease or cessation of infusion rate. Central vein thrombosis is indicated by a slow flow rate and no blood return. Symptoms of phlebitis are pain, swelling, and redness.

TEST-TAKING STRATEGY: Use your knowledge of anatomy and physiology to determine the correct answer.

614. A client has recently undergone central line placement. The client complains of shortness of breath and right-sided chest pain. Vital signs are blood pressure 98/50 mm Hg, pulse rate 110 beats/minute, and respiratory rate 36 breaths/minute. Which action should the nurse take first?

A. Gather supplies for chest-tube insertion.

B. Notify the physician immediately.

C. Order a chest x-ray.

D. Administer oxygen.

Answer: D. Administering oxygen is the first priority. Notifying the physician and preparing

for chest-tube insertion are appropriate after oxygen is administered. The nurse cannot order a chest x-ray; the physician must do this.

TEST-TAKING STRATEGY: Remember your ABCs, and care for the client's airway first.

615. A client complains of pain at the insertion site of an implanted venous port device during infusion of a medication. Which is the most likely explanation for this problem?

A. Extravasation.

B. Malpositioned catheter.

C. Occlusion.

D. Chylothorax.

Answer: A. Pain or "a funny feeling" at the insertion site during administration of fluids or medications can indicate extravasation. A malpositioned catheter is difficult to irrigate and may cause ear or neck pain. An occlusion is indicated by cessation of the infusion. A chylothorax occurs during insertion and indicates an interruption or transaction of the thoracic duct, which allows chyle (lymph fluid) to enter the thoracic cavity.

TEST-TAKING STRATEGY: Use the process of elimination to rule out incorrect answer selections to help choose the correct answer.

616. A client who takes warfarin sodium (Coumadin) requires blood testing to guide treatment. The client requests the implanted venous access device be utilized. Which test should not be drawn from the device?

A. Complete blood count.

B. Metabolic panel.

C. Lipid profile.

D. Protime.

Answer: D. Because the implanted venous access device requires flushing with heparin, this site should not be used to guide anticoagulant therapy. If the device does have to be used, the first blood drawn should be discarded and the laboratory notified. The complete blood count, metabolic panel, and lipid profile are safe to be drawn from the device.

TEST-TAKING STRATEGY: Use the process of elimination to rule out incorrect answer selections to help choose the correct answer.

617. When drawing blood from a central venous access device, how many milliliters of blood should the nurse discard before drawing the laboratory specimen?

   A. 3 mL.

   B. 10 mL.

   C. 20 mL.

   D. 30 mL.

   Answer: B. The nurse should draw 10 mL of blood and discard it when accessing a central venous access device in an adult.

   TEST-TAKING STRATEGY: If the age of the client does not appear in the question, it is safe to assume the client is an adult.

618. The nurse knows a true statement regarding intra-arterial catheters is:

   A. There is no such thing as an intra-arterial catheter. Central lines are only placed in the venous system.

   B. Intra-arterial lines are used to provide chemotherapeutic agents in high concentrations.

   C. Intra-arterial catheters are always placed in the large femoral artery for any treatment.

   D. An intra-arterial line can cause a tear in the adventitia of the artery.

   Answer: B. Intra-arterial lines are placed for oncology clients so that high concentrations of chemotherapeutic agents can be given in close proximity to the tumor. Also, there is less dilution within the circulatory system. It also decreases the amount of metabolization that occurs. Intra-arterial catheters are placed in several different arteries depending on the location of the tumor. A complication that can occur is a tear in the intima (innermost layer) of the artery.

   TEST-TAKING STRATEGY: Use the process of elimination to rule out incorrect answer selections to help choose the correct answer.

619. An infant is in need of intravenous access. The nurse makes an observation about scalp veins. Which statement indicates that the nurse is knowledgeable about this type of venous access?

   A. "The vein has to be cannulated in a downward fashion toward the neck."

   B. "These veins are good to have, but I can't give anything very fast through them."

   C. "I remember that you are not supposed to use a tourniquet on these veins."

   D. "Once I see a flash of blood, I need to advance the needle and cannula 1/8 inch."

   Answer: B. It is difficult to administer increased amounts of intravenous fluids or medications through a scalp vein. Blood flow in scalp veins goes in either direction. The vein is "milked" to determine which way the flow goes in that particular vein. Once the direction has been determined, the needle is inserted in that direction. A rubber band is used as a tourniquet to distend the vein. The cannula is advanced once a flash of blood is noted.

   TEST-TAKING STRATEGY: Questions that ask for "knowledgeable" information require you to choose the answer that states accurate information.

620. An 8-year-old client needs to have an intravenous line placed peripherally. The parents request "that cream be used to help deaden the area." Which information is correct regarding prilocaine (EMLA) cream?

   A. If rapid access is necessary, prilocaine (EMLA) cream is not used because it must be on the skin for 20 to 60 minutes.

   B. Prilocaine (EMLA) cream is only approved for use in the geriatric population and therefore cannot be used in this situation.

   C. Prilocaine (EMLA) cream causes a stinging type of pain at the site and can cause children to become frightened.

   D. Children can absorb increased amounts of the prilocaine (EMLA) cream through their skin with significant negative outcomes.

Answer: A. EMLA cream must be placed 20 to 60 minutes prior to intravenous access insertion in order for the desired effect to occur. EMLA is approved for use with the pediatric population. It does not cause any discomfort when applied to the skin nor is there any significant absorption of the medication that can cause negative outcomes.

TEST-TAKING STRATEGY: Use the process of elimination to rule out incorrect answer selections to help choose the correct answer.

621. The nurse starts an intravenous line on an 81-year-old client. Which statement is accurate for this client population? Select all that apply.

   A. Not using a tourniquet helps to avoid hematomas associated with a "blown" vein.

   B. Blood draws from an intravenous line are best performed with a syringe and not vacuum bottles.

   C. Veins in older clients are more likely to roll when attempts are made to cannulate the veins.

   D. Lower-extremity veins on older clients should not be accessed due to impaired circulation.

   Answer: A, B, C, & D. Tourniquets are not always needed on the older client and may actually increase chances of "blowing" the vein. Vacuum tubes also contribute to hematomas from blown veins. The older client has decreased subcutaneous fat and collagen, and therefore the veins are more prone to roll. Many older clients have impaired lower-extremity circulation, making the use of these vessels a poor choice.

   TEST-TAKING STRATEGY: When answering "Select all that apply" questions, be sure and treat each answer as a true or false statement. There may be one correct answer or more.

622. A client with an intravenous line complains of pain at the insertion site. The area appears reddened and the vein feels slightly hard to the touch for approximately 2 inches of the length of the vein. Which is an appropriate action for the nurse to take?

   A. Apply ice to the area.

   B. Apply pressure to the vein.

   C. Apply warm moist packs.

   D. Apply antibiotic ointment.

   Answer: C. Manifestations of phlebitis are pain at the insertion site, redness, warmth, and a hard, tortuous vein. Treatment for this involves removal of the catheter, and the application of warm, moist packs. Ice is appropriate for an early infiltration. Pressure is used to decrease hematoma formation. Antibiotic ointment does not help phlebitis.

   TEST-TAKING STRATEGY: Use the process of elimination to rule out incorrect answer selections to help choose the correct answer.

623. Which nursing action helps to prevent the occurrence of phlebitis due to intravenous line insertion?

   A. Change intravenous sites every 48 hours.

   B. Use large veins to infuse irritating medications.

   C. Utilize veins over areas of flexion.

   D. Carefully advance the catheter during insertion.

   Answer: B. Medications or fluids that are irritating to the vein should be infused into the largest vein possible. Recommendations are to change intravenous sites every 72 hours in the adult client. Veins over areas of flexion increase the chances of infiltration and phlebitis. Carefully inserting the catheter during the insertion process is a prevention technique associated with hematoma formation.

   TEST-TAKING STRATEGY: Use the process of elimination to rule out incorrect answer selections to help choose the correct answer.

624. When inserting an intravenous needle peripherally, the nurse should insert the needle at which angle?

   A. 30 degrees.

   B. 45 degrees.

   C. 60 degrees.

   D. 90 degrees.

Answer: A. Insertion of the needle during intravenous access should be at a 10-degree to 30-degree angle.

TEST-TAKING STRATEGY: Visualize the procedure in your mind in order to determine the correct answer.

625. A 6-year-old female client is in need of an intravenous line and fluid infusion. Which over-the-needle intravenous catheter is an appropriate size for this client?

A. 14 gauge.

B. 16 gauge.

C. 18 gauge.

D. 20 gauge.

Answer: D. The larger the number on the over-the-needle intravenous catheters, the smaller the size. A 20-gauge or smaller (e.g., 22-gauge) needle is most appropriate for this age group depending on the size of the vein. An 18-gauge, 16-gauge, or 14-gauge needle is too large for this age group.

TEST-TAKING STRATEGY: Look for similar answer choices and eliminate them.

626. A client diagnosed with a contusion to the brain has an intravenous line. Which solution should be contraindicated for this client?

A. 0.9% normal saline.

B. Lactated Ringer's.

C. 5% dextrose and water.

D. Hartmann's solution.

Answer: C. In clients with head injuries or neurosurgical processes, 5% dextrose and water is contraindicated. Infusion of this fluid can cause cerebral edema. Maintenance solutions should include 0.9% normal saline or lactated Ringer's (also known as Hartmann's solution).

TEST-TAKING STRATEGY: Look for similar answer choices and eliminate them.

627. A client receives a nitroglycerin drip. Which is a true statement regarding the use of this medication in intravenous therapy?

A. Vented tubing is needed to administer this medication.

B. A glass bottle and vented tubing are needed to administer this medication.

C. Admixture must be done under a laminar flow hood with proper handling techniques.

D. This medication cannot be given through small diameter catheters in elderly clients.

Answer: B. Nitroglycerin adheres to the plastic of the IV bag, so the medication must be mixed in a bottle instead. Bottles must have vents in them to make them drip well. It is not necessary to mix this medication under a laminar flow hood. Any sized catheter can be used to administer this medication.

TEST-TAKING STRATEGY: Look for similar answer choices and eliminate them.

628. A client receives an intravenous fluid infusion at a rate of 20 milliliters per hour. The tubing attached to the bag of fluid is microdrip tubing. How many drops per milliliter does this tubing provide?

A. 10.

B. 12.

C. 15.

D. 60.

Answer: D. Microdrip tubing provides 60 drops per milliliter. This number is important when setting drip rates. Macrodrip tubing provides a variety of drops per milliliter depending on the manufacturer. It may deliver 10, 12, or 15 drops per milliliter.

TEST-TAKING STRATEGY: Use the process of elimination to rule out incorrect answer selections to help choose the correct answer.

629. A client is to receive an intravenous line and has requested that lidocaine hydrochloride 1% (lidocaine) be used to locally anesthetize the area. Which is a potential complication that can occur with the use of this technique?

A. Obliteration of the vein.

B. Thrombosis.

C. Phlebitis.

D. Fluid infiltration.

Answer: A. The use of lidocaine hydrochloride 1% (lidocaine) for local anesthetic purposes can cause obliteration of the vein as well as allergic reactions and anaphylaxis. Thrombosis, phlebitis, and fluid infiltration are all complications of intravenous therapy.

TEST-TAKING STRATEGY: Utilize concepts of anatomy and physiology to help select the correct answer.

630. An elderly client who receives intravenous therapy has a history of a fractured femur, acute myocardial infarction, glaucoma, and hypothyroidism. Which of these conditions most likely influences the rate at which fluids should be infused for this client?

A. Fractured femur.

B. Acute myocardial infarction.

C. Glaucoma.

D. Hypothryroidism.

Answer: B. Decreased cardiac function can influence the rate at which fluids are delivered. Faster rates can predispose the client to develop circulatory overload. Decreased renal functioning can do the same. A past history of a fractured femur does not influence present intravenous flow rates. A fresh femur fracture could influence the decision, especially if trauma related. If that were the case, the client would most likely need increased fluids. Glaucoma and hypothyroidism are not indicators that flow rates need to be adjusted.

TEST-TAKING STRATEGY: Terms like *most likely* and *most accurately* mean that the undeniable correct answer is most likely not present. Therefore, you must select the best answer choice.

631. The median vein is often used in the placement of intravenous access. Which is a true statement regarding the use of this vein?

A. There is increased difficulty with maintaining an intact system due to constant flexion of the site.

B. This is a difficult vein to utilize in the older client due to decreased amounts of collagen and fatty tissue.

C. This is a good vein to use because it provides stability and anatomical splinting of the area.

D. This is not recommended in the adult patient due to decreased lower extremity circulation.

Answer: A. The median vein is located in the antecubital space. Constant movement by the client can cause occlusion and the development of phlebitis. Decreased amounts of collagen and fatty tissue are problematic for the metacarpal veins in the dorsum of the hand. The cephalic vein, which runs along the radial aspect of the arm, provides for added support in anatomical splinting. The median vein is not located in the lower extremity.

TEST-TAKING STRATEGY: Utilize your knowledge of anatomy and physiology to help select the correct answer.

632. A client who receives intravenous fluid therapy and an intravenous injection of diphenhydramine (Benadryl) suddenly complains of chest tightness and light-headedness. The nurse notes that the client has a flushed face and an irregular pulse of 120 beats/minute. Which is the most likely cause of this reaction in this client?

A. Circulatory overload.

B. Sepsis.

C. Speed shock.

D. Chylothorax.

Answer: C. Speed shock occurs when medications are given too quickly and toxic levels are reached. The manifestations are chest pain, light-headedness, flushing, dizziness, and irregular pulse. Cardiac arrest can occur. Circulatory overload happens with too rapid infusion of fluids, especially in the older client. Manifestations include dyspnea and other symptoms of pulmonary edema. Sepsis occurs from an infection and includes fever. Chylothorax is a complication of inserting a central venous access catheter when the thoracic duct is injured.

TEST-TAKING STRATEGY: Rule out obvious incorrect answers first.

633. A client who has difficulty taking medications requests that the tablet be crushed and mixed with applesauce. Which medication is appropriate for the nurse to crush?

    A. Enteric-coated aspirin.

    B. Diltiazem hydrochloride (Cardizem SR).

    C. Omeprazole (Prilosec).

    D. Levothyroxine sodium (Levothroid).

    Answer: D. Levothyroxine sodium (Levothroid) can be crushed and mixed with food. Enteric-coated medications (enteric-coated aspirin), those that are sustained release (diltiazem hydrochloride [Cardizem SR]), and capsules (omeprazole [Prilosec]) should not be crushed, split, broken, or chewed. This can cause irritation to the stomach, rapid absorption, or inactivation of the medication.

    TEST-TAKING STRATEGY: Use the process of elimination to rule out incorrect answer selections to help choose the correct answer.

634. Nitroglycerin is ordered for an elderly client who is having an episode of chest pain. Which is a correct statement regarding the use of nitroglycerin spray instead of nitroglycerin tablets in this age group?

    A. There is increased absorption in the older client with the spray.

    B. Older clients attempt to chew the tablet.

    C. Tablets dissolve slower in this population.

    D. The spray lasts longer in the system.

    Answer: A. Due to dry mouth experienced by many older clients, the spray is preferred because it absorbs faster and more completely. Older adults generally are able to understand not to chew the tablet. Tablets do not dissolve slower just because they are taken by older clients. The spray is absorbed faster, but does not have a longer half-life in the body.

    TEST-TAKING STRATEGY: Use the process of elimination to rule out incorrect answer selections to help choose the correct answer.

635. An infant client who takes oral medication can be encouraged to swallow the medication by which method?

    A. Place the liquid in an empty nipple.

    B. Add the liquid to the infant's bottle of formula.

    C. Lay the infant with the head lower than the feet.

    D. Use a syringe and give 1 milliliter with each swallow.

    Answer: A. By placing the needed medication in an empty nipple, the infant will most likely swallow it without difficulty. Adding the medication to a full bottle of formula or other liquid can pose problems when the infant does not take the entire feeding and the complete dose of medication is not taken. Anyone who is taking oral medications should be held in an upright position to prevent the possibility of aspiration. Only small amounts of medication should be given to an infant at each time. Giving 1 milliliter can be too much for an infant to take and may cause choking.

    TEST-TAKING STRATEGY: Consider the cause and effect of actions when selecting the correct answer.

636. A client has several medications administered via nasogastric tube. Which statement made by the nurse indicates proper knowledge about this form of medication administration?

A. "I crushed the medications and gave them together to cut down on the amount of liquid I have to use."

B. "The feeding in the nasogastric tube was running well, so I didn't have to interrupt that to check the tube."

C. "I left the client sitting up in the bed so that aspiration would not be a problem."

D. "I had to push really hard to get those medications to go in, but they finally went in."

Answer: C. Clients should be placed in semi-Fowler's position and left there for at least 30 minutes to prevent aspiration. Each medication should be given separately. If the medications are given together, they cannot be checked and identified appropriately. If spillage occurs, there can be problems determining which medications the patient received. Prior to giving medications via nasogastric tube, the tube should be checked for placement. If medications do not flow easily or with gentle pressure, they should not be forced.

TEST-TAKING STRATEGY: The words "proper knowledge" means you are looking for a true statement.

637. A child client who has vomiting, high fever, and cough is prescribed acetaminophen (Tylenol) 325 mg by suppository. The medication on hand is acetaminophen (Tylenol) 650 mg suppository. Which action should the nurse take to provide the proper dose?

A. Give the child the oral elixir instead.

B. Break the suppository in half and administer.

C. Wait for the pharmacy to send a 325-mg suppository.

D. Contact the physician for a change in dosage order.

Answer: C. The nurse should have the appropriate dose on hand. Suppositories are not supposed to be broken in half. The distribution of the ingredients is not always equal. Giving oral elixir to this client could be contraindicated due to the vomiting. The dose should not be changed to accommodate the medication on hand, especially when children are involved.

TEST-TAKING STRATEGY: Use the process of elimination to rule out incorrect answer selections to help choose the correct answer.

638. An infant client weighs 18.5 pounds. The physician orders ibuprofen (Motrin) 10 mg/kg. The medication on hand is 100 mg/5 mL. Which is the proper dose of medication for this client?

A. 37 mg.

B. 84 mg.

C. 185 mg.

D. 407 mg.

Answer: B. A child weighing 18.5 pounds requires 84 milligrams of ibuprofen (Motrin). Dividing 18.5 pounds by 2.2 pounds equals 8.4 kilograms. Multiplying 8.4 kilograms by the recommended dose of 10 milligrams per kilogram equals 84 milligrams. The amount of 37 milligrams is not correct, because this is simply doubling the child's weight. The 185 milligrams would be correct if the pounds were not changed into kilograms. The 407 milligrams would be correct if the 18.5 pounds is multiplied (instead of divided) by 2.2. All children should be weighed and their weight recorded in kilograms to avoid problems with medication administration.

TEST-TAKING STRATEGY: When asked to figure mathematical equations regarding medication administration, be sure that weights are transferred to kilograms.

639. A client has eye ointment instilled in both eyes. Which action should the nurse take immediately after medication administration?

A. Have the client squeeze the eyes shut tightly.

B. Apply some of the ointment to the eyelid.

C. Apply gentle pressure to the nasolacrimal duct.

D. Have the client lie flat for 10 minutes.

Answer: C. Applying gentle pressure to the nasolacrimal duct keeps the medication from being absorbed systemically and can prevent the client from tasting the medication. Shutting the eyes tightly is contraindicated because it can cause the medication to extrude out of the eye. Applying ointment to the outside of the eyelid is not useful. Lying flat is not necessary.

TEST-TAKING STRATEGY: Use the process of elimination to rule out incorrect answer selections to help choose the correct answer.

640. A 2-year-old client has an order for instillation of antipyrine and benzocaine otic (Auralgan) into the external ear canal. Which action by the nurse is correct?

A. Pull the ear backward and down.

B. Pull the ear upward and in.

C. Pull the ear backward and up.

D. Pull the ear upward and lateral.

Answer: A. The ear of a child or infant should be pulled downward and back to open the canal. Pulling upward and lateral will open the adult canal. Pulling either upward and in or backward and up will not open the canal of either the adult or the pediatric client.

TEST-TAKING STRATEGY: Go through each option carefully when they contain two pieces of information.

641. Which statement by the client indicates that further education is necessary regarding the administration of ear drops? Select all that apply.

A. "I will push a cotton ball into the canal once I have finished putting in the medication."

B. "I will lie on my side for an hour after putting in the drops."

C. "I will warm up the medicine in my hand before putting the drops in my ear."

D. "I will use a cotton tip applicator to make sure the drops go far enough in."

Answer: A, B, & D. Ear drops must be warmed if they are kept refrigerated. Cold drops placed in the ear can cause nausea and dizziness. A cotton ball can be used but it should be placed gently into the ear canal and not pushed in too far. Lying on the side after instillation is recommended for approximately 5 to 10 minutes. Cotton-tipped applicators should not be used.

TEST-TAKING STRATEGY: The phrase "further teaching is necessary" tells you to select an answer with inaccurate information.

642. Prior to instilling nasal medications, it is important for the client to have clear nasal passages. The client can blow the nose to clear the nasal passages. Which client should not perform this preliminary intervention?

A. 55-year-old client recovering from a closed head injury.

B. 22-year-old client who has a fractured mandible.

C. 44-year-old client status post-myocardial infarction.

D. 82-year-old client with a history of chronic obstructive pulmonary disease (COPD).

Answer: A. Blowing the nose can increase intracranial pressure, which is not recommended for clients who have a closed head injury. A fractured mandible should not interfere with this practice. Myocardial infarction and chronic obstructive pulmonary disease should not cause patients to refrain from blowing their nose.

TEST-TAKING STRATEGY: Think about cause and effect in questions that ask about disease processes.

643. A client has the following medications ordered: Albuterol sulfate (Proventil) inhaler 2 puffs every 4 hours and fluticasone propionate (Flovent) one puff in each nostril twice a day. Which is a true statement regarding the use of these two medications?

A. They should not be used together.

B. The fluticasone propionate (Flovent) should be used first.

C. The albuterol sulfate (Proventil) should be used first.

D. The nurse should ask the pharmacist to combine them into one medication.

Answer: C. Albuterol sulfate (Proventil) should be used first because it is a bronchodilator. This will open the passageways and allow the fluticasone propionate (Flovent), a steroid, to be well absorbed into the lungs. Fluticasone propionate (Flovent) and albuterol sulfate (Proventil) can be used together. The pharmacist cannot combine the two into one medication.

TEST-TAKING STRATEGY: Use the process of elimination to rule out incorrect answer selections to help choose the correct answer.

644. A client uses budesonide (Pulmocort Turbuhaler) twice a day. Why should the nurse give instruction for the client to rinse the mouth out after each use?

A. To aid in the absorption of the medication.

B. To prevent the development of oral fungal infections.

C. To decrease the negative taste of medication.

D. To enhance the effects of the medication.

Answer: B. Steroid medications can decrease defense mechanisms and allow oral fungal infections to occur. Rinsing out the mouth does not help with absorption of the medication, decrease in the taste of the medication, or enhance the effects of the medication.

TEST-TAKING STRATEGY: Consider the action of medications when answering questions about drugs.

645. Alpha-adrenergic blocking agents include medications such as doxazosin (Cardura) and prazosin hydrochloride (Minipress). The mechanism of action for these medications is to:

A. Inhibit the parasympathetic system.

B. Stimulate the sympathetic system.

C. Inhibit the sympathetic system.

D. Stimulate the parasympathetic system.

Answer: C. Alpha-adrenergic blocking agents work by suppressing the action of the sympathetic nervous system. When this system is blocked, vasodilation occurs. Anti-hypertensives

are one type of medication that works via this system. Alpha-adrenergic blocking agents do not work by inhibiting or stimulating the parasympathetic system or by stimulating the sympathetic system.

TEST-TAKING STRATEGY: Look for similar answer choices and eliminate them.

646. A medication is said to have inotropic, chronotropic, or dromotropic effects on cardiac tissue. The nurse knows medications that have a chronotropic effect can cause:

A. A change in heart rate.

B. A change in force of cardiac contraction.

C. A change in conduction of cardiac impulses.

D. A change in valvular strength.

Answer: A. Chronotropic effects cause a change in heart rate. The term *inotropic* has to do with the force of contraction of the heart. Dromotropic effects involve changes in conduction of electrical impulses from the heart. Change in valvular strength does not have a term or medication action.

TEST-TAKING STRATEGY: Use the process of elimination to rule out incorrect answer selections to help choose the correct answer.

647. One of the side effects that can occur in nitrates is a process called reflex tachycardia. What is the mechanism of action that causes this effect?

A. Venoconstriction occurs in the coronary arteries, causing the heart to beat more rapidly in response to the stress it is experiencing.

B. Oxygen demand on the heart increases and causes the heart to respond with an increasing rate and force of contraction.

C. Rapid vasodilation causes an increase of blood volume in the venous system, which makes the heart react to a perceived low blood volume.

D. An increase in venous blood flow to the cardiac tissue causes a parasympathetic response, which increases the heart rate.

Answer: C. When a nitrate works too quickly, there is a shift in the blood flow to the venous system. The heart perceives this as low blood volume. The heart rate then increases due to this false "low blood volume." Nitrates do not cause venoconstriction in the coronary arteries. Nitrates increase the supply of oxygen to the heart, not decrease it. The parasympathetic system does not cause an increase in heart rate, but rather bradycardia.

TEST-TAKING STRATEGY: If you have problems with a question regarding medications, use your knowledge of the basics of that medication to select the correct answer.

648. A client is diagnosed with hypovolemia following surgery evidenced by low blood pressure and tachycardia. The physician orders albumin 5% 500 milliliters intravenously. The nurse knows the administration of this medication causes a change in:

   A. Hydrostatic pressure.

   B. Colloidal osmotic pressure.

   C. Peripheral capillary pressure.

   D. Central venous pressure.

Answer: B. Instilling colloids such as albumin 5% causes a change in the colloidal osmotic pressure. When more colloids are added to the system, it causes hypertonicity in the vascular system, which by the process of osmosis (the movement of water) pulls fluid into the vascular system (from the extravascular space into the intravascular space). Water is pulled from an area of low concentration to an area of high concentration in order to attempt to make it isotonic. Hydrostatic pressure is a pushing pressure in the arterial end of the capillary system. Central venous pressure and hydrostatic pressure elevate when the vascular system fills back up, but this happens because of increased colloidal osmotic pressure. Peripheral capillary pressure is not a measurement in health care.

TEST-TAKING STRATEGY: Use the process of elimination to rule out incorrect answer selections to help choose the correct answer.

649. Propylthiouracil (Proypyl-Thyracil, PTU) is useful in the treatment of hyperthyroidism. Which is the mechanism of action for this medication? Select all that apply.

   A. Propylthiouracil works by inactivating thyroid hormone, which is already present in the body.

   B. Propylthiouracil increases the amount of thyrotropin-releasing hormone in the hypothalamus.

   C. Propylthiouracil inhibits the action of iodine when the iodine combines with tyrosine to create thyroid hormone.

   D. Propylthiouracil stops the conversion of T_4 to T_3 at the cellular level throughout the body.

Answer: C & D. The mechanism of action for propylthiouracil is to stop iodine from combining with tyrosine (an amino acid). This combination is an important step in creating both T_4 and T_3. Propylthiouracil also inhibits the conversion of T_4 to T_3. T_3 is the form in which thyroid hormone is utilized by the cells. Propylthiouracil does not inactivate thyroid hormone, which the body has already created. It also does not increase the amount of thyrotropin-releasing hormone (TRH) in the hypothalamus. If it did increase the amount of TRH, that would increase the amount of circulating thyroid hormone.

TEST-TAKING STRATEGY: When answering "Select all that apply" questions, be sure and treat each answer as a true or false statement. There may be one correct answer or more.

650. A nurse caring for a client with Alzheimer's disease administers tacrine hydrochloride (Cognex) to the client four times a day. The nurse knows this medication works by binding to:

   A. Acetylcholine.

   B. Cholinesterase.

   C. Norepinephrine.

   D. Epinephrine.

Answer: B. Tacrine hydrochloride (Cognex) is a cholinergic medication that works by binding to cholinesterase. Once the cholinesterase is bound, aceylcholine levels increase. Tacrine hydrochloride (Cognex) does not bind with norepinephrine or epinephrine.

TEST-TAKING STRATEGY: Look for similar answer choices and eliminate them.

651. Cholinergic agents are also known as parasympathomimetics. Why is this type of medication useful in the treatment of glaucoma?

A. It causes miosis.

B. It increases anhidrosis.

C. It decreases lacrimation.

D. It causes mydriasis.

Answer: **A.** In the treatment of glaucoma, cholinergic agents cause the pupil to constrict, which helps decrease intraocular pressure. Because cholinergics are parasympathomimetics, they mimic the parasympathetic system. Miosis is a characteristic of this system. Anhidrosis is the inability to sweat. Cholinergics increase this activity. Increased lacrimation is a manifestation of parasysmpathetic stimulation. Mydriasis, which is an enlarged or dilated pupil, is a manifestation of the sympathetic nervous system.

TEST-TAKING STRATEGY: Review basic terminology and physiology, if you had difficulty answering this question.

652. Clients diagnosed with Alzheimer's disease respond to cholinergic medications. Why do these medications help these clients?

A. Cholinergics increase acetylcholine in the brain.

B. Parasympathetic stimulation helps the Alzheimer's client to function at a higher level.

C. Sympathetic stimulation is inhibited when cholinergic medications are used.

D. The vasodilation caused by the cholinergics increases the amount of oxygen available.

Answer: **A.** In Alzheimer's disease, levels of acetylcholine (ACH) are decreased. When the medication binds with the cholinesterase enzyme, acetylcholine increases. Parasympathetic stimulation does not help the Alzheimer's client. Sympathetic stimulation does not occur with these medications. Vasodilation occurs but does not impact the Alzheimer's client.

TEST-TAKING STRATEGY: Use the process of elimination to rule out incorrect answer selections to help choose the correct answer.

653. Bronchodilators are classified as adrenergic drugs. In addition to this classification, bronchodilators work by stimulating which receptor?

A. $Alpha_1$-adrenergic receptor sites.

B. $Alpha_2$-adrenergic receptor sites.

C. $Beta_1$-adrenergic receptor sites.

D. $Beta_2$-adrenergic receptor sites.

Answer: **D.** $Beta_2$-adrenergic receptor sites are found in the pulmonary system. Stimulation of these receptor sites causes bronchodilation. $Alpha_1$-adrenergic receptor sites are located throughout the body, and cause vasoconstriction. $Alpha_2$-adrenergic receptor site stimulation causes an inhibition of sympathetic activity. $Beta_1$-adrenergic receptor sites are located in the heart.

TEST-TAKING STRATEGY: Utilize your knowledge of anatomy and physiology to answer medication questions.

654. A client diagnosed with hypertensive crisis develops the following symptoms: headache, muscle twitching, chest pain, nausea, vomiting, and confusion. Which medication should the nurse administer?

A. Dobutamine hydrochloride (Dobutrex).

B. Sodium nitrite.

C. Pralodoxime chloride (2-PAM).

D. Edetate calcium disodium (calcium EDTA).

Answer: **B.** Clients treated for hypertensive crisis can develop cyanide toxicity from the infusion of nitroprusside (Nipride). Sodium nitrite (and amyl nitrite) is the first drug of choice to correct cyanide toxicity. Sodium thiosulfate is used after sodium nitrite as part of the cyanide toxicity kit. Dobutamine hydrochloride (Dobutrex) is not indicated in the treatment of cyanide poisoning. Pralodoxime chloride (2-PAM) is used to treat organophosphate poisoning. Edetate calcium disodium (calcium EDTA) is used in the treatment of lead poisoning.

TEST-TAKING STRATEGY: Use the process of elimination to rule out incorrect answer selections to help choose the correct answer.

655. Warfarin (Coumadin) works by obstructing certain clotting factors in the clotting cascade. Which information is correct regarding this mechanism of action?

A. Interference with calcium occurs within the clotting cascade.

B. Increased solubility of vitamin D occurs in the mucosal lining of the stomach.

C. Decreased functioning of vitamin K occurs within the production sites.

D. Binding with magnesium occurs in the hepatic cells.

Answer: C. Fat-soluble vitamin K works with certain clotting factors within the clotting cascade. When its functionality is interfered with, the clotting factors cannot produce the effect required for blood clotting. Warfarin (Coumadin) does not work through interference of calcium, solubility of vitamin D, or binding with magnesium.

TEST-TAKING STRATEGY: Have in mind the correct answer before looking at the answer selection.

656. Which medication provides artificially acquired passive immunity?

A. Diptheria and tetanus toxoid.

B. Snakebite antivenin.

C. *Haemophilus influenzae* type B conjugate vaccine.

D. Influenza virus vaccine.

Answer: B. Snakebite antivenin is a type of artificially acquired passive immunity. Diptheria and tetanus toxoid, *haemophilus influenzae* virus type B conjugate vaccine, and the influenza virus vaccine are examples of active immunity.

TEST-TAKING STRATEGY: Look for the one answer that is different from the other options to help you select the correct answer.

657. A client receives rabies immunization after being bitten by a bat. Which statement is correct?

A. Active immunity occurs when the rabies immune globulin helps the body build up antibodies.

B. Passive immunity from the rabies vaccine provides antibodies to inactivate the virus.

C. Active immunity takes time to increase and is measured by the antibody titer.

D. Passive immunity requires the client to promote an immune response within the humoral immune system.

Answer: C. Active immunity works with the humoral immune system to help the client develop antibodies through the activation of immunoglobulins. Antibody titers are used to measure the active immunity response. Rabies immune globulin is a form of passive immunity, which provides the antibodies necessary to inactivate the virus. Active immunity works with the humoral immune system, not passive immunity.

TEST-TAKING STRATEGY: Read the options in their entirety. They may have one piece of information that is correct and one that is incorrect.

658. Pain control is an important aspect of client care. Which theory most accurately addresses a client's pain?

A. Endorphin-releasing theory.

B. Nociceptor-reversal theory.

C. Gate-control theory.

D. Open-door theory.

Answer: C. The most popular theory that is discussed in pain control is the gate-control theory. The endorphin-releasing theory, nociceptor-reversal theory, and open-door theory do not exist.

TEST-TAKING STRATEGY: If you encounter an answer selection that contains information you've never heard before, the information is most likely incorrect.

659. Within the understanding of pain control, nociceptors play an important role. What is this role?

A. Nociceptors are nerve endings, which have receptors that respond to painful stimuli.

B. Nociceptors are blocking agents that decrease the amount of pain a client experiences.

C. Nociceptors are neurotransmitters that increase nerve-cell membrane activity.

D. Nociceptors allow the client experiencing pain to relax.

Answer: A. Nociceptors are free nerve endings that perceive and respond to painful stimuli. Nociceptors are not blocking agents that decrease pain. Neurotransmitters on the nerve-cell membranes are acetylcholine, norepinephrine, epinephrine, and dopamine. Nociceptors do not work to dissipate pain because they are responsible for feeling pain.

TEST-TAKING STRATEGY: Use the process of elimination to rule out incorrect answer selections to help choose the correct answer.

660. A Native-American client experiences chronic pain associated with rheumatoid arthritis. The nurse is aware that culture is an important factor in the perception and treatment of pain. Without stereotyping, the nurse knows many Native-Americans employ which practice to combat pain?

A. Moxibustion.

B. Sweat baths.

C. Yin and yang.

D. Acupuncture.

Answer: B. Many Native Americans practice the use of sweat baths, massage, heat, and herbal teas and potions. Moxibustion, yin and yang, and acupuncture are often used by individuals of Chinese descent.

TEST-TAKING STRATEGY: Group options together if they seem to belong together. This will help with the process of elimination when there is only one correct answer.

661. The Wong-Baker FACES scale is useful in determining pain level. In which population is this scale most useful? Select all that apply.

A. Pediatric.

B. Developmentally disabled.

C. Language challenged.

D. Geriatric.

Answer: A, B, C, & D. The Wong-Baker FACES scale is used in clients who are children, developmentally disabled, language challenged, and the elderly.

TEST-TAKING STRATEGY: When answering "Select all that apply" questions, be sure and treat each answer as a true or false statement. There may be one correct answer or more.

662. An 82-year-old female client is prescribed meperidine (Demerol) to be given every 4 hours as needed for pain. Why should the nurse question this order?

A. The older adult cannot rate their pain well, and therefore may overdose on the medication.

B. The older adult may not excrete metabolites of this medication easily due to the normal aging process.

C. The older adult always has a decrease in liver function and will not metabolize the medication readily.

D. The older adult has sensory deprivations and may not tolerate normal side effects of this medication.

Answer: B. The normal aging process may cause decreased excretion of many medications including the metabolites of meperidine (Demerol). Any patient with decreased renal function has the same risk. Older adults may be very capable of rating pain. Decreased liver functioning does not always occur in every older adult. Sensory deprivations do not occur with every older adult.

TEST-TAKING STRATEGY: Be cautious of options that use definitive terms like "always" or "never."

663. When meperidine (Demerol) is used too often for chronic pain, a metabolite known as normeperidine can build up in the body. The nurse knows that one of the effects of this metabolite is:

A. Hypertension.

B. Hyperthermia.

C. Diplopia.

D. Seizures.

Answer: D. Seizures can occur with a buildup of the metabolite normeperidine. Other effects include psychiatric disturbances such as hallucinations, paranoia, and depression. Memory loss can also occur. Hypertension, hyperthermia, and diplopia are not effects associated with normeperidine.

TEST-TAKING STRATEGY: Use the process of elimination to rule out incorrect answer selections to help choose the correct answer.

664. Which statement made by the nurse to the client who is given hydrocodone bitartrate (Vicodin) for pain control indicates knowledge of possible side effects of this medication?

A. "It is important that you avoid bananas and green, leafy vegetables while on this medication."

B. "You will need to stay close to a bathroom while taking this medication because it can cause urinary incontinence."

C. "Drink plenty of liquids and increase your intake of high-fiber foods while on this medication."

D. "Report any muscle twitching, muscle cramping, or numbness and tingling that may occur."

Answer: C. Constipation is a common side effect of hydrocodone bitartrate (Vicodin). Increasing fluids and fiber in the diet can alleviate constipation. Bananas and green, leafy vegetables do not interact with Vicodin. Vicodin can cause urinary retention but not incontinence. Muscle twitching and cramping could indicate hypocalcemia, and numbness or tingling could indicate potassium imbalances, neither of which are side effects of Vicodin.

TEST-TAKING STRATEGY: Rely on your knowledge of pharmacology to determine the correct answer.

665. The nurse is concerned that an elderly home care client may overdose on prescribed opiod analgesics. Which set of symptoms indicate the classic triad of opiate overdose?

A. Miosis, decreased respiratory rate, coma.

B. Diplopia, decreased respiratory rate, hyperactivity.

C. Hallucinations, hypertension, Kussmaul respirations.

D. Seizures, decreased respiratory rate, dilated pupils.

Answer: A. Miosis (pinpoint pupils), decreased respiratory rate, and coma represent the classic triad of symptoms associated with opioid overdose. Diplopia, hyperactivity, hallucinations, hypertension, dilated pupils, and Kussmaul respirations (deep, increased respiratory rate and effort) do not occur as classic symptoms of opioid overdose. Seizures could occur, but not as a classic symptom.

TEST-TAKING STRATEGY: When given a list in the answer choice, every word in the list must be correct in order for that answer to be correct.

666. A client experiences an opioid overdose. Which medication antagonizes the effects of opioids?

A. Flumazenil (Romazicon) 0.2 mg IV up to total of 1 mg.

B. Naloxone (Narcan) 0.4 mg IV up to a total of 10 mg.

C. Dimercaprol (BAL in oil) 4 mg/kg IM.

D. Atropine sulfate (Atropine) 1 to 2 mg IV.

Answer: B. Naloxone (Narcan) is the drug of choice for opioid overdose. Flumazenil (Romazicon) is used for benzodiazepine overdoses. Dimercaprol (BAL in oil) is used to treat heavy metal poisonings. Activated charcoal should not be used in the treatment of opioid overdose due to the depressant effects on the central nervous system. Atropine is used to treat anticholinergic poisonings, such as insecticide spray.

TEST-TAKING STRATEGY: Make sure that the doses of medication are accurate when selecting the correct answer.

667. The nurse notes that a client has a blood pressure of 102/56 mm Hg, pulse of 94 beats/minute, and respiratory rate of 6 breaths/minute. The client is pale with cyanotic lips and nail beds. The nurse suspects a reaction to medication. Which medication is most likely the cause of these symptoms?

A. Morphine sulfate (morphine).

B. Nalmefene (Revex).

C. Acetylsalicylic acid (aspirin).

D. Methylphenidate hydrochloride(Ritalin).

Answer: A. Morphine and other opioids can cause respiratory depression, pallor, and cyanosis. Nalemefene (Revex) is a narcotic antagonist with a long duration of action. Acetylsalicylic acid (aspirin) causes increased respiratory rate. Methylphenidate hydrochloride (Ritalin) does not cause a depressed respiratory rate.

TEST-TAKING STRATEGY: Use the process of elimination to rule out incorrect answer selections to help choose the correct answer.

668. A client with a closed head injury requests pain medication for headache. Which medication is most likely contraindicated in this client?

A. Acetaminophen with codeine (Tylenol with codeine #3).

B. Acetaminophen (Tylenol).

C. Hydrocodone bitartrate (Vicodin).

D. Ibuprofen (Motrin).

Answer: C. Hydrocodone bitartrate (Vicodin) binds with opiate receptors located in the central nervous system. This medication can mask manifestations of increased intracranial pressure and should not be used in clients with head injuries. Acetaminophen with codeine (Tylenol with codeine #3), acetaminophen (Tylenol), and ibuprofen (Motrin) can be used for headache associated with minor head injuries.

TEST-TAKING STRATEGY: Home in on key words in the stem such as *contraindicated*. Then eliminate the incorrect answers while focusing on the answer that provides information or an action that is the most important.

669. A client who has difficulty rating pain is noted to have the following vital signs. Which of these indicates to the nurse that pain may be present?

A. Blood pressure 124/72 mm Hg.

B. Pulse 120 beats/minute.

C. Respiratory rate 8 breaths/minute.

D. Pulse oximetry 92%.

Answer: B. Tachycardia is often seen in clients who experience pain. Increased pulse due to pain is a sympathetic nervous response. Blood pressure of 124/72 mm Hg is within normal range. A respiratory rate of 8 indicates respiratory depression, not pain. The pulse oximetry reading of 92% is not indicative of pain.

TEST-TAKING STRATEGY: Rely on your knowledge of "normal" vital sign findings to select the correct answer.

670. A client who takes morphine sulfate (morphine) for pain control may have which potential nursing diagnose as part of the care plan?

A. Impaired gas exchange.

B. Disturbed body image.

C. Imbalanced nutrition.

D. Excess fluid volume.

Answer: A. Impaired gas exchange can occur if respiratory depression takes place. Disturbed body image, imbalanced nutrition, and excess fluid volume are not nursing diagnoses associated with the use of morphine sulfate (morphine).

TEST-TAKING STRATEGY: Think of the potential problems that may occur with the medication prior to reading the answer selections.

671. Which nursing diagnosis is the highest priority for the client taking analgesic agents?

A. Risk for infection.

B. Risk for injury.

C. Risk for impaired gas exchange.

D. Risk for constipation.

Answer: C. Risk for impaired gas exchange is the highest priority for the client taking analgesic agents. Risk for infection could occur due to urinary retention, but is not the highest priority. Risk for injury could occur due to possible overdose and decreased sensorium. Risk for constipation can occur due to the decrease in intestinal motility, but again is not the highest priority.

TEST-TAKING STRATEGY: When choosing a nursing diagnosis priority, choose the one that brings the most harm to the client.

672. A variation of total parenteral nutrition (TPN) is partial parenteral nutrition (PPN). Which is a characteristic of PPN? Select all that apply.

A. PPN is used for short-term therapy.

B. Clients must be able to accept large amounts of fluids.

C. Clients are not allowed to eat during this therapy.

D. Calories delivered are greater than 2000 calories per day.

Answer: A & B. PPN (partial parenteral nutrition) is used for clients who need supplementation on a short-term basis. Large amounts of fluids are used in this form. PPN is used as a supplement and oral feeding can still take place. Calories delivered with PPN are less than 2000 calories per day.

TEST-TAKING STRATEGY: When answering "Select all that apply" questions, be sure and treat each answer as a true or false statement. There may be one correct answer or more.

673. A client receives partial parenteral nutrition (PPN). The nurse notes the fluid has a dextrose content of 30%. Which nursing action takes priority?

A. This fluid content is normal, and no action is necessary.

B. Notify the physician and ask for clarification of the order.

C. Slow the drip rate to a keep open rate.

D. Stop the infusion immediately.

Answer: D. An infusion of parenteral nutrition containing 30% dextrose is meant for central line infusion or total parenteral nutrition and is too hypertonic for the peripheral vein. PPN uses an isotonic solution. The physician should be notified after the nurse cares for the client. Slowing the drip rate still infuses the hyperosmolar solution.

TEST-TAKING STRATEGY: Never delay treatment. Choose an answer that addresses the client's problem immediately.

674. A client who receives total parenteral nutrition (TPN) will most likely require which medication on a routine basis?

A. Sodium supplementation.

B. Furosemide (Lasix).

C. Insulin.

D. Ceftriaxone (Rocephin).

Answer: C. Clients who require TPN receive large amounts of dextrose. Blood sugar testing is required, and insulin injections are necessary. Electrolytes are included in the solution, so sodium supplementation is not necessary. Furosemide (Lasix) may be needed if complications occur. Ceftriaxone (Rocephin) is not needed.

TEST-TAKING STRATEGY: Use the process of elimination to rule out incorrect answer selections to help choose the correct answer.

675. A client who receives total parenteral nutrition (TPN) has an increase in urinary output. The client's pulse is 130 beats/minute and blood pressure is 98/50 mm Hg. The client's mucous membranes are dry. Which circumstance is most likely responsible for the client's symptoms?

A. Excess insulin.

B. Increased rate of administration.

C. Hypocalcemia.

D. Hypermagnesemia.

Answer: B. Increased rate of administration provides an excess of dextrose quickly. Osmotic diuresis occurs, which causes dehydration. Not having enough insulin can also lead to an osmotic diuresis because the dextrose load is still present. Hypocalcemia and hypermagnesemia do not contribute to the osmotic diuresis effect.

TEST-TAKING STRATEGY: Look for similar answer choices and eliminate them.

676. A home health client receives total parenteral nutrition (TPN) and complains of weakness, nausea, intermittent vomiting, and malaise. Which laboratory value should the nurse most likely expect to see?

A. Positive glucosuria.

B. Decreased pH.

C. Decreased calcium.

D. Increased ketones.

Answer: A. Clients receiving total parenteral nutrition (TPN) therapy can develope hyperosmolar hyperglycemic nonketotic (HHNK) coma because of the body's inability to metabolize the excess dextrose. Glucose levels will be high in the serum and in the urine. The client is not acidotic, so a decreased pH is unlikely. A decreased calcium level does not lead to weakness, nausea, intermittent vomiting, and malaise. Increased ketones should not be present.

TEST-TAKING STRATEGY: Terms like *most likely* and *most accurately* mean that the undeniably correct answer is probably not present. Therefore you must select the best answer choice from the selections provided.

677. The nurse making rounds prior to shift change realizes the total parenteral nutrition (TPN) on one client is behind by about 200 mL. Which action should the nurse take?

A. Increase the rate so that it will catch up faster.

B. Run in 200 mL of the TPN solution so it will be on time.

C. Leave the solution running as is and notify the physician.

D. Slow the rate in an effort to keep the patient from needing more insulin.

Answer: C. Drip rates for TPN should never be changed. Rates should not be increased, decreased, or "run in" to catch up when fluids fall behind. The reason for the discrepancy should be sought.

TEST-TAKING STRATEGY: Notify the physician when there is nothing more that the nurse can do to fix the problem.

678. Partial parenteral nutrition (PPN) should not be implemented in a client with:

A. Hepatitis C.

B. Emphysema.

C. Mesenteric occlusion.

D. Chronic renal failure.

Answer: D. Clients receiving partial parenteral nutrition (PPN) should be able to handle large volumes of fluid. Renal failure and cardiac failure clients are not able to accommodate large volumes, which results in circulatory overload. Hepatitis C, emphysema, and mesenteric occlusion are not contraindicated.

TEST-TAKING STRATEGY: Be aware of the word *not* in the stem.

679. The purpose of total parenteral nutrition (TPN) is to maintain nutrition. Varied energy sources supply different amounts of calories for the body's use. How many kilocalories does 1 gram of fat yield?

A. 3.4 kcal.

B. 4 kcal.

C. 9 kcal.

D. 15 kcal.

Answer: C. One gram of fat supplies 9 kilocalories of energy. One gram of sugar supplies 3.4 kilocalories. One gram of protein supplies 4 kilocalories. Fifteen kilocalories is not a measurement that is utilized.

TEST-TAKING STRATEGY: Use the process of elimination to rule out incorrect answer selections to help choose the correct answer.

680. Trace elements are found in total parenteral nutrition (TPN). Which is a trace element found in TPN?

   A. Iodine.

   B. Potassium.

   C. Magnesium.

   D. Sodium.

Answer: A. Iodine is a trace element found in TPN and partial parenteral nutrition (PPN). Others include chromium, copper, manganese, selenium, zinc, and molybdenum. Potassium, magnesium, and sodium are electrolytes, not trace elements found in TPN and PPN.

TEST-TAKING STRATEGY: Read the question twice to ensure that you understand what the question is asking, especially if the question is tricky or confusing. Focus on what the question is asking: identify a trace element, not an electrolyte, from the answer selections provided.

681. Lipid emulsions are part of the total parenteral nutrition (TPN) and partial parenteral nutrition (PPN). What do lipid emulsions supply?

   A. Proteins.

   B. Carbohydrates.

   C. Electrolytes.

   D. Fats.

Answer: D. Lipid emulsions supply calories in the form of fatty acids, which are essential to nutrition and energy production. Lipid emulsions do not contribute proteins, carbohydrates, or electrolytes.

TEST-TAKING STRATEGY: Read the stem carefully to locate a key word, such as *lipid,* to help determine the correct answer.

682. Lipid emulsions for total parenteral nutrition (TPN) and partial parenteral nutrition (PPN) originate from different fat products. Which is a true statement regarding lipid emulsions?

   A. Intralipid originates from safflower oil.

   B. Liposyn III is created from safflower oil.

   C. Liposyn II is a combination of safflower and soybean oil.

   D. Interlipid comes from soybean oil.

Answer: C. Liposyn II is a combination of safflower and soybean oil. Intralipid comes from soybean oil, as does Liposyn III. There is no such lipid emulsion as interlipid.

TEST-TAKING STRATEGY: When there are two parts to an answer selection, read each part carefully to help determine the correct answer.

683. Essential and nonessential amino acids are found in total parenteral nutrition (TPN) and partial parenteral nutrition (PPN). Which statement is true regarding these two types of amino acids? Select all that apply.

   A. An essential amino acid is recreated by the body on a daily basis.

   B. A nonessential amino acid is not needed by the body.

   C. An essential amino acid must be taken in through the diet.

   D. A nonessential amino acid is produced in the body.

Answer: C & D. Essential amino acids are not produced by the body and must be taken in through the diet. Essential amino acids are not recreated by the body. Nonessential amino acids are produced in the body and are needed by the body on a daily basis.

TEST-TAKING STRATEGY: When answering "Select all that apply" questions, be sure and treat each answer as a true or false statement. There may be one correct answer or more.

684. A physician writes an order for total parenteral nutrition (TPN) to be discontinued for a client who has been receiving it for 1 month. The nurse knows which statement is true regarding this order?

A. Stopping total parenteral nutrition (TPN) can cause hyperglycemia in the client.

B. Reducing the drip rate gradually is necessary for client safety.

C. Weighing the client before and immediately after the feeding ensures nutrition.

D. Assessing the client for cerebral edema is important after discontinuing the feeding.

Answer: B. Gradually reducing the drip rate when total parenteral nutrition (TPN) is discontinued is imperative. If it is stopped suddenly, hypoglycemia can occur. Clients should always be weighed at the same each day with the same clothing on, but this is unnecessary after TPN is discontinued. Cerebral edema is not a side effect of discontinuing TPN.

TEST-TAKING STRATEGY: Use the process of elimination to rule out incorrect answer selections to help choose the correct answer.

685. A client is diagnosed with malnutrition secondary to cirrhosis. Which laboratory study supports a diagnosis of malnutrition?

A. Decreased serum transferrin level.

B. Increased serum albumin level.

C. Normal cholesterol level.

D. Elevated BUN.

Answer: A. Decreased serum transeferrin level is an indicator of malnutrition. It is more sensitive than albumin level because it has a shorter half-life. Serum albumin levels are decreased in malnutrition. Cholesterol levels are decreased in malnutrition. An elevated BUN is indicative of dehydration, but not necessarily malnutrition.

TEST-TAKING STRATEGY: Read the answer options closely when they use the words decreased, increased, elevated, depressed, or anything similar.

686. A key nursing task is to administer injections to clients. This requires the nurse's knowledge of needle sizes and lengths. Which needle size is the largest?

A. 25 gauge.

B. 22 gauge.

C. 20 gauge.

D. 18 gauge.

Answer: D. The 18-gauge needle is the largest of these listed. The larger the gauge number, the smaller the needle. The 25-gauge, 22-gauge, and 20-gauge needles are smaller than the 18-gauge needle.

TEST-TAKING STRATEGY: Use your knowledge of nursing fundamentals to determine the correct answer.

687. The nurse prepares to administer a subcutaneous injection of 0.3 mL of epinephrine to a client. Which syringe should the nurse use?

A. 3-mL syringe.

B. Tuberculin syringe.

C. Insulin syringe.

D. Carpuject syringe.

Answer: B. To draw up a small amount (0.3 mL) of medication, a 1-mL tuberculin syringe should be used. A 3-mL syringe is too big for smaller amounts—anything less than 1 mL. An insulin syringe does not have the proper markings for medications other than insulin. Carpuject syringes are used with special prefilled medications; epinephrine is not one of these.

TEST-TAKING STRATEGY: Use the process of elimination to rule out incorrect answer selections to help choose the correct answer.

688. An ampule of promethazine hydrochloride (Phenergan) is opened by the nurse. Why should the nurse choose to use a filter needle to draw this medication into the syringe?

A. Light can change this medication chemically and cause precipitates.

B. Rapidly shaking the vial to bring the medication to the bottom can cause physical property changes.

C. Very small particles of the glass vial can be drawn through a regular needle.

D. Particles from the nurse's hands can drop into the vial when it is opened.

Answer: C. A filter needle is used to guard against drawing small particles of glass into the syringe. The filter needle is not used to administer the medication. Many medications are light sensitive, but the chemical changes that occur do not usually cause precipitates. Physical property changes do not occur with the rapid shaking of the vial. Particles from the nurse's hands do not enter the vial.

TEST-TAKING STRATEGY: Use the process of elimination to rule out incorrect answer selections to help choose the correct answer.

689. A client receives an injection of hydroxyzine hydrochloride (Vistaril). Which is a true statement regarding the use of the Z-track method of injection for this medication? Select all that apply.

   A. A ¹/₂-inch skin fold at the injection site should be pinched between the fingers.

   B. The injection site should be massaged for 15 seconds after administration of the medication.

   C. The Z-track method keeps the medication from leaking and absorbing into the subcutaneous tissues.

   D. The Z-track method is used to decrease client discomfort associated with pain and irritation at the injection site.

Answer: C & D. The Z-track method is used for administering irritating medications. When used correctly, this method keeps the medication from leaking into the surrounding subcutaneous tissues and will help to reduce pain and irritation at the injection site. The Z-track method requires the nurse to pull skin at the site tautly in a laterally downward direction, maintaining that position throughout the injection. Once the medication is administered, the needle is left in place for a count of 10 seconds. As soon as the needle is withdrawn, the skin is released.

TEST-TAKING STRATEGY: When answering "Select all that apply" questions, be sure and treat each answer as a true or false statement. There may be one correct answer or more.

690. The nurse uses an intradermal injection to administer a tuberculin test. Which statement indicates that the injection is administered correctly?

   A. An area of redness is present at the injection site.

   B. A small bleb or wheal is seen at the site of injection.

   C. The client states the site itches slightly.

   D. The bevel of the needle points downward as it is withdrawn.

Answer: B. The presence of a bleb or wheal at the injection site indicates that an intradermal injection was properly administered. Redness and itching are not indicators of proper technique. The bevel of the needle must be inserted and withdrawn pointing upward.

TEST-TAKING STRATEGY: Use the process of elimination to rule out incorrect answer selections to help choose the correct answer.

691. The nurse prepares to give an intramuscular injection to a client. Which is considered the safest and preferred site for intramuscular injections?

   A. Vastus lateralis.

   B. Dorsogluteal.

   C. Ventrogluteal.

   D. Deltoid.

Answer: C. The ventrogluteal area is the safest injection site and is preferred for both the adult and pediatric client over the age of 7 months. The vastus lateralis, dorsogluteal, and deltoid are used, but are not the safest due to the proximity of nerves and blood vessels.

TEST-TAKING STRATEGY: If the age of the client does not appear in the question, it is safe to assume the client is an adult.

692. A 2-month-old child receives a dose of ceftriaxone (Rocephin) intramuscularly. Which is the preferred site of injection for this client?

   A. Vastus lateralis.

   B. Dorsogluteal.

C. Ventrogluteal.

D. Deltoid.

Answer: A. The vastus lateralis is the safest injection site in children under the age of 7 months. The dorsogluteal, ventrogluteal, and deltoid are not preferred sites. The ventrogluteal can be used, but it is not preferred.

TEST-TAKING STRATEGY: Use the process of elimination to rule out incorrect answer selections to help choose the correct answer.

693. A client receiving an injection of morphine requests that "my buttocks be used for the injection." The nurse explains that this site is not preferred because it is in close proximity to:

A. The femoral nerve.

B. The peroneal nerve.

C. The phrenic nerve.

D. The sciatic nerve.

Answer: D. The sciatic nerve runs in close proximity to the dorsogluteal site. The femoral nerve runs alongside the femoral artery in the inner groin area. The peroneal nerve runs in the lower leg. The phrenic nerve is situated between the diaphragm and the neck.

TEST-TAKING STRATEGY: Utilize your knowledge of anatomy to help determine the correct answer.

694. A client is to receive an injection of methylprenisolone sodium succinate (Solu-Medrol) 125 mg. The vial on hand has 125 mg per 2 mL. Which is the least likely site to use for this medication?

A. Vastus lateralis.

B. Dorsogluteal.

C. Ventrogluteal.

D. Deltoid.

Answer: D. The deltoid should not be used for medication amounts greater than 1 milliliter or for irritating medications. The vastus lateralis, dorsogluteal, and ventroglueteal sites are preferred.

TEST-TAKING STRATEGY: The phrase "least likely" means you are looking for the answer choice with incorrect information.

695. A nurse gives a subcutaneous injection of heparin sodium (heparin). Which is a true statement regarding this injection?

A. Massage the area after heparin is administered subcutaneously.

B. Aspiration before injection can cause hematoma formation.

C. Give the injection each time in the same general area.

D. Hold the skin taut when giving the injection.

Answer: B. Aspiration before injecting the heparin sodium (heparin) can cause a hematoma to form. Massaging the area is contraindicated. Subcutaneous injection sites should be rotated. The skin should be pinched upward when giving a subcutaneous injection.

TEST-TAKING STRATEGY: Use the process of elimination to rule out incorrect answer selections to help choose the correct answer.

696. A client who is being discharged home will be giving his own enoxaparin sodium (Lovenox) subcutaneously. Which statement by the client indicates the need for further education?

A. "I remember that I need to hold the needle at a 45-degree angle."

B. "I know to pinch the skin up for the injection."

C. "I will not pull back on the plunger before injecting the medicine."

D. "I am going to use the right side of my lower abdomen all the time."

Answer: D. Injection sites should be rotated on the client's body. When giving subcutaneous injections, the needle should be held at a 45-degree angle. Skin should be pinched around the area of the injection. Heparin should not be aspirated.

TEST-TAKING STRATEGY: The phrase *further teaching is necessary* tells you to select an answer with inaccurate information.

697. A client informs the nurse that the abdomen is used for every insulin injection. The nurse informs the client that other body sites may be used for injection. Which area is considered appropriate for subcutaneous injection? Select all that apply.

A. Lower abdomen.

B. Anterior and lateral thighs.

C. Lower back.

D. Scapular region.

Answer: A, B, C, & D. The lower abdomen, anterior and lateral thighs, lower back, and scapular regions as well as the lower upper arms are appropriate areas for subcutaneous injections.

TEST-TAKING STRATEGY: When answering "Select all that apply" questions, be sure and treat each answer as a true or false statement. There may be one correct answer or more.

698. The nurse teaches an elderly client about the use of subcutaneous therapy (hypodermoclysis) for fluid infusion. Which statement by the client indicates an understanding of the therapy?

A. "I understand this therapy can be used for extended periods of time."

B. "I don't have any bleeding problems, so that should make it OK for me to have this therapy."

C. "I will be getting massive amounts of fluids through this injection."

D. "I was told that large-sized needles have to be used for this therapy."

Answer: B. Clients receiving subcutaneous therapy (hypodermoclysis) should not have bleeding or coagulation problems. Subcutaneous therapy is used for short-term fluid infusion and is used when less than 3000 mL of fluid is infused per day. The needles used for the injection of the fluid are smaller, usually around 25 to 27 gauge.

TEST-TAKING STRATEGY: The phrase *understanding of the therapy* tells you to select the answer with accurate information.

699. The medication hyaluronidase is sometimes added to the fluid used for subcutaneous therapy (hypodermoclysis). What is the action of this medication?

A. Hyaluronidase increases absorption of the fluids being given.

B. Hyaluronidase decreases pain at the injection site.

C. Hyaluronidase provides protection against an allergic reaction to the fluid administration.

D. Hyaluronidase prevents infectious processes from developing when the fluids are infused.

Answer: A. Hyaluronidase is added to the subcutaneous fluids being infused, so the absorption is improved. Hyaluronidase does not decrease pain, protect against allergic reactions, or prevent infectious processes.

TEST-TAKING STRATEGY: Use the process of elimination to rule out incorrect answer selections to help choose the correct answer.

700. The nurse prepares to give an injection to an elderly client. When the nurse aspirates prior to injecting, a small amount of blood is noted in the syringe. Which action is most appropriate for the nurse to take?

A. Pull back slightly on the needle and attempt aspiration again.

B. Push the needle into the muscle at least 1 cm and give the injection.

C. Withdraw the needle and restart the process with new medication and equipment.

D. Administer the medication more slowly than normal.

Answer: C. If blood is noted with aspiration after the needle has been inserted, the needle should be withdrawn, and the syringe, needle, and medication should be discarded. The nurse needs to restart the process with new equipment and medication. It is not appropriate to pull the needle back and attempt to aspirate again. It is also incorrect to push the needle into the tissue further or to proceed with giving the medication at a slower rate.

TEST-TAKING STRATEGY: Use the process of elimination to rule out incorrect answer selections to help choose the correct answer.

701. A client presents to the emergency department with complaint of severe indigestion. The physician orders diagnostic tests to confirm cholecystitis. The nurse anticipates the physician will order which test?

    A. Abdominal computed tomography (CT) scan.

    B. Abdominal ultrasound.

    C. Barium swallow.

    D. Colonoscopy.

    Answer: B. An ultrasound can detect an enlarged gallbladder, the presence of gallstones, thickening of the gallbladder wall, and distension of the lumen of the gallbladder. A CT scan can also detect these things but it is more expensive. A barium swallow looks at the stomach and duodenum, and a colonoscopy looks at the lower colon and small intestines.

    TEST-TAKING STRATEGY: Eliminate answers that do not look at the gallbladder (barium swallow and colonoscopy). Then choose the answer that is most convenient for the client, least invasive, and least expensive (abdominal ultrasound).

702. Which test is most commonly used to determine the area of myocardial damage during or after a myocardial infarction (MI)?

    A. Cardiac catheterization.

    B. Cardiac enzymes.

    C. Echocardiogram.

    D. Electrocardiogram.

    Answer: D. An electrocardiogram is the quickest and most accurate way to determine the location of myocardial damage. Cardiac catheterization is an invasive procedure that can determine coronary artery disease and may also locate damage, but this is usually performed after other tests are completed. Cardiac enzymes can diagnose a MI but cannot determine the location of damage. An echocardiogram is used to detect heart wall abnormalities after a MI.

TEST-TAKING STRATEGY: Choose the test that is least invasive, gives the quickest results, and provides the desired information.

703. The nurse collects a urine specimen from a client's indwelling urinary catheter. Which method is the correct procedure for obtaining a urine specimen from an indwelling urinary catheter?

    A. Place a new drainage bag on the catheter and collect the specimen from the bag.

    B. Disconnect the catheter tubing from the drainage bag and drain urine from the tubing into a specimen cup.

    C. Remove the catheter and insert a straight catheter to collect the specimen.

    D. Clean the sampling port on the catheter with an alcohol pad and insert a sterile needle with syringe into the port.

    Answer: D. When obtaining a urine sample from an indwelling urinary catheter, the sampling port must be cleaned with alcohol so that bacteria are not introduced into the catheter. A urine sample must be fresh, and urine in the drainage bag may have been sitting for several hours allowing for bacterial growth. To prevent contamination, the drainage system should never be disconnected.

    TEST-TAKING STRATEGY: Eliminate answer choices that are harmful to the client. From the remaining answers, choose the one that allows the nurse to collect the best specimen.

704. A client undergoes a bone marrow biopsy. The nurse understands the purpose of the biopsy is to determine (select all that apply):

    A. The type of leukemia the client has.

    B. The number of platelets the client has.

    C. The number of red blood cells the client has.

    D. The type of leukemia treatment the client needs.

Answer: A & D. A bone marrow biopsy is performed to determine the type and amount of immature white blood cells in the body. This helps to diagnose the type of leukemia the client has as well as guide treatment for the leukemia. A platelet and red blood cell count is performed through a blood test.

TEST-TAKING STRATEGY: Eliminate similar answers (B and C); these answers refer to components of the blood. Then choose the answer that is related to bone marrow—white blood cells are produced in the marrow. Leukemia is an excess of white blood cells.

705. The nurse cares for a client who is scheduled for an upper GI series. The nurse teaches the client about the test. Which statement by the client indicates an understanding of the nurse's teaching?

A. "I'll have to take a strong laxative the night before the test."

B. "I'll have to drink contrast while x-rays are taken."

C. "I'll have a CT scan after I'm injected with a radiopaque contrast dye."

D. "The doctor will pass an instrument through my mouth to my stomach."

Answer: B. In an upper GI series, the client swallows barium contrast while x-rays are taken. Laxatives are taken the night before a colonoscopy to ensure stool is cleared from the colon. Radiopaque dye injected before a CT (computed tomography) scan is not part of a GI series. In a gastroscopy, a scope is passed through the mouth to the stomach.

TEST-TAKING STRATEGY: Use the process of elimination to determine the correct answer.

706. The nurse prepares a client for a bedside thoracentesis. The nurse helps the client into a sitting position with a pillow placed on top of the over-bed table in front of the client for support. The nurse understands this is the correct client position for a thoracentesis because:

A. It is less painful for the client.

B. It allows for maximal lung expansion.

C. Fluid will accumulate at the base of the pleural cavity.

D. There is a risk of a pneumothorax.

Answer: C. A thoracentesis is performed to aspirate fluid or air from the pleural space. With the client in an upright position, fluid will accumulate at the base of the pleural cavity allowing for maximal fluid removal. This position does not relieve pain. It does allow for maximal lung expansion, but this is not the reason why the client is placed in this position. Regardless of position, a pneumothorax is always a potential risk.

TEST-TAKING STRATEGY: Visualize the position the client is placed in and why this might be beneficial when performing a throacentesis.

707. A client comes to the emergency department with sudden onset of shortness of breath. The client's condition deteriorates quickly. The physician suspects a pulmonary embolism. The nurse can expect the physician to order which test?

A. Chest x-ray.

B. Ultrasound of chest.

C. Pulmonary function tests.

D. Ventilation perfusion (VQ) scan.

Answer: D. A ventilation perfusion scan shows perfusion defects in normally ventilated areas due to pulmonary embolism. Chest x-ray, chest ultrasound, and pulmonary function tests are not beneficial in the diagnosis of pulmonary embolism.

TEST-TAKING STRATEGY: Use the process of elimination to choose the correct answer.

708. The nurse is preparing a client for a lumbar puncture. Which is the appropriate position for the client?

A. Prone with a pillow under the abdomen.

B. Side-lying.

C. Side-lying with chin to chest and knees pulled up to chest.

D. Side-lying in semi-Fowler's position.

Answer: C. A side-lying position with chin to chest and knees pulled up to the chest allows the space between the vertebrae to open for easier needle insertion. The other options do not allow for easier insertion.

TEST-TAKING STRATEGY: Visualize the listed positions and determine which would facilitate needle insertion.

709. The nurse is preparing a client for a colonoscopy the following morning. The nurse should expect to administer which medication to the client?

   A. Vitamin K.

   B. Warfarin (Coumadin).

   C. Polyethylene glycol electrolyte solution (GoLytely).

   D. Calcium carbonate (Tums).

Answer: C. A colonoscopy is performed to visualize the colon. In order to perform the test effectively, the bowel must be clear of stool. Polyethylene glycol electrolyte solution (GoLytely) acts as a potent laxative to clear stool form the colon. Vitamin K and warfarin facilitate and inhibit clotting, respectively. Calcium carbonate is an antacid and is not effective in clearing the bowel.

TEST-TAKING STRATEGY: Focus on answers that are directly related to the gastrointestinal tract. This narrows your choices to two: polyethylene glycol electrolyte solution and calcium carbonate. You would not give calcium carbonate the night before to prepare for a colonoscopy, but you would administer a laxative the night before to allow it time to be effective in clearing the colon of stool.

710. The nurse teaches a client how to collect urine for a 24-hour urine collection for protein and creatinine clearance. The nurse knows the client understands how to collect urine when the client states:

   A. "I will throw out my first void of the morning and then start my collection."

   B. "I will collect all of my urine for 24 hours."

   C. "If I don't collect some of my urine, the test results will still be accurate."

   D. "I must collect urine midstream."

Answer: A. At the start time of the 24-hour urine collection, a client must discard the first void. For results of a 24-hour urine collection to be accurate, all urine must be collected, except for the first void (first void is the start time of the collection). Only urine for a urine culture and sensitivity must be collected midstream.

TEST-TAKING STRATEGY: The phrase *the client understands* signals you to select the answer with the most accurate information.

711. The nurse checks the results of a urinalysis performed on a client with dehydration. Which results should the nurse expect to find?

   A. Increased white blood cells.

   B. Presence of protein.

   C. Presence of ketones.

   D. Increased specific gravity.

Answer: D. Specific gravity is an indicator of hydration status. In a dehydrated client, specific gravity is increased indicating highly concentrated urine. Ketones should not be present and are found in clients with poorly controlled diabetes or hyperglycemia. Protein should also not be found. Presence of protein indicates renal disease. White blood cells should not be found in the urine unless an infection is present.

TEST-TAKING STRATEGY: Eliminate answer choices that do not pertain directly to hydration status.

712. The nurse working in the emergency department is caring for a client with suspected acute myocardial infarction. STAT blood tests are ordered. About which test result should the nurse be most concerned?

   A. CK-MB 3%.

   B. Hematocrit 42%.

   C. Erythrocyte sedimentation rate 10 mm/h.

   D. Glucose 115 mg/dL.

Answer: A. CK-MB, or creatine kinase-MB, is an enzyme that is specific for damage due to myocardial injury. The level rises 3 to 6 hours after a myocardial infarction; otherwise none should be detected. The erythrocyte sedimentation rate is within normal limits, although it is a nonspecific indicator of myocardial infarction. Hematocrit and glucose are within normal limits and are not useful in detecting myocardial infarction.

TEST-TAKING STRATEGY: Eliminate answer choices that are not specific in detecting myocardial infarction.

713. The nurse instructs a client with newly diagnosed diabetes mellitus that hypoglycemia occurs when the blood sugar level is less than:

    A. 100 mg/dL.

    B. 58 mg/dL.

    C. 75 mg/dL.

    D. 140 mg/dL.

    Answer: B. A blood sugar level less than 60 mg/dL is considered hypoglycemia. A normal blood sugar is between 60 and 120 mg/dL. Anything over this is considered hyperglycemia.

    TEST-TAKING STRATEGY: Eliminate similar choices, in this case, 75 and 100 mg/dL: both are within the normal range. Examine the remaining two choices. Anything less than normal is hypo-, and anything above the normal is hyper-. Because the question asks about hypoglycemia, the correct answer is the lower of the two.

714. A nurse cares for a client with hyperthyroidism whose serum calcium level is 11.7 mg/dL. Which medication should the nurse anticipate being ordered for this client?

    A. Vitamin D.

    B. Calcium chloride.

    C. Calcium gluconate.

    D. Calcitonin.

    Answer: D. Normal calcium levels are 9 to 10.5 mg/dL. The client is hypercalcemic, which is a symptom of hyperthyroidism. Both calcium chloride and calcium gluconate increase calcium

levels. Vitamin D is used to facilitate calcium absorption in clients with hypoparathyroidism. The nurse wishes to lower calcium levels by administering calcitonin.

TEST-TAKING STRATEGY: Eliminate similar answer choices. In this case, answers that increase calcium are eliminated, leaving only one answer.

715. The nurse reviews arterial blood gas results for her client with chronic obstructive pulmonary disease (COPD). The pH is 7.3; $PaCO_2$ is 56 mm Hg; and HCO_3 is 24 mEq/L. Which acid–base imbalance is this client experiencing?

    A. Respiratory acidosis.

    B. Metabolic acidosis.

    C. Respiratory alkalosis.

    D. Metabolic alkalosis.

    Answer: A. Normal arterial blood gas values are as follows: pH 7.5 to 7.45; $PaCO_2$ 35 to 45 mm Hg; and HCO_3 22 to 26 mEq/L. The pH alone indicates an acid imbalance. The $PaCO_2$ (represents respiratory influence on acid–base involvement) and HCO_3 (represents metabolic influence on acid–base balance) determine whether the imbalance is respiratory or metabolic. In the question, the $PaCO_2$ is elevated and the HCO_3 is within normal limits. This indicates a respiratory imbalance. In a client with chronic obstructive pulmonary disease (COPD), respiratory acidosis related to ineffective ventilation and air trapping is expected.

    TEST-TAKING STRATEGY: Even if you did not remember your normal blood gas values, you could still correctly answer this question by looking at the client's disease: COPD. You would expect a respiratory imbalance. This narrows down your choices to two. Using your knowledge of pathophysiology, you know that clients with COPD have inadequate ventilation and air trapping leading to an excess of CO_2. High levels of CO_2 indicate a respiratory imbalance.

716. A client's sodium is 122 mEq/L. Which action is a priority nursing intervention?

    A. Obtaining vital signs every 15 minutes.

    B. Increasing fluid intake.

C. Initiating seizure precautions.

D. Implementing cardiac monitoring.

Answer: C. Clients with hyponatremia are at risk for seizures. Vital signs are important, but not as important as the client's safety. The nurse should increase fluid intake in a client who is hypernatremic. Cardiac monitoring is important in clients with hypo- or hyperkalemia.

TEST-TAKING STRATEGY: Eliminate similar answer choices (A and D); both choices deal with client monitoring. Then choose the action the nurse can take immediately to ensure the client's safety.

717. A client's absolute neutrophil count (ANC) is 750/mm³. Which measure should the nurse take to protect the client? Select all that apply.

A. Prohibit the client from shaving.

B. Instruct the client to wear a mask when leaving the hospital room.

C. Remove fresh flowers and plants from the client's room.

D. Ask visitors to perform hand hygiene before entering the client's room.

Answer: B, C, & D. If a client's ANC is less than 1000/mm³, the client is at risk for infection. Instructing the client to wear a mask outside of the hospital room protects the client from infection. The soil in fresh flowers and plants can carry bacteria and fungi, which can cause infection. Performing hand hygiene is the best way to prevent the spread of infection. Not allowing the client to shave would be an appropriate intervention for someone with a low platelet count.

TEST-TAKING STRATEGY: Recognize that neutrophils are part of the immune system and help prevent infection. A low ANC indicates that the client is at risk for infection. Choose answers that will help prevent infection in the client.

718. Which sign or symptom should a nurse most likely assess in a client with a magnesium level of 2.9 mEq/L?

A. Positive Homan's sign.

B. Tetany.

C. Loss of deep tendon reflexes.

D. Twitching.

Answer: C. A normal magnesium level is 1.2 to 2 mEq/L. This client is suffering from hypermagnesemia. Signs and symptoms of hypermagnesemia include decreased neurological functioning, lethargy, drowsiness, decreased respirations, bradycardia, hypotension, and loss of deep tendon reflexes. Tetany and twitching are seen in hypomagnesemia. A positive Homan's sign is found in clients with a deep vein thrombosis.

TEST-TAKING STRATEGY: Recognize that a client with hypermagnesemia exhibits decreased neurological activity. Next eliminate similar answer choices (B and D); these answer choices indicate increased neurological activity.

719. After reviewing morning laboratory data belonging to a trauma client, the nurse notices that the client's potassium is 5.6 mEq/L. The nurse should immediately:

A. Attach the client to a heart monitor and obtain vital signs.

B. Call the physician.

C. Call the emergency response team.

D. Begin chest compressions.

Answer: A. Tissue damage releases potassium from the damaged cells, casing hyperkalemia. A client with hyperkalemia is at risk for ventricular tachycardia (VT), a potentially lethal dysrhythmia. The nurse should attach the client to a cardiac monitor to watch for the dysrhythmia. The nurse may want to call the physician to notify her of the client's hyperkalemia, but not before attaching the client to the cardiac monitor. The emergency response team is not warranted at this time unless the client is in VT. If the client had no pulses, chest compressions would be appropriate.

TEST-TAKING STRATEGY: Eliminate similar answer choices (B and C); both answers deal with calling for help. The question does not actually say the client is in VT, so there would be no reason to call for help. Eliminate answer D, because again, the question does not say that the client does not have any pulses.

720. A client experiences nausea and vomiting for over 24 hours. The nurse notices that the client is becoming confused and lethargic. As the nurse goes to call the physician, the client has a seizure. Which electrolyte abnormality should the nurse expect to see?

A. Hypocalcemia.

B. Hyponatremia.

C. Increased lipase.

D. Hyperkalemia.

Answer: **B.** Signs and symptoms of hyponatremia include headaches, lethargy, confusion, and seizures. Hypocalcemia is usually manifested by increased neurological activity. Hyperkalemia is characterized by dysrhythmias. Lipase is not an electrolyte; it is a test of liver function.

TEST-TAKING STRATEGY: Eliminate obvious incorrect answers like C (increased lipase). To answer this question, you have to know the general signs and symptoms of electrolyte disturbances. If you had trouble with this question, review electrolyte abnormalities.

721. A client's platelet count is 70,000/mm³. The nurse instructs the client to:

A. Avoid crowds.

B. Use an electric razor to shave.

C. Increase calcium intake.

D. Drink plenty of fluids.

Answer: **B.** A normal platelet count is between 150,000 and 400,000/mm³. This client is thrombocytopenic and is at risk for bleeding. For this client, the nurse should recommend actions that decrease the risk of bleeding, like using an electric razor. The client should avoid crowds in the presence of a low absolute neutrophil count. A client should increase calcium intake if the serum calcium is low or if the client is at risk for osteoporosis. A client who is dehydrated should drink fluids.

TEST-TAKING STRATEGY: You must first recognize the function of platelets in the body: clotting. Then determine what to do for a client who is at risk for bleeding.

722. A client starts filgrastim (Neupogen) injections 11 days after completing a course of chemotherapy. Which lab value indicates the neupogen is effective?

A. Absolute neutrophil count 1100/mm³.

B. Absolute neutrophil count 750/mm³.

C. Hemoglobin 10 g/dL.

D. Hemoglobin 6.5 g/dL.

Answer: **A.** A normal neutrophil count is between 2200 and 7000/mm³. Filgrastim is a colony-stimulating factor given after chemotherapy to stimulate white blood cell production. Neutrophils are a type of white blood cell. Indication of a response to filgrastim is an increase of absolute neutrophil count.

TEST-TAKING STRATEGY: The client's recent chemotherapeutic treatment should clue you in to the fact that the client's white blood count is low to nonexistent. Filgrastim increases the client's white blood count, specifically the absolute neutrophil count. Based on this information, you should eliminate answers C and D. You then need to choose a count that is within normal limits.

723. A client's potassium level is 5.38 mEq/L. Which drug should the nurse expect the physician to order?

A. Furosemide (Lasix).

B. Sodium polystyrene sulfonate (Kayexalate).

C. Potassium (K-Dur).

D. Magnesium citrate (Citroma).

Answer: **B.** A normal potassium level is 3.5 to 5 mEq/L. The client in this question is hyperkalemic. Kayexalate is used to bind excess potassium. Lasix is a diuretic, which causes fluid loss as well as potassium. K-Dur is a potassium supplement, which increases potassium levels. Magnesium citrate is used as a laxative.

TEST-TAKING STRATEGY: Use the process of elimination to rule out incorrect answer selections to help choose the correct answer.

724. The nurse reviews a client's arterial blood gas results. The results are as follows: pH is 7.6; PaCO$_2$ is 37 mm Hg; and HCO$_3$ is 32 mEq/L. Which acid–base imbalance is this client experiencing?

A. Metabolic acidosis.

B. Metabolic alkalosis.

C. Respiratory acidosis.

D. Respiratory alkalosis.

Answer: B. Normal arterial blood gas values are as follows: pH 7.5 to 7.45; PaCO$_2$ 35 to 45 mm Hg; and HCO$_3$ 22 to 26 mEq/L. The pH alone indicates a base imbalance. To determine whether or not it is a metabolic or respiratory acidosis, examine the PaCO$_2$ level (represents respiratory influence on acid–base involvement) and HCO$_3$ level (represents metabolic influence on acid–base balance). In the question, the PaCO$_2$ is within normal limits and the HCO$_3$ is above the normal range. This indicates a metabolic imbalance.

TEST-TAKING STRATEGY: First determine if there is an acid or base imbalance, then determine if the imbalance is due to a respiratory or metabolic disturbance.

725. Which is not a component of intravenous conscious sedation? Select all that apply.

A. The client has the ability to independently maintain a patent airway.

B. The client has the ability to respond to verbal commands.

C. The client has the ability to respond to physical stimulation.

D. The client is given oral analgesics and anxiolytics.

Answer: A, B, & C. The client undergoing conscious sedation receives intravenous analgesics and anxiolytics. The definition of conscious sedation states that the client is able to independently maintain a continuous patent airway and is able to respond to verbal commands and physical stimulation.

TEST-TAKING STRATEGY: Note the word "conscious" in the question. This indicates that the client maintains some level of consciousness in order to answer questions/commands and maintain an airway.

726. The nurse is caring for a client who is receiving intravenous conscious sedation. Which is the nurse's priority?

A. Monitoring level of consciousness.

B. Monitoring urine output.

C. Monitoring for lower extremity edema.

D. Monitoring temperature.

Answer: A. The nurse's priority during conscious sedation is to monitor the client's level of consciousness. If the level of consciousness decreases, the client may not be able to maintain a patent airway. Monitoring urine output, temperature, and for the presence of lower extremity edema would not be a priority during this time.

TEST-TAKING STRATEGY: Remember the ABCs. Maintaining a patent airway is crucial in a client receiving conscious sedation. Loss of airway is an emergency. Monitoring the level of consciousness allows the nurse to determine if the client can properly maintain an airway.

727. The nurse is discharging a client who has just been diagnosed with chronic pancreatitis. The nurse's teaching regarding diet should include which information? Select all that apply.

A. Avoidance of foods high in fat.

B. Abstinence from alcohol.

C. Limiting intake of green, leafy vegetables.

D. Limiting intake of carbohydrates.

Answer: A, B, & D. A high-fat diet and alcohol consumption can cause further irritation to the pancreas. Because clients with chronic pancreatitis have difficulty controlling their blood sugar, a low-carbohydrate diet is recommended. Limiting the intake of green, leafy vegetables would be recommended to a client on warfarin to prevent further anticoagulation.

TEST-TAKING STRATEGY: Use the process of elimination to rule out incorrect answer selections to help choose the correct answer.

728. The physician orders a continuous positive airway pressure (CPAP) mask for a client. The nurse explains to the client that CPAP provides:

A. Extra oxygen.

B. A constant flow of oxygen.

C. Pressurized oxygen at the end of expiration to open collapsed alveoli.

D. Pressurized oxygen so the client can breathe more easily.

Answer: D. CPAP provides pressurized oxygen so the client can breathe more easily; the mask can be set to deliver any amount of oxygen. CPAP may provide the client with extra oxygen and a constant flow of oxygen, but these features are not exclusive to CPAP. Positive end-expiratory pressure (PEEP) provides pressurized oxygen at the end of expiration to open collapsed alveoli.

TEST-TAKING STRATEGY: Eliminate answers that are found in other oxygen-delivery devices (A and B); these features can be found with a simple mask or nasal cannula. Next, focus on the word *continuous* in CPAP. You can eliminate answer C, because pressurized oxygen is only delivered at end-expiration, not continuously.

729. The nurse changes a wet-to-dry dressing for a client who has a pressure ulcer with infected, necrotic tissue. The nurse knows the purpose of the wet-to-dry dressing is to:

A. Prevent extensive infection.

B. Reduce pain.

C. Debride the wound.

D. Keep the wound moist.

Answer: C. A wet-to-dry dressing placed over a necrotic area adheres to the necrotic tissue as the dressing dries, debriding the wound as the dressing is removed. Antibiotics prevent and help to control infection. Keeping a wound moist does not allow for debridement, and a dressing does not provide analgesics.

TEST-TAKING STRATEGY: Focus on the words *necrotic tissue* in the question. This tells you that the dressing is used to remove the necrotic tissue (debride) so the wound can continue to heal.

730. A client experiences partial-thickness burns to both lower extremities and portions of the trunk. Which intravenous fluids should the nurse expect to administer to this client?

A. Albumin.

B. Dextrose 5% in water (D5W).

C. Normal saline with potassium.

D. Lactated Ringer's (LR) solution.

Answer: D. LR solution replaces sodium loss and corrects metabolic acidosis common after a burn. Albumin may be used as an adjunctive therapy. D5W within the first 24 hours causes psuedodiabetes. Normal saline with potassium is not necessary since the client is most likely hyperkalemic secondary to massive tissue injury, which releases potassium into the blood.

TEST-TAKING STRATEGY: Determine what type of physiologic alterations you would see in a burn client: fluid and electrolyte imbalances and acid–base imbalances secondary to tissue injury. Use the process of elimination to eliminate incorrect answers to help choose the correct answer.

731. Hyperosmolar hyperglycemic nonketotic syndrome (HHNS) can be differentiated from diabetic ketoacidosis (DK) by which physiologic finding?

A. Increased serum osmolarity.

B. Hypokalemia.

C. Hyperglycemia.

D. Absence of ketosis.

Answer: D. HHNS is hyperglycemia in the absence of ketosis. Enough insulin is released but not enough to prevent hyperglycemia. Just as the name of the syndrome implies, no ketosis is present in HHNS. Clients with HHNS and DK both show increased serum osmolarity, hypokalemia, and hyperglycemia.

TEST-TAKING STRATEGY: Look for similar words in the question and the answer. HHNS actually has the word *nonketotic* in it, while DK actually has the word *ketoacidosis* in it. This should lead you to the conclusion that the difference between HHNS and DK is the absence of ketosis.

732. A nurse is caring for a client with a central line catheter that is attached to a monitor to observe central venous pressure (CVP). The client's wife asks what the CVP measures. The nurse states:

A. "The CVP measures the pressure within the lungs."

B. "The CVP is a measure of blood volume status."

C. "The CVP measures how much blood the heart pumps."

D. "The CVP measures the heart rate."

Answer: B. Normal CVP ranges from 2 to 5 mm Hg. The CVP is a measure of blood volume status in the body. A higher value indicates fluid overload. Pulmonary artery pressure is a measure of pressure within the lungs, and cardiac output is a measure of the amount of blood the heart pumps. Heart rate is measured by palpation, auscultation, or through a machine.

TEST-TAKING STRATEGY: The venous side of the heart deals with preload, or volume. It follows that central venous pressure would measure volume status.

733. The nurse is instructing a client with chronic obstructive pulmonary disease (COPD) how to perform pursed-lip breathing. The nurse determines that the client understands the instructions when the nurse observes the client:

A. Lying flat and inhaling deeply and exhaling slowly.

B. Sitting in an upright position, inhaling deeply and exhaling slowly through slightly closed lips.

C. Sitting with arms draped over the over-bed table and breathing normally.

D. Inhaling, holding the breath, and then exhaling forcefully.

Answer: B. Pursed-lip breathing involves sitting upright, inhaling deeply, and prolonging expiration though pursed, or slightly closed lips to prevent alveolar collapse.

TEST-TAKING STRATEGY: Visualize the client's actions and determine which one prevents alveolar collapse.

734. A client's echocardiogram indicates vegetation on the heart valves. The nurse knows that the vegetation may be caused by which condition?

A. Diabetes mellitus.

B. Myocardial infarction.

C. Bacterial infection.

D. Hypertension.

Answer: C. A bacterial infection can produce vegetative growths on the valve, endocardial lining, and endothelium of blood vessels. The growths can embolize to other parts of the body.

TEST-TAKING STRATEGY: Use the process of elimination to rule out incorrect answer selections to help choose the correct answer.

735. The nurse is helping a client to bed when the client begins having a generalized seizure. Which action should the nurse take first?

A. Place a tongue blade in the client's mouth.

B. Assist the client to the floor into a side-lying position.

C. Restrain the client.

D. Notify the physician.

Answer: B. By assisting the client to the floor, the nurse prevents harm to the client. The side-lying position prevents aspiration should the client vomit. When a client is experiencing a seizure, nothing should be placed in the client's mouth. In addition, the client should not be restrained. However, linens or a pillow should be placed around the client to prevent injury. The physician may be notified after the client is safe.

TEST-TAKING STRATEGY: Determine which action will bring the most harm or help to the client. This helps determine the highest nursing priority.

736. A 24-year-old female client is diagnosed with acute lymphoblastic leukemia and requires an allogeneic bone marrow transplant. The nurse determines the client understands the treatment when the client states:

A. "I'll have to stay in the hospital for at least 2 weeks after the transplant."

B. "I'll finally be able to have children after my disease is cured."

C. "I'll have to have chemotherapy before my transplant."

D. "I usually don't have nausea, so I shouldn't have a problem with it during my treatment."

Answer: C. Prior to a bone marrow transplant, the client undergoes chemotherapy to make space for the new marrow and to ensure that all cancer cells are removed from the body. After transplant, the client may remain hospitalized from 1 to 3 months or longer. After chemotherapy and bone marrow transplant, both male and female clients are sterile; egg and sperm banking are encouraged. Regardless of whether or not a client has nausea before chemotherapy and transplant, the client will likely experience some nausea during treatment.

TEST-TAKING STRATEGY: The phrase *client understands the treatment* tells you to select the answer with accurate information.

737. An elderly client diagnosed with pneumonia most likely exhibits which symptom first?

A. Dyspnea.

B. Productive cough.

C. Altered mental status.

D. Fever.

Answer: C. Elderly clients who develop pneumonia usually show signs of mental status changes before they develop clinical manifestations like dyspnea, cough, and fever. Eliminate similar answer choices (A, B, and D); these answers refer to typical signs of pneumonia. Because the question specifies a certain population—the elderly—the question is asking you to identify an atypical symptom.

738. The nurse cares for a client suspected of having hypothyroidism. Which test can the nurse expect the physician to order?

A. Complete blood count.

B. T4 and thyroid-stimulating hormone.

C. Serum electrolytes.

D. Liver function tests.

Answer: B. T4 and thyroid-stimulating hormone levels are ordered when hypothyroidism is suspected. The nurse should expect normal or low levels of T4 and high levels of thyroid-stimulating hormone in primary hypothyroidism. A complete blood count is ordered for leukemias, anemias, or if hemorrhage is suspected. Electrolytes are ordered for fluid and electrolyte imbalances, and liver function tests are ordered if liver dysfunction is suspected.

TEST-TAKING STRATEGY: Look for similar concepts or words in the question and the answer choices to determine the correct answer.

739. The nurse cares for a client with a pulmonary embolism. The nurse's care should focus on which intervention?

A. Assessing oxygenation status.

B. Ensuring that oxygen-delivery devices are functioning.

C. Monitoring for deep vein thrombosis.

D. Drawing arterial blood gases (ABGs).

Answer: A. Although assessing for deep vein thromboses is important, assessing the client's oxygenation status is top priority for the nurse. If the client's oxygen status deteriorates, the nurse should make sure that the oxygen-delivery devices are working correctly. ABGs are drawn per physician's orders.

TEST-TAKING STRATEGY: Remember the ABCs. Monitoring a client's breathing is top priority.

740. A client has a chest tube placed for treatment of a pneumothorax. Which statement indicates that the chest tube is ready to be removed?

A. Drainage from the tube is serous.

B. The client is not short of breath.

C. When suction is removed, no fluctuation is noted in the water seal chamber.

D. Arterial blood gases are within normal limits.

Answer: **C.** The chest tube should not be removed until the lung has re-expanded. One indication of re-expansion is lack of fluctuation in the water seal chamber. When the lung re-expands, the chest tube may be removed. Type of drainage is not an indicator of whether or not to remove the drain, although the amount of drainage may influence the decision. The client's subjective feeling of shortness of breath, and arterial blood gases within normal limits, are not used to determine removal of the chest tube.

TEST-TAKING STRATEGY: Use the process of elimination to rule out incorrect answer selections to help choose the correct answer.

741. A client presents to the emergency department with a cough. The nurse's assessment reveals that the client is also experiencing chills, fever, night sweats, and hemoptysis. The nurse suspects the client may have which illness?

A. Active tuberculosis (TB).

B. Bronchitis.

C. Upper respiratory infection.

D. Pneumonia.

Answer: **A.** Classic signs and symptoms of active TB infection include fever, chills, night sweats, and hemoptysis. The nurse may see cough, fever, and chills in bronchitis, an upper respiratory infection, and pneumonia, but would not see hemoptysis and drenching night sweats.

TEST-TAKING STRATEGY: Look for similar answer choices and eliminate them.

742. A 33-year-old client complains of fatigue, anorexia, and a low-grade fever. The client also complains of joint pain. Which condition does the nurse suspect?

A. Osteoarthritis (OA).

B. Rheumatoid arthritis (RA).

C. Systemic lupus erythematosus (SLE).

D. Anemia.

Answer: **B.** Fatigue, anorexia, weight loss, and a low-grade fever are common in RA, SLE, and anemia. However, joint pain is exclusive to RA. Clients with osteoarthritis complain of joint pain, but not signs of systemic inflammation.

TEST-TAKING STRATEGY: Use the process of elimination to rule out incorrect answer selections to help choose the correct answer.

743. The nurse cares for a client with a diagnosis of diabetes mellitus type 1 who is admitted to hospital for treatment of ketoacidosis. Which client behavior most likely contributed to the development of ketoacidosis?

A. Taking too much insulin.

B. Failing to take insulin regularly.

C. Not following sick-day instructions.

D. Exercising too vigorously.

Answer: **B.** Ketoacidosis results from insufficient endogenous insulin and hyperglycemia, which occur from not taking insulin. Taking too much insulin, not following sick-day instructions, and exercising too vigorously are likely to result in hypoglycemia.

TEST-TAKING STRATEGY: Even if you were unclear what causes ketoacidosis, you know that it would have to do with blood sugar levels because the question mentions diabetes. Review each answer and determine if is more likely to cause hyper- or hypoglycemia. This would leave you with one answer.

744. A client comes to the clinic for a blood pressure check-up. The client takes anti-hypertensive medications at home. The nurse knows the medication is most likely not effective in controlling the client's blood pressure if the client complains of which common symptom of hypertension?

A. Blurred vision.

B. Decreased urine output.

C. Lower extremity edema.

D. Headache.

Answer: D. Headache is a typical symptom of hypertension due to continued increased pressure in the cerebral vasculature. Blurred vision, decreased urine output, and edema related to fluid and sodium retention are also possible, but are not as common as headache.

TEST-TAKING STRATEGY: Think of which complaint you would most likely associate with hypertension. Clients generally complain of pain (headache) more frequently than other symptoms.

745. A client who is rushed to the emergency department is diagnosed with a ruptured aortic aneurysm. Which intervention should the nurse expect for this client?

A. Administration of beta-blockers.

B. Administration of anti-hypertensives.

C. Areteriogram.

D. Surgical repair.

Answer: D. Surgical repair is the only treatment for a ruptured aneurysm. Administration of drugs could prevent rupture. An arteriogram is used to detect an aneurysm.

TEST-TAKING STRATEGY: Look for similar answer choices and eliminate them.

746. The nurse admits a client to the hospital for a carotid endarterectomy. The nurse should expect to find which condition documented in the client's history?

A. End-stage liver disease.

B. Chronic kidney disease.

C. Cancer.

D. Atherosclerosis.

Answer: D. Arterial occlusive disease, which can narrow the carotid artery, is a complication of atherosclerosis. End-stage liver disease, chronic kidney disease, and cancer are not involved in the narrowing of the carotid artery.

TEST-TAKING STRATEGY: From the word "end-arterectomy" you know that the disease must be related to vasculature. Atherosclerosis is a narrowing of arteries.

747. A client diagnosed with end-stage liver disease notices a decrease in ascites. The nurse should expect which finding to accompany the decrease in ascites?

A. Increased urine output.

B. Increased ankle edema.

C. Shiny abdominal skin.

D. Shallow respirations.

Answer: A. As excess fluid is removed, the nurse expects urine output to increase. Ankle edema decreases or stays the same while abdominal skin becomes less shiny. Respirations deepen, because the diaphragm has more room to expand as excess fluid is removed.

TEST-TAKING STRATEGY: Use the process of elimination to rule out incorrect answer selections to help choose the correct answer.

748. The nurse cares for a client diagnosed with peptic ulcer disease. Which finding most likely explains the client's peptic ulcer disease?

A. Family history of cancer.

B. Ingestion of ibuprofen twice a day for chronic back pain.

C. Computer use for at least 4 hours a day.

D. Avoidance of eating vegetables.

Answer: B. Ibuprofen is a nonsteroidal anti-inflammatory drug that can erode the stomach lining, leading to peptic ulcer disease. Cancer, computer use, and lack of vegetables in the diet do not predispose the client to a peptic ulcer.

TEST-TAKING STRATEGY: Use the process of elimination to rule out incorrect answer selections to help choose the correct answer.

749. A client with left-sided heart failure is to be maintained on bed rest. What is the rationale for maintaining the client on bed rest?

A. To reduce the workload of the heart.

B. To increase blood pressure.

C. To increase oxygenation of tissue.

D. To improve the heart's pumping action.

Answer: A. Bed rest reduces the workload of the heart by decreasing the body's demand for oxygen. Increasing blood pressure increases the heart's workload. Bed rest does not improve oxygenation. Drugs can be used to improve the heart's pumping action.

TEST-TAKING STRATEGY: Use the process of elimination to rule out incorrect answer selections to help choose the correct answer.

750. The nurse cares for a postoperative mastectomy client. A wound drain is attached to a Hemovac drainage system. Which action should the nurse take?

   A. Apply pressure around the drain insertion site to promote drainage.

   B. Clamp the catheter when emptying the Hemovac drain.

   C. Flush the drainage catheter if it becomes obstructed.

   D. Assess the color and amount of drainage in the Hemovac chamber.

Answer: D. The nurse should frequently assess the color and amount of drainage coming from the wound. If the drain output is excessive and the drainage is bloody, this may indicate a hemorrhage. Suction from the Hemovac promotes drainage and is also responsible for keeping the catheter patent. Clamping the catheter to drain the Hemovac is not necessary.

TEST-TAKING STRATEGY: Look for similar answer choices and eliminate them.

751. The nurse performs tracheal suctioning through a client's nose. Which is the correct method for suctioning the client?

   A. Rotate the catheter while inserting it.

   B. Apply suction while inserting the catheter.

   C. Lubricate the catheter before insertion.

   D. Suction for 45 seconds.

Answer: C. Lubricating the catheter prior to insertion eases its passage through the nasal cavity. As the catheter is removed, it is rotated while suction is applied to ensure secretion removal. Suctioning for greater than 10 seconds can lead to hypoxia.

TEST-TAKING STRATEGY: Look for similar answer choices and eliminate them.

752. The nurse cares for a client diagnosed with left-sided heart failure. The nurse knows that one of the symptoms of left-sided heart failure is:

   A. Pulmonary edema.

   B. Hepatomegaly.

   C. Jugular venous distension.

   D. Abdominal pain.

Answer: A. Pulmonary edema, dyspnea, orthopnea, and paroxysmal nocturnal dyspnea are all symptoms of left-sided heart failure. Right-sided heart failure is characterized by dependent edema, hepatomegaly, abdominal pain, bloating, nausea, anorexia, and cool extremities.

TEST-TAKING STRATEGY: Look for similar answer choices and exclude them—hepatomegaly (answer B) causes abdominal pain (answer D).

753. The nurse is discharging a client who is diagnosed with gout. The nurse recognizes further teaching is necessary when the client states:

   A. "I'll have to tell my wife that I can't eat too much beef."

   B. "If I lose weight, I may have fewer gout attacks."

   C. "The doctor gave me medication to keep my uric acid levels down."

   D. "I shouldn't drink too many fluids."

Answer: D. Decreasing the amount of red meat and organ meat, losing weight, and taking anti-gout medication can decrease gout attacks. Increasing fluid intake also decreases the likelihood of an attack by flushing uric acid from the body.

TEST-TAKING STRATEGY: The phrase "further teaching is necessary" tells you to select an answer with inaccurate information.

754. The nurse cares for a client diagnosed with a brainstem injury. Which is the nurse's priority assessment?

A. Intake and output.

B. Heart rate.

C. Blood pressure.

D. Respiratory rate and rhythm.

Answer: D. The brainstem regulates respiratory rate and rhythm. The nurse should also assess and monitor intake and output, heart rate, and blood pressure; but respiratory rate and rhythm are a priority.

TEST-TAKING STRATEGY: Questions that ask you to prioritize your nursing actions use terms like *priority, first, best, initial, most important, immediate,* and *next.*

755. A nurse cares for a client with an intracranial pressure reading of 10 mm Hg. The nurse knows that this reading:

A. Is normal.

B. Is elevated.

C. Requires the nurse to notify the physician.

D. Needs to be treated immediately.

Answer: A. Normal intracranial pressure ranges from 0 to 15 mm Hg.

TEST-TAKING STRATEGY: Eliminate similar answer choices (B, C, and D). If the intracranial pressure was elevated, it requires treatment as well as notification of the physician.

756. The nurse cares for a client with a hip fracture. The nurse understands that it is important for the client to ambulate frequently because:

A. Weight-bearing exercise causes calcium to be absorbed into the bone, facilitating bone growth and repair.

B. Weight-bearing exercise stimulates red blood cell production, preventing anemia.

C. Ambulation prevents skin breakdown.

D. Ambulation stimulates the bone marrow to produce more white blood cells to prevent infection.

Answer: A. Weight-bearing exercise causes calcium to be absorbed into the bone so that the bone can repair itself. Weight-bearing exercise does not increase red or white blood cell production. Although ambulation prevents skin breakdown, this is not the main reason for ambulating a client with a hip fracture.

TEST-TAKING STRATEGY: Look for similar answer choices and eliminate them.

757. The nurse assesses a client who has a vitamin K deficiency. What should the nurse expect to find upon assessment of this client?

A. Eccymosis.

B. Anemia.

C. Hypertension.

D. Mental status changes.

Answer: A. Vitamin K is an important component in coagulation. A deficiency causes bleeding and eccymosis. Anemia occurs due to a red blood cell or red blood cell component deficiency. Hypertension and metal status changes are not symptoms of vitamin K deficiency.

TEST-TAKING STRATEGY: Remembering that vitamin K is the antidote for warfarin (Coumadin) will help you choose the correct answer.

758. The nurse cares for a client with Addison's disease. Which should the nurse expect to observe when assessing the client?

A. Anorexic appearance.

B. Tachycardia.

C. Edema.

D. Dry skin.

Answer: A. Addison's disease is caused by hyposecretion of the adrenal hormones (mineralocorticoids, glucocorticoids, and androgens). Signs and symptoms of Addison's disease include anorexia, loss of appetite, weight loss, abdominal cramps, syncope, dehydration, hypotension from fluid loss, muscle weakness, depression, and irritability. Dry skin and hair is a symptom of hypothyroidism, and tachycardia is a symptom of hyperthyroidism.

TEST-TAKING STRATEGY: To answer this question, you must know the signs and symptoms of Addison's disease, or recognize the signs and symptoms produced by the hyposecretion of adrenal hormones.

759. The nurse cares for a client following a modified left radical mastectomy in the treatment of breast cancer. Which is the proper position for the nurse to place the client's left arm?

A. Elevated above the shoulder.

B. Elevated on a pillow.

C. Dependent to right atrium.

D. Level with the right atrium.

Answer: **B.** Elevating the arm on the pillow allows for optimal drainage from the limb without impairing circulation to the arm. If the arm is dependent or level to the right atrium, this could increase edema.

TEST-TAKING STRATEGY: Visualize the position in each answer to determine which one promotes drainage and circulation.

760. The nurse cares for a client diagnosed with atelectasis. Which intervention should be included in the client's plan of care?

A. Administer oxygen at 2 L/min.

B. Encourage use of incentive spirometry every hour.

C. Cough and deep breathe every 4 hours.

D. Have the client ambulate once a day.

Answer: **B.** The incentive spirometer (IS) is used to prevent and treat atelectasis. Using the IS forces the client to inhale deeply, which helps to open collapsed alveoli. Coughing and deep breathing does not encourage as deep of an inspiratory effort as the IS. Oxygen does not promote deep inspiration. Ambulation helps expand the lungs and stimulate deep breathing, but because it is done less often than IS, it is less effective.

TEST-TAKING STRATEGY: Determine which action will bring the most help to the client. This determines the highest nursing priority.

761. The nurse cares for a client who has a continuous passive motion (CPM) machine in place after a total knee replacement. The physician writes orders for the degree of flexion and hours per day of CPM use. Which intervention should the nurse perform?

A. Turn off the CPM machine when the client is eating.

B. Check the flexion settings every morning.

C. Educate the family on how to change the degree of flexion.

D. Increase the degree of flexion per the client's tolerance.

Answer: **A.** The CPM machine should be turned off while the client is eating to improve the client's comfort. The CPM setting should be checked every shift. The family should not manipulate the CPM machine. Only the physician or physical therapist should make changes to the degree of flexion.

TEST-TAKING STRATEGY: Eliminate incorrect answer choices, and then choose the answer that is least harmful to or provides the most comfort to the client.

762. A client arrives in the emergency department after a motor vehicle accident. The client has sinus tachycardia, is hypotensive, and has muffled heart sounds. There is no apparent sign of hemorrhage. Which condition does the nurse suspect?

A. Cor pulmonale.

B. Pneumothorax.

C. Cardiac tamponade.

D. Pulmonary embolism.

Answer: **C.** Cardiac tamponade produces muffled heart sounds and signs and symptoms of shock (hypotension and tachycardia). Cor pulmonale (right heart failure in the absence of left heart failure) produces liver enlargement, abdominal pain, and jugular venous distension. Pneumothorax causes diminished breath sounds, respiratory distress, and tracheal displacement. In clients with pulmonary embolism, shortness of breath, apprehension, and hemoptysis are present.

TEST-TAKING STRATEGY: Use the process of elimination to rule out incorrect answer selections to help choose the correct answer.

763. The nurse cares for a client with a diagnosis of chronic kidney disease. Which nursing intervention is appropriate for this client?

A. Weigh the client at the same time every day.

B. Serve the client three large meals and a bedtime snack.

C. Offer food high in calcium and phosphorus.

D. Encourage fluid intake.

Answer: A. Fluid retention can be monitored by obtaining daily weights taken at the same time everyday. Small meals and snacks should be offered to improve intake. Calcium intake is encouraged, but clients with chronic kidney disease have difficulty excreting phosphorus. Fluid intake is usually restricted in clients with chronic kidney disease.

TEST-TAKING STRATEGY: Think about the goal of treatment for a client with chronic kidney disease: fluid balance and appropriate nutrition. Then, use the process of elimination to rule out incorrect answer selections to help choose the correct answer.

764. The nurse cares for a client with the syndrome of inappropriate antidiuretic hormone (SIADH). Which should the nurse find consistent with the diagnosis?

A. Urinary output of 2600 mL in 24 hours; sodium 120 mEq/L.

B. Urinary output of 750 mL in 24 hours; sodium 154 mEq/L.

C. Urinary output of 2800 mL in 24 hours; sodium 160 mEq/L.

D. Urinary output of 600 mL in 24 hours; sodium 116 mEq/L.

Answer: D. A client who secretes too much antidiuretic hormone (ADH) will have decreased urine output, because ADH signals the body to hold on to fluid. Because of the increased blood volume, the nurse expects to see dilutional hyponatremia (normal sodium level is 136 to 145 mEq/L).

TEST-TAKING STRATEGY: First examine the sodium level and eliminate levels that are higher than normal or within normal lights. This leaves you with two answer choices (A and D). From these two choices, pick the one with the lowest urine output.

765. A client comes to the clinic complaining of sensitivity to cold, weight gain, and dry skin. The nurse recognizes that the client may be suffering from:

A. Hypothyroidism.

B. Hyperthyroidism.

C. Hyperparathyroidism.

D. Hypoparathyroidism.

Answer: A. Sensitivity to cold, weight gain, dry skin, alopecia, constipation, and decreased ability to perspire are all signs and symptoms of hypothyroidism. Hyperthyroidism signs and symptoms are the exact opposite. Parathyroid disease involves calcium imbalances and signs and symptoms that are caused by hypo- or hypercalcemia.

TEST-TAKING STRATEGY: To eliminate incorrect answers, determine which gland is causing the signs and symptoms. Then determine if underactivity or overactivity is the cause of the signs and symptoms.

766. The nurse admits a client to the hospital who was involved in a motor vehicle accident. The client sustained a skull fracture. The nurse knows this client is at risk for increased intracranial pressure and therefore avoids placing the client in which position?

A. Head turned to the side.

B. Head of bed at 30 to 45 degrees.

C. Head midline.

D. Neck in neutral position.

Answer: A. Keeping the head elevated, midline, and in a neutral position promotes venous return from the head, preventing a rise in intracranial pressure. Turning the head to the side may obstruct venous outflow, causing an increase in pressure.

TEST-TAKING STRATEGY: Visualize each position and identify which would be most likely to inhibit or reduce flow to or from the head.

767. A client presents to the emergency department complaining of large amounts of bright red blood in the stool. The client is currently in no apparent distress. Which intervention should be the nurse's first action?

    A. Perform a thorough health history.

    B. Examine the abdomen.

    C. Assess vital signs.

    D. Insert a nasogastric tube.

    Answer: C. The priority intervention for this client is to assess vital signs. This gives the health care team an estimate of blood loss (based on blood pressure and heart rate) and a baseline. Although a health history and abdominal exam are important, they are not the most important interventions to take. Inserting a nasogastric tube is not indicated in a lower gastrointestinal bleed.

    TEST-TAKING STRATEGY: Remember the ABCs: airway, breathing, and circulation. Interventions involving the assessment or support of the ABCs are always priorities. Assessment of vital signs allows the nurse to assess for adequacy of circulation.

768. Which client is least likely to develop third spacing?

    A. The client with a diagnosis of cirrhosis.

    B. The client with a diagnosis of diabetes mellitus.

    C. The client with a diagnosis of chronic kidney disease.

    D. The client with a diagnosis of end-stage liver disease.

    Answer: B. Third spacing occurs when fluid accumulates in cavities that do not support circulation. This fluid accumulation usually occurs in the abdomen, pleural cavity, peritoneal cavity, or pericardial sac. Liver and kidney disease, trauma, cancer, and sepsis can lead to third spacing. Diabetes mellitus is not a cause of third spacing.

TEST-TAKING STRATEGY: Use the process of elimination to rule out incorrect answer selections to help choose the correct answer.

769. An elderly client complains of difficulty beginning a urine stream and sensing a full bladder even after urination. The physician performs a digital rectal exam and has the nurse draw blood for prostate specific antigen (PSA). The nurse knows the physician ordered a PSA because:

    A. The physician wanted to determine if the client's prostate was enlarged.

    B. Although the client is describing symptoms of benign prostatic hyperplasia (BPH), the physician wants to be sure a prostatic malignancy is not present.

    C. The physician wants to confirm the diagnosis of benign prostatic hyperplasia (BPH).

    D. Based on the client's complaints, the PSA test will indicate if the client has a urinary tract infection.

    Answer: B. To differentiate between BPH and prostate cancer, the physician orders a PSA. An elevated PSA can indicate a malignancy. Only a digital rectal exam determines if the prostate is enlarged. A PSA does not confirm the diagnosis of BPH. A PSA does not determine if a client has a urinary tract infection; a urine culture needs to be obtained to confirm a urinary tract infection.

    TEST-TAKING STRATEGY: Use the process of elimination to rule out incorrect answer selections to help choose the correct answer.

770. The nurse knows that a symptom of right-sided heart failure is:

    A. Pulmonary edema.

    B. Hepatomegaly.

    C. Orthopnea.

    D. Rales.

    Answer: B. Right-sided heart failure is characterized by dependent edema, hepatomegaly, abdominal pain, bloating, nausea, anorexia, and cool extremities. Pulmonary edema, dyspnea, orthopnea, and paroxysmal nocturnal dyspnea are all symptoms of left-sided heart failure.

TEST-TAKING STRATEGY: Look for similar answer choices and eliminate them.

771. A client returns from a bone marrow biopsy. Which post-procedure complications should the nurse assess for? Select all that apply.

A. Bleeding from the puncture site.

B. Pain.

C. Bone fracture.

D. Ecchymosis around the puncture site.

Answer: A, B, & D. During a bone marrow biopsy, a needle is inserted through the skin into the bone. Bleeding from the puncture site could likely occur. Ecchymosis around the puncture site could indicate hemorrhage. Bone marrow biopsies are painful due to the puncture and the actual bone marrow aspiration. A bone marrow biopsy does not cause a bone fracture.

TEST-TAKING STRATEGY: When answering "Select all that apply" questions, be sure and treat each answer as a true or false statement. There may be one correct answer or more.

772. The nurse cares for a client who returns from a cystoscopy. The nurse knows that which assessment finding is within normal limits for this client?

A. Blood-tinged urine.

B. Decreased urine output.

C. Severe abdominal or pelvic pain.

D. Fever.

Answer: A. During a cystoscopy, a cystoscope is used to directly visualize the bladder and urethra. The nurse should expect the appearance of blood-tinged urine after this invasive procedure. The nurse should be concerned if the following abnormal assessment findings appear: decreased urine output (indicates blockage), abdominal or pelvic pain (indicates substantial trauma to urinary structures), or fever (indicates infection secondary to the invasive procedure).

TEST-TAKING STRATEGY: Use the process of elimination to rule out incorrect answer selections to help choose the correct answer.

773. The nurse cares for a client with chronic obstructive pulmonary disease (COPD). The physician orders oxygen via nasal cannula for this client. Which action should the nurse take?

A. Teach the client to adjust the oxygen rate.

B. Change the oxygen tubing each shift.

C. Increase oxygen to 6 L per minute as needed.

D. Maintain oxygen at 3 L per minute or less.

Answer: D. A client with chronic obstructive pulmonary disease should not receive more than 3 L per minute of oxygen. Anything over 3 L per minute may cause the client to lose respiratory drive. The client should not adjust the oxygen. Changing the oxygen tubing every shift is unnecessary.

TEST-TAKING STRATEGY: Use the process of elimination to rule out incorrect answer selections to help choose the correct answer.

774. The nurse cares for a client receiving a blood transfusion. The nurse notes that the client has become hypotensive and febrile since the transfusion began. Which is the most appropriate nursing action?

A. Stop the transfusion.

B. Notify the physician.

C. Decrease the rate of the transfusion.

D. Continue to monitor for signs and symptoms of a transfusion reaction.

Answer: A. The client is experiencing symptoms of a transfusion reaction. In order to stop or limit the reaction, the transfusion must be stopped. Then the physician should be notified to determine the next course of action. Symptoms could become worse if the transfusion is continued whether or not the rate is decreased.

TEST-TAKING STRATEGY: Determine which action will bring the most harm or help to the client. This helps determine the highest nursing priority.

775. The nurse cares for a client with a chest tube. Which symptom would indicate to the nurse the presence of subcutaneous emphysema?

A. Dyspnea.

B. Shortness of breath.

C. Increased heart rate.

D. A crackling sensation upon palpation of the chest tube insertion site.

Answer: D. Subcutaneous emphysema—also called subcutaneous crepitus—is assessed by palpating around the insertion site of the chest tube. Assessment reveals a puffy, crackling sensation around the insertion site. Dyspnea, shortness of breath, and increased heart rate are not signs of subcutaneous emphysema.

TEST-TAKING STRATEGY: Look for similar answer choices and eliminate them.

776. A client is to receive an intravenous injection of radiopaque dye for a diagnostic procedure. The nurse knows which action is most important to take before administering the dye?

A. Obtaining baseline vital signs.

B. Obtaining height and weight.

C. Asking the client about allergies to iodine or shellfish.

D. Reviewing the client's intake and output.

Answer: C. Although obtaining baseline vital signs and height and weight and reviewing intake and output are important, the most important information is determining if the client has an allergy to the dye. Clients who are allergic to iodine or shellfish are also allergic to readiopaque dye.

TEST-TAKING STRATEGY: Determine which action will bring the most harm or help to the client. This helps determine the highest nursing priority.

777. A client expectorates pink-tinged sputum after returning from a bronchoscopy. Which action is most appropriate for the nurse to take?

A. Notify the physician.

B. Obtain the client's vital signs and then call the physician.

C. Auscultate the client's lungs for rhonchi.

D. Continue to monitor the client's condition.

Answer: D. After a bronchoscopy, pink-tinged sputum is normal secondary to the irritation of the bronchial tree by the scope. Because this is a normal finding, the physician does not need to be notified. The nurse should explain to the client that the symptoms are normal while continuing to monitor the client's condition. The signs and symptoms of pulmonary edema include shortness of breath, anxiety, and pink, frothy sputum expectoration.

TEST-TAKING STRATEGY: Recognize what is a normal finding after bronchoscopy, and then eliminate answers that do not support the actions to take for a normal finding.

778. The nurse cares for a client following cardiac catheterization. The nurse assesses the insertion site and notices that the client is bleeding. What is the best action for the nurse to take?

A. Obtain the client's vital signs.

B. Assess pedal pulses of the affected extremity.

C. Don sterile gloves and place pressure on the insertion site with sterile gauze.

D. Notify the physician.

Answer: C. The best action to take is to stop the bleeding. Notifying the physician, obtaining vital signs, and assessing pulses should occur after the client's bleeding is controlled.

TEST-TAKING STRATEGY: Notify the physician when there is nothing more the nurse can do to fix the problem. The nurse should always take action prior to calling the physician.

779. The nurse cares for a client in skin traction. The nurse knows to assess the client frequently for:

A. Signs of infection around the pin sites.

B. Skin breakdown.

C. Bowel incontinence.

D. Bowel sounds.

Answer: B. Ace wraps, boots, and slings that apply a direct force on the client's skin are used to achieve skin traction. Traction is maintained by the use of weights, which may cause skin breakdown. No pins are involved in skin traction. Although constipation can occur because of immobility, bowel sounds do not need to be frequently assessed.

TEST-TAKING STRATEGY: Look for similar answer choices and eliminate them.

780. The nurse checks gastric residual prior to administering an intermittent tube feeding through a nasogastric tube. The nurse understands that this is necessary to:

A. Confirm tube placement.

B. Remove undigested tube feed formula.

C. Assess fluid and electrolyte status.

D. Evaluate absorption of the last feeding.

Answer: D. Before administering a bolus tube feeding, it is important to evaluate gastric residuals to determine if the last tube feeding is absorbed. If too much tube feeding was not absorbed and more formula is administered, this could cause gastric distension and possible aspiration. Placement is confirmed through air auscultation, chest x-ray, or measuring pH of gastric contents. Residual tube feeding formula should not be removed as this can upset the acid–base and electrolyte balance. Fluid and electrolyte balance cannot be assessed by measuring gastric residuals.

TEST-TAKING STRATEGY: Focus in on the words *gastric residual*. This gives you a clue as to what the question is asking: how much of the last tube feeding formula is undigested.

781. While the nurse performs nasopharyngeal suction, the client's oxygen saturation measures 86%. Which action should the nurse take?

A. Stop suctioning until oxygen saturation returns to normal.

B. Stop suctioning, remove the suction catheter, and administer oxygen.

C. Leave the catheter in place and wait several seconds before resuming suction.

D. Continue suctioning until saturation decreases to 80%.

Answer: B. Not only should suctioning be discontinued, the catheter should be removed from the nasal cavity so that the air passages are clear. Oxygen should be administered until the client's saturation returns to baseline. Discontinuing suction temporarily while leaving the catheter in place does not allow for the free passage of air. Allowing oxygen saturation to decrease below 90% can be harmful to the client.

TEST-TAKING STRATEGY: Determine which action will bring the most help to the client. This determines the highest nursing priority.

782. The nurse cares for a client receiving bolus tube feedings through a Dobhoff tube. The bolus has just been completed. Which position is best for the client?

A. Side-lying with the head of bed flat.

B. Right lateral position with head of bed elevated 30 degrees.

C. Semi-Fowler's position with head of bed at negative 30 degrees.

D. Supine position with head of bed elevated 90 degrees.

Answer: B. The head of bed should be elevated between 30 and 45 degrees to prevent aspiration. In addition, placing the client in a right lateral position uses gravity to facilitate gastric retention and prevent aspiration. The head of bed should not be flat or on a decline immediately following a tube feeding.

TEST-TAKING STRATEGY: Visualize the positions presented in the answer choices and determine which facilitates tube absorption and prevents aspiration.

783. The nurse assesses a client who is in an arm cast. The client complains of severe pain, decreased motion and sensation, and swelling in the fingers. Which action should the nurse take first?

A. Notify the physician.

B. Remove the cast.

C. Elevate the arm.

D. Administer analgesics.

Answer: A. In this situation, the nurse should notify the physician first. The client is most likely experiencing compartment syndrome, which is an emergency situation. The physician can assess the client to determine if the cast should be removed. The arm should already be elevated. Although pain management is important, notifying the physician takes precedence, as permanent loss of function and sensation is imminent.

TEST-TAKING STRATEGY: Questions that ask you to prioritize your nursing actions use terms like *priority, first, best, initial, most important, immediate,* and *next.*

784. The nurse assesses a client who is in an arm cast for compartment syndrome. Which is a late symptom of compartment syndrome?

A. Sudden decrease in pain.

B. Swelling of the fingers.

C. Inability to move the fingers.

D. Change in skin color.

Answer: D. Compartment syndrome is a complication of cast placement. In compartment syndrome, the cast places pressure on vessels and nerves, which can cause pain, numbness, and swelling. A late complication is a change in color of the extremity as well as decreased pulses in the affected limb.

TEST-TAKING STRATEGY: Use the process of elimination to rule out incorrect answer selections to help choose the correct answer.

785. A client develops stomatitis status post-chemotherapeutic treatment. Which nursing action is most appropriate to reduce pain and irritation in the mouth?

A. Using a toothbrush to frequently clean the teeth.

B. Avoiding taking oral temperatures.

C. Rinsing the mouth with a water and hydrogen peroxide solution.

D. Encouraging intake of hot liquids.

Answer: B. In a client with stomatitis, oral temperatures should be avoided. Oral care should involve the use of a soft-sponge swab or gauze-wrapped finger. In addition, salt and soda rinses can be used to soothe the mouth—hydrogen peroxide is too harsh and irritating.

TEST-TAKING STRATEGY: Questions that ask you to prioritize your nursing actions use terms like *priority, first, best, initial, most important, immediate,* and *next.*

786. The nurse inserts an indwelling urinary catheter in a client. Which nursing intervention is most likely to prevent a urinary tract infection?

A. Restricting fluid intake.

B. Cleaning the perineal area and urinary meatus twice a day and as needed.

C. Obtaining specimens by disconnecting the tube form the drainage bag.

D. Irrigating the catheter with saline twice a day and as needed.

Answer: B. Ensuring that the perineal area and urinary meatus are clean can prevent urinary tract infections. Restricting fluid intake can increase the risk of infection, as can opening up the drainage system when collecting specimens. Irrigating the catheter prevents obstruction, but requires a physician's order.

TEST-TAKING STRATEGY: Terms like *most likely* mean that the undeniably correct answer is probably not present. Therefore, you must select the best answer choice from the answer selections provided.

787. The nurse cares for a client with cervical cancer when the nurse notices the radium implant has been dislodged. Which action should the nurse take first?

A. Contact the radiology department.

B. Wrap the implant in a blanket and place it behind a lead shield.

C. Pick up the implant with long-handled forceps and place it in a lead container.

D. Contact the physician.

Answer: **C.** Although contacting the radiology department and the physician are important, the safety of the client and the staff needs to be maintained by placing the implant in a lead container. To do this, the nurse should use long-handled forceps. The implant should then be placed in a lead box.

TEST-TAKING STRATEGY: Determine which action brings the most help to the client. This determines the highest nursing priority.

788. The nurse working in an outpatient clinic cares for a client immediately after a sigmoidoscopy. Which sign and symptom should be most concerning to the nurse?

A. Abdominal fullness and pressure.

B. Grogginess and thirst.

C. Mild abdominal pain and cramping.

D. Light-headedness and dizziness.

Answer: **D.** Light-headedness and dizziness could indicate hypovolemic shock secondary to a bowel perforation. The nurse should expect to find abdominal fullness, pressure, and mild pain from this invasive procedure. Grogginess and thirst are also expected as the sedation and analgesia given during the procedure wear off.

TEST-TAKING STRATEGY: Remember the ABCs. Hemorrhage leading to hypovolemic shock would severely impair circulation, making this a medical emergency.

789. Which nursing diagnosis is most important for a client receiving enteral tube feedings?

A. Diarrhea.

B. Risk for fluid volume deficit.

C. Risk for aspiration.

D. Knowledge deficit.

Answer: **C.** When gastrointestinal motility is decreased or esophageal reflux is possible, aspiration is a risk. Although diarrhea may develop and the client may have a knowledge deficit, these are not the most important diagnoses in this client. A fluid volume deficit is unlikely to occur.

TEST-TAKING STRATEGY: Remember the ABCs. In this case, aspiration could inhibit breathing making risk for aspiration the most important diagnosis.

790. The nurse cares for a client who experienced an endoscopic examination. Which is the least important nursing intervention post-endoscopy?

A. Maintain NPO status until the gag reflex returns.

B. Observe for hematemesis.

C. Monitor intake and output.

D. Monitor respirations and oxygen saturation.

Answer: **C.** An endoscopic procedure uses a flexible, fiber-optic tube to visualize the esophagus and/or stomach. The throat is numbed before the procedure to inhibit the gag reflex and to allow the scope to pass freely. Therefore, it is important to maintain NPO status until the gag reflex returns. The nurse should monitor for hematemesis, respirations, and oxygen saturation to ensure that the scope did not damage any structures like the esophagus or lungs. Because the kidneys are not affected during this procedure, monitoring intake and output is the least important intervention.

TEST-TAKING STRATEGY: Home in on the key words in the stem like *least important*. Then eliminate the answers that provide the *most important* interventions while focusing on the answer that provides information or an action that is the least important.

791. A client is sent for a computed tomography (CT) scan with dye injection. The nurse explains to the client:

A. The test will take 3 hours.

B. The client cannot eat 12 hours prior to the procedure.

C. The client will be unconscious during the procedure.

D. The client may feel a warm, flushing sensation when the dye is injected.

Answer: D. A CT scan is usually performed in less than an hour. Clients are not sedated to unconsciousness prior to this procedure. Because the test is noninvasive, there are no eating restrictions before or after the test. However, the dye will cause a warm, flushing feeling when injected.

TEST-TAKING STRATEGY: Use the process of elimination to rule out incorrect answer selections to help choose the correct answer.

792. A client received a radioisotope bone scan yesterday. The client had no adverse reactions to the radioisotope. This morning, the physician orders another bone scan using a radioisotope because the results from yesterday's scan are inconclusive. The nurse calls the physician to question his order because:

A. A second bone scan is too costly.

B. The client refuses another invasive procedure.

C. The client develops an allergy to the radioisotope.

D. The client could develop acute renal failure.

Answer: D. Radioisotopes are difficult for the kidneys to process, which could result in renal failure if administered for 2 consecutive days. The nurse should assess the client's creatinine level from the past few days to determine if there is an increase in creatinine. If creatinine is increased, it could mean the client is not tolerating the radioisotope.

TEST-TAKING STRATEGY: Eliminate answers that do not focus on the client (cost of the bone scan). Next, use the process of elimination to rule out incorrect answer selections to help choose the correct answer.

793. The nurse provides education to a client after the client receives an initial external beam radiation treatment for melanoma. The nurse should instruct the client to:

A. Avoid close contact with others for at least 2 weeks to reduce exposure to radiation.

B. Apply cold to the irradiated area to decrease discomfort.

C. Wash off all body markings applied by the radiologist.

D. Limit the use of creams or lotions to those approved by the oncologist.

Answer: D. Many over-the-counter creams and lotions contain alcohol, drying agents, or perfume, which may cause damage to the irradiated area. Only creams or lotions recommended by the oncologist should be used. Markings should not be removed until therapy is completed. Cold may damage the irradiated area. Because this is an external therapy, not an internal therapy like bracytherapy, radiation precautions are not needed.

TEST-TAKING STRATEGY: Use the process of elimination to rule out incorrect answer selections to help choose the correct answer.

794. The nurse provides discharge instructions to a client going home with furosemide (Lasix) and potassium (K-Dur). The client asks the nurse why potassium is indicated. Which statement by the nurse is most appropriate?

A. "Your potassium level is low."

B. "Because Lasix causes potassium loss, you need a potassium supplement."

C. "Potassium is needed for your heart to work."

D. "Lasix does not work unless you have a high potassium level."

Answer: B. Lasix is a non–potassium-sparing diuretic, so it is important to supplement the client with potassium. The client's potassium level is not mentioned in the question. Potassium is needed to prevent dysrhythmias, but this is not the direct reason for giving the potassium supplement. Lasix is effective regardless of potassium level.

TEST-TAKING STRATEGY: Terms like *most appropriately* and *most accurately* mean that the undeniably correct answer is most likely not present. Therefore, you must select the best answer choice from the selections provided.

795. The nurse cares for a client who has a chest tube that is connected to suction. Which interventions should the nurse perform?

A. Monitor the client for respiratory distress and check the tube connections and drainage system for an air leak.

B. Monitor the client for absence of breath sounds and check the tube connections.

C. Monitor the client's condition and assess the dressing over the chest tube insertion site.

D. Monitor the client for signs and symptoms of respiratory distress.

Answer: A. The nurse should monitor for respiratory distress, check the tube connections, and monitor the drainage system for an air leak. The nurse should also check breath sounds and assess the dressing over the insertion site.

TEST-TAKING STRATEGY: Choose the umbrella answer, or the answer that has the most correct interventions.

796. The nurse cares for a client in Buck's traction. The nurse understands that it is important to ensure that the weights hang free to:

A. Relieve muscle spasms of the legs and back.

B. Prevent skin breakdown.

C. Maintain the client's ability to move freely.

D. Maintain proper bone alignment.

Answer: A. Buck's traction is used to relieve muscle spasms of the legs and back, not to maintain alignment of fractures for healing. Buck's traction inhibits the client's mobility. Skin assessment is important, but freely hanging weights do not prevent skin breakdown.

TEST-TAKING STRATEGY: Use the process of elimination to rule out incorrect answer selections to help choose the correct answer.

797. The nurse provides teaching to a client who is status post-laminectomy with fusion. The nurse understands further teaching is necessary when the client states:

A. "I should keep my back straight when I am walking."

B. "It is OK for me to sleep on my stomach."

C. "I should exercise daily but avoid strenuous activities."

D. "I should avoid sitting or standing for too long."

Answer: B. Sleeping in a prone position causes curvature of the spine. Post-laminectomy, the spine must remain in alignment. Walking with a straight back maintains alignment. In addition, clients who are status post-laminectomy should exercise daily and avoid sitting, standing, driving, or walking for extended periods of time.

TEST-TAKING STRATEGY: The phrase *further teaching is necessary* tells you to select an answer with inaccurate information.

798. Which client is at least risk for acquiring pneumonia during hospitalization?

A. A client diagnosed with human immunodeficiency virus (HIV).

B. A postoperative client who ambulates frequently.

C. A client in Buck's traction.

D. An older client diagnosed with diabetes mellitus.

Answer: B. The postoperative client who ambulates frequently is at lowest risk for acquiring pneumonia during hospitalization. Clients diagnosed with respiratory illnesses, chronic diseases (diabetes), or immunosuppression (HIV) are at highest risk for acquiring pneumonia during hospitalization. Clients who are immobile are also at high risk.

TEST-TAKING STRATEGY: Home in on the key words in the stem like *least risk*. Then eliminate the incorrect answers while focusing on the answer that provides information or an action that is the least risk.

799. A client with pneumonia complains of chest pain. The nurse knows that this pain is pleuritic in nature because it (select all that apply):

A. Decreases when the client leans forward.

B. Resolves with rest.

C. Is not present during vigorous activity.

D. Increases with deep inspiration.

Answer: A & D. Pleuritic chest pain increases with deep inspiration and decreases when the client leans forward. Leaning forward pulls the heart away from the diaphragmatic pleurae of the lungs. Pain associated with stable angina resolves with rest.

TEST-TAKING STRATEGY: Look for similar answer choices and eliminate them.

800. A client with a spinal cord injury complains of severe headache. The nurse finds the client to be diaphoretic, hypertensive, and bradycardiac. The nurse suspects the client is experiencing autonomic dysreflexia. Which is the nurse's first action?

A. Elevate the head of the bed.

B. Check vital signs.

C. Notify the physician.

D. Check the client's bladder for distension.

Answer: A. Autonomic dysreflexia occurs in clients with spinal cord injuries. This disorder is characterized by exaggerated autonomic responses to stimuli that are innocuous in normal individuals. A distended bowel or bladder or stimulation of the skin can trigger a response. When autonomic dysreflexia occurs, the client is immediately placed in a sitting position to lower the blood pressure. The nurse then performs an assessment and removes the stimulus. Vital signs can then be rechecked and the physician notified.

TEST-TAKING STRATEGY: Choose the answer which provides immediate relief of the physiological disturbance. In this case, elevating the head of the bed reduces blood pressure until the stimulus can be detected and removed.

801. The nurse cares for a client who returns from gastric resection surgery. Which nursing intervention is a priority?

A. Assessing for flatus.

B. Monitoring for symptoms of hemorrhage.

C. Monitoring patency of the nasogastric tube.

D. Encouraging ambulation.

Answer: B. In the immediate gastric resection postoperative period, the nurse should monitor for signs and symptoms of hemorrhage: bloody drainage form the nasogastric tube, tachycardia, and hypotension. Although the other interventions are important, the priority is to monitor for hemorrhage, which could be life threatening.

TEST-TAKING STRATEGY: Remember the ABCs. In the immediate postoperative period, monitoring the ABCs is crucial.

802. The nurse plans to turn a client who just returned from surgery where the client's fractured hip was repaired. Which item should the nurse use to help position the client?

A. A drawsheet.

B. A backboard.

C. An overhead trapeze.

D. An abductor splint.

Answer: D. An abductor splint is used to keep the hip in proper alignment with the rest of the body when a client is turned from side to side. A backboard is used to move the client between beds. An overhead trapeze is used so the client can reposition independently. Although a drawsheet is used to turn a client, it does allow for proper alignment of the hips.

TEST-TAKING STRATEGY: Use the process of elimination to rule out incorrect answer selections to help choose the correct answer.

803. The nurse cares for a client after a transphenoidal hypophysectomy. The nurse should monitor for which sign of hemorrhage?

A. Hematuria.

B. Hemoptysis.

C. Frequent swallowing.

D. Ear drainage.

Answer: C. Frequent swallowing after transphenoidal hypophysectomy may indicate fluid or blood is leaking from the sinuses into the oropharynx. Hematuria is a sign of cystitis. Hemoptysis is a sign of pulmonary embolism or tuberculosis. Ear drainage results from a basilar skull fracture.

TEST-TAKING STRATEGY: Look for similar answer choices and eliminate them (hematuria and hemoptysis)—both involve bloody drainage.

804. A client has a nasogastric (NG) tube placed after abdominal surgery. Which finding indicates that the NG tube may be removed?

A. Drainage volume decreases.

B. The client experiences flatus.

C. The client no longer feels nauseous.

D. The client is burping.

Answer: B. NG tubes are placed after abdominal surgery to prevent distension secondary to decreased peristalsis and retention of gas in the bowel. Passing flatus indicates that the bowel has returned to its normal functioning, at which point the NG tube can be removed.

TEST-TAKING STRATEGY: Use the process of elimination to rule out incorrect answer selections to help choose the correct answer.

805. The nurse cares for a client post-thyroidectomy. The nurse notices the client experiences muscle twitches. Upon questioning, the client complains of numbness and tingling of the mouth and fingertips. The nurse suspects which electrolyte disturbance?

A. Hyponatremia.

B. Hyperkalemia.

C. Hypocalcemia.

D. Hypermagnesemia.

Answer: C. Hypocalcemia may occur if the parathyroid glands are accidentally removed with the thyroid. Hyponatremia can result if the surgical client receives too much intravenous fluid. Hyperkalemia and hypermagnesemia are usually associated with reduced renal function.

TEST-TAKING STRATEGY: Read the question twice to ensure that you understand what the question is asking, especially if the question is tricky or confusing. Focus on what the question is asking: the electrolyte disturbance that causes muscle twitching and tingling of the mouth and fingertips.

806. A client returns to the nursing unit after a transurethral prostatic resection. The client has an indwelling urinary catheter with a continuous bladder irrigation system in place. The client complains of bladder spasms. Which priority action should the nurse take?

A. Remove the indwelling catheter per the physician's order.

B. Assess the client's vital signs.

C. Notify the physician per the physician's order.

D. Flush the catheter per the physician's order.

Answer: D. The bladder spasms are caused by bladder distension. The distension is most likely caused by a clot that is obstructing urinary outflow. Removing the catheter is not the priority action. Assessing vital signs does not relieve bladder spasms. The nurse should notify the physician if the flush does not remove the obstruction and/or relieve the client's bladder spasms.

TEST-TAKING STRATEGY: Determine which action will bring the most help to the client. This determines the highest nursing priority.

807. Which chronic complications are associated with diabetes mellitus?

A. Angina and dyspnea on exertion.

B. Leg ulcers and pulmonary infarcts.

C. Retinopathy and neuropathy.

D. Fatigue, nausea, and cardiac dysrhythmias.

Answer: C. Retinopathy, neuropathy, and coronary artery disease are complications of diabetes. Angina and dyspnea on exertion are complications of aortic valve stenosis. Leg ulcers and pulmonary infarcts are complications of sickle-cell anemia. Fatigue, nausea, and cardiac dysrhythmias are complications of hyperparathyroidism.

TEST-TAKING STRATEGY: Choose the answer that lists all of the correct complications.

808. A client is admitted to the hospital with a decubitus ulcer in the sacral area. The client is bedridden and refuses to eat. The nurse realizes that the client is at risk for which complication?

   A. Knowledge deficit related to nutritional status.

   B. Impaired wound healing.

   C. Fluid volume deficit.

   D. Hemorrhage.

   Answer: B. The client is at risk for impaired wound healing due to skin breakdown, immobility, and poor nutrition. The question does not indicate that the client has a knowledge deficit, fluid deficit, or risk for hemorrhage.

   TEST-TAKING STRATEGY: Eliminate answers that do not directly relate to the question (fluid volume deficit and hemorrhage). Although the client does have nutritional issues, the question does not mention that the client has a knowledge deficit related to this.

809. A client returns from surgery after an abdominal perineal resection. The client has a nasogastric (NG) tube in place that is connected to low suction. After several hours, drainage from the NG tube stops. Which action should the nurse take first?

   A. Advance the NG tube into the nasopharynx.

   B. Check the suction tubing for kinks.

   C. Increase the amount of suction.

   D. Irrigate the NG tube.

   Answer: B. The first action the nurse should take is to check if the suction tubing is kinked. Advancing the tube, increasing the amount of suction, and irrigating the tube may occur if no kinks are found. A physician's order is required for these interventions.

TEST-TAKING STRATEGY: Choose the simplest, most noninvasive method of restoring patency to the tube.

810. The nurse instructs the client how to perform foot pumps (extension and flexion of the foot at the ankle). The nurse knows that contracting the leg muscles helps to prevent which postoperative complication?

   A. Pneumonia.

   B. Deep vein thrombosis.

   C. Dehydration.

   D. Muscle atrophy.

   Answer: B. Postoperative clients are often immobile, and encouraging foot pumps can decrease venous stasis and subsequent deep vein thrombosis (DVT). An incentive spirometer or coughing and deep-breathing exercises prevent pneumonia. Foot pumps do not prevent dehydration. More vigorous exercise is required to prevent muscle atrophy.

   TEST-TAKING STRATEGY: Use the process of elimination to rule out incorrect answer selections to help choose the correct answer.

811. A client status post-cholecystectomy has a T-tube placed during the surgery. Which action should the nurse take when caring for the T-tube?

   A. Irrigate the tube as needed.

   B. Aspirate the tube every shift.

   C. Attach the tube to low intermittent suction.

   D. Connect the tube to a drainage bag.

   Answer: D. T-tubes are connected to a simple drainage bag and allowed to drain via gravity. The tube should not be irrigated, aspirated, or attached to suction.

   TEST-TAKING STRATEGY: Use the process of elimination to rule out incorrect answer selections to help choose the correct answer.

812. Heart failure post myocardial infarction is most commonly caused by:

A. Impaired contractile function secondary to the damaged myocardium.

B. Increased workload on the myocardium.

C. Increased oxygen demands of the myocardium.

D. Ventricular hypertrophy.

Answer: A. Myocardial infarction (MI) causes damage to the myocardium secondary to decreased or lack of blood flow and oxygen to the heart. The myocardial cells affected by MI lose the ability to contract or contract in a coordinated manner. After an MI resolves, oxygen and workload demands should decrease. Ventricular hypertrophy is a sign of heart failure.

TEST-TAKING STRATEGY: Use the process of elimination to rule out incorrect answer selections to help choose the correct answer.

813. The nurse instructs a client diagnosed with chronic obstructive disease (COPD) about positions to use during times of dyspnea. The nurse recognizes that further teaching is necessary when the client states:

A. "I will lie flat on my back."

B. "I will sit up and rest my elbows on my knees."

C. "I will lean up against a wall."

D. "I will sit up and lean over a table."

Answer: A. Sitting in the tripod position—sitting up while leaning over a table—allows for maximal chest expansion, which helps the client during periods of dyspnea. Leaning against a wall allows the accessory muscles to work to facilitate breathing, thus relieving episodes of dyspnea. Lying down reduces movement of the client's chest wall.

TEST-TAKING STRATEGY: The phrase *further teaching is necessary* tells you to select an answer with inaccurate information.

814. The nurse cares for a client with end-stage liver disease due to cirrhosis secondary to alcohol abuse. The nurse monitors the client for which potentially life-threatening complication of cirrhosis?

A. Ascites.

B. Hepatomegaly.

C. Ruptured esophageal varices.

D. Epistaxis.

Answer: C. Esophageal varices are a result of congested portal circulation, which cause fragile collateral vessels to form. Ruptured esophageal varices are a serious complication of end-stage liver disease (ESLD). The client is at risk for hemorrhage that can cause hypotension and internal bleeding. Although ascites, hepatomegaly, and epistaxis are symptoms of ESLD, they are not life-threatening.

TEST-TAKING STRATEGY: Review the ABCs. Impaired circulation is a medical emergency. Hemorrhage severely impairs circulation and is the most life threatening of the answer choices.

815. The nurse cares for a client who experienced a cerebral vascular accident. The client's husband asks why his wife has a splint on her hand. The nurse explains that the splint is needed to prevent:

A. Skin breakdown.

B. Deformity of the hand.

C. Edema.

D. Muscle wasting.

Answer: B. After a stroke, fingers of the affected hand should be extended to prevent deformity and loss of function. A splint could cause skin breakdown, not prevent it. Edema may occur regardless of the splint. Muscle wasting could occur if range-of-motion exercises are not performed routinely.

TEST-TAKING STRATEGY: You may find the question does not offer a distinct correct answer. In this case, choose the most correct answer.

816. A client is admitted to the emergency department with a diagnosis of sickle-cell crisis. The nurse anticipates which priority nursing intervention to be ordered by the physician?

A. Administer oxygen.

B. Perform laboratory tests.

C. Conduct genetic counseling.

D. Administer transfusion of platelets.

Answer: A. Administering oxygen, fluids, and analgesics is the priority intervention when treating a sickle-cell crisis. Laboratory tests will be ordered, but it is not a primary intervention. Genetic counseling is recommended, but not during a crisis. Transfusion of platelets would not be ordered, but transfusion of red blood cells may be ordered.

TEST-TAKING STRATEGY: Questions that ask you to prioritize your nursing actions use terms like *priority, first, best, initial, most important, immediate,* and *next.*

817. A client has a history of left-sided heart failure. The nurse knows that one of the complications of this type of heart failure is pulmonary congestion. What should the nurse expect to find upon assessment?

A. Tenting of the skin.

B. Pulmonary hypertension.

C. Increased jugular vein distension.

D. Hypotension.

Answer: B. During left-sided heart failure, the heart's left ventricle loses its ability to pump effectively. Blood backs up into the pulmonary vasculature. Meanwhile, blood returns from the right ventricle into the pulmonary vasculature. The two forces create and elevate pressure in the lungs, leading to pulmonary hypertension. Tenting of the skin is caused by dehydration, and hypotension can be due to a myriad of conditions. However, in left-sided heart failure, the nurse should expect hypertension. Jugular vein distension occurs in right-sided heart failure as blood backs up into the systemic circulation.

TEST-TAKING STRATEGY: Look for similar words in the question and answer. Also, eliminate non-specific answers like hypotension, which can occur in many diseases.

818. A client is admitted to the nursing unit after experiencing a cerebral vascular accident. The client is unconscious. What is the nurse's priority intervention?

A. Preventing skin breakdown.

B. Maintaining a patent airway.

C. Preventing muscle atrophy.

D. Promoting fluid intake.

Answer: B. Maintaining a patent airway is a priority in the unconscious client. Although preventing skin breakdown and muscle atrophy and promoting fluid intake are important, they are not the nurse's first priority in caring for this client.

TEST-TAKING STRATEGY: Remember the ABCs. Maintaining an airway is the nurse's first priority.

819. A client underwent an abdominal hysterectomy 6 hours ago. The nurse teaches the client to avoid which position?

A. Side-lying.

B. High Fowler's.

C. Supine.

D. Lateral recumbent.

Answer: B. High Fowler's position can lead to pelvic congestion, while side-lying, supine, and lateral recumbent positions do not.

TEST-TAKING STRATEGY: Visualize the positions and determine which is detrimental to a client who just had abdominal surgery.

820. The nurse cares for a client who underwent abdominal surgery 2 days ago. Which symptom suggests the client has developed complications?

A. Muscle soreness.

B. Incisional pain.

C. Abdominal distension.

D. Serous wound drainage.

Answer: C. Abdominal distension after abdominal surgery could indicate paralytic ileus. Muscle soreness, incisional pain, and serous wound drainage are expected findings postoperatively.

TEST-TAKING STRATEGY: Eliminate answer choices that are a normal part of recovery after a surgical procedure.

821. The nurse cares for a client recovering from a subdural hematoma. Which nursing intervention should the nurse perform to prevent foot drop and contractures?

    A. Apply high-top sneakers.

    B. Administer low-molecular-weight heparin (LMWH).

    C. Encourage the client to ambulate.

    D. Apply sequential compression devices (SCDs).

    Answer: A. High-top sneakers prevent contractures and foot drop in clients with neurological disease processes by keeping the feet flexed and toes extended. LMWH, SCDs, and ambulation prevent deep vein thrombosis (DVT).

    TEST-TAKING STRATEGY: You may find that the question does not offer a distinct correct answer. In this case, choose the most correct answer.

822. The nurse cares for a client who recently underwent surgery to create a stoma for colostomy. The nurse notes that the stoma is dark and dusky in color. What action should the nurse immediately take?

    A. Notify the physician.

    B. Change the ostomy bag.

    C. Irrigate the colostomy.

    D. Remove the ostomy bag.

    Answer: A. A healthy stoma looks red and beefy. A dark and dusky colored stoma may indicate ischemia. This is an emergency, and the physician should be notified immediately. Changing or removing the ostomy bag or irrigating the colostomy will do nothing to relieve the ischemia.

    TEST-TAKING STRATEGY: Notify the physician when there is nothing more the nurse can do to fix the problem.

823. A client underwent a cholecystectomy and is now complaining of cramping and pain in the left calf. Which action is the nurse's first priority?

    A. Administer pain medication.

    B. Notify the physician.

    C. Assess the client for Homan's sign.

    D. Elevate the client's legs.

    Answer: C. Pain and cramping is a possible symptom of a deep vein thrombosis, which is a common complication of surgical procedures. Before notifying the physician, the nurse needs to gather more data, which would include assessment for Homans' sign. Elevating the client's legs would further decrease arterial blood flow to the lower extremities. Although administering pain medications is important, assessing for potential life-threatening complications should occur first.

    TEST-TAKING STRATEGY: Questions that ask you to prioritize your nursing actions use terms like *priority, first, best, initial, most important, immediate,* and *next.*

824. The nurse cares for a client who is 2 days postop femoral popliteal bypass. While assessing the client, the nurse notes that the client's right leg is cool and pale. Which action should the nurse take first?

    A. Notify the physician.

    B. Assist the client to a chair.

    C. Position the client flat.

    D. Check dorsalis pedis pulses.

    Answer: D. The client has the bypass surgery due to arterial disease. A complication of bypass surgery is clot formation. To assess for a potential clot, the nurse should check distal pulses. After the nurse assesses the pulses, the physician should be notified. Lying the client flat is of no benefit. Ambulating a client could cause a clot to dislodge.

    TEST-TAKING STRATEGY: Look for similar answer choices and eliminate them.

825. A client is admitted to the hospital due to complications of cardiomyopathy. The client states, "I am always being admitted to the hospital for the same problem." The nurse knows that which recurring condition develops in clients with cardiomyopathy?

A. Heart failure.

B. Hypertension.

C. Myocardial infarction.

D. Anemia.

Answer: A. Heart failure is the most commonly recurring complication of cardiomyopathy. Hypertension is not a common complication. If a client with heart failure does have hypertension, it can usually be controlled with medication on an outpatient basis. Myocardial infarction and anemia are not complications of cardiomyopathy.

TEST-TAKING STRATEGY: Use the process of elimination to rule out incorrect answer selections to help choose the correct answer.

826. The nurse cares for a client who recently underwent a colon resection. The nurse notes that arterial blood gas results show metabolic alkalosis. The nurse expects this finding because:

A. The client is hyperventilating.

B. The client is complaining of severe pain.

C. The client has a nasogastric tube connected to suction.

D. The client is receiving normal saline maintenance fluids.

Answer: C. Nasogastric suction removes acidic gastric secretions. This causes metabolic alakalinization of the blood pH. Hyperventilation causes respiratory alkalosis. Pain could cause an acid–base imbalance if the client is hypoventilating. The nurse should expect to see respiratory acidosis in this case. Normal saline has no effect on blood pH.

TEST-TAKING STRATEGY: To answer this question, go through each answer choice to determine whether you would expect to see an acid or base imbalance. Eliminate choices that indicate an acid imbalance (hyperventilation and complaint of severe pain). Normal saline has the same pH as the blood, so it does not cause an acid–base imbalance.

827. A client is postoperative day one after a thoracotomy. The client complains of incisional pain.

Vital signs are temperature 100.9°F (38.3°C), heart rate 94 beats/minute, blood pressure 138/90 mm Hg, and respirations 22 breaths/minute. Physical assessment reveals shallow respirations and rhonchi at the bases. Which intervention should the nurse perform first?

A. Encourage the client to cough and deep-breathe.

B. Administer pain medication.

C. Assist the client into a chair.

D. Administer ibuprofen to reduce the client's fever.

Answer: B. The priority intervention is to relieve the client's pain. By relieving the client's pain, the client will be able to ambulate (this will resolve the rhonchi) and cough and deep-breathe. In addition, by breathing more deeply, the fever will decrease.

TEST-TAKING STRATEGY: Determine which intervention is most helpful to the client. In this case, treating the client's pain enables ambulation and deep breathing, which will decrease the fever and clear the lungs.

828. The nurse cares for a client with a history of diabetes mellitus. The nurse notes that the client's skin is cool and clammy and that the client is difficult to arouse. Which action should the nurse take first?

A. Check the client's blood sugar.

B. Ask the client to drink a cup of orange juice.

C. Administer an intravenous dose of 50% dextrose.

D. Administer subcutaneous insulin.

Answer: A. The nurse suspects that the client is experiencing hypoglycemia. Before administering any kind of treatment, the nurse needs to verify her suspicions by checking the client's glucose level. If the client is found to be hypoglycemic, the nurse should administer 50% dextrose, not orange juice. Giving a client who is difficult to arouse a glass of orange juice could cause the client to aspirate. Insulin is given for hyperglycemia or to maintain a diabetic in a euglycemic state.

TEST-TAKING STRATEGY: Eliminate similar answer choices (administering orange juice, 50% dextrose, or insulin). These answers have the nurse administering a treatment.

829. A client is diagnosed with iron-deficiency anemia. The nurse expects which complaint from the client?

   A. "I am short of breath even while I am sitting."

   B. "My face is always flushed."

   C. "I always feel like eating."

   D. "I can't taste anything."

   Answer: **A.** Iron-deficiency anemia causes decreased hemoglobin in the blood. This reduces the amount of oxygen transported to body tissues. The client may complain of experiencing shortness of breath, pallor, chills, loss of appetite, and faintness.

   TEST-TAKING STRATEGY: Use the process of elimination to rule out incorrect answer selections to help choose the correct answer.

830. A client is status post-thyroidectomy. The client complains of paresthesia and leg cramps. The nurse reviews the client's lab results and notes hypocalcemia. The nurse realizes the reason for the hypocalcemia is:

   A. Decreased intake of dairy products due to postoperative nausea.

   B. Removal of the thyroid gland.

   C. Inadvertent removal of the parathyroid gland with thyroidectomy.

   D. Hyperphosphatemia.

   Answer: **C.** Because the parathyroid gland is in close proximity to the thyroid, the parathyroid gland may be inadvertently removed during a thyroidectomy. Decreased intake of dairy products in the immediate postoperative period does not cause such a marked decline in calcium levels. Hyperphosphatemia can also cause a decrease in calcium; however, there is no indication in the question that the client has high phosphorus levels.

   TEST-TAKING STRATEGY: Use the process of elimination to rule out incorrect answer selections to help choose the correct answer.

831. The nurse cares for a client who is status post right above-knee amputation. The client complains of severe pain below the level of the amputation. The nurse realizes that the client is experiencing:

   A. Narcotic withdrawal.

   B. Phantom pain.

   C. Hallucinations.

   D. Denial.

   Answer: **B.** Phantom pain can occur immediately after surgery up to 2 to 3 months post-amputation. The pain is real, and is not a hallucination. It is also not related to denial of the lost limb or due to narcotic withdrawal.

   TEST-TAKING STRATEGY: Use the process of elimination to rule out incorrect answer selections to help choose the correct answer.

832. A nurse cares for a client who underwent a liver transplant 2 days prior. The Jackson–Pratt (JP) drain drains serosanguinous fluid. The nurse now notes the drainage is a greenish-brown color. The nurse suspects (select all that apply):

   A. A bile leak due to a ruptured bile duct anastamosis.

   B. A hepatic artery clot.

   C. Cholelithiasis.

   D. Recurrence of cirrhosis.

   Answer: **A, B, & C.** A ruptured bile duct anastamosis, created between a donor and recipient liver, can sometimes rupture, leading to a bile leak. The nurse is seeing bile drainage in this scenario. A hepatic artery clot manifests as hepatic vasculature congestion, which is observed on ultrasound. Cholelithiasis is not a risk in the immediate postoperative period, but is observed on ultrasound. Recurrence of cirrhosis is seen in elevated liver function tests, but is not usually present at the second postoperative day.

   TEST-TAKING STRATEGY: When answering "Select all that apply" questions, be sure and treat each answer as a true or false statement. There may be one correct answer or more.

833. A client completes a course of chemotherapy. During this time of nadir, which assessment finding may the nurse encounter?

A. Hypokalemia.

B. Elevated platelets.

C. Elevated serum creatinine level.

D. Decreased absolute neutrophil count (ANC).

Answer: D. Nadir occurs when the client's blood counts reach their lowest level. ANC represents the absolute amount of neutrophils, a type of WBC found in the blood. The nurse should not expect hypokalemia or elevated creatinine levels. A decreased platelet count, not an elevated one, is common during nadir.

TEST-TAKING STRATEGY: Choose an answer that directly relates to the complications of chemotherapy. Chemotherapy destroys rapidly dividing cells, like white blood cells.

834. The nurse cares for client who is status post-lung transplant. The client has a double thoracotomy incision. Which drug may impair healing of the incision?

A. Corticosteriod (Dexamethasone).

B. Furosemide (Lasix).

C. Potassium (K-Dur).

D. Docusate sodium (Colace).

Answer: A. Dexamethasone is used as an immunosuppressant. Any type of immunosuppressant impedes the function of white blood cells, which are needed for healing. Lasix is a diuretic, K-Dur is a potassium supplement, and Colace is a stool softener. None of these drugs impede healing.

TEST-TAKING STRATEGY: Use the process of elimination to rule out incorrect answer selections to help choose the correct answer.

835. A client has pinpoint, pink-to-purple, non-blanching macular lesions 1 to 3 mm in diameter. Which term best describes the lesions?

A. Eccymosis.

B. Petechiae.

C. Purpura.

D. Hematoma.

Answer: B. Petechiae are pinpoint, pink-to-purple, nonblanching macular lesions 1 to 3 mm in diameter. Ecchymosis is a purple-to-brown bruise, macular or papular, and varies in size. Purpura is purple macular lesions larger than 1 cm. A hematoma is a collection of ruptured blood vessels more than 1 cm in diameter.

TEST-TAKING STRATEGY: Look for similar answer choices and eliminate them. Ecchymoses, purpura, and hematomas are all larger lesions.

836. A client develops hepatic encephalopathy. The nurse expects which assessment finding? Select all that apply.

A. Lethargy.

B. Asterixis.

C. Improved concentration.

D. Improved coordination.

Answer: A & B. Asterixis, or liver flap, is elicited by applying a blood pressure cuff. When the cuff is deflated, the client's hands flap. This is a sign of hepatic encephalopathy. Lethargy, decreased energy, decreased concentration, and a decline in coordination are signs and symptoms of hepatic encephalopathy. Hepatic encephalopathy occurs due to an increase in ammonia levels. Ammonia is toxic to the brain, thus causing a decrease in cognitive function and level of consciousness.

TEST-TAKING STRATEGY: Look for similar answer choices and eliminate them (improved concentration and improved coordination).

837. A client is suspected of having an abdominal aortic aneurysm. Which would the nurse expect to hear while auscultating the middle lower abdomen to the left of midline?

A. Bruit.

B. Thrill.

C. Crackles.

D. Friction rub.

Answer: A. A bruit is distinctly heard over an abdominal aortic aneurysm. It suggests a partial arterial occlusion. A thrill is palpated over an aneurysm. Crackles are heard in the lungs. A friction rub indicates inflammation of the peritoneum, pleura, and mediastinum.

TEST-TAKING STRATEGY: Eliminate the answer that involves palpation (thrill) and not auscultation. Think of the sound you might hear if listening to a vessel with an obstruction. It would be a swishing sound. Crackles indicate fluid, and a friction rub indicates two surfaces rubbing together.

838. Which best describes Babinski's reflex?

A. Flexion of the arm at the elbow when the biceps tendon is tapped.

B. Extension of the leg when the patellar tendon is tapped.

C. Dorsiflexion of the great toe and fanning of the other toes when a sharp object is moved along the sole of the foot.

D. Plantar flexion of the foot when the Achilles tendon is tapped.

Answer: C. Babinski's reflex is characterized by dorsiflexion of the great toe and fanning of the other toes when a sharp object is moved across the sole of the foot. This response should be absent in children over 2 years of age and in adults. If the reflex is present, this could indicate damage to the pyramidal tracts. Flexion of the arm at the elbow when the biceps tendon is tapped describes the biceps reflex. Extension of the leg when the patellar tendon is tapped describes the patellar reflex. Plantar flexion of the foot when the Achilles tendon is tapped describes ankle or Achilles reflex.

TEST-TAKING STRATEGY: Look for similar answer choices and eliminate them.

839. Jugular vein distension (JVD) is most prominent in:

A. Heart failure.

B. Myocardial infarction (MI).

C. Pneumothorax.

D. Abdominal aortic aneurysm (AAA).

Answer: A. JVD is prominent in heart failure as a result of increased venous pressure. An MI can lead to heart failure and subsequent JVD, but it is not responsible for JVD on its own. Pneumothorax and AAA do not cause JVD.

TEST-TAKING STRATEGY: Use the process of elimination to rule out incorrect answer selections to help choose the correct answer.

840. A heart murmur is heard at the second left intercostal space along the left sternal border. Which heart valve is found in this area?

A. Aortic.

B. Mitral.

C. Pulmonic.

D. Tricuspid.

Answer: C. Pulmonic abnormalities are heard at the second left intercostal space along the left sternal border. Aortic valve abnormalities are heard at the second intercostal space to the right of the sternum. Mitral valve abnormalities are heard at the fifth intercostal space at the midclavicular line. Tricuspid valve abnormalities are heard at the third and fourth intercostal spaces along the sternal border.

TEST-TAKING STRATEGY: Visualize where the heart is located within the chest. Picture where the outflow from the valves occurs.

841. Which landmarks are used to obtain an apical pulse?

A. Left fifth intercostal space, midaxillary line.

B. Left fifth intercostal space, midclavicular line.

C. Left second intercostal space, midclavicular line.

D. Left seventh intercostal space, midclavicular line.

Answer: B. The left fifth intercostal space at the midclavicular line is the point of maximal impulse and the location of the left ventricular apex. The second intercostal space at the midclavicular line is where pulmonic sounds are auscultated. No heart sounds are heard at the midaxillary line or at the seventh intercostal space.

TEST-TAKING STRATEGY: Eliminate answer A (left fifth intercostal space, midaxillary line), because no heart sounds are auscultated at the midaxillary line. Next, visualize where the heart sits in the chest and the point where the heart is closest to the chest wall. The second intercostal space is too high, and the seventh intercostal space is too low to auscultate the apical pulse.

842. A client returns from surgery after having a transurethral prostatic resection (TURP) due to benign prostatic hyperplasia. The client has an indwelling urinary catheter in place. Which type of drainage should the nurse expect to see during the immediate postoperative period?

A. Scant urinary drainage.

B. Serous urinary drainage.

C. Bloody urinary drainage.

D. Clear, yellow urinary drainage.

Answer: C. During a TURP, the surgeon removes prostate tissue through the urethra. The urethra is removed in slices via a resecto-scope. This is traumatic to the urethra, and the nurse should expect to see bloody drainage in the immediate postoperative period. Urine gradually turns to a serous color and then to clear yellow after the TURP. The nurse should expect to see normal to increased amounts of urine secondary to intravenous fluids given intra- and postoperatively.

TEST-TAKING STRATEGY: Use the process of elimination to rule out incorrect answer selections to help choose the correct answer.

843. The nurse checks the carotid pulses in a client. The nurse knows to check the carotid pulse one side at a time:

A. So that the client does not feel like he is being choked.

B. Because the rate will be easier to count.

C. To prevent a syncopal episode.

D. To obtain a more accurate description of the quality of the pulse.

Answer: C. Applying pressure to the carotid arteries simultaneously causes the client to experience a syncopal episode (decreased heart rate and blood pressure that could lead to loss of consciousness).

TEST-TAKING STRATEGY: Use the process of elimination to rule out incorrect answer selections to help choose the correct answer.

844. The nurse performs an assessment on an elderly client. The nurse notes the client performs pill movement of the hand. The nurse suspects which disorder?

A. Myasthenia gravis.

B. Huntington's chorea.

C. Parkinson's disease.

D. Residual effect of a cerebral vascular accident (CVA).

Answer: C. An early symptom of Parkinson's disease is a pill-rolling movement of the hands. Myasthenia gravis is characterized by a progressive muscle weakness, while Huntington's chorea is characterized by progressive loss of muscle control. Residual effects of a CVA are loss of function in the extremities and facial droop.

TEST-TAKING STRATEGY: Use the process of elimination to rule out incorrect answer selections to help choose the correct answer.

845. The nurse auscultates breath sounds in a client. The nurse knows an incorrect method for auscultation is:

A. Using the diaphragm of the stethoscope.

B. Placing the diaphragm directly on the client's skin.

C. Asking the client to breathe deeply and slowly through the mouth.

D. Ask the client to lie flat in bed.

Answer: D. The best way to auscultate breath sounds is to have the client sit up and breathe slowly and deeply through the mouth. This allows for chest expansion and better assessment of the lung fields. The diaphragm of the stethoscope, which should be placed directly on the client's skin to prevent artifact, should be used for auscultation.

TEST-TAKING STRATEGY: The question asks you to identify incorrect information. Eliminate answer selections that contain correct assessment information.

846. The nurse monitors a client who receives treatment for an asthma attack. The nurse knows the client's respiratory status has worsened if which occurs?

  A. Clear breath sounds.

  B. Diminished breath sounds.

  C. Wheezing throughout all lung fields.

  D. Rhonchi.

Answer: B. Diminished breath sounds can indicate obstruction, which may lead to respiratory distress. Clear breath sounds indicate improvement while rhonchi are an indication of fluid in the lungs. Wheezing is not a reliable indicator of worsening respiratory status related to asthma.

TEST-TAKING STRATEGY: Eliminate obvious incorrect answers (clear breath sounds and diminished breath sounds). Although wheezing is often associated with asthma, it can occur with allergies as well, making this an incorrect answer.

847. The nurse assesses for cyanosis in a dark-skinned client. Which is the best site to assess for cyanosis in this client?

  A. Soles of the feet.

  B. Palms of the hands.

  C. Conjunctiva.

  D. Earlobes.

Answer: C. In dark-skinned clients, cyanosis is best assessed in places where the epidermis is thin and skin color is lighter. These lighter areas include the conjunctiva, mucous membranes, and nailbeds. In light-skinned clients, cyanosis is best assessed for in nailbeds, earlobes, lips, mucous membranes, palms of the hands, and soles of feet.

TEST-TAKING STRATEGY: Eliminate soles of the feet (A) and palms of the hands (B), because they refer to areas of the body where the epidermis is

thick. Next, visualize the remaining body areas and determine where the nurse would best find changes in coloration.

848. The nurse assesses her client's dorsalis pedis and posterior tibial pulses. The nurse understands that this assessment is an important part of the physical exam because:

  A. It determines heart rate.

  B. It examines pulse rate.

  C. It monitors perfusion of the lower extremities.

  D. It assesses adequacy of oxygenation.

Answer: C. Assessing the dorsalis pedis and posterior tibial pulses helps to determine adequacy of lower extremity perfusion. Weak or absent pulses indicate inadequate perfusion of the lower extremities. Heart rate, also known as pulse rate, is assessed through apical or radial pulses. Although poor perfusion can indicate poor oxygenation, assessing the lower extremity pulses is used to monitor perfusion.

TEST-TAKING STRATEGY: First eliminate similar answer choices (heart rate and pulse rate). Then, use the process of elimination to rule out incorrect answer selections to help choose the correct answer.

849. The nurse cares for a client diagnosed with bronchial obstruction. Which assessment finding should the nurse expect to find?

  A. Productive cough.

  B. Normal breath sounds.

  C. Rust colored sputum.

  D. Decreased use of accessory muscles.

Answer: A. Productive cough usually indicates presence of mucus, which causes obstruction of the bronchial passageways. The nurse should expect to find increased breath sounds and use of accessory muscles. Rust colored sputum is produced in pneumococcal pneumonia.

TEST-TAKING STRATEGY: Use the process of elimination to rule out incorrect answer selections to help choose the correct answer.

850. The nurse finds a client to have increased tactile fremitus. Which condition is associated with increased tactile fremitus?

A. Atelectasis.

B. Chronic obstructive pulmonary disease (COPD).

C. Pneumothorax.

D. Pneumonia.

Answer: D. Pneumonia causes the consolidation of mucous in the lungs. Mucous results in increased tactile fremitus. Atelectasis, COPD, and pneumothorax involve air, which decreases tactile fremitus.

TEST-TAKING STRATEGY: Look for similar answer choices and eliminate them.

851. The nurse examines a client's external auditory canal and tympanic membrane with an otoscope. Which is the best way to position the ear for the examination?

A. Pull the auricle downward.

B. Pull the auricle up and back.

C. Pull the ear lobe downward.

D. Pull the tragus forward.

Answer: B. To perform an otoscopic exam in an adult, the auricle should be pulled up and back before the otoscope is introduced. The auricle is pulled down when examining a child. Pulling the ear lobe or tragus does not open up the ear canal for better visualization.

TEST-TAKING STRATEGY: If the age of the client does not appear in the question, it is safe to assume the client is an adult.

852. The nurse examines the client's extraocular muscle movements (cranial nerve VI). Which equipment is used for this examination?

A. Piece of cotton to test corneal sensitivity.

B. Finger to test cardinal positions of gaze.

C. Snellen's chart to test visual acuity.

D. Ophthalmoscope to examine red reflex.

Answer: B. The six cardinal positions of gaze tests the extraocular muscles. This can be done using a finger or another object, such as a pen or pencil. To test the function of the optic nerve (cranial nerve II), the Snellen chart is used. To examine the structure of the optic disk and retina, an ophthalmoscopic examination is required. To test the trigeminal nerve (cranial nerve IV), a wisp of cotton is touched to the eye. This test is usually not performed in conscious clients, as it could cause damage to the cornea.

TEST-TAKING STRATEGY: Think about what the extraocular muscles do. They help the eye move in all directions or change the position, or gaze, of the eye.

853. The nurse cares for a client with chronic kidney disease. The client has an arteriovenous fistula that is being used for dialysis. As part of the assessment, the nurse should:

A. Listen for a bruit and palpate for a thrill over the fistula.

B. Measure urine output.

C. Observe for signs of edema.

D. Monitor creatinine level.

Answer: A. Although the client does have chronic kidney disease, this fact is a distractor. The question is really asking which type of assessment is appropriate for a client with a fistula. For clients with an arteriovenous fistula, assessing the patency of the fistula is important. To assess for patency, the nurse must listen for a bruit and palpate for a thrill over the fistula. Measuring urine output, monitoring creatinine level, and observing for signs of edema are assessments performed for a client with chronic kidney disease, but the question is not asking about assessment of kidney disease.

TEST-TAKING STRATEGY: You may find that the question does not offer a distinct correct answer. In this case, choose the most correct answer from the answer selections provided.

854. The nurse cares for a client who is complaining of nausea, vomiting, and back pain. Upon assessment, the nurse notices a pulsation left of midline in the upper abdomen. The nurse auscultates a bruit at this same site. Which illness does the nurse suspect?

A. Urolithiasis.

B. Cholecystitis.

C. Abdominal aortic aneurysm (AAA).

D. Pancreatitis.

Answer: C. A pulsation and bruit located left of midline in the upper abdomen usually indicates an AAA. Urolithiasis, cholecystitis, and pancreatitis are not vascular disease, so a bruit is not present in these diseases.

TEST-TAKING STRATEGY: Use the process of elimination to rule out incorrect answer selections to help choose the correct answer.

855. The nurse notices that a client is jaundiced upon physical assessment. The nurse also notes dark colored urine in the client's Foley bag. The nurse suspects the client has:

A. An intestinal obstruction.

B. A urinary tract infection.

C. Cholelithiasis.

D. Benign prostatic hyperplasia (BPH).

Answer: C. Gallstones from cholelithiasis impede bile flow. This results in excess bilirubin in the circulation, which is then excreted through the kidneys, causing dark colored urine. An intestinal obstruction, urinary tract infections, and BPH do not cause dark-colored urine.

TEST-TAKING STRATEGY: Use the process of elimination to rule out incorrect answer selections to help choose the correct answer.

856. The nurse observes white patches and ulcerations in a client's oral cavity. The client tells the nurse the sores developed during chemotherapy treatment even though the client performed oral care regularly. The nurse suspects which complication?

A. Low hemoglobin level.

B. Thrush.

C. Mucositis

D. Infection due to poor oral hygiene.

Answer: C. Chemotherapy causes damage to rapidly regenerating epithelial cells, like those found in the lower and upper gastrointestinal tract. This causes epithelial thinning, inflammation, and decreased cell production. Low hemoglobin does not cause mouth sores. Thrush is characterized by a white or black plaque on the tongue. The question states that the client performed regular oral hygiene, so infection is not likely the answer.

TEST-TAKING STRATEGY: Eliminate obvious incorrect answers (low hemoglobin level and thrush). Then choose the answer that is most closely related to the information given in the question. Chemotherapy is known to cause mucositis.

857. Which treatment is used to manage hyperthyroidism? Select all that apply.

A. Irradiation of the thyroid.

B. Administration of oral thyroid hormones.

C. Thyroidectomy.

D. Nephrectomy.

Answer: A & C. Irradiation destroys the thyroid gland while a thyroidectomy involves completely removing the gland. Oral thyroid hormones treat hypothyroidism. A nephrectomy involves removal of the kidney.

TEST-TAKING STRATEGY: Eliminate answers that do not have to do with the thyroid gland (nephrectomy). This answer is easily eliminated based on the root word of *nephr*—meaning kidney. Would you want to give a client more thyroid hormone if they are already producing too much? No. So administering oral thyroid hormones may be eliminated. This leaves the correct answers: irradiation of the thyroid and thyroidectomy.

858. A percutaneous transluminal coronary angioplasty (PTCA) is performed on the client with a myocardial infarction to:

A. Open coronary arteries blocked by plaque in order to improve blood flow to the myocardium.

B. Bypass obstructed coronary arteries that are preventing blood flow to the myocardium.

C. Ablate conduction pathways to prevent tachycardia that can cause increased workload.

D. Prevent heart failure related to increased workload on the myocardium.

Answer: A. PTCA uses a balloon tipped catheter to compress the obstructing plaque against the wall of the vessel. This opens the obstructed vessel and restores blood flow to the myocardium. A coronary artery bypass graft (CABG) uses the saphenous vein or mammary artery to bypass obstructed coronary arteries. This is also an intervention for clients suffering form a severe myocardial infarction. An ablation disrupts conduction pathways that are causing dysrhythmias. Decreased blood flow to the heart can cause ischemia, which damages the myocardium, causing it to pump ineffectively. However, both PTCA and CABG restore blood flow.

TEST-TAKING STRATEGY: Any intervention performed in a client who has had a myocardial infarction is aimed at restoring blood flow.

859. A transjugular intrahepatic portosystemic shunt (TIPS) is performed for which condition?

A. Portal hypertension.

B. Ruptured esophageal varices.

C. Jaundice.

D. Jugular venous distension.

Answer: A. In a TIPS procedure, a catheter is introduced into the jugular vein and threaded into a branch of the portal vein. A stent is then inserted, which connects the portal vein with the hepatic vein. This allows blood returning from the digestive tract via the portal vein to be returned directly to the heart via the hepatic vein, thus bypassing the sclerosed and scarred liver.

This relieves portal hypertension. Esophageal banding or sclerotherapy prevents rupture of esophageal varices. Jaundice and jugular venous distension are not prevented by TIPS.

TEST-TAKING STRATEGY: Focus on key terms like *intrahepatic portosystemic shunt*. This tells you that the procedure involves placement of a stent into the liver (*intrahepatic*). *Portosystemic* tells you that the shunt is from the portal liver circulation (portal vein) to the systemic circulation (hepatic vein). Shunts are usually placed to bypass an obstruction; in this case, the obstruction is the scarred and sclerosed vessels of the liver.

860. A nurse cares for a postoperative client who has become tachycardiac and tachypneic. The client's blood pressure is 88/60 mm Hg. Which action should the nurse immediately take? Select all that apply.

A. Monitor hourly urine output.

B. Elevate the client's feet.

C. Draw blood for laboratory testing.

D. Recheck vital signs.

Answer: B & D. The client is experiencing signs of shock. Placing the client in a supine position (with the head slightly elevated) and elevating the feet increase venous blood return to the heart. This decreases the heart rate and normalizes the blood pressure. Monitoring hourly output and drawing blood for laboratory tests should be performed, but they are not a priority.

TEST-TAKING STRATEGY: Choose the answer that brings immediate help to the client. In this case, elevating the client's legs helps to normalize the client's vital signs. This is confirmed by rechecking vital signs.

861. The nurse cares for a client with a heart rate of 112 beats/minute. Which could be the cause of this condition?

A. Straining during a bowel movement.

B. Suctioning.

C. Fear, anger, or pain.

D. Stress, pain, or vomiting.

Answer: C. Fear, anger, or pain can cause a client to become tachycardiac. Straining during a bowel movement, vomiting, or suctioning can cause vagal stimulation, which causes bradycardia.

TEST-TAKING STRATEGY: You may find that the question does not offer a distinct correct answer. In this case, choose the most correct answer from the selections provided.

862. The nurse cares for a client who sustained serious injuries from a motor vehicle accident. In assessing client needs, the nurse knows that a client's response to stressors depends on individual differences such as:

   A. Gender.

   B. Number of roommates.

   C. Room assignment.

   D. Time of day.

   Answer: A. A client's response to stressors depends on individual differences such as age, gender, social support, cultural background, medical diagnosis, current hospital course, and prognosis. Room assignment, number of roommates, and time of day are not individual differences that will necessarily impact coping.

   TEST-TAKING STRATEGY: Look for similar answer choices and eliminate them.

863. In order to be effective, nursing interventions should consider the client's wholeness. The human self-concept is a major concern for all nurses and comprises attitudes about:

   A. A child.

   B. A neighbor.

   C. A spouse.

   D. Oneself.

   Answer: D. The self-concept comprises attitudes about oneself: perceptions of personal abilities, body image, and identity; and a general sense of worth. The stressors imposed by physical illness, trauma, and surgical procedures can cause disturbances in the self-concept.

   TEST-TAKING STRATEGY: Look for similar answer choices and eliminate them.

864. When reviewing a client's morning laboratory results, the nurse knows that potassium is important because it can alter:

   A. Myocardial muscle function.

   B. Myocardial ventricular function.

   C. Pulmonary artery function.

   D. Pulmonary muscle function.

   Answer: A. During depolarization and repolarization of nerve and muscle fiber, potassium and sodium exchange occur intracellularly and extracellularly. The potassium gradient across the cell membrane determines conduction velocity and helps confine pacing activity to the sinus node. Thus either an excess or a deficiency of potassium can alter myocardial muscle function. Pulmonary muscle function, myocardial ventricular function, and pulmonary artery function are not affected by potassium imbalances.

   TEST-TAKING STRATEGY: Use the process of elimination to rule out incorrect answer selections to help choose the correct answer.

865. The nurse cares for a client with hypokalemia. The nurse knows that hypokalemia is commonly caused by (select all that apply):

   A. Chronic steroid therapy.

   B. Diuretic therapy with insufficient replacement.

   C. GI losses.

   D. Muscle twitching.

   Answer: A, B, & C. A low serum potassium level, called hypokalemia, is commonly caused by GI losses, diuretic therapy with insufficient replacement, or chronic steroid therapy. Muscle twitching is a side effect, not a cause of hypokalemia.

   TEST-TAKING STRATEGY: When answering "Select all that apply" questions, be sure and treat each answer as a true or false statement. There may be one correct answer or more.

866. A client undergoes an electrocardiogram (EKG) to assess the impact of hypokalemia. The earliest EKG changes that are most often seen in hypokalemia are:

A. Atrial-ventricular blocks.

B. Junctional rhythms.

C. Premature atrial contractions (PACs).

D. Premature ventricular contractions (PVCs).

Answer: D. Hypokalemia is reflected by the EKG. The earliest EKG change is often premature ventricular contractions (PVCs), which can deteriorate into ventricular tachycardia or fibrillation (VT/VF) without appropriate potassium replacement. Junctional rhythms, PACs, and PVCs are not often seen initially with hypokalemia.

TEST-TAKING STRATEGY: Read the questions twice to ensure that you understand what the question is asking, especially if the question is tricky or confusing. Focus on what the question is asking: early EKG changes most often seen in hypokalemia.

867. The nurse studies an electrocardiogram (EKG) and notices a U-wave. The nurse suspects that this is caused by:

A. Hypermagnesemia.

B. Hypocalcemia.

C. Hypokalemia.

D. Hyponatremia.

Answer: C. Hypokalemia impairs myocardial conduction and prolongs ventricular repolarization. This can be seen by a prominent U-wave (a positive deflection following the T-wave on the EKG). The U-wave is not totally unique to hypokalemia, but its presence is a signal for the clinician to check the serum potassium level. Hypermagnesemia, hypocalcemia, and hyponatremia do not result in the appearance of a U-wave on the EKG.

TEST-TAKING STRATEGY: Read the questions twice to ensure that you understand what the question is asking, especially if the question is tricky or confusing. Focus on what the question is asking: the cause for a U-wave on an EKG.

868. A client is diagnosed with hypokalemia. The nurse knows the electrolyte that must be corrected in this situation is:

A. Calcium.

B. Magnesium.

C. Manganese.

D. Zinc.

Answer: B. If concomitant hypomagnesemia exists, successful replenishment of potassium deficit cannot be accomplished until the hypomagnesemia is reversed. Deficits of calcium, manganese, and zinc have no impact on potassium deficits.

TEST-TAKING STRATEGY: Read the questions twice to ensure that you understand what the question is asking, especially if the question is tricky or confusing. Focus on what the question is asking: the electrolyte required to assist in reversing low potassium levels.

869. A client with osteoporosis requires regular monitoring of serum calcium levels. The nurse knows that the biologically active portion of the total calcium is called the:

A. Binding calcium

B. Bound calcium.

C. Ionized calcium.

D. Nonionized calcium.

Answer: C. Although the most commonly performed blood test for calcium levels is total serum calcium, the biologically active portion of the total calcium is called the ionized calcium. The inactive forms of plasma calcium are bound to protein (primarily albumin) and complexed to anions such as chloride and phosphate. Ionized calcium is primarily responsible for the pathophysiologic effects of hypercalcemia and hypocalcemia. The normal serum concentration of ionized calcium is maintained within very narrow limits (4 to 5 mg/dL), and direct measurement is the most accurate method of assessment. Binding calcium, bound calcium, and nonionized calcium are not the biologically active portion of total calcuim.

TEST-TAKING STRATEGY: Read the questions twice to ensure that you understand what the question is asking, especially if the question is tricky or confusing. Focus on what the question is asking: the biologically active portion of total calcium.

870. A client's electrocardiogram (EKG) shows a shortened QT interval. Which electrolyte deficiency is most likely the cause of this EKG change?

   A. Hypercalcemia.

   B. Hyperkalemia.

   C. Hypocalcemia.

   D. Hypokalemia.

   Answer: A.   Serum calcium levels are increased by bone tumors, some endocrine disorders, hypomagnesemia, and excessive intake of vitamin D. This condition has a cardiovascular effect of strengthening contractility and shortening ventricular repolarization. The EKG demonstrates the shortened repolarization with a shortened QT interval. Rhythm disturbances may include bradycardia; first-, second-, and third-degree heart block; and bundle branch block. Hyperkalemia usually results in ST elevation. Hypocalcemia usually does not result in any EKG changes. Hypokalemia usually results in U-waves.

   TEST-TAKING STRATEGY: Use the process of elimination to rule out incorrect answer selections to help choose the correct answer.

871. A postsurgical client requires a blood transfusion. Which disorder is common in critically ill and postsurgical clients requiring blood transfusions?

   A. Hypercalcemia.

   B. Hyperkalemia.

   C. Hypocalcemia.

   D. Hypokalemia.

   Answer: C.   Hypocalcemia is common in critically ill and postsurgical clients because of blood transfusions (the citrate used as an anticoagulant in bank blood binds to the calcium), magnesium imbalances, shock, or alkalosis.

Hypercalcemia, hyperkalemia, and hypokalemia are not found secondary to blood transfusions.

   TEST-TAKING STRATEGY: Use the process of elimination to rule out incorrect answer selections to help choose the correct answer.

872. Client incidence of hypermagnesemia is rare in comparison with hypomagnesemia. Hypermagnesemia generally occurs secondary to:

   A. Cardiac contractility.

   B. Hypokalemia.

   C. Liver failure.

   D. Renal insufficiency.

   Answer: D.   The incidence of hypermagnesemia is rare in comparison with hypomagnesemia, and it occurs secondary to renal insufficiency or iatrogenic overtreatment. Hypermagnesemia does not occur secondary to liver failure, cardiac contractility, or hypokalemia.

   TEST-TAKING STRATEGY: Use the process of elimination to rule out incorrect answer selections to help choose the correct answer.

873. Chronic alcohol abuse, rapid administration of citrated blood products, or treatment with total parenteral nutrition puts the client at risk for which condition?

   A. Hyperkalemia.

   B. Hypermagnesemia.

   C. Hypokalemia.

   D. Hypomagnesemia.

   Answer: D.   Hypomagnesemia can be caused by insufficient intake in the diet, chronic alcohol abuse, rapid administration of citrated blood products, or treatment with total parenteral nutrition (TPN).

   TEST-TAKING STRATEGY: Read the question carefully. Consider the potential deficiencies that are associated with each condition.

874. The nurse is caring for a patient who is experiencing a cardiac dysrhythmia. The nurse knows that cardiac dysrhythmias are often caused by an electrolyte imbalance. Which electrolyte

imbalance can cause the cardiac dysrhythmia known as torsades de pointes?

A. Hypomagnesemia.

B. Hypokalemia.

C. Hyperkalemia.

D. Hypermagnesemia.

Answer: A. Hypomagnesemia, a magnesium deficiency, may cause cardiac dysrhythmias. Cardiac dysrhythmias may be supraventricular or ventricular and include torsades de pointes. Dysrhythmias associated with hypomagnesemia may not respond to pharmacological interventions but often respond well to magnesium infusions. Magnesium (IV) is the treatment of choice for torsades de pointes.

TEST-TAKING STRATEGY: Read the question twice to ensure that you understand what the question is asking, especially if the question is tricky or confusing. Focus on what the question is asking: X not Y.

875. Cardiac enzymes can be divided into cardiac-specific enzymes and nonspecific enzymes. Which nonspecific cardiac enzyme indicates myocardial damage?

A. Creatine kinase (CK).

B. Troponin I.

C. CK-MB.

D. Creatinine.

Answer: A. Creatine kinase (CK) is a nonspecific cardiac enzyme that is indicative of myocardial damage. Nonspecific muscle enzymes include myoglobin, creatine kinase, and troponin T. Cardiac-specific muscle enzymes include troponin I and CK-MB. Creatinine is neither a nonspecific or cardiac-specific enzyme.

TEST-TAKING STRATEGY: Read the questions twice to ensure that you understand what the question is asking, especially if the question is tricky or confusing. Focus on what the questions is asking: X not Y.

876. The nurse is caring for a client in the emergency department (ED) who is experiencing chest pain. The physician suspects that the client has suffered a myocardial infarction. If the client has had a myocardial infarction, when should the nurse anticipate an initial rise in the cardiac-specific enzymes troponin and CK-MB?

A. Two days after the acute myocardial damage has occurred.

B. Four to six hours after the acute myocardial damage has occurred.

C. As soon as the individual has blood drawn in the emergency department.

D. After reperfusion therapy has occurred.

Answer: B. The nurse should anticipate an initial rise of troponin and CK-MB 4 to 6 hours after an acute myocardial damage has occurred. If a client presents in the ED as soon as chest pain is experienced, the enzymes will not have risen.

TEST-TAKING STRATEGY: Use the process of elimination to rule out incorrect answer selections to help choose the correct answer.

877. The nurse is assisting the physician with the placement of a central line. Which catheter, when properly positioned, is in the superior vena cava?

A. Central venous catheter.

B. Left atrial catheter.

C. Pulmonary artery catheter.

D. Right atrial catheter.

Answer: A. The central venous catheter is used for central venous pressure measurement and venous access. Proper placement of the central venous catheter is in the superior vena cava. The left atrial (LA) catheter is used to measure atrial pressure. A left atrial catheter is properly placed in the left atrium. The pulmonary artery catheter (Swan-Ganz) is used to measure PAOP and right heart pressures. Proper positioning for the pulmonary artery catheter is in the right or left pulmonary artery. There is no right atrial catheter.

TEST-TAKING STRATEGY: Use the process of elimination to rule out incorrect answer selections to help choose the correct answer.

878. The nurse is caring for a client in the intensive care unit with acute cardiopulmonary problems. The client is receiving mechanical ventilation for cardiopulmonary support. How often is a chest x-ray indicated for clients receiving mechanical ventilation?

A. Hourly.

B. Once daily.

C. Twice daily.

C. Weekly.

Answer: B. The American College of Radiology recommends a daily chest x-ray for clients with acute cardiopulmonary problems and those receiving mechanical ventilation. A chest x-ray is performed whenever a new device is placed or whenever there is a specific question about the client's cardiopulmonary status that the chest x-ray could address.

TEST-TESTING STRATEGY: Read the questions twice to ensure that you understand what the question is asking, especially if the question is tricky or confusing. Focus on what the question is asking: X not Y.

879. Which is a potential complication of central line placement?

A. Hemothorax.

B. Liver laceration.

C. Pneumothorax.

D. Spleen laceration.

Answer: C. Pneumothorax is a potentially life-threatening complication of central line placement. The placement of a central line into the right atrium or right ventricle could cause dysrhythmias, endocrinal damage, cardiac perforation, and pericardial tamponade. Arterial cannulation would result in an inaccurate CVP measurement and would be unsafe for fluid infusion. Other potential complications of central line placement include ectopic placement in the pleural space, infection, and catheter knotting or fragmentation. Hemothorax, liver laceration, and splenic laceration are not complications of central line placement.

TEST-TAKING STRATEGY: Read the questions twice to ensure that you understand what the question is asking, especially if the question is tricky or confusing. Focus on what the question is asking: X not Y.

880. The pulmonary artery catheter, also known as a Swan–Ganz catheter, is commonly used to obtain specific hemodynamic measurements. What is the usual insertion site for a pulmonary artery catheter?

A. Radial artery.

B. Radial vein.

C. Subclavian artery.

D. Subclavian vein.

Answer: D. The pulmonary artery catheter, also known as a Swan–Ganz catheter, is commonly used to obtain specific hemodynamic measurements. The insertion site is generally in the subclavian or internal jugular vein. The radial artery, radial vein, and subclavian artery are not insertion sites for Swan–Ganz catheters.

TEST-TAKING STRATEGY: Read the questions twice to ensure that you understand what the question is asking, especially if the question is tricky or confusion. Focus on what the question is asking: X not Y.

881. A nurse in the intensive care unit is caring for a critically ill client with an intra-aortic balloon pump (IABP). An IABP provides mechanical support for the client's failing heart. Even when inserted properly, the client is at risk for complications. Which complication can result from the use of an IABP?

A. Aortic dissection.

B. Cardiac tamponade.

C. Pneumothorax.

D. Splenic rupture.

Answer: A. The client with the IABP is at risk for an aortic dissection. An IABP is a 26- to 28-mm inflatable balloon surrounding a catheter that is inserted into the descending aorta. Even when inserted properly, there is a risk of aortic dissection, especially when there is pre-existing aortic disease. Cardiac tamponade, pneumothorax, and splenic rupture are not risks associated with IABP insertion.

TEST-TAKING STRATEGY: Use the process of elimination to rule out incorrect answer selections to help choose the correct answer.

882. The nurse in the intensive care unit is caring for a client receiving hemodynamic monitoring. When planning for the client's care, which nursing diagnoses associated with hemodynamic monitoring may be used by the nurse? Select all that apply.

    A. Decreased cardiac output.

    B. Fluid volume deficit.

    C. Fluid volume excess.

    D. Ineffective tissue perfusion.

    Answer: A, B, C, & D.   Nursing diagnoses associated with hemodynamic monitoring that may be used by the nurse include decreased cardiac output, fluid volume deficit, fluid volume excess, and ineffective tissue perfusion. These nursing diagnoses relate to the pathophysiologic processes that alter one of the four hemodynamic mechanisms that support normal cardiovascular function: preload, afterload, heart rate, and contractility.

    TEST-TAKING STRATEGY: When answering "Select all that apply" questions, be sure and treat each answer as a true or false statement. There may be one correct answer or more.

883. Which medication is added to the client's central line infusion/flush setup to maintain the patency of the hemodynamic monitoring system?

    A. Aspirin.

    B. Heparin.

    C. Normal saline.

    D. Zantac.

    Answer: B.   Heparin is added to the infusion/flush setup to maintain catheter patency. Arterial monitoring lines maintained with a heparin flush solution have a greater probability of remaining patent than do lines maintained with nonheparinized solutions, such as normal saline.

Aspirin, normal saline, and Zantac are not used to maintain the patency of a hemodynamic monitoring system.

TEST-TAKING STRATEGY: Read the questions twice to ensure that you understand what the question is asking, especially if the question is tricky or confusing. Focus on what the question is asking.

884. To ensure the accuracy of hemodynamic pressure readings, two baseline measurements are necessary. The first pressure reading is used to calibrate the system to atmospheric pressure, also known as "zeroing" the transducer. Which axis is the second pressure reading used to determine?

    A. Geometric axis.

    B. Hemodynamic axis.

    C. Phlebostatic axis.

    D. Hemodynamic axis.

    Answer: C.   The second pressure reading is used to determine the phlebostatic axis. The phlebostatic axis is a physical reference point on the chest that is used as a baseline for consistent transducer height placement. This point approximates the level of the atria. It is used as the reference mark for both CVP and pulmonary artery catheter transducers.

    TEST-TAKING STRATEGY: Read the questions twice to ensure that you understand what the question is asking, especially if the question is tricky or confusing. Focus on what the question is asking: X not Y.

885. Nurse researchers have determined that the central venous pressure (CVP), pulmonary artery pressure (PAP), and pulmonary artery wedge pressure (PAWP) can be reliably measured at head-of-bed positions. From which position can these pressures be accurately measured?

    A. 0 to 60 degrees if the client is lying prone.

    B. 0 to 60 degrees if the client is lying supine.

    C. 60 to 90 degrees if the client is lying prone.

    D. 60 to 90 degrees if the client is lying supine.

Answer: B. Nurse researchers have determined that the CVP, PAP, and PAWP can be reliably measured at head-of-bed positions from 0 to 60 degrees if the client is lying in a supine position. In general, the majority of clients do not need the head of the bed to be lowered to "0" to obtain accurate CVP, PAP, or PAWP readings.

TEST-TAKING STRATEGY: Read the questions twice to ensure that you understand what the question is asking, especially if the question is tricky or confusing. Focus on what the question is asking: X not Y.

886. If the central venous pressure (CVP) or pulmonary artery pressure (PAP) transducer is placed below the phlebostatic axis, which readings would be obtained? Select all that apply.

   A. Accurate reading.

   B. False high reading.

   C. False low reading.

   D. Inaccurate reading.

   Answer: B & D. An inaccurate, false high reading would be obtained. Error in measurement can occur if the transducer is placed below the phlebostatic axis because the fluid in the system will weigh on the transducer (hydrostatic pressure) and produce a false high reading. If the transducer is placed above the atrial level, gravity and lack of fluid pressure will give an erroneously low reading.

   TEST-TAKING STRATEGY: Read the questions twice to ensure that you understand what the question is asking, especially if the question is tricky or confusing. Focus on what the question is asking: X not Y. "Select all that apply" indicates that there may be more than one correct answer.

887. A client has been diagnosed with mononucleosis. Which statements made by the client let you know that further teaching is needed? Select all that apply.

   A. I can share my spoon while eating with my daughter.

   B. I cannot kiss my spouse and pass saliva for at least 10 weeks.

   C. I cannot play basketball for at least 10 weeks.

   D. I cannot ride my bike for at least 10 weeks.

   Answer: A. Treatment for mononucleosis is supportive with special instructions to avoid saliva contact with any person for at least 10 weeks (no kissing, shared glasses, etc.). Clients should also be advised to avoid any activity that may increase risk for splenic rupture.

   TEST-TAKING STRATEGY: The phrase *further teaching is necessary* tells you to select an answer with inaccurate information.

888. Which factors should the nurse include when teaching a parent about risk factors for otitis media? Select all that apply.

   A. Breast feeding.

   B. Contact with siblings.

   C. Day-care attendance.

   D. Season of the year.

   Answer: B, C, & D. Contact with siblings, day-care attendance, and season of the year all increase a child's risk of developing otitis media. Breast feeding decreases the incidence of acute otitis media.

   TEST-TAKING STRATEGY: When answering "Select all that apply" questions, be sure and treat each answer as a true or false statement. There may be one correct answer or more.

889. Which prevention measures should the nurse include when instructing a client on how to avoid otitis externa?

   A. Avoidance of any activity that may increase risk for splenic rupture.

   B. Simple hand washing and safe food preparation techniques.

   C. Ear canal drying and use of astringent drops after swimming or bathing.

   D. Taking preventative antibiotics prior to dental or other invasive procedures.

   Answer C. Prevention and avoidance measures for otitis externa include thorough ear canal drying and use of acidifying or astringent drops after swimming or bathing. Avoidance of any activity that may increase risk for splenic rupture is a measure taken with mononucleosis. Simple hand-washing and safe food preparation techniques are ways to avoid infectious diarrhea. Avoidance of any activity that may increase risk for splenic rupture is a prevention measure for mononucleosis. Taking preventative antibiotics prior to dental or other invasive procedures is a preventative measure for pericarditis and myocarditis.

TEST-TAKING STRATEGY: Use the process of elimination to rule out incorrect answer selections to help choose the correct answer.

890. A client has been diagnosed with Ludwig's angina. This client has profound brawny edema of the entire superior-anterior neck, dysphagia, and tongue retropulsion and elevation. Which symptoms are also associated with Ludwig's angina? Select all that apply.

A. Bradycardia.

B. Fever.

C. "Tripod" sitting.

D. Toxic appearance.

Answer: C & D. Clients with Ludwig's angina are usually toxic in appearance and frequently insist on a "tripod" sitting position to help open their narrowing upper airway. Bradycardia and fever are not classic signs of Ludwig's angina.

TEST-TAKING STRATEGY: When answering "Select all that apply" questions, be sure and treat each answer as a true or false statement. There may be one correct answer or more.

891. Which are accepted methods of treatment for routine infectious conjunctivitis? Select all that apply.

A. Broad-spectrum antibiotics.

B. Cool compresses.

C. Temporary cessation of contact lens use.

D. Topical antibiotics.

Answer: A, B, C, & D. Broad-spectrum antibiotics, cool compresses, temporary cessation of contact lens use, and topical antibiotics are all used in the treatment of routine infectious conjunctivitis.

TEST-TAKING STRATEGY: When answering "Select all that apply" questions, be sure and treat each answer as a true or false statement. There may be one correct answer or more.

892. Which is the most frequent etiologic agent of bacterial meningitis?

A. *Haemophilus influenzae.*

B. Methacillin-resistant *Staphylococcus aureus.*

C. *Moraxella.*

D. *Streptococcus pneumoniae.*

Answer: D. *Streptococcus pneumoniae* is the leading etiologic agent of bacterial meningitis and responsible for almost half of all episodes. Before the advent of the *Haemophilus influenzae* type B (Hib) vaccine, *H. influenzae* type B accounted for 70% of cases of bacterial meningitis among children under 5 years of age.

TEST-TAKING STRATEGY: Use the process of elimination to rule out incorrect answer selections to help choose the correct answer.

893. A client presents in the emergency department with acute onset of fever, headache, stiff neck, nausea/vomiting, and mental status changes. From which condition is the client most likely suffering?

A. Bacterial meningitis.

B. Peritonsillar abscess.

C. Pharyngitis.

D. Rhinosinusitis.

Answer: A. An acute onset of fever, headache, stiff neck, nausea/vomiting, and mental status changes are consistent with bacterial meningitis.

TEST-TAKING STRATEGY: Use the process of elimination to rule out incorrect answer selections to help choose the correct answer.

894. The nurse is performing a physical assessment on a client. The nurse places the client in a sitting position and observes that the extension of the knee is limited due to pain. Which sign is associated with limited extension of the knee when the hip is flexed?

A. Brudzinski's sign.

B. Homan's sign.

C. Kernig's sign.

D. Peter's sign.

Answer: C. Kernig's sign is described as limited extension of the knee secondary to pain and is elicited by positioning the client in a sitting position with the hip flexed and extending the knee. Extension of the knee is limited secondary to pain.

TEST-TAKING STRATEGY: Use the process of elimination to rule out incorrect answer selections to help choose the correct answer.

895. The nurse is performing a physical assessment on a client. The nurse asks the client to flex the neck. The neck flexion results in flexion of the hip and knee, which is known as Brudzinski's sign. Which condition is associated with Brudzinski's sign?

A. Meningitis.

B. Peritonsillar abscess.

C. Pharyngitis.

D. Rhinosinusitis.

Answer: A. Brudzinski's sign is suggestive of meningitis.

TEST-TAKING STRATEGY: Use the process of elimination to rule out incorrect answer selections to help choose the correct answer.

896. The nurse is performing a physical assessment on a client. The physical assessment is positive for Kernig's sign, Brudzinski's sign, and nuchal rigidity. Which condition is associated with these symptoms?

A. Meningitis.

B. Otitis media.

C. Pharyngitis.

D. Sinusitis.

Answer: A. Kernig's sign, Brudzinski's sign, and nuchal rigidity are all suggestive of meningitis.

TEST-TAKING STRATEGY: Use the process of elimination to rule out incorrect answer selections to help choose the correct answer.

897. Which illness typically presents with headache, fever, and altered mental status?

A. Encephalitis.

B. Meningitis.

C. Pharyngitis.

D. Sinusitis.

Answer: A. Encephalitis is defined as inflammation of the brain parenchyma. Clients with encephalitis present with headache, fever, and altered mental status. The clinical presentation of encephalitis is similar to bacterial meningitis. Clients with bacterial meningitis often present with headache, fever, and nuchal rigidity. Clients with encephalitis present with headache, fever, and altered mental status, ranging from mood disorders to focal neurological deficits to coma.

TEST-TAKING STRATEGY: Use the process of elimination to rule out incorrect answer selections to help choose the correct answer.

898. Encephalitis is defined as an inflammation of the brain parenchyma. Which acute infections may cause encephalitis? Select all that apply.

A. Enterovirus.

B. Herpesviruses.

C. Paramyxoviruses.

D. Rabies.

Answer: A, B, C, & D. Acute infections that may cause encephalitis include enteroviruses, herpesviruses, the paramyxoviruses (measles, mumps), and rabies. The arenaviruses, rubella, and yellow fever may also cause encephalitis.

TEST-TAKING STRATEGY: When answering "Select all that apply" questions, be sure and treat each answer as a true or false statement. There may be one correct answer or more.

899. Which encephalitis is found predominantly west of the Mississippi River and occurs most often during the months of June and July?

A. Eastern equine encephalitis.

B. Saint Louis encephalitis.

C. Venezuelan equine encephalitis.

D. Western equine encephalitis.

Answer: D. Western equine encephalitis is found predominately west of the Mississippi River and occurs most often during the months of June and July. Eastern equine encephalitis occurs along the Eastern seaboard, in the Midwest, and on the Gulf Coast. Saint Louis Encephalitis is distributed throughout the continental US. Venezuelan Equine encephalitis occurs in Central and South America.

TEST-TAKING STRATEGY: Use the process of elimination to rule out incorrect answer selections to help choose the correct answer.

900. The nurse is caring for a client with an opportunistic infection of the central nervous system. The nurse knows that opportunistic infections affecting the central nervous system are extremely likely once the CD4 count drops below which level?

A. $50/mm^3$.

B. $75/mm^3$.

C. $100/mm^3$.

D. $200/mm^3$.

Answer: D. Opportunistic infections affecting the central nervous system are extremely likely once the CD4 count drops below $200/mm^3$.

TEST-TAKING STRATEGY: Look for similar answer choices and eliminate them.

901. A virus exists that has the potential to cause significant morbidity and mortality globally, killing more Americans every year than any other infectious disease, including AIDS. This virus causes acute viral respiratory illness that is usually self-limited. Which virus does this describe?

A. Adenovirus.

B. Enterovirus.

C. Influenza.

D. Paramyxoviruses.

Answer: C. Influenza kills more Americans every year than any other infectious disease, including AIDS. Adenovirus, enterovirus, and paramyxoviruses do not have this impact.

TEST-TAKING STRATEGY: Use the process of elimination to rule out incorrect answer selections to help choose the correct answer.

902. Which are risk factors for post-influenza complications? Select all that apply.

A. Age over 65 years.

B. Chronic cardiopulmonary disease.

C. Diabetes.

D. Renal disease.

Answer: A, B, C, & D. Clients who are over the age of 65, or who have chronic cardiopulmonary disease, diabetes, or renal disease, are all at risk for post-influenza complications. In addition, clients who reside in a closed community, such as a nursing home, are also at risk.

TEST-TAKING STRATEGY: When answering "Select all that apply" questions, be sure and treat each answer as a true or false statement. There may be one correct answer or more.

903. The live intranasal vaccine (FluMist) is indicated for use only in healthy persons. For which age group is the vaccine appropriate?

A. 6 months to 5 years of age.

B. 5 to 49 years of age.

C. 49 to 65 years of age.

D. 65 and older.

Answer: B. The live intranasal vaccine is indicated for use only in healthy persons aged 5 to 49 years of age.

TEST-TAKING STRATEGY: Use the process of elimination to rule out incorrect answer selections to help choose the correct answer.

904. To which groups of clients should the live intranasal vaccine be administered?

A. Clients undergoing chemotherapy.

B. Clients with HIV.

C. Healthy persons aged 5 to 49 years of age.

D. Pregnant women.

Answer: C. Healthy persons aged 5 to 49 years of age are appropriate candidates for live intranasal vaccination. Intranasal administration poses a risk to pregnant mothers and to immunocompromised clients, such as those undergoing chemotherapy and those with HIV.

TEST-TAKING STRATEGY: Use the process of elimination to rule out incorrect answer selections to help choose the correct answer.

905. Which are signs of community-acquired pneumonia? Select all that apply.

A. Cough.

B. Crackles.

C. Egophany.

D. Tactile fremitus.

Answer: A, B, C, & D. Signs of community-acquired pneumonia include cough, crackles, egophany, tactile fremitus, fever, dyspnea, sputum production, and myalgias.

TEST-TAKING STRATEGY: When answering "Select all that apply" questions, be sure and treat each answer as a true or false statement. There may be one correct answer or more.

906. Which atypical pathogens are associated with community-acquired pneumonia? Select all that apply.

A. *Chlamydia pneumoniae.*

B. *Legionella pneumophila.*

C. *Mycoplasma pneumoniae.*

D. *Streptococcus pneumoniae.*

Answer: A, B, & C. Atypical pathogens in community acquired-pneumonia include *Chlamydia pneumoniae*, *Legionella pneumophila*, and *Mycoplasma pneumoniae*. The most commonly isolated etiology of community-acquired pneumonia is *Streptococcus pneumoniae*.

TEST-TAKING STRATEGY: Use the process of elimination to rule out incorrect answer selections to help choose the correct answer.

907. A client is diagnosed with pneumonia. What signs of this disease process should the nurse anticipate? Select all that apply.

A. Cough.

B. Dyspnea.

C. Fever.

D. Leukocytosis.

Answer: A, B, C, & D. Clients with pneumonia usually complain of cough, dyspnea, a sudden onset of chills followed by fever, and leukocytosis resulting in purulent sputum production.

TEST-TAKING STRATEGY: When answering "Select all that apply" questions, be sure and treat each answer as a true or false statement. There may be one correct answer or more.

908. Which diseases are often incorrectly diagnosed as community-acquired pneumonia? Select all that apply.

A. Acute myocardial infarction.

B. Aortic dissection.

C. Congestive heart failure.

D. Pulmonary embolism.

Answer: C & D. Two diseases often incorrectly diagnosed as community-acquired pneumonia are congestive heart failure and pulmonary embolism. In any of these diseases, clients can experience leukocytosis, fever, constitutional symptoms, chest radiograph changes, hypoxia, adventitial lung sounds on auscultation, cough, and minor hemoptysis.

TEST-TAKING STRATEGY: Read the questions twice to ensure that you understand what the question is asking, especially if the question is tricky or confusing. "Select all that apply" indicates that there may be more than one answer option.

909. The nurse asks the client to say "EEE" and hears "AYE" over an area of consolidation. Which term is used to describe this phenomenon?

A. Egophony.

B. Percussion.

C. Tactile fremitus.

D. Whispered pectroliliquy.

Answer: A. This phenomenon described is called egophony. Percussion that produces dullness indicates that fluid occupies formerly air-filled spaces. Tactile fremitus is performed by asking a client to repeat "99" and comparing each hemithorax for pleural effusion (decreased or absent fremitus) or infiltrate (increased fremitus). Whispered pectroliliquy can be performed by asking the client to whisper. The spoken words are clearer and louder over areas of consolidation than over unaffected areas of the lung.

TEST-TAKING STRATEGY: Use the process of elimination to rule out incorrect answer selections to help choose the correct answer.

910. A newly recognized corona virus has been identified as the causative agent of which disease?

A. Bronchitis.

B. Influenza.

C. Pneumonia.

D. SARS.

Answer: D. The newly recognized corona virus has been identified as the causative agent of SARS, a highly contagious and deadly disease. This illness should be suspected in those who have recently traveled to an area where SARS is present, or have had contact with someone who has traveled to these areas, has the disease, or has symptoms of a respiratory illness and fever. Bronchitis, influenza, and pneumonia are not caused by corona virus.

TEST-TAKING STRATEGY: Use the process of elimination to rule out incorrect answer selections to help choose the correct answer.

911. What infectious agents cause tuberculosis (TB)? Select all that apply.

A. *Mycobacterium africanum.*

B. *Mycobacterium bovis.*

C. *Mycobacterium microti.*

D. *Mycobacterium tuberculosis.*

Answer: A, B, C, & D. Tuberculosis is defined as a disease caused by members of the *Mycobacterium tuberculosis* complex, which includes *M. tuberculosis*, *M. bovis*, *M. africanum*, and *M. microti*. The cell-wall components give the mycobacterium its characteristic staining properties. The organism stains gram positive. The mycolic acid structure confers the ability to resist destaining by acid alcohol after being stained by certain aniline dyes, hence the term acid-fast bacillus (AFB).

TEST-TAKING STRATEGY: When answering "Select all that apply" questions, be sure and treat each answer as a true or false statement. There may be one correct answer or more.

912. Which are immunosuppressive conditions associated with reactivation TB? Select all that apply.

A. AIDS.

B. End-stage renal disease.

C. Diabetes mellitus.

D. HIV infection.

Answer: A, B, C, & D. Immunosuppressive conditions associated with reactivation TB include HIV infection and AIDS, end-stage renal disease, diabetes mellitus, malignancies, chronic immunosuppressive drug use, and age-related immune deficiencies. In general, individuals who become infected with *M. tuberculosis* have approximately a 10% risk for developing active TB during their lifetimes. This risk is greatest during the first 2 years after infection. Immuno-compromised persons have greater risk for the progression of latent TB infection to active TB diseases.

TEST-TAKING STRATEGY: When answering "Select all that apply" questions, be sure and treat each answer as a true or false statement. There may be one correct answer or more.

913. A nurse is caring for a client who complains of fatigue, weight loss, afternoon fevers, night sweats, cough, and hemoptysis. The nurse immediately puts the client in isolation. The nurse suspects that the client is suffering from which condition?

A. Bronchitis.

B. Pneumonia.

C. Pneumothorax.

D. Tuberculosis.

Answer: D. The nurse suspects that the client is suffering from tuberculosis. Early pulmonary tuberculosis is asymptomatic. When the bacterial load increases, nonspecific constitutional symptoms of fatigue, weight loss, afternoon fevers, and night sweats may set in. As disease burden advances, cough, sputum production, and localized symptoms such as hemoptysis may appear. This client has the classic symptoms of tuberculosis and should be placed in respiratory isolation. Bronchitis, pneumonia, and pneumothorax do not classically present with the symptoms listed and are not on respiratory isolation.

TEST-TAKING STRATEGY: Use the process of elimination to rule out incorrect answer selections to help choose the correct answer.

914. Which segments of the population are at increased risk for tuberculosis? Select all that apply.

A. Current and former residents of correctional facilities.

B. Elderly in long-term facilities.

C. Foreign-born persons from areas with high TB prevalence.

D. Homeless persons.

Answer: A, B, C, & D. Certain segments of the population are at increased risk for TB. These include foreign-born persons from areas with high TB prevalence, homeless persons, those residing in underserved sections of inner cities, current and former residents of correctional facilities, persons with history of substance abuse, and the elderly in long-term facilities.

TEST-TAKING STRATEGY: When answering "Select all that apply" questions, be sure and treat each answer as a true or false statement. There may be one correct answer or more.

915. About 80% of all tuberculosis is pulmonary. Which other areas are affected by tuberculosis? Select all that apply.

A. Bone.

B. Genitourinary tract.

C. Lymph nodes.

D. Pleura.

Answer: A, B, C, & D. Bone, the genitourinary tract, lymph nodes, and the pleura are all affected by tuberculosis. Of these areas, TB affects the pleura 30% of the time, the lymph nodes 30% of the time, and the remaining 40% involves the genitourinary tract, bone, the central nervous system, and miliary disease.

TEST-TAKING STRATEGY: When answering "Select all that apply" questions, be sure and treat each answer as a true or false statement. There may be one correct answer or more.

916. Many persons with active tuberculosis often first present in ambulatory care settings. What is the first action that should be taken in caring for a client with symptoms of tuberculosis?

A. Identify and evaluate the client promptly.

B. Instruct the client to cover the mouth and nose with tissues when sneezing or coughing.

C. Isolate the client in a negative pressure room.

D. Place a surgical mask on the client.

Answer: A. The *first* action that should be taken is to identify and evaluate the client promptly.

TEST-TAKING STRATEGY: Read the question carefully. Questions that ask you to prioritize your nursing actions use terms like *priority, first, best, initial, most important,* and *next.*

917. When teaching tuberculosis containment issues to the staff at the local hospital, the nurse educator emphasizes the use of personal protective equipment (PPE) in caring for clients with TB. Under which circumstances should a respiratory protective mask be worn? Select all that apply.

A. When entering a TB isolation room when the client is present.

B. When administrative and engineering controls are unlikely to be protective.

C. When an aerosol-inducing procedure is being performed, such as during the administration of aerosolized drugs.

D. When a cough-inducing procedure is being performed, such as induced sputum collection.

Answer: A, B, C, & D.   When caring for a client who may have TB, a respiratory protective mask should be worn under all circumstances.

TEST-TAKING STRATEGY: When answering "Select all that apply" questions, be sure and treat each answer as a true or false statement. There may be one correct answer or more.

918. Which hepatitis virus is most likely to be transmitted through the fecal–oral route?

A. Hepatitis A.

B. Hepatitis B.

C. Hepatitis C.

D. Hepatitis D.

Answer: A.   Hepatitis A virus is transmitted through the fecal–oral route either by ingestion of contaminated food or water or by direct contact with an infected individual. Hepatitis B virus is transmitted percutaneously and more rarely by body fluid exposures. Hepatitis C virus is transmitted percutaneously and sexually. Hepatitis D virus is transmitted percutaneously and generally occurs only in the presence of hepatitis B infections.

TEST-TAKING STRATEGY: Use knowledge and the process of elimination to rule out incorrect answer options.

919. Which hepatitis virus has only one serotype, stimulates antibodies that are thought to result in lifelong immunity, has an incubation period of approximately 28 days, and can unknowingly be passed by the host?

A. Hepatitis A.

B. Hepatitis B.

C. Hepatitis C.

D. Hepatitis D.

Answer: A.   Hepatitis A virus has only one serotype, stimulates antibodies that are thought to result in lifelong immunity, has an incubation period of approximately 28 days, and can be passed from the host without detection. The viral shedding occurs during the 14 days that precede the onset of jaundice. Infectivity declines during the week after symptom onset. Therefore, clients will pass the virus without knowing they are infected. Hepatitis B, C, and D do not share these characteristics.

TEST-TAKING STRATEGY: Use the process of elimination to rule out incorrect answer selections to help choose the correct answer.

920. Which hepatitis virus begins with nonspecific symptoms such as low-grade fever, nausea, vomiting, diarrhea, myalgias, anorexia, and malaise? Select all that apply.

A. Hepatitis A.

B. Hepatitis B.

C. Hepatitis C.

D. Hepatitis D.

Answer: A, B, & C.   Hepatitis A infection begins with nonspecific symptoms such as low-grade fever, nausea, vomiting, diarrhea, myalgias, anorexia, and malaise. Symptoms such as jaundice, light-colored stools, dark urine, right upper quadrant pain, or general abdominal discomfort might follow in a few days or be present at onset. Hepatitis B and C infections can also clinically present with the same constitutional symptoms. Hepatitis D is a concomitant infection found with hepatitis B.

TEST-TAKING STRATEGY: When answering "Select all that apply" questions, be sure and treat each answer as a true or false statement. There may be one correct answer or more.

921. A nurse is working triage in an emergency department (ED). A client presents in the ED complaining of stomach pain. The nurse palpates the abdomen and discovers that the client has right upper quadrant tenderness. The physician suspects cholecystitis. Which symptoms should the nurse anticipate when caring for a client with cholecystitis? Select all that apply.

A. Chills.

B. Fever.

C. Nausea and vomiting.

D. Right upper quadrant pain.

Answer: A, B, C, & D. Many clients with acute cholecystitis present with acute onset of right upper quadrant pain associated with nausea and vomiting. Epigastric pain may also be present. Additional symptoms may include fever, chills, and anorexia. A physical examination often reveals right upper quadrant tenderness. Rebound and guarding are present in some cases.

TEST-TAKING STRATEGY: When answering "Select all that apply" questions, be sure and treat each answer as a true or false statement. There may be one correct answer or more.

922. Which aerobic gram-negative bacillus is the most common pathogen for all manifestations of urinary tract infection in all groups of clients?

A. *Escherichia coli.*

B. *Klebsiella.*

C. *Pseudomonas aeruginosa.*

D. *Staphylococcus aureus.*

Answer: A. The aerobic gram-negative bacillus, *Escherichia coli*, remains the most common pathogen for all manifestations of urinary tract infections and in all groups of clients. It is the causative pathogen in approximately 80% to 90% of clients diagnosed with acute uncomplicated cystitis or acute uncomplicated pyelonephritis. *Klebsiella, Pseudomonas aeruginosa,* and *Staphylococcus aureus* are causative factors in urinary tract infections but are not the most common pathogens.

TEST-TAKING STRATEGY: Use the process of elimination to rule out incorrect answer selections to help choose the correct answer.

923. The nurse is caring for a client with a suspected urinary tract infection. Which symptoms are associated with urinary tract infections? Select all that apply.

A. Abdominal pain.

B. Dysuria.

C. Frequency.

D. Hematuria.

Answer: A, B, C, & D. Most clients with a urinary tract infection will have some combination of dysuria, frequency, or hematuria.

TEST-TAKING STRATEGY: When answering "Select all that apply" questions, be sure and treat each answer as a true or false statement. There may be one correct answer or more.

924. The client has been diagnosed with an uncomplicated urinary tract infection and prescribed the medication levofloxacin (Levaquin). The nurse knows that this medication is a quinolone. Which information should be given to the client regarding quinolones? Select all that apply.

A. Antacids can affect absorption.

B. Children 18 and under can safely take this medication.

C. The medication may cause gastrointestinal and dermatologic side effects.

D. They can increase the effects of warfarin.

Answer: A, C, & D. Quinolones are generally well tolerated with once-daily dosing. Aluminum and magnesium-containing antacids can affect the absorption of quinolones. Quinolones may cause gastrointestinal and dermatologic side effects and can increase the effects of warfarin. Other side effects may include central nervous system effects, torsades de pointes, and QT prolongation. Quinolones are not safely used in children under age 18 or in women who are pregnant or nursing.

TEST-TAKING STRATEGY: When answering "Select all that apply" questions, be sure and treat each answer as a true or false statement. There may be one correct answer or more.

925. The nurse is caring for a child who has a fever. Which factors should be included in the nurse's assessment of the child? Select all that apply.

    A. Age.

    B. Behavior.

    C. General appearance.

    D. Magnitude of the fever.

    Answer: A, B, C, & D. The child's age, magnitude of fever, general appearance, and behavior should all be evaluated by the nurse.

    TEST-TAKING STRATEGY: When answering "Select all that apply" questions, be sure and treat each answer as a true or false statement. There may be one correct answer or more.

926. The nurse is caring for a client with sepsis. Which symptoms should the nurse expect to see in a client with sepsis? Select all that apply.

    A. Cool extremities.

    B. Decreased systolic arterial blood pressure.

    C. Mottled skin.

    D. Tachycardia.

    Answer: A, B, C, & D. Cardiovascular derangements due to sepsis may include cool extremities, decreased systolic and/or diastolic arterial blood pressure, mottled skin, and tachycardia.

    TEST-TAKING STRATEGY: When answering "Select all that apply" questions, be sure and treat each answer as a true or false statement. There may be one correct answer or more.

927. The nurse knows varicella is a highly infectious agent that is spread primarily by (select all that apply):

    A. Direct contact.

    B. Fecal contact.

    C. Oral contact.

    D. Respiratory droplets.

Answer: A & D. Varicella is a highly infectious agent that is spread primarily via respiratory droplets. Direct contact with infectious lesions is also another route of infection.

TEST-TAKING STRATEGY: When answering "Select all that apply" questions, be sure and treat each answer as a true or false statement. There may be one correct answer or more.

928. The nurse knows which illness represents a reactivation of the latent varicella zoster virus? Select all that apply.

    A. Hepatitis.

    B. Herpes simplex.

    C. Herpes zoster.

    D. Shingles.

    Answer: C & D. Herpes zoster, or shingles, represents a reactivation of the latent varicella zoster virus. Clients must have prior exposure and infection with chickenpox or have received the varicella vaccine. The eruption is sporadic, there is no seasonal prevalence, and an increasing incidence of disease is seen with increasing age. Hepatitis and herpes simplex are not caused by reactivation of the latent varicella zoster virus.

    TEST-TAKING STRATEGY: When answering "Select all that apply" questions, be sure and treat each answer as a true or false statement. There may be one correct answer or more.

929. The nurse cares for client with diabetes mellitus type 2. The nurse knows diabetics are prone to foot ulcerations due to (select all that apply):

    A. Infection.

    B. Ischemia.

    C. Neuropathy.

    D. Nutritional dysfunction.

    Answer: A, B, C, & D. Diabetics are more susceptible to foot ulcerations than clients without diabetes because of ischemia, neuropathy, infection, and nutritional dysfunction.

    TEST-TAKING STRATEGY: When answering "Select all that apply" questions, be sure and treat each answer as a true or false statement. There may be one correct answer or more.

930. The nurse who works in the emergency department cares for a client who was bitten by a stray cat. Which gram-negative causative organism is found in 75% of cat bite wound infections?

A. *Bacteroides.*

B. *Fusobacterium.*

C. *Pasteurella.*

D. *Prevotella.*

Answer: C. *Pasteurella* species are found in 75% of cat bite wound infections and 50% of dog bite infections. *Bacteroides, Fusobacterium,* and *Prevotella* are not found in the majority of cat bite wounds.

TEST-TAKING STRATEGY: Use the process of elimination to rule out incorrect answer selections to help choose the correct answer.

931. *Clostridium tetani* is an anaerobic, gram-positive bacillus that forms spores. It is found in soil, dust, rust, and the feces of animals and humans. These spores are highly resilient to extremes in temperatures, moisture, and chemical substances. Once exposed to anaerobic conditions, such as the environment associated with wounds, tissue necrosis, or foreign bodies, the spores can germinate. Which organism is this?

A. Folliculitis.

B. Osteomyelitis.

C. Rabies.

D. Tetanus.

Answer: D. Tetanus is found in the environment and waste products of animals and humans. The spores can germinate and cause illness to humans.

TEST-TAKING STRATEGY: Use the process of elimination to rule out incorrect answer selections to help choose the correct answer.

932. A client complains of being stung by a yellow jacket, which caused "whelps" on the skin and light-headedness. The nurse knows first-line treatment consists of:

A. Cool compresses.

B. Intravenous access.

C. Supplemental oxygen therapy.

D. Tetanus injection.

Answer: C. This client exhibits signs of anaphylactic shock. First-line treatment consists of supplemental oxygen therapy, intravenous access, epinephrine administration, albuterol or another beta-agonist nebulizer, hydrocortisone or methylprednisolone administration, and histamine H2 and H1 administration.

TEST-TAKING STRATEGY: Always pick that answer that is most life threatening or the nursing intervention that is most lifesaving.

933. A client complains of crushing chest pain 3 hours prior to arrival in the emergency department. Initial vital signs show hypotension: a weak, thready pulse; cool, clammy skin; and confusion. Which intervention should the nurse perform first?

A. Airway management.

B. Intravenous access.

C. Obtaining an EKG.

D. Preparing for an intra-aortic balloon pump.

Answer: A. This client exhibits signs of cardiogenic shock, a complication of myocardial infarction. Hypotension accompanied by clinical signs of increased peripheral resistance (weak, thready pulse and cool, clammy skin) and inadequate organ perfusion (altered mental status and decreased urine output) are found in this client. Airway management is always the most important intervention. Intravenous access, obtaining an EKG, and possible preparation for an intra-aortic balloon pump are interventions that occur after the initial intervention of airway management.

TEST-TAKING STRATEGY: Always pick the answer that is most life threatening or the nursing intervention that is most lifesaving.

934. Which type of shock is known for decreased intravascular volume resulting from loss of blood or plasma?

A. Cardiogenic shock.

B. Hypovolemic shock.

C. Neurogenic shock.

D. Obstructive shock.

Answer: **B.** Hypovolemic shock results in decreased intravascular volume resulting from loss of blood or plasma. Obstructive shock occurs when impaired filling of the ventricles causes a fall in cardiac output. Neurogenic shock occurs when hypotension is present in the presence of spinal cord injury. Cardiogenic shock is shock in the setting of cardiac outflow obstruction or pump failure.

TEST-TAKING STRATEGY: Use the process of elimination to rule out incorrect answer selections to help choose the correct answer.

935. A client complains of wheezing, cough, and chest tightness. The client has a history of asthma, but has been out of medications for this condition for the past 3 weeks. Which is a priority nursing intervention?

    A. Prepare to administer an inhaled corticosteroid.

    B. Prepare to administer an oral steroid.

    C. Prepare to administer a parenteral steroid.

    D. Prepare to administer a short-acting bronchodilator.

Answer: **D.** The first-line therapy for acute asthma is the administration of an inhaled short-acting bronchodilator. All of the choices are correct, but the most important action to take first is administering a bronchodilator to open the air passages.

TEST-TAKING STRATEGY: Questions that ask you to prioritize your nursing actions use terms like *priority, first, best, initial, most important,* and *next.*

936. A client complains of acute onset of periumbilical pain that is well localized over McBurney's point. This pain is accompanied by a low-grade fever. As the client is triaged, the nurse palpates the left lower quadrant causing, the client to complain of right lower quadrant pain. Which sign does this best describe?

    A. Homans' sign.

    B. Kernig's sign.

C. Ludwig's sign.

D. Rovsing's sign.

Answer: **D.** The signs this client is exhibiting are characteristic of appendicitis. Pain in the right lower quadrant when the left lower quadrant is palpated is characteristic of Rovsing's sign. Homans' sign is pain on passive dorsiflexion of the ankle. Kernig's sign is pain in the hamstrings upon extension of the knee with the hip at 90-degree flexion. There is no such thing as Ludwig's sign.

TEST-TAKING STRATEGY: Use the process of elimination to rule out incorrect answer selections to help choose the correct answer.

937. In a client with ulcerative colitis, the nurse should expect to find (select all that apply):

    A. Acute abdominal pain.

    B. Bloody diarrhea.

    C. Fever.

    D. Vomiting.

Answer: **B, C, & D.** Ulcerative colitis is characterized by an idiopathic inflammatory disorder involving the submucosa of the rectum and spreading proximally without skipping areas. This condition usually has chronic recurrent abdominal pain, bloody diarrhea, tenesmus, vomiting, and fever.

TEST-TAKING STRATEGY: Read the questions twice to ensure that you understand what the question is asking, especially if the question is tricky or confusing. Also, in "select all that apply" questions, there may be one or more than one correct answers.

938. Which condition is caused by arterial bleeding from tears in the distal esophagus or promixal stomach?

    A. Appendicitis.

    B. Gastritis.

    C. Ischemic colitis.

    D. Mallory–Weiss syndrome.

Answer: D. Mallory–Weiss syndrome occurs with arterial bleeding from tears in the distal esophagus or proximal stomach. It is believed to arise from large pressure gradient between the chest and stomach. Patients usually present with acute hematemesis but can present with melena, hematochezia, abdominal pain, or syncope. Appendicitis, gastritis, and ischemic colitis are not caused by arterial bleeding from tears in the distal esophagus or proximal stomach.

TEST-TAKING STRATEGY: Read the questions twice to ensure that you understand what the question is asking, especially if the question is tricky or confusing.

939. Which tinea is best described by an annular erythematous patch on the body, hands, or face?

   A. Tinea capitus.

   B. Tinea corporis.

   C. Tinea cruris.

   D. Tinea pedis.

Answer: B. Tinea corporis is characterized by an annular erythematous patch with leading edge of scale and varying degrees of central clearing on the body, hands, or face. Tinea pedis is characterized by a scale on the lateral aspects of the feet or maceration between the toes. Tinea capitus is characterized by circumscribed patches of slopecia with varying degrees of scale and erythema. Tinea cruris involves the moist areas of groin and buttocks with scrotal sparing.

TEST-TAKING STRATEGY: Use the process of elimination to rule out incorrect answer selections to help choose the correct answer.

940. Which skin condition is characterized by erythematous plaques with an adherent silvery scale usually appearing over the extensor surfaces of the extremities, including lesions on the palms, soles, scalp, umbilicus, and genital areas?

   A. Impetigo.

   B. Molluscum contagiosum.

   C. Pityriasis rosea.

   D. Psoriasis.

Answer: D. Psoriasis is characterized by erythematous plaques with adherent silvery scale usually appearing over the extensor surfaces of the extremities, including lesions on the palms, soles, scalp, umbilicus, and genital areas. Pityriasis rosea consists of pruritic brownish to erythematous oval patches with a collarette of scale, classically in a Christmas-tree distribution of the trunk. Molluscum contagiosum is discrete flesh-colored to pink, dome-shaped, umbilicated papules singly or in groups; they are smooth, and shiny, some may have a keratotic plug. Impetigo starts as small, erythematous macules, which progress to fragile blisters that break, releasing a serous discharge that dries to form a honey-colored crust.

TEST-TAKING STRATEGY: Use the process of elimination to rule out incorrect answer selections to help choose the correct answer.

941. A client suffers from a right radial fracture. The client now complains of severe pain in the right arm accompanied with edema in the fingers. The nurse suspects:

   A. Carpal tunnel syndrome.

   B. Compartment syndrome.

   C. Subsequent ulnar fracture.

   D. Ulnar nerve palsy.

Answer: B. This situation best describes compartment syndrome. Compartment syndrome is when edema within a closed space may result in vascular compromise and decreased blood flow with eventual neurologic compromise. There are five P's of compartment syndrome: pallor, pulselessness, pain, paresthesias, and poikilothermia. This does not describe carpal tunnel syndrome, ulnar fracture, or ulnar nerve palsy. The key to this question is that this client has recently sustained a right radial fracture.

TEST-TAKING STRATEGY: Use the process of elimination to rule out incorrect answer selections to help choose the correct answer.

942. A client is involved in a horseback riding accident. The client complains of right upper quadrant pain and radiation to the right shoulder. In which injury is this most compatible?

A. Diaphragmatic hernia.

B. Liver injury.

C. Pancreatic injury.

D. Splenic injury.

Answer: B. The symptoms of this injury are most compatible with liver injury. This type of injury alone can be the cause of hemodynamic instability. The spleen and pancreas are located in the left upper quadrant.

TEST-TAKING STRATEGY: Use the process of elimination to rule out incorrect answer selections to help choose the correct answer.

943. A client presents with a right tension pneumothorax. The nurse expects to find which sign and symptom?

A. Diminished breath sounds on the left.

B. Hypertension.

C. Hypoxia.

D. Tracheal deviation to the right.

Answer: C. Tension pneumothorax presents with absent or decreased breath sounds, hyper-resonance to chest wall percussion, tracheal deviation (away from the side of the pneumothorax) in the presence of respiratory distress, and hypotension. Respiratory distress, tachypnea, hypotension, and hypoxia are signs of this condition. Tension pneumothorax results in hemodynamic instability and death unless treated promptly.

TEST-TAKING STRATEGY: Read the questions twice to ensure that you understand what the question is asking, especially if the question is tricky or confusing.

944. A client experiences a nosebleed. The nurse documents this as:

A. Epistaxis.

B. Miosis.

C. Hematoma.

D. Myalgia.

Answer: A. Epistaxis is the medical term for nosebleed. Epistaxis may be caused by nasal trauma, nose picking, dry environmental conditions, warfarin or platelet-inhibiting drug use, renal failure, or other bleeding disorders. Miosis is pin-point pupils, hematoma is a bruise, and myalgia is muscle pain.

TEST-TAKING STRATEGY: Use the process of elimination to rule out incorrect answer selections to help choose the correct answer.

945. The nurse cares for a client diagnosed with angina. Which type of angina is caused by coronary artery spasm?

A. Variant angina.

B. Silent angina.

C. Stable angina.

D. Unstable angina.

Answer: A. Variant, or Prinzmetal angina is caused by coronary artery spasm. It results from spasm with or without atherosclerotic lesions. There is no such thing as silent angina. Stable angina is predictable and caused by similar precipitating factors each time, such as exercise, emotional upset, and tachycardia. Unstable angina is defined as a change in a previously established stable pattern of angina or a new onset of severe angina. It is usually more intense than stable angina, may awaken the client from sleep, or may necessitate more than nitrates for pain relief. A change in the level or frequency of symptoms requires immediate medical evaluation.

TEST-TAKING STRATEGY: Use the process of elimination to rule out incorrect answer selections to help choose the correct answer.

946. A client is diagnosed with emphysema. Which clinical sign should the nurse expect to see? Select all that apply.

A. Atelectasis.

B. Barrel chest.

C. Tachypnea.

D. Use of accessory muscles with respiration.

Answer: B, C, & D. Emphysema is described as a permanent hyperinflation of lung beyond the bronchioles with destruction of alveolar walls. Airway resistance is increased, especially on expiration. Inspection reveals dyspnea on exertion, barrel chest, tachypnea, and use of accessory muscles with respiration. Atelectasis is collapse of alveolar lung tissue, and findings reflect presence of a small, airless lung; this condition is caused by complete obstruction of a draining bronchus by a tumor, thick secretions, or an aspirated foreign body, or by compression of lung.

TEST-TAKING STRATEGY: Use the process of elimination to rule out incorrect answer selections to help choose the correct answer. Also, in "select all that apply" questions, there may be more than one correct answer.

947. The nurse cares for a client with thromboembolism. Which is a predisposing factor for pulmonary thromboembolism? Select all that apply.

A. Atrial fibrillation.

B. Hypercoagulability.

C. Immobility.

D. Injury to vascular endothelium.

Answer: A, B, C, & D. Predisposing factors for pulmonary thromboembolism include venous stasis—atrial fibrillation, decreased cardiac output, immobility; injury to vascular endothelium—local vessel injury, infection, incision, atherosclerosis; and hypercoagulability—polycythemia.

TEST-TAKING STRATEGY: When answering "Select all that apply" questions, be sure and treat each answer as a true or false statement. There may be one correct answer or more.

948. Which nursing diagnosis relates to self-concept disturbances imposed by critical stages of illness? Select all that apply.

A. Disturbed body image.

B. Ineffective coping.

C. Ineffective role performance.

D. Situational low self-esteem.

Answer: A, B, C, & D. Nursing diagnoses related to self-concept disturbances imposed by critical stages of illness include disturbed body image, situational low self-esteem, ineffective role performance, ineffective coping, and compromised family coping.

TEST-TAKING STRATEGY: When answering "Select all that apply" questions, be sure and treat each answer as a true or false statement. There may be one correct answer or more.

949. Client experiences of critical illness and care vary. Which is a stressor that a critically ill client may experience? Select all that apply.

A. Lack of sleep.

B. Loss of dignity.

C. Pain or discomfort.

D. Threat of death.

Answer: A, B, C, & D. The following stressors may be experienced by a critically ill client: threat of death; threat of survival, with significant residual problems related to the illness/injury; pain, or discomfort; lack of sleep; loss of autonomy over most aspects of life and daily functioning; loss of control over environment, such as loss of privacy and exposure to light, noise, and general activity of the critical care unit, including the care of other clients; daily hassles or common frustrations; loss of usual role and, with that, the arena in which usual coping mechanisms serve the client; separation from family and friends; loss of dignity; boredom broken only by brief visits, threatening stimuli, and frightening thoughts; and loss of ability to express self verbally when intubated.

TEST-TAKING STRATEGY: When answering "Select all that apply" questions, be sure and treat each answer as a true or false statement. There may be one correct answer or more.

950. The nurse knows that the causes of powerlessness a client may feel are due to (select all that apply):

A. Illness-related regimen.

B. Interpersonal interactions.

C. One's culture.

D. One's religious beliefs.

Answer: A, B, C, & D. Powerlessness is defined as the perception of the individual that one's own action will not significantly affect an outcome. Unrelieved powerlessness may result in hopelessness. The causes of powerlessness include factors in the health care environment, interpersonal interactions, one's culture and religious beliefs, illness-related regimen, and a life-style of helplessness.

TEST-TAKING STRATEGY: When answering "Select all that apply" questions, be sure and treat each answer as a true or false statement. There may be one correct answer or more.

951. Which nursing diagnosis may critically ill clients experience? Select all that apply.

   A. Powerlessness.

   B. Hopelessness.

   C. Spiritual distress.

   D. Mental status changes.

   Answer: A, B, C, & D. Powerlessness, hopelessness, spiritual distress, and mental status changes can all be experienced by critically ill clients.

   TEST-TAKING STRATEGY: When answering "Select all that apply" questions, be sure and treat each answer as a true or false statement. There may be one correct answer or more.

952. A client faced with an intolerable situation may (select all that apply):

   A. Be suspicious of motives and methods of the caregivers.

   B. Display behavior that distorts reality.

   C. Exhibit excessive demands.

   D. Panic.

   Answer: A, B, C, & D. Any event with unpredictable body changes and functions requires adjustments in the self-concept as well as a realistic readjustment to the role limitations that are imposed. These adjustment stages are complex and highly individualized. A person faced with an intolerable situation may panic, may display behavior that distorts reality, and may exhibit excessive demands or be suspicious of motives and methods of the caregivers.

TEST-TAKING STRATEGY: When answering "Select all that apply" questions, be sure and treat each answer as a true or false statement. There may be one correct answer or more.

953. Anxiety elicits changes in the neurohumoral-release patterns involving the neurotransmitters, including:

   A. Acetylcholine.

   B. Epinephrine.

   C. Insulin.

   D. Sodium.

   Answer: A. Anxiety elicits changes in the neurohumoral release patterns involving the neurotransmitters, including acetylcholine, norepinephrine, dopamine, serotonin, and their corresponding receptors. Epinephrine, insulin, and sodium are not hormones that are initially impacted by anxiety.

   TEST-TAKING STRATEGY: Use the process of elimination to rule out incorrect answer selections to help choose the correct answer.

954. Which reaction is common as the client experiences a loss of control and worries over outcomes? Select all that apply.

   A. Anxiety.

   B. Depression.

   C. Fatigue.

   D. Happiness.

   Answer: A & B. Any event with unpredictable body changes and functions requires adjustments in the self-concept as well as a realistic readjustment to the role limitations that are imposed. These adjustments are complex and highly individualized. A person faced with an intolerable situation may panic, display behavior that distorts reality, exhibit excessive demands, or be suspicious of motives and methods of the caregivers. Depression and anxiety are common reactions as the person experiences a loss of control and worries over outcomes. Fatigue and happiness are not common reactions to loss of control.

TEST-TAKING STRATEGY: Use the process of elimination to rule out incorrect answer selections to help choose the correct answer.

955. Clients who have extended stays in the critical care unit will often experience delirium. The known predisposing contributors to the development of delirium are (select all that apply):

   A. Age 60 years and under.

   B. Presence of brain damage.

   C. Presence of chronic brain disorder.

   D. Presence of family.

   Answer: B & C. Three predisposing contributors to the development of delirium include age 60 years or older, presence of brain damage, and presence of a chronic brain disorder such as Alzheimer's disease.

   TEST-TAKING STRATEGY: When answering "Select all that apply" questions, be sure and treat each answer as a true or false statement. There may be one correct answer or more.

956. A client is using a leaf blower near an old campfire. Glass debris from a broken bottle flies everywhere. The client comes to the emergency room complaining of a foreign body sensation in his right eye, watery eyes, and photophobia. Which nursing action takes priority?

   A. Evert eyelid and examine for foreign body.

   B. Measure visual acuity.

   C. Notify immediately for transfer.

   D. Place an eye shield over eye.

   Answer: D. If a foreign body is the result of explosion or blunt or sharp trauma, the eye should be protected from further damage by placing an eye shield over the eye (or if a shield is not available, a paper cup to prevent rubbing of the eye). After this is done, arrangements should be made to transport the client for emergency care by an ophthalmologist. Everting of the eyelid, examining for foreign body, and measuring visual acuity are not measures that should be performed immediately.

TEST-TAKING STRATEGY: Questions that ask you to prioritize your nursing actions use terms like *priority, first, best, initial, most important,* and *next.*

957. A client comes to the emergency department following a motor vehicle collision with questionable loss of consciousness. To quickly rule out a serious injury, the nurse should first:

   A. Assess airway patency, breathing, and circulation.

   B. Assess level of consciousness.

   C. Measure vital signs.

   D. Stabilize neck and check for signs of neck injury.

   Answer: A. The nurse should always assess airway patency, breathing, and circulation first. Assessing level of consciousness, measuring vital signs, and stabilizing the neck, and checking for signs of neck injury are all measures that are taken after the nurse initially assesses airway patency, breathing, and circulation.

   TEST-TAKING STRATEGY: Questions that ask you to prioritize your nursing actions use terms like *priority, first, best, initial, most important,* and *next.* ABCs are always a nursing priority.

958. Signs of increased intracranial pressure (ICP) include:

   A. Increased pulse.

   B. Lowered systolic pressure.

   C. Narrowed pulse pressure.

   D. Papilledema.

   Answer: D. Signs of increased intracranial pressure include papilledema, elevated systolic pressure, wide pulse pressure, decreased pulse, and slow respirations.

   TEST-TAKING STRATEGY: Use the process of elimination to rule out incorrect answer selections to help choose the correct answer.

959. A client is diagnosed with second-degree burns. The nurse expects the physician to order:

   A. Application of cool water or saline-soaked gauze to the burn.

   B. Application of ice to the burn.

C. Cleansing with betadine.

D. Cleansing with hydrogen peroxide.

Answer: A. Treatment of superficial burns from all causes except radiation includes applying cool water- or saline-soaked gauze to the burn (do not apply ice or immerse wound in fluid), and cleansing with water or saline with or without mild soap. Do not use agents such as hydrogen peroxide or alcohol. Hibiclens and betadine are discouraged because they can delay healing. A topical anesthetic such as dibucaine cream or benzocaine spray may be used 3 to 4 times a day as needed for pain.

TEST-TAKING STRATEGY: Use the process of elimination to rule out incorrect answer selections to help choose the correct answer.

960. The nurse knows which burn involves the entire thickness of the skin?

A. First degree.

B. Second degree.

C. Third degree.

D. Fifth degree.

Answer: C. Full-thickness (third-degree) burns involve the entire thickness of the skin, and may involve subcutaneous fat, connective tissue, muscle, and even bone. Superficial (first-degree) burns have minimal epithelial damage and cause no skin loss. Partial-thickness (superficial second-degree) burns involve the upper layers of the epidermis, but spare epidermal appendages such as hair follicles, nails, sweat and sebaceous glands, and sensory nerve cells. Deep dermal partial-thickness (deep second-degree) burns typically have patchy areas of injury varying from superficial partial thickness to full thickness; wounds may progress to full thickness. There is no fifth-degree burn classification.

TEST-TAKING STRATEGY: Use the process of elimination to rule out incorrect answer selections to help choose the correct answer.

961. Which type of burn is very painful and heals without scarring or contractures in approximately 7 to 14 days?

A. First degree.

B. Third degree.

C. Fourth degree.

D. Deep second degree.

Answer: A. First-degree burns heal without scarring or contractures in about 7 to 14 days. Third-degree burns take months to heal because the dermal elements needed to regenerate new skin are destroyed and surgical management with excision and grafting is needed. There is no fourth-degree burn classification. Deep second-degree burns may take more than 21 days to heal, and may have contracture formation and hypertrophic scarring.

TEST-TAKING STRATEGY: Use the process of elimination to rule out incorrect answer selections to help choose the correct answer.

962. If a client has an avulsed tooth, the nurse should store the tooth (select all that apply):

A. In cold milk.

B. In Hank's balanced salt solution.

C. In saline.

D. Under the tongue.

Answer: A, B, C, & D. An avulsed tooth should be replanted immediately if possible. If the tooth is displaced from the mouth and has collected debris from the ground or floor, rinse gently with sterile water holding the tooth by the crown. If the avulsed tooth cannot be placed into the socket for transport, store the tooth in a physiologic medium to preserve vitality of the tooth. The best medium is a commercially available kit containing Hank's balanced salt solution. Cold milk is also a good storage medium. Saline and saliva are acceptable as storage media, and are preferable to allowing the tooth to become dry. If milk, saline, or Hank's balanced solution are not available, placement of the tooth under the patient's tongue or in the buccal vestibule between the gums and teeth is better than allowing it to air dry, which is destructive to the tooth (irreversible damage to the periodontal cells occurs in 30 minutes of air drying).

TEST-TAKING STRATEGY: When answering "Select all that apply" questions, be sure and treat each answer as a true or false statement. There may be one correct answer or more.

963. Ionizing radiation is the only form of radiation proven to cause human cancer. Which are examples of ionizing radiation?

    A. Cell phones.

    B. Microwaves.

    C. Radio waves.

    D. X-rays.

    Answer: D. Examples of ionizing radiation are x-rays, radon, cosmic rays, and ultraviolet (UV) radiation. Radiation produced by radio waves, cell phones, microwaves, computer screens, televisions, electric blankets, and other products are examples of nonionizing radiation.

    TEST-TAKING STRATEGY: Use the process of elimination to rule out incorrect answer selections to help choose the correct answer.

964. Which diagnostic test utilizes a huge electromagnet that detects hidden tumors by mapping the vibrations of the various atoms in the body on a computer screen?

    A. Computerized axial tomography (CAT scan).

    B. Magnetic resonance imaging (MRI).

    C. Radiotherapy.

    D. Ultrasound.

    Answer: B. MRI is a device that uses magnetic fields, radio waves, and computers to generate an image of internal tissues of the body for diagnostic purposes without the use of radiation.

    TEST-TAKING STRATEGY: Use the process of elimination to rule out incorrect answer selections to help choose the correct answer.

965. Which form of therapy uses radiation to kill cancerous cells?

    A. Chemotherapy.

    B. Chirotherapy.

    C. Radiotherapy.

    D. Ultratherapy.

Answer: C. Radiotherapy is the use of radiation to kill cancerous cells. Radiation works by destroying malignant cells or stopping cell growth. It is most effective in treating localized cancer masses. Unfortunately, in the process of destroying malignant cells, radiotherapy also destroys some healthy cells. It may also increase the risk for other types of cancer.

TEST-TAKING STRATEGY: Use the process of elimination to rule out incorrect answer selections to help choose the correct answer.

966. Thyroid radioactive iodine uptake and scan is usually performed on clients with an established diagnosis of:

    A. Hypothyroidism.

    B. Myxedema.

    C. Thyroid storm.

    D. Thyrotoxicosis.

    Answer: D. Thyroid radioactive iodine uptake and scan is usually performed on clients with an established diagnosis of thyrotoxicosis. This procedure is not usually performed with hypothyroidism, myxedema, or thyroid storm.

    TEST-TAKING STRATEGY: Use the process of elimination to rule out incorrect answer selections to help choose the correct answer.

967. The nurse knows irradiation may cause (select all that apply):

    A. Destruction of fingernails.

    B. Edema.

    C. Erythema.

    D. Fever.

    Answer: A & C. Irradiation may cause erythema, epilation, destruction of fingernails, or epidermolysis. Ionizing radiation burns appear similar to thermal burns but usually have a slower onset and course. Edema and fever are not typically seen with irradiation.

    TEST-TAKING STRATEGY: When answering "Select all that apply" questions, be sure and treat each answer as a true or false statement. There may be one correct answer or more.

968. The type of damage due to radiation exposure depends on (select all that apply):

A. The dose rate.

B. The organs exposed.

C. The technician.

D. The time of day.

Answer: A & B. The extent of damage due to radiation exposure depends on the quantity of radiation delivered to the body, dose rate, organs exposed, type of radiation (x-rays, neutrons, gamma rays, alpha or beta particles), duration of exposure, and energy transfer from the radioactive wave or particle to the exposed tissue. The technician and time of day have no bearing on the type of damage due to radiation exposure.

TEST-TAKING STRATEGY: When answering "Select all that apply" questions, be sure and treat each answer as a true or false statement. There may be one correct answer or more.

969. Which are side effects of radiation? Select all that apply.

A. Injury to the bone marrow.

B. Mucositis.

C. Pericarditis with effusion.

D. Permanent sterility.

Answer: A, B, C, & D. Side effects of radiation include injury to the bone marrow, which causes diminished production of blood elements. Pericarditis with effusion or constrictive pericarditis may occur after a period of months or even years. In males, small single doses may cause temporary aspermatogenesis, and larger doses may cause permanent sterility. In females, small single doses may cause temporary cessation of menses and larger doses may cause permanent castration. Moderate to heavy irradiation of the embryo results in injury to the fetus or in embryonic death and abortion. High or repeated moderate doses may cause pneumonitis. Mucositis with edema and painful swallowing of food may occur within hours or days after exposure. Inflammation and ulceration of the intestines may follow moderately large doses of radiation. Hepatitis and nephritis may be delayed effects of therapeutic radiation.

TEST-TAKING STRATEGY: When answering "Select all that apply" questions, be sure and treat each answer as a true or false statement. There may be one correct answer or more.

970. The nurse caring for a client diagnosed with cancer knows that radiation sickness (systemic reaction) symptoms include (select all that apply):

A. Anorexia.

B. Nausea.

C. Vomiting.

D. Weakness.

Answer: A, B, C, & D. The basic mechanisms of radiation sickness are not known. Anorexia, nausea, vomiting, weakness, exhaustion, lassitude, and in some cases prostration may occur singly or in combination. Dehydration, anemia, and infection may follow. Radiation sickness is most likely to occur when the therapy is given in large dosage to large areas over the abdomen, less often when given over the thorax, and rarely when therapy is given over the extremities.

TEST-TAKING STRATEGY: When answering "Select all that apply" questions, be sure and treat each answer as a true or false statement. There may be one correct answer or more.

971. The success of treatment of local radiation depends upon:

A. Extent of tissue injury.

B. Rate of therapy.

C. The designated area.

D. Use of systemic medications.

Answer: A. The success of treatment of local radiation effects depends upon the extent, degree, and location of tissue injury. Rate of therapy, designated area, and use of systemic medications do not directly impact the success of treatment.

TEST-TAKING STRATEGY: Use the process of elimination to rule out incorrect answer selections to help choose the correct answer.

972. Nurses handling radiation sources can minimize exposure to radiation by recognizing the importance of:

A. Area.

B. Density.

C. Time.

D. Volume.

Answer: C. Nurses handling radiation sources can minimize exposure to radiation by recognizing the importance of time, distance, and shielding. Area, density, and volume are not variables that impact radiation exposure.

TEST-TAKING STRATEGY: Use the process of elimination to rule out incorrect answer selections to help choose the correct answer.

973. Which electrolyte imbalance will the nurse find with hyperparathyroidism, Paget's disease, adrenal insufficiency, and prolonged immobilization?

A. Hypercalcemia.

B. Hypermagnesemia.

C. Hypocalcemia.

D. Hypomagnesemia.

Answer: A. Hypercalcemia is found in hyperparathyroidism, Paget's disease, adrenal insufficiency, and prolonged immobilization. Hypermagnesemia, hypocalcemia, and hypomagnesemia are not found with these processes.

TEST-TAKING STRATEGY: Use the process of elimination to rule out incorrect answer selections to help choose the correct answer.

974. Which is manifested by an increase in weight and peripheral edema or ascites?

A. Dehydration.

B. Hyperosmolality.

C. Volume depletion.

D. Volume overload.

Answer: D. Volume overload is manifested by an increase in weight and peripheral edema or ascites. Edema from local obstruction of venous return must be differentiated from systemic process (congestive heart failure, cirrhosis, and nephritic syndrome). A history of increased dietary sodium intake and use of medications that affect the renin–angiotensin system should be sought. Dehydration, hyperosmolality, and volume depletion are not manifested by weight increase, peripheral edema, or ascites.

TEST-TAKING STRATEGY: Use the process of elimination to rule out incorrect answer selections to help choose the correct answer.

975. Which condition is characterized by weight loss, excessive thirst, and dry mucous membranes?

A. Hyperosmolality.

B. Hypoosmolality.

C. Volume depletion.

D. Volume overload.

Answer: C. Volume depletion is characterized by weight loss, excessive thirst, and dry mucous membranes. Dehydration, or pure water deficit, should be distinguished from volume depletion, in which both water and salt are lost. There may be resting tachycardia, orthostatic hypotension, or shock. Causes include vomiting or diarrhea, diuretic use, renal disease, diabetes mellitus or diabetes insipidus, inadequate oral intake associated with altered mental status, and excessive insensible losses from sweating or fever. Hyperosmolality, hypoosmolality, and volume overload are not characterized by weight loss, excessive thirst, and dry mucous membranes.

TEST-TAKING STRATEGY: Use the process of elimination to rule out incorrect answer selections to help choose the correct answer.

976. Treatment of fluid and electrolyte disorders is based on:

A. Assessment of total body water and its distribution.

B. Serum water concentrations.

C. Total body electrolyte concentrations.

D. Urine osmolality.

Answer: A. Treatment of fluid and electrolyte disorders is based on assessment of total body water and its distribution, serum electrolyte concentrations, urine electrolyte concentrations, and serum osmolality. Serial changes in body weight constitute the best way of knowing if there has been an acute change in body water balance.

TEST-TAKING STRATEGY: Use the process of elimination to rule out incorrect answer selections to help choose the correct answer.

977. A client's arterial blood gases (ABG) reveal the following values: pH 7.0, HCO_3 24 mEq/L, $PaCO_2$ 56 mm Hg. Which illness does this indicate?

A. Metabolic acidosis.

B. Metabolic alkalosis.

C. Respiratory acidosis.

D. Respiratory alkalosis.

Answer: C. Respiratory acidosis reveals a pH less than 7.35, $PaCO_2$ greater than 45 mm Hg, and HCO_3 22 to 26 mEq/L. Metabolic acidosis reveals a pH less than 7.35, $PaCO_2$ 35 to 45mm Hg, and HCO_3 22 mEq/L. Metabolic alkalosis reveals a pH less than 7.45, $PaCO_2$ 35 to 45 mm Hg, and HCO_3 26 mEq/L. Respiratory alkalosis reveals a pH less than 7.45, $PaCO_2$ less than 35 mm Hg, and HCO_3 22 to 26 mEq/L.

TEST-TAKING STRATEGY: Read the questions twice to ensure that you understand what the question is asking, especially if the question is tricky or confusing.

978. A client's arterial blood gases (ABG) reveal the following values: pH 7.2, HCO_3 22 mEq/L, and $PaCO_2$ 40 mm Hg. Which illness does this indicate?

A. Metabolic acidosis.

B. Metabolic alkalosis.

C. Respiratory acidosis.

D. Respiratory alkalosis.

Answer: A. Metabolic acidosis reveals a pH less than 7.35, $PaCO_2$ 35 to 45 mm Hg, and HCO_3 22 mEq/L. Respiratory acidosis reveals a pH less than 7.35, $PaCO_2$ greater than 45 mm Hg, and HCO_3 22 to 26 mEq/L. Metabolic alkalosis reveals a pH greater than 7.45, $PaCO_2$ 35 to 45 mm Hg, and HCO_3 26 mEq/L. Respiratory alkalosis reveals a pH greater than 7.45, $PaCO_2$ less than 35 mm Hg, and HCO_3 22 to 26 mEq/L.

TEST-TAKING STRATEGY: Read the questions twice to ensure that you understand what the question is asking, especially if the question is tricky or confusing. Focus on what the question is asking.

979. A client's arterial blood gases (ABG) reveal the following values: pH 7.6, HCO_3 26 mEq/L, and $PaCO_2$ 38 mm Hg. Which illness does this indicate?

A. Metabolic acidosis.

B. Metabolic alkalosis.

C. Respiratory acidosis.

D. Respiratory alkalosis.

Answer: B. Metabolic alkalosis reveals a pH greater than 7.45, $PaCO_2$ 35 to 45 mm Hg, and HCO_3 26 mEq/L. Metabolic acidosis reveals a pH less than 7.35, $PaCO_2$ 35 to 45 mm Hg, and HCO_3 22 mEq/L. Respiratory acidosis reveals a pH less than 7.35, $PaCO_2$ greater than 45 mm Hg, and HCO_3 22 to 26 mEq/L. Respiratory alkalosis reveals a pH greater than 7.45, $PaCO_2$ less than 35 mm Hg, and HCO_3 22 to 26 mEq/L.

TEST-TAKING STRATEGY: Read the questions twice to ensure that you understand what the question is asking, especially if the question is tricky or confusing.

980. A client's arterial blood gases (ABG) reveal the following values: pH 7.8, HCO_3 26 mEq/L, and $PaCO_2$ 28 mm Hg. Which illness does this indicate?

A. Metabolic acidosis.

B. Metabolic alkalosis.

C. Respiratory acidosis.

D. Respiratory alkalosis.

Answer: B. Respiratory alkalosis reveals a pH greater than 7.45, $PaCO_2$ less than 35 mm Hg, and HCO_3 22 to 26 mEq/L. Metabolic alkalosis reveals a pH greater than 7.45, $PaCO_2$ 35 to 45 mm Hg, and HCO_3 26 mEq/L. Metabolic acidosis reveals a pH less than 7.35, $PaCO_2$ 35 to 45 mm Hg, and HCO_3 22 mEq/L. Respiratory acidosis reveals a pH less than 7.35, $PaCO_2$ greater than 45 mm Hg, and HCO_3 22 to 26 mEq/L.

TEST-TAKING STRATEGY: Read the questions twice to ensure that you understand what the question is asking, especially if the question is tricky or confusing.

981. The nurse knows respiratory acidosis occurs in:

    A. Diuretic therapy.

    B. Hypoxia.

    C. Oversedation.

    D. Potassium deficit.

    Answer: C. Respiratory acidosis occurs in hypoventilation resulting from COPD, oversedation, head trauma, anesthesia, drug overdose, neuromuscular disease, and hypoventilation with mechanical ventilation. Respiratory alkalosis occurs in hypoxia, anxiety, pulmonary embolism, and hyperventilation with mechanical ventilation. Metabolic acidosis occurs in diabetic or alcoholic ketoacidosis, renal failure, rhabdomyolysis, toxin ingestion, methanol or salicylate ingestion, diarrhea, renal tubular acidosis, ureterosigmoidoscopy, and illeostomy. Metabolic alkalosis occurs in steroid therapy, vomiting, gastrointestinal suction, diuretic therapy, potassium deficit, and sodium bicarbonate intake.

    TEST-TAKING STRATEGY: Use the process of elimination to rule out incorrect answer selections to help choose the correct answer.

982. The nurse knows respiratory alkalosis occurs in (select all that apply):

    A. Anxiety.

    B. Hyperventilation with mechanical ventilation.

    C. Hypoxia.

    D. Pulmonary embolism.

    Answer: A, B, C, & D. Respiratory alkalosis occurs in hypoxia, anxiety, pulmonary embolism, and hyperventilation with mechanical ventilation. Respiratory acidosis occurs in hypoventilation resulting from COPD, oversedation, head trauma, anesthesia, drug overdose, neuromuscular disease, and hypoventilation with mechanical ventilation. Metabolic acidosis occurs in diabetic or alcoholic ketoacidosis, renal failure, rhabdomyolysis, toxin ingestion, methanol or salicylate

ingestion, diarrhea, renal tubular acidosis, ureterosigmoidoscopy, and illeostomy. Metabolic alkalosis occurs in steroid therapy, vomiting, gastrointestinal suction, diuretic therapy, potassium deficit, and sodium bicarbonate intake.

TEST-TAKING STRATEGY: When answering "Select all that apply" questions, be sure and treat each answer as a true or false statement. There may be one correct answer or more.

983. The nurse cares for a client diagnosed with metabolic acidosis. The nurse knows metabolic acidosis occurs in (select all that apply):

    A. Diabetic ketoacidosis.

    B. Diarrhea.

    C. Renal failure.

    D. Rhabdomyolysis.

    Answer: A, B, C, & D. Metabolic acidosis occurs in diabetic or alcoholic ketoacidosis, renal failure, rhabdomyolysis, toxin ingestion, methanol or salicylates, diarrhea, renal tubular acidosis, ureterosigmoidoscopy, illeostomy. Respiratory alkalosis occurs in hypoxia, anxiety, pulmonary embolism, and hyperventilation with mechanical ventilation. Respiratory acidosis occurs in hypoventilation resulting from COPD, oversedation, head trauma, anesthesia, drug overdose, neuromuscular disease, and hypoventilation with mechanical ventilation. Metabolic alkalosis occurs in steroid therapy, vomiting, gastrointestinal suction, diuretic therapy, potassium deficit, and sodium bicarbonate intake.

TEST-TAKING STRATEGY: When answering "Select all that apply" questions, be sure and treat each answer as a true or false statement. There may be one correct answer or more.

984. The nurse cares for a client diagnosed with metabolic alkalosis. Metabolic alkalosis occurs in:

    A. Head trauma.

    B. Hypoxia.

    C. Steroid therapy.

    D. Uremia.

    Answer: C. Metabolic alkalosis occurs in steroid therapy, vomiting, gastrointestinal suction, diuretic therapy, potassium deficit, and sodium bicarbonate intake. Respiratory acidosis occurs in hypoventilation resulting from COPD, oversedation, head trauma, anesthesia, drug overdose, neuromuscular disease, and hypoventilation with mechanical ventilation. Respiratory alkalosis occurs in hypoxia, anxiety, pulmonary embolism, and hyperventilation with mechanical ventilation. Metabolic acidosis occurs in diabetic or alcoholic ketoacidosis, renal failure, rhabdomyolysis, toxin ingestion, methanol or salicylate ingestion, diarrhea, renal tubular acidosis, ureterosigmoidoscopy, and illeostomy.

TEST-TAKING STRATEGY: Use the process of elimination to rule out incorrect answer selections to help choose the correct answer.

985. The nurse cares for a post bronchoscopy client. The nurse knows to assess this client for (select all that apply):

A. Bronchospasm.

B. Epistaxis.

C. Fever.

D. Hypoxemia.

Answer: A, B, C, & D. Complications of a bronchoscopy may be related to the procedure itself, the anesthetic, or an ancillary procedure. Minor complications include laryngospasm, bronchospasm, epistaxis, fever, vomiting, altered pulmonary mechanics, and hemodynamic instability. Major complications include anaphylaxis, infection, hypotension, cardiac dysrhythmias, pneumothorax, hemorrhage, respiratory failure, hypoxemia, and cardiopulmonary arrest.

TEST-TAKING STRATEGY: When answering "Select all that apply" questions, be sure and treat each answer as a true or false statement. There may be one correct answer or more.

986. The nurse asks a client about an upcoming medical procedure. The client will be undergoing a thoracentesis for a large right pleural effusion. The nurse knows further teaching is necessary when the client states:

A. "I cannot cough during the procedure."

B. "I will be on the ventilator during the procedure."

C. "I will be in a sitting position leaning forward."

D. "The doctor knows where the fluid is from the x-ray."

Answer: B. During a thoracentesis, the client is placed in a sitting position with legs over the side of the bed and hands and arms supported on a padded overbed table. If the client's condition precludes sitting, the side-lying position with the back flush with the edge of the bed and the affected side down can be used. The client is cautioned not to move or cough during the procedure. During the thoracentesis, the site of the needle insertion is usually determined by previous chest x-ray examination, computed tomography (CT) scan, or chest percussion.

TEST-TAKING STRATEGY: The phrase *further teaching is necessary* tells you to select an answer with inaccurate information.

987. Nursing management of a client undergoing a diagnostic procedure includes (select all that apply):

A. Assessing the client after the procedure.

B. Monitoring the client's responses to the procedure.

C. Positioning the client for the procedure.

D. Teaching the client about the procedure.

Answer: A, B, C, & D. Nursing management of a client undergoing a diagnostic procedure involves a variety of interventions, which include preparing the client psychologically and physically for the procedure, maintaining the client's responses to the procedure, and assessing the client after the procedure. Preparing the client includes teaching the client about the procedure, answering any questions, and positioning the client for the procedure. Monitoring the client's responses to the procedure includes observing the client for signs of pain, anxiety, or respiratory distress, and monitoring vital signs, breath sounds, and oxygen saturation. Assessing the client after the procedure includes observing for complications of the procedure and medicating the client for any postprocedural discomfort.

TEST-TAKING STRATEGY: When answering "Select all that apply" questions, be sure and treat each answer as a true or false statement. There may be one correct answer or more.

988. Pulse oximetry is a noninvasive method for monitoring oxygen saturation. The pulse oximeter is considered very accurate. However, several physiologic and technical factors limit the monitoring system. Physiologic limitations in pulse oximetry include:

A. Bright lights.

B. Excessive motion.

C. Incorrect placement of the probe.

D. Poor tissue perfusion.

Answer: **D.** Physiologic limitations include elevated levels of abnormal hemoglobins, presence of vascular dyes, and poor tissue perfusion. Technical limitations include bright lights, excessive motion, and incorrect placement of the probe.

TEST-TAKING STRATEGY: Read the questions twice to ensure that you understand what the question is asking, especially if the question is tricky or confusing.

989. Which sedation is typically achieved by administering a single, non-IV dose of a long-acting agent?

A. Conscious sedation.

B. General anesthesia.

C. Light sedation.

D. Regional anesthesia.

Answer: **C.** Light sedation is typically achieved by administering a single, non-IV dose of a long-acting agent. Conscious sedation is the condition produced by the administration of a drug or combination of drugs to relieve anxiety or pain during diagnostic or therapeutic procedures. General anesthesia and regional anesthesia are achieved by administration of IV agents.

TEST-TAKING STRATEGY: Use the process of elimination to rule out incorrect answer selections to help choose the correct answer.

990. The goals and effects of conscious sedation include the following:

A. Alteration of personality.

B. Cooperation.

C. Lowering of pain threshold.

D. Major variation of vital signs.

Answer: **B.** The goals and effects of conscious sedation include the following: alteration of mood, maintenance of consciousness, cooperation, elevation of pain threshold, minor variation of vital signs, and some degree of amnesia.

TEST-TAKING STRATEGY: Use the process of elimination to rule out incorrect answer selections to help choose the correct answer.

991. The "stir-up" regimen is probably the most important aspect of perianesthesia nursing management. The basics of the regimen include the prevention of complications, primarily atelectasis and venous stasis. The five major activities of the "stir-up" regimen include (select all that apply):

A. Coughing.

B. Deep-breathing exercises.

C. Mobilization.

D. Pain management.

Answer: **A, B, C, & D.** Five major activities— deep-breathing exercises, coughing, positioning, mobilization, and pain management—constitute the stir-up regimen.

TEST-TAKING STRATEGY: When answering "Select all that apply" questions, be sure and treat each answer as a true or false statement. There may be one correct answer or more.

992. Aspiration is defined as the passage of regurgitated gastric contents or other foreign materials into the trachea and down to the smaller air units. The most common and severest form of aspiration is the aspiration of gastric contents. If aspiration is suspected, the nurse should:

A. Contact the physician.

B. Elevate the foot of the bed.

C. Initiate oxygen via a nonrebreather mask.

D. Lower the client's head of bed.

Answer: D. If aspiration is suspected, nursing management begins with lowering the client's head, if possible. The client is positioned with the head turned to the side to permit gravity to pull secretions from the trachea.

TEST-TAKING STRATEGY: Use the process of elimination to rule out incorrect answer selections to help choose the correct answer.

993. Clients recovering from anesthesia usually experience some form of thermoregulatory imbalance. Management of these alterations is important because they are associated with other physiologic alterations that may interfere with recovery. These types of thermoregulatory imbalance include (select all that apply):

A. Hyperthermia.

B. Hyperkalemia.

C. Hypothermia.

D. Hypokalemia.

Answer: A & C. Both hypothermia and hyperthermia can occur in the postoperative client. Management of these alterations is important because they are associated with other physiologic alterations that may interfere with recovery following anesthesia. Hyperkalemia and hypokalemia have nothing to do with thermoregulatory imbalance.

TEST-TAKING STRATEGY: When answering "Select all that apply" questions, be sure and treat each answer as a true or false statement. There may be one correct answer or more.

994. The nurse cares for a postoperative client who has a temperature of 103°F. The nurse knows the causes of postoperative fever include:

A. Abscess formation.

B. Blood transfusion.

C. Endocrine disorders.

D. Warm environment.

Answer: A. Causes of postoperative fever include abscess formation, atelectasis, wound infection, fat emboli after bone trauma, drug reactions, malignancy, silent aspiration, dehydration, central nervous system damage, urinary tract infections, phlebitis/deep vein thrombosis, and pulmonary emboli. Causes of elevated core temperature include blood transfusion, drug-induced fever, overuse of techniques to prevent hypothermia, hypothalamic injury, malignant hyperthermia, warm environment, use of anti-cholinergics, endocrine disorders, and neurogenic hyperthermia.

TEST-TAKING STRATEGY: Use the process of elimination to rule out incorrect answer selections to help choose the correct answer.

995. The medulla oblongata contains groups of neurons, or "centers," that control involuntary functions such as (select all that apply):

A. Coughing.

B. Hiccoughing.

C. Respirations.

D. Vasoconstriction.

Answer: A, B, C, & D. The medulla oblongata contains neurons that control involuntary functions such as swallowing, vomiting, hiccoughing, coughing, vasoconstriction, and respirations.

TEST-TAKING STRATEGY: When answering "Select all that apply" questions, be sure and treat each answer as a true or false statement. There may be one correct answer or more.

996. In the unconscious client, noxious stimuli may elicit an abnormal motor response. When assessing a client, the nurse finds that in response to painful stimuli, the upper extremities exhibit flexion of the arm, wrist, and fingers with adduction of the limb. The lower extremity exhibits extension, internal rotation, and plantar flexion. This is known as:

A. Decerebrate posturing.

B. Decorticate posturing.

C. Reflex posturing.

D. Superficial posturing.

Answer: B. This describes decorticate posturing. Decerebrate posturing occurs when the client is stimulated, and teeth clench and the arms are stiffly extended, adducted, and hyperpronated. The legs are stiffly extended with plantar flexion of the feet. Abnormal extension occurs with lesions in the area of the brain stem. There is no such condition as reflex posturing or superficial posturing.

TEST-TAKING STRATEGY: Use the process of elimination to rule out incorrect answer selections to help choose the correct answer.

997. The nurse performs a follow-up assessment of a client who was involved in a motor vehicle accident and sustained massive head injuries. The client is weaned off the ventilator and is breathing independently. The nurse notices the client's respirations have a rhythmic crescendo and decrescendo of rate and depth of respiration and include brief periods of apnea. This type of respiratory pattern is:

A. Apneustic.

B. Ataxic.

C. Cheyne–Stokes.

D. Cluster.

Answer: C. This type of respiratory pattern is characteristic of Cheyne–Stokes. Apneustic respirations have a prolonged inspiratory and/or expiratory pause of 2 to 3 seconds. Ataxic respirations have an irregular, random pattern of deep and shallow respirations with irregular apneic periods. Cluster breathing involves clusters of irregular, gasping respirations separated by long periods of apnea.

TEST-TAKING STRATEGY: Read the questions twice to ensure that you understand what the question is asking, especially if the question is tricky or confusing.

998. A client complains of progressively worsening shortness of breath since cutting the grass 3 days ago. The client has a history of asthma. The nurse knows that this client is having a severe exacerbation and should immediately receive:

A. High doses of inhaled short-acting beta$_2$-agonists.

B. Intravenous fluids.

C. Oxygen.

D. Systemic corticosteroids.

Answer: C. Owing to the life-threatening nature of severe exacerbations of asthma, treatment should be started immediately once the exacerbation is recognized. All clients with a severe exacerbation should immediately receive oxygen. High doses of inhaled short-acting beta$_2$-agonists and systemic corticosteroids are secondary interventions. Asphyxia is a common cause of death, and oxygen therapy is therefore very important. Intravenous fluids are not indicated for asthma exacerbation.

TEST-TAKING STRATEGY: Always pick the answer that is most life threatening or the nursing intervention that is most life-saving.

999. Pulmonary embolism and deep venous thrombosis (DVT) are two manifestations of the same disease. The risk factors for pulmonary embolism are the risk factors for thrombus formation within the venous circulation. These risk factors, known as Virchow's triad, include:

A. Decreased central venous pressures.

B. Hypocoagulability.

C. Injury to the bone.

D. Venous stasis.

Answer: D. The risk factors known as Virchow's triad include venous stasis, injury to the vessel wall, and hypercoagulability. Venous stasis increases with immobility (bed rest, immobility, stroke), hyperviscosity (polycythemia), and increased central venous pressures (low cardiac output states, pregnancy).

TEST-TAKING STRATEGY: Use the process of elimination to rule out incorrect answer selections to help choose the correct answer.

1000. Thrombolytic therapy reduces mortality and limits infarct size in clients with acute myocardial infarction associated with ST segment elevation or with left bundle branch block. The greatest benefit occurs if treatment is initiated:

A. Within the first 3 days.

B. Within the first 30 days.

C. Within the first 3 hours.

D. Within 30 minutes.

Answer: C. The greatest benefit for thrombolytic therapy occurs if treatment is initiated within the first 3 hours, when up to a 50% reduction in mortality rate can be achieved.

TEST-TAKING STRATEGY: Use the process of elimination to rule out incorrect answer selections to help choose the correct answer.

1001. The major risk factors for intracranial bleeding in clients who receive thrombolytic therapy are:

A. Age greater than 65 years.

B. Hypotension at presentation.

C. Obesity.

D. Race.

Answer: A. The major risk factors for intracranial bleeding in clients who receive thrombolytic therapy are age over 65 years, hypertension at presentation, low body weight (less than 70 kg), and the use of clot-specific thrombolytic agents (alteplase, reteplase, tenecteplase). Race is not a factor.

TEST-TAKING STRATEGY: Use the process of elimination to rule out incorrect answer selections to help choose the correct answer.

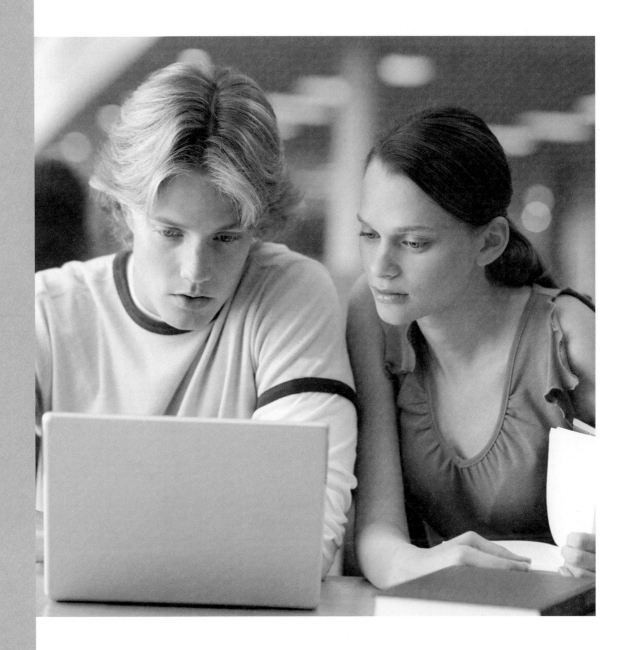

CHAPTER

18 Directory of State Boards of Nursing

LET'S GET THE NORMAL STUFF STRAIGHT FIRST

The only thing you have to get straight in this chapter is to locate your state in the directory listed below and read through the state licensing requirements! Easy enough!

Isn't it nice of me to provide you with all of this useful information? OK, OK . . . yes, I did have some help, but still here it all is at your fingertips! Just remember that although all of the information is current at the time of this writing, it very well may change in the future. Boards of Nursing are known to change locations, increase fees, and change renewal requirements.

This chapter concludes our time together. I have thoroughly enjoyed working with you, and know without a doubt and without hesitation that you will pass NCLEX® the **FIRST TIME!**

✚ Alabama

Board of Nursing

RSA Plaza, Ste. 250

770 Washington Avenue

Montgomery, AL 36130-3900

Phone: (334) 242-4060

Fax: (334) 242-4360

www.abn.state.al.us/

Temporary Permit: 90 days by exam; 3 months if by endorsement; $50

State Board Application Fee: $85

Additional State Endorsement: $85

NCLEX-PN® Test Fee: $200

Re-Examination Limitations: Every 45 days; $85; number unlimited

License Renewal: December 31, per biennial renewal period; $75

CEU Requirements: 24 contact hours per biennial renewal period. Nurses licensed by examination are required to have four contact hours of Board-provided continuing education for the first renewal (included in the total number of hours to be earned). MEDCEU contact hours are no longer accepted.

Results: Mail within 4 weeks

✚ Alaska

Board of Nursing

Department of Community and Economic Development

Division of Occupational Licensing

P.O. Box 110806

333 Willoughby Avenue, 9th Floor

Juneau, AK 99811-0806

Phone: (907) 465-2544 (last names A–K); (907) 269-8401 (last names L–Z)

(907) 269-8402

Fax: 1-(907)-465-2974

www.dced.state.ak.us/occ/pnur.htm

Temporary Permit: 4 months by exam or by endorsement; $50

State Board Fee: $215 permanent license fee; $50 application fee plus $59 fingerprint fee

Additional State Endorsement: $374 license fee; $50 application fee plus $59 fingerprint fee

NCLEX-PN® Test Fee: $200

Re-Examination Limitations: Every 91 days. Must pass within 5 years, then retake with remediation.

License Renewal: November 30, every even year; $215

CEU Requirements: Method 1: Two of the three required for renewal: (1) 30 contact hours of CE, (2) 30 hours of professional nursing activities, (3) 320 hours of nursing employment.

Method 2: Completed a board-approved nursing refresher course. Method 3: Attained a degree or certificate in nursing, beyond the requirements of the original license, by successfully completing at least two required courses. Method 4: Successfully completed the National Council Licensing Examination.

Results: Mail

✛ Arizona

Board of Nursing

1651 E. Morten Avenue, Ste. 210

Phoenix, AZ 85020

Phone: (602) 889-5150

Fax: (602) 889-5155

www.azboardofnursing.org

Temporary Permit: 4 months pending results of fingerprint check, must have already passed the exam; $25

State Board Fee: $220, plus $43 fingerprint fee

Additional State Endorsement: $150, plus $43 fingerprint fee

NCLEX-PN® Test Fee: $263

Re-Examination Limitations: Every 45 days; $60

License Renewal: June 30, every four years; $120

CEU Requirements: None

Maximum Number Attempts: Unlimited

Notification: Internet

✚ Arkansas

State Board of Nursing

University Tower Building

1123 South University, Ste. 800

Little Rock, AR 72204-1619

Phone: (501) 686-2700

Fax: (501) 686-2714

www.arsbn.org

Temporary Permit: Up to 90 days if by endorsement; $25

State Board Fee: $75

Additional State Endorsement: $100

NCLEX-PN® Test Fee: $200

Re-Examination Limitations: Every 90 days

License Renewal: Birthday, every 2 years; $55

CEU Requirements: 15 contact hours or certification/recertification during renewal period

Maximum Number Attempts: Unlimited

Notification: Mail (5–7 business days)

✚ California

Board of Registered Nursing

400 R Street, Ste. 4030

P.O. Box 944210

Sacramento, CA 94244-2100

Phone: (916) 322-3350

Fax: (916) 327-4402

www.rn.ca.gov/

Temporary Permit: Interim license pending results of first exam; 6 months if by endorsement; $30

State Board Fee: $85 application fee, plus $32 fingerprint fee

Additional State Endorsement: $50, plus $56 fingerprint fee

NCLEX-PN® Test Fee: $200

Re-Examination Limitations: Every 91 days; $75

License Renewal: Last day of the month following birth month, every two years; $85

CEU Requirements: 30 contact hours every 2 years.

Maximum Number Attempts: Unlimited

Notification: Mail (4–6 weeks)

✚ Colorado

Board of Nursing

1560 Broadway, Ste. 880

Denver, CO 80202

Phone: (303) 894-2430

Fax: (303) 894-2821

www.dora.state.co.us/nursing/

Temporary Permit: 90 days; 4 months if by endorsement; Fee is included in application fee.

State Board Fee: $87 initial exam

Additional State Endorsement: $37

NCLEX-PN® Test Fee: $200

Re-Examination Limitations: Every 45 days; $75

License Renewal: September 30, every 2 years; $102

CEU Requirements: None

Maximum Number Attempts: Unlimited

Notification: Mail (3 weeks) and Internet

✚ Connecticut

Board of Examiners for Nursing

Department of Public Health

RN Licensure

410 Capitol Avenue

MS# 12 APP

P.O. Box 340308

Hartford, CT 06134-0308

Phone: (860) 509-7603

Fax: (860) 509-8457

www.dph.state.ct.us/licensure/licensure.htm#R

Temporary Permit: 4 months (120 days) from completion of nursing program. Temporary permit also available for endorsement applicants, valid for 120 days, nonrenewable; must hold valid license in another state. Fee is included in application fee.

State Board Fee: $83 (RN, LPN)

Additional State Endorsement: $90

NCLEX-PN® Test Fee: $200

Re-Examination Limitations: Every 91 days, no more than four times in 1 year

License Renewal: Last day of birth month, every year; $50

CEU Requirements: None

Notification: Internet

✚ Delaware

Division of Professional Regulation

Board of Nursing

861 Silver Lake Boulevard

Cannon Building, Ste. 203

Dover, DE 19904-2467

Phone: (302) 744-4516

Fax: (302) 739-2711

www.professionallicensing.dpr.state.de.us/boards/nursing/index.shtml

Temporary Permit: 90 days by endorsement or pending results of first exam; $25

State Board Fee: $77

Additional State Endorsement: $20–$94

NCLEX-PN® Test Fee: $200

Re-Examination Limitations: Every 45 days; $10

License Renewal: February 28, May 31, and September 30, every odd year; $67

CEU Requirements: 30 contact hours every 2 years. Nurses licensed by exam are exempt from CE requirements for the first renewal after initial licensure. Minimum practice requirement of 1000 hours in 5 years or 400 hours in 2 years.

Maximum Number: Unlimited within 2 years of graduation. Greater than 2 years, must request from board to attempt. Board will individualize their requirements.

Notification: Mail (7 business days)

✚ District of Columbia

Board of Nursing

Department of Health

825 N. Capitol Street, N.E., Room 2224

Washington, DC 20002

Phone: (202) 442-4778

Fax: (202) 442-9431

dchealth.dc.gov/prof_license/services/main.asp

Temporary Permit: None

State Board Fee: $78 license fee; $65 application fee

Additional State Endorsement: $111 license fee; $65 application fee

NCLEX-PN® Test Fee: $200

Re-Examination Limitations: Every 91 days; $65

License Renewal: June 30, every 2 years; $60

CEU Requirements: Applicants for reinstatement of a license must submit 12 contact hours for each year after 6/30/90 that the applicant was not licensed, up to a maximum of 24 contact hours.

Notification: Internet

✚ Florida

Board of Nursing

4052 Bald Cypress Way, BIN C02

Tallahassee, FL 32399

Phone: (850) 245-4125

Fax: (850) 245-4172

www.doh.state.fl.us/mqa/nsglink

Temporary Permit: 90 days pending results of first exam; 60 days if by endorsement. Fee is included in licensure fee.

State Board Fee: $190 initial exam

Additional State Endorsement: $212

NCLEX-PN® Test Fee: $200

Re-Examination Limitations: Every 45 days; remedial training program is required after three attempts; $105

License Renewal: Every odd year; $65

CEU Requirements: 25 contact hours every 2 years. One hour per month. Two hours in the prevention of medical errors and one hour each in HIV and domestic violence by a provider approved by the state of Florida; proof of training in latter two prior to licensure. Nurses licensed by examination are exempt from CE requirements in the period following first licensure.

Notification: Internet

✚ Georgia

Board of Nursing

237 Coliseum Drive

Macon, GA 31217-3858

Phone: (478) 207-1640

Fax: (478) 207-1660

www.sos.state.ga.us/plb/rn/

Temporary Permit: 6 months if by endorsement. Fee is included in application fee

State Board Fee: $40

Additional State Endorsement: $60

NCLEX-PN® Test Fee: $200, plus $12 when registering by telephone

Re-Examination Limitations: Every 91 days, three years maximum from graduation.

License Renewal: January 31, every even year. $45 if paid before November 30, $65 after November 30

CEU Requirements: None

Maximum Number: Unlimited within 3 years from graduation. Return to nursing school to begin as a new student if not successful in 3 years

Notification: Internet, mail. Time varies. May pay "extra" fee to obtain results earlier

✚ Hawaii

DCCA—PVL

Board of Nursing

P.O. Box 3469

Honolulu, HI 96801

Phone: (808) 586-3000

Fax: (808) 586-2689 – (2874)

www.state.hi.us/dcca/pvl/areas_nurse.html

Temporary Permit: By endorsement with employment verification

State Board Fee: $40

Additional State Endorsement: $135 or $180, depending on the year license is issued. Noted on application information sheet

NCLEX-PN® Test Fee: $200

Re-Examination Limitations: Every 91 days

License Renewal: June 30, every odd year (deadline May 31); $90

CEU Requirements: None

✚ Idaho

Board of Nursing

280 North 8th Street, Ste. 210

P.O. Box 83720

Boise, ID 83720-0061

Phone: (208) 334-3110

Fax: (208) 334-3262

www.2.state.id.us/ibn/ibnhome.htm

Temporary Permit: 90 days if by endorsement, $25

State Board Fee: $90

Additional State Endorsement: $85

NCLEX-PN® Test Fee: $200

Re-Examination Limitations: Every 46 days for 12 months from graduation

License Renewal: August 31, every odd year; $50

CEU Requirements: None

Maximum Number: Unlimited 1 year. After 1 year, must complete "form" for Board to decide on necessary recommendations

Notification: 48 hours per phone and/or mail, Internet

✚ Illinois

Department of Professional Regulation

320 West Washington Street, 3rd Floor

Springfield, IL 62786

Phone: (217) 782-8556

Fax: (217) 782-7645

www.dpr.state.il.us/WHO/nurs.asp

Temporary Permit: 3-month approval letter by examination; six months by endorsement; $25

State Board Fee: $73

Additional State Endorsement: $50

NCLEX-PN® Test Fee: $200

Re-Examination Limitations: Every 45 days, 3 years from first writing to board

License Renewal: May 31, every even year; $40

CEU Requirements: None

Maximum Number: >3 years—Return to nursing school or remediation

Notification: Mail (time varies), Internet

✚ Indiana

State Board of Nursing

Health Professions Bureau

402 West Washington Street, Room W066

Indianapolis, IN 46204

Phone: (317) 234-2043

Fax: (317) 233-4236

www.state.in.us/hpb/boards/isbn

Temporary Permit: 90 days if by endorsement; $10

State Board Fee: $50

Additional State Endorsement: $50

NCLEX-PN® Test Fee: $200

Re-Examination Limitations: Every 91 days

License Renewal: October 31, every odd year; $50

CEU Requirements: None

Maximum Number: Unlimited

Notification: Mail (7–10 business days), Internet

✚ Iowa

Board of Nursing

Riverpoint Business Park

400 SW 8th Street, Ste. B

Des Moines, IA 50309-4685

Phone: (515) 281-3255

Fax: (515) 281-4825

www.state.ia.us/government/nursing/

Temporary Permit: 30 days if by endorsement. Fee is included in application fee

Background Check: $50; good for 1 year

State Board Fee: $93

Additional State Endorsement: $119

NCLEX-PN® Test Fee: $200

Re-Examination Limitations: Every 45 days

License Renewal: 30 days prior to the 15th of month of birth, every 3 years; $99

CEU Requirements: 36 contact hours or 3.6 CEUs every 3 years

Maximum Number: Unlimited

Notification: Mail (within 2 weeks), Internet

✚ Kansas

State Board of Nursing

Landon State Office Building

900 SW Jackson, Ste. 1051

Topeka, KS 66612-1230

Phone: (785) 296-4929

Fax: (785) 296-3929

www.ksbn.org

Temporary Permit: Pending results of first exam, or no longer than 90 days from graduation; 120 days if by endorsement. Fee is included in application fee

State Board Fee: $75

Additional State Endorsement: $75

NCLEX-PN® Test Fee: $200

Re-Examination Limitations: Every 45 days, unlimited number of times; after 2 years the applicant must provide an approved study plan

License Renewal: Month of birth, every 2 years; $60

CEU Requirements: 30 contact hours every 2 years

Maximum Number: After 2 years must submit written action plan and receive approval.

Notification: Mail (3–5 business days), Internet

✚ Kentucky

Board of Nursing

312 Whittington Parkway, Ste. 300

Louisville, KY 40222-5172

Phone: (502) 429-3300

Fax: (502) 329-7011

www.kbn.state.ky.us/

Temporary Permit: No temporary work permits are issued to new graduates. Six months by endorsement. Fee included in application fee

After January 1, 2006 all applicants must complete 120 hours of clinical internship prior to NCLEX or obtaining license.

State Board Fee: $110

Background Check: $10

Additional State Endorsement: $120

NCLEX-PN® Test Fee: $200

Re-Examination Limitations: Every 45 days

License Renewal: October 31, every even year; $105

CEU Requirements: 30 contact hours every 2 years; 2 of the 30 hours must be AIDS CE-approved by the Kentucky Cabinet for Health Services. A one-time, 3-hour domestic violence requirement must be completed within 3 years of the date of initial licensing.

Maximum Number: Unlimited

Notification: Mail only (within 2 weeks)

✚ Louisiana

Board of Nursing

3510 North Causeway Boulevard, Ste. 601

Metairie, LA 70002

Phone: (504) 838-5332

Fax: (504) 838-5349

www.lsbn.state.la.us/

Temporary Permit: Pending results of first exam; 90 days if by endorsement. Fee is included in application fee. Permit becomes void when exam results received

State Board Fee: $130

Additional State Endorsement: $100, plus $50 fingerprint fee

NCLEX-PN® Test Fee: $200

Re-Examination Limitations: Every 91 days, up to four times

License Renewal: January 31, every year; $45

CEU Requirements: For all RNs: 5, 10, or 15 contact hours every year, based on employment

✚ Maine

Board of Nursing

24 Stone Street

#158 State House Station

Augusta, ME 04333

Phone: (207) 287-1133

Fax: (207) 287-1149

www.state.me.us/boardofnursing

Temporary Permit: 90 days. Fee is included in application fee. Does not routinely issue permit

State Board Fee: $60

Additional State Endorsement: $60

NCLEX-PN® Test Fee: $200

Re-Examination Limitations: Every 91 days

License Renewal: Birthday, every 2 years; $40

CEU Requirements: None

Maximum Number: Unlimited

Notification: Mail (within 2 weeks), Internet

✚ Maryland

Board of Nursing

4140 Patterson Avenue

Baltimore, MD 21215-2254

Phone: (410) 585-1900

Fax: (410) 358-3530

www.mbon.org

Temporary Permit: 90 days by endorsement, not renewable; $25

State Board Fee: $75

Additional State Endorsement: $75

NCLEX-PN® Test Fee: $200

Re-Examination Limitations: Every 91 days

License Renewal: 28th day of month of birth, every year; $62

CEU Requirements: None

Notification: Internet

✚ Massachusetts

Division of Professional Licensure

Board of Registration in Nursing

239 Causeway Street, Ste. 500

Boston, MA 02114

Phone: (617) 973-0800

Fax: (617) 727-1630

www.state.ma.us/reg/boards/rn/

Temporary Permit: Not granted

State Board Fee: $350, includes test fee

Additional State Endorsement: $130

NCLEX-PN® Test Fee: $200, included in state board fee

Re-Examination Limitations: Every 45 days

License Renewal: Birthday, every even year; $80

CEU Requirements: 15 contact hours every 2 years

Maximum Number Attempts: Unlimited.

Notification: Internet within 5 days; Mail within 10 days. May obtain "unofficial" results next day for additional fee

✛ Michigan

Bureau of Health Professions

Michigan Department of Community Health

Board of Nursing

Ottowa Towers North

611 West Ottowa, 1st Floor

Lansing, MI 48933

Phone: (517) 335-0918

Fax: (517) 373-2179

www.michigan.gov/healthlicense

Temporary Permit: No longer available

State Board Fee: $48

Additional State Endorsement: $48

NCLEX-PN® Test Fee: $200

Re-Examination Limitations: Every 91 days, up to six attempts within 3 years. Must pass exam within 6 months of first attempt or attend another RN education program/remedial program

License Renewal: March 31, every 2 years; $48

CEU Requirements: 25 credits every 2 years

Maximum Number: 6 times within 3 years. After 3 years, must complete nursing school again

Notification: Mail; online if passed but results not always entered promptly in Website

✛ Minnesota

Board of Nursing

2829 University Avenue, SE #500

Minneapolis, MN 55414-3253

Phone: (612) 617-2270

Fax: (612) 617-2190

www.nursingboard.state.mn.us/

Temporary Permit: 60 days, license by exam; $60. One year if by endorsement, no fee

State Board Fee: $105 initial exam

Additional State Endorsement: $105

NCLEX-PN® Test Fee: $200

Re-Examination Limitations: Every 45 days. Must retake within 1 year or application becomes null; $60

License Renewal: Birth month, every 2 years; $85

CEU Requirements: 24 contact hours every 2 years

Maximum Number Attempts: Unlimited

Notification: Online (within 3–5 days after exam)

+ Mississippi

Board of Nursing

1935 Lakeland Drive, Ste. B

Jackson, MS 39216

Phone: (601) 987-4188

Fax: (601) 364-2352

www.msbn.state.ms.us/

Temporary Permit: 90 days by endorsement; $25

State Board Fee: $60

Additional State Endorsement: $60

NCLEX-PN® Test Fee: $200

Re-Examination Limitations: Every 91 days

License Renewal: December 31, every even year; $50

CEU Requirements: None

+ Missouri

Board of Nursing

3605 Missouri Boulevard

P.O. Box 656

Jefferson City, MO 65102-0656

Phone: (573) 751-0681

Fax: (573) 751-0075

www.pr.mo.gov/nursing.asp

Temporary Permit: months. Fee is included in application fee

State Board Fee: $83 initial exam

Additional State Endorsement: $93

NCLEX-PN® Test Fee: $200

Re-Examination Limitations: Retake after 45 days; $40

License Renewal: April 30, every odd year; $80 (plus additional fee for renewing online)

CEU Requirements: None

Maximum Number: Unlimited

Notification: Mail, telephone, Internet

✚ Montana

Department of Labor and Industry

Board of Nursing

301 South Park, Rm. 430

P.O. Box 200513

Helena, MT 59620-0513

Phone: (406) 841-2340/2345

Fax: (406) 841-2343

https://app.discoveringmontana.com/cgi-bin/bsdrnw.cgi

dlibsdnur@mt.gov

Temporary Permit: Yes for recent graduates for 90 days until either pass or fail.

State Board Fee: $100

Additional State Endorsement: $200

NCLEX-PN® Test Fee: $200

Re-Examination Limitations: Every 91 days, up to five attempts in 3 years. After failing twice, must present a plan of study to the Board before next retake. If one doesn't pass within 3 years, must take Nursing Program before sixth retake. (If do not pass on fifth attempt, must return to nursing school.)

License Renewal: December 31, every 2 years; $100

CEU Requirements: None

Notification: Internet

✚ Nebraska

Department of HHS Regulation and Licensure

Nursing and Nursing Support Section

State Office Building

301 Centennial Mall South, 3rd Floor

P.O. Box 94986

Lincoln, NE 68509-4986

Phone: (402) 471-4376

Fax: (402) 471-1066

www.hhs.state.ne.us/crl/nursing/

Temporary Permit: 60 days if by endorsement. Fee is included in licensing fee

State Board Fee: $75 plus $2 LAP fee

Additional State Endorsement: $75 plus $2 LAP fee

NCLEX-PN® Test Fee: $200

Re-Examination Limitations: Every 91 days

License Renewal: October 31, every even year; $40 plus $2 LAP fee. If 90 days prior to expiration, $10

CEU Requirements: 20 contact hours every 2 years with 500 practice hours every 5 years, or a refresher course of study in previous 5 years. New graduates are exempt from CEU requirements for the first renewal period for 2 years from graduation.

Maximum Number: No limit on number of times to test. May retake after 45 days

Notification: Internet

✚ Nevada

Board of Nursing

2500 W. Sahara Avenue, Ste. 207

Las Vegas, NV 89102-4392

Phone: (888) 590-NSBN or (702) 486-5800

Fax: (702) 486-5803

www.nursingboard.state.nv.us/

Temporary License: Four months, not renewable. Fee is included in application fee; $50 if not seeking permanent license. Application by endorsement.

State Board Fee: $100

Additional State Endorsement: $105

NCLEX-PN® Test Fee: $200

Re-Examination Limitations: Every 91 days, up to three times, then only with remediation. If fail after third time, conduct plan of study.

License Renewal: Birthday, every 2 years; $100

CEU Requirements: 30 contact hours every 2 years at renewal. New grads may be exempt from CE requirements for their first renewal period.

Notification: Internet

✚ New Hampshire

Board of Nursing

78 Regional Drive, Building B

P.O. Box 3898

Concord, NH 03302-3898

Phone: (603) 271-2323

Fax: (603) 271-6605

www.state.nh.us/nursing/

Temporary Permit: 6 months or until results of first exam are received and license is issued; $20

State Board Fee: $80

Additional State Endorsement: $70 plus $10 Criminal Release Authorization form

NCLEX-PN® Test Fee: $200

Re-Examination Limitations: Every 45 days

License Renewal: Birthday, every 2 years; $60

CEU Requirements: 30 contact hours every 2 years

Notification: Internet, mail; obtaining results by phone discouraged. Usually given test results within 24 hours

+ New Jersey

Board of Nursing

P.O. Box 45010

Newark, NJ 07101

Phone: (973) 504-6430

Fax: (973) 648-3481

www.state.nj.us/lps/ca/medical.htm

Temporary Permit: Not available

State Board Fee: $75 application fee plus $65 initial license fee

Additional State Endorsement: $75 application fee; $65 license certificate fee

NCLEX-PN® Test Fee: $200

Re-Examination Limitations: Every 45 days; only with remediation after three attempts.

License Renewal: May 31, every 2 years, $65

CEU Requirements: None

Notification: Internet, mail, telephone

+ New Mexico

Board of Nursing

4206 Louisiana NE, Ste. A

Albuquerque, NM 87109

Phone: (505) 841-8340

Fax: (505) 841-8347

www.state.nm.us/nursing

Temporary Permit: 24 weeks from graduation if application process is completed within 12 weeks of graduation; 6 months if by endorsement. Fee is included in application fee; must have NM employment verified

State Board Fee: $110 initial exam

Additional State Endorsement: $110

NCLEX-PN® Test Fee: $200

Re-Examination Limitations: Every 45 days; $55

License Renewal: Every 2 years from date of issue; $93

CEU Requirements: 30 contact hours every 2 years

Maximum Number: Unlimited

Notification: Mail, telephone, Internet

✚ New York

Board of Nursing

NYS Education Department

Office of the Professions

Division of Professional Licensing Services, Nurse Unit

89 Washington Avenue

Albany, NY 12234-1000

Phone: (518) 474-3817, ext. 280

Fax: (518) 474-3398

www.op.nysed.gov/nurse.htm

Temporary Permit: Must have completed all other requirements for licensure except the licensing examination. Valid for one year from date of issue or until 10 days after the applicant is notified of failure on the licensing examination, whichever occurs first. Graduates of New York state nursing programs may be employed without permit for 90 days immediately following graduation; $35

State Board Fee: $135 (includes first license and 3-year registration)

Additional State Endorsement: $135

NCLEX-PN® Test Fee: $200

Re-Examination Limitations: Every 45 days

License Renewal: Every 3 years; $65

CEU Requirements: None

Maximum Number: Unlimited

Notification: Internet, mail.

✚ North Carolina

Board of Nursing

P.O. Box 2129

Raleigh, NC 27602-2129

Phone: (919) 782-3211

Fax: (919) 781-9461

www.ncbon.com

Temporary Permit: None for new graduates. By endorsement: 6 months or until the endorsement is approved, whichever occurs first; not renewable. Fee is included in application fee

State Board Fee: $50

Additional State Endorsement: $135, plus $38 fingerprint fee

NCLEX-PN® Test Fee: $200

Re-Examination Limitations: Every 45 days; $35

License Renewal: Month of birth, every 2 years; $60

CEU Requirements: None

Maximum Number: Unlimited

Notification: Mail only

✛ North Dakota

Board of Nursing

919 South 7th Street, Ste. 504

Bismarck, ND 58504-5881

Phone: (701) 328-9778

Fax: (701) 328-9785

www.ndbon.org

Work Authorization: By endorsement: 90 days; fee is included in endorsement fee. By exam: 90 days after the date of issue or upon notification of exam results, whichever occurs first. No limit on test-taking

You are not eligible for licensure in ND if your primary state of residence is AZ, AR, DE, ID, IA, ME, MD, MS, NM, NC, SD, TN, TX, UT, or WI. (Nurse Licensure Compact, 1/1/04)

State Board Fee: $110

Additional State Endorsement: $110

NCLEX-PN® Test Fee: $200

Re-Examination Limitations: Every 91 days, up to five attempts in 3 years

License Renewal: December 31, every even year; $90

Maximum Attempts: Unlimited

CEU Requirements: Nursing practice for relicensure must meet or exceed 12 hours within preceding 2 years.

Notification: Internet

✛ Ohio

Board of Nursing

17 South High Street, Ste. 400

Columbus, OH 43215-7410

Phone: (614) 466-3947

Fax: (614) 466-0388

www.state.oh.us/nur/

Temporary Permit: 180 days if by endorsement, not renewable. Fee is included in endorsement application fee

State Board Fee: $75

Additional State Endorsement: $75

NCLEX-PN® Test Fee: $200

Re-Examination Limitations: Every 45 days; $75

License Renewal: August 31, every odd year; $65

CEU Requirements: 24 hours in a 2-year period, except in the case of first renewal after licensure by examination.

Maximum Number: Unlimited until 1 year, then contact Board and complete new application

Notification: Official results by mail; Internet

✚ Oklahoma

Board of Nursing

2915 North Classen Boulevard, Ste. 524

Oklahoma City, OK 73106

Phone: (405) 962-1800

Fax: (405) 962-1821

www.youroklahoma.com/gov/nursing

Temporary Permit: Not applicable to new graduates. 90 days if by endorsement. Fee is included in application fee.

State Board Fee: $75

Additional State Endorsement: $75

NCLEX-PN® Test Fee: $200

Re-Examination Limitations: Every 91 days. After 2 years, forced to return to school; retest after 45 days until 2 years, then return to school with approved remedial course

License Renewal: Last day of birth month, every even year

Notification: Internet

✚ Oregon

Board of Nursing

800 NE Oregon Street, Ste. 465

Portland, OR 97232-2162

Phone: (503) 731-4745

Fax: (503) 731-4755

www.welcomeoregon.gov/OSBN/

Search Division 31 Nurse Practice Act

Temporary Permit: None

State Board Fee: $100

Additional State Endorsement: $115

NCLEX-PN® Test Fee: $200

Re-Examination Limitations: Every 45 days, up to 3 years from the date of graduation

License Renewal: Birthday, every 2 years; $85

CEU Requirements: Nursing practice for re-licensure must exceed 960 hours within preceding 5 years.

Maximum Number: Unlimited up to 3 years from graduation, then return to repeat nursing school

Notification: Internet, mail. Telephone notification discouraged

✚ Pennsylvania

Board of Nursing

P.O. Box 2649

Harrisburg, PA 17105-2649

Phone: (717) 783-7142

Fax: (717) 783-0822

www.dos.state.pa.us/nurse

Temporary Permit: One year maximum; examination results preempt permit; $35

State Board Fee: $35

Additional State Endorsement: $100

NCLEX-PN® Test Fee: $200

Re-Examination Limitations: Every 45 days

License Renewal: Renewal date by license number every 2 years; $45

CEU Requirements: None

Maximum Number: Unlimited

Notification: Mail, telephone

✚ Rhode Island

Board of Nurse Registration and Nursing Education

3 Capitol Hill, Rm. 105

Providence, RI 02908

Phone: (401) 222-5700

Fax: (401) 222-3352

www.health.ri.org

Temporary Permit: Pending results of first exam but no longer than 90 days after graduation; 90 days if by endorsement. Not renewable. No fee

State Board Fee: $93.75

Additional State Endorsement: $93.75

NCLEX-PN® Test Fee: $200

Re-Examination Limitations: Every 45 days

License Renewal: March 1, every two years by license number; $62.50

CEU Requirements: Beginning in March 2006, 10 contact hours in preceding 2 years.

Maximum Number: Unlimited

Notification: Mail, Internet

✚ South Carolina

Board of Nursing

P.O. Box 12367

Columbia, SC 29211-2367

Phone: (803) 896-4550

Fax: (803) 896-4525

www.llr.state.sc/pol/nursing

Temporary Permit: 90 days by endorsement only.

State Board Fee: $97

Additional State Endorsement: $114; with permit $124

NCLEX-PN® Test Fee: $200

Re-Examination Limitations: Every 45 days, up to four times in 1 year; then must remediate. $97

License Renewal: January 31, every year; $84

CEU Requirements: Minimum practice requirement of 960 hours in preceding 5 years.

Maximum Number: Must pass within 3 years of graduation; if fail, return to school or apply in another state

Notification: Internet, mail, telephone

✚ South Dakota

Board of Nursing

4305 S. Louise Avenue, Ste. 201

Sioux Falls, SD 7106-3115

Phone: (605) 362-2760

Fax: (605) 362-2768

www.state.sd.us/dcr/nursing/

Temporary Permit: 90 days from graduation pending results of first exam; 90 days if by endorsement; $25

State Board Fee: $100

Additional State Endorsement: $100

NCLEX-PN® Test Fee: $200

Re-Examination Limitations: Every 45 days, maximum of four times per year in 3 years; then must requalify

License Renewal: Birthday, every 2 years; $90

CEU Requirements: Continuing employment 140 hours in one year or 480 hours in 6 years.

Maximum Number: Unlimited

Notification: Mail

✛ Tennessee

Board of Nursing

425 Fifth Avenue North

Cordell Hull Building, 3rd Floor

Nashville, TN 37247-1010

Phone: (615) 532-5156

Fax: (615) 741-7899

www.tennessee.gov/health

Temporary Permit: 6 months if by endorsement. Fee included in application fee

State Board Fee: $140

Additional State Endorsement: $140

NCLEX-PN® Test Fee: $200

Re-Examination Limitations: Every 45 days up to 3 years, then only with remediation

License Renewal: Last day of month of birth, every 2 years; $50

CEU Requirements: Continued practice requirement over a 5-year period

Maximum Number: Pass within 3 years from graduation

Notification: Mail (within 5 business days), Internet, telephone

✛ Texas

Board of Nurse Examiners

333 Guadalupe #3-460

P.O. Box 430

Austin, TX 78701

Phone: (512) 305-7400

Fax: (512) 305-7401

www.bne.state.tx.us/

Temporary Permit: By endorsement: 12 weeks. By exam: 60 days or pending results of first exam. Fee included in application fee

State Board Fee: $109

Additional State Endorsement: $169

NCLEX-PN® Test Fee: $200

Re-Examination Limitations: Every 45 days; unlimited testing within four years of eligibility; $70 retake fee

License Renewal: Every even year for those born in even years; every odd year for those born in odd years (initial licensure period ranges from 6 months to 29 months depending on birth year); $53

CEU Requirements: 20 contact hours (2 CEUs) every 2 years. Nurses licensed by exam or by endorsement are exempt from CE requirements for the first renewal after initial licensure.

Notification: Mail (within 3 weeks), Internet

✛ Utah

Board of Nursing

Division of Occupational and Professional Licensing

P.O. Box 146741

Salt Lake City, UT 84114-6628

Phone: (801) 530-6597

Fax: (801) 530-6511

www.commerce.utah.gov/licensing/nurse.html

Temporary Permit: 4 months; $50

State Board Fee: $99

Additional State Endorsement: $99

NCLEX-PN® Test Fee: $200

Re-Examination Limitations: Every 45 days; those who fail to pass exam within 2 years after completing educational program must submit plan of action for approval before retaking

License Renewal: January 31, every odd year; $43

CEU Requirements: Must have practiced not less than 400 hours during 2 years preceding application for renewal, or have completed 30 contact hours, or have practiced not less than 200 hours and completed 15 contact hours during 2 years preceding application for renewal.

Maximum Number: Unlimited

Notification: Mail, Internet. Phone notification discouraged

✛ Vermont

Board of Nursing

Office of the Secretary of State

81 River Street

Montpelier, VT 05609-1106

Phone: (802) 828-2396

Fax: (802) 828-2484

www.vtprofessionals.org/

Temporary Permit: 90 days if by endorsement; $25

State Board Fee: $90

Additional State Endorsement: $150

NCLEX-PN® Test Fee: $200

Re-Examination Limitations: Every 45 days; Board of Nursing approval is needed after two attempts; $30

License Renewal: March 31, every odd year; $85

CEU Requirements: Minimum practice requirement of 960 hours in 5 years or 400 hours in 2 years.

Maximum Number: After two failures, take NCLEX® review and appear before Board.

Notifications: Mail (7–14 days), Internet

✚ Virginia

Board of Nursing

6603 West Broad Street, 5th Floor

Richmond, VA 23230-1712

Phone: (804) 662-9909

Fax: (804) 662-9512

www.dhp.state.va..us/nursing

Temporary Permit: 90 days pending results of exam

State Board Fee: $130

Additional State Endorsement: $130

NCLEX-PN® Test Fee: $200

Re-Examination Limitations: Every 45 days; $25

License Renewal: Last day of month of birth, every even year for those born in even years; every odd year for those born in odd years; $95

CEU Requirements: None

Maximum Number: Unlimited

Notification: Mail, telephone

✚ Washington

Nursing Care Quality Assurance Commission

310 Israel Road

P.O. Box 47860

Tumwater, WA 98501-7860

Phone: (360) 236-4706

Fax: (360) 236-4738

www.doh.wa.gov/

Temporary Permit: None

State Board Fee: $65

Additional State Endorsement: $65

NCLEX-PN® Test Fee: $200

Re-Examination Limitations: Every 91 days, up to three times in 2 years, then must requalify

License Renewal: Birthday, every year; $50

CEU Requirements: Not mandatory

Maximum Number: Four times in a 2-year period. After fourth failure, must complete approved program of study and then may retake four more times.

Notification: Mail, Internet. Telephone notification discouraged

+ West Virginia

Board of Examiners for Registered Professional Nurses

101 Dee Drive

Charleston, WV 25311-1620

Phone: (304) 558-3595

Fax: (304) 558-3666

www.wvrnboard.com

Temporary Permit: 90 days pending results of first exam; 90 days if by endorsement; $10

State Board Fee: $51.50

Additional State Endorsement: $30

NCLEX-PN® Test Fee: $200

Re-Examination Limitations: Every 45 days; additional requirements are needed after two attempts

License Renewal: December 31, every year; $25

CEU Requirements: 30 contact hours every odd year. If initial licensure occurs during the first half of any 2-year reporting period, must complete 12 contact hours before the end of that reporting period. If initial licensure occurs during the second half of any 2-year reporting period, exempt from CE requirements for the entire reporting period.

Maximum Number: Unlimited

Notification: Internet with online verification (updated every night), mail

+ Wisconsin

Bureau of Health Service Professions—RN

Department of Regulation and Licensing

1400 East Washington Avenue

P.O. Box 8935

Madison, WI 53708-8935

Phone: (608) 266-0145

www.drl.wi.gov/index.htm

Temporary Permit: 3 months pending results of exam; 3 months if by endorsement; $10

State Board Fee: $68

Additional State Endorsement: $66

NCLEX-PN® Test Fee: $200

Re-Examination Limitations: Every 45 days; $15

License Renewal: February 28 or 29, every even year; $66

CEU Requirements: None

Notification: Internet

✚ Wyoming

Board of Nursing

2020 Carey Avenue, Ste. 110

Cheyenne, WY 82001

Phone: (307) 777-7601

Fax: (307) 777-3519

www.nursing.state.wy.us/

Temporary Permit: 90 days by endorsement or by exam. Fee is included in application fee.

State Board Fee: $190

Additional State Endorsement: $195

NCLEX-PN® Test Fee: $200

Re-Examination Limitations: Every 45 days, maximum of 10 times within 5 years of graduation; then return to school

License Renewal: December 31, every even year; $110

CEU Requirements: Minimum practice requirement of 1600 hours in 5 years or 500 hours in 2 years.

Notification: Mail, Internet, telephone

INDEX